Understanding Your Health

Understanding Your Health

Tenth Edition

Wayne A. Payne, Ed.D.

Dale B. Hahn, Ph.D.

Ellen B. Lucas, Ph.D.

All of Ball State University
Muncie, Indiana

Boston   Burr Ridge, IL   Dubuque, IA   Madison, WI   New York   San Francisco   St. Louis
Bangkok   Bogotá   Caracas   Kuala Lumpur   Lisbon   London   Madrid   Mexico City
Milan   Montreal   New Delhi   Santiago   Seoul   Singapore   Sydney   Taipei   Toronto

*To all our students, with the hope that the
decisions they make will be healthy ones.*

Higher Education

Published by McGraw-Hill, an imprint of The McGraw-Hill Companies, Inc., 1221 Avenue of the Americas, New York, NY 10020. Copyright © 2009. All rights reserved. No part of this publication may be reproduced or distributed in any form or by any means, or stored in a database or retrieval system, without the prior written consent of The McGraw-Hill Companies, Inc., including, but not limited to, in any network or other electronic storage or transmission, or broadcast for distance learning.

This book is printed on acid-free paper.

2 3 4 5 6 7 8 9 0 QPD/QPD 1 0 9 8

ISBN: 978-0-07-340464-6
MHID: 0-07-340464-0

Editor in Chief: *Michael Ryan*
Publisher: *William Glass*
Sponsoring Editor: *Joseph Diggins*
Executive Marketing Manager: *Nick Agnew*
Director of Development: *Kathleen Engelberg*
Senior Developmental Editor: *Kirstan Price*
Development Editor, Technology: *Julia D. Akpan*
Lead Media Project Manager: *Ron Nelms, Jr.*
Production Editor: *Karol Jurado*
Production Service: *Melanie Field, Strawberry Field Publishing*
Manuscript Editor: *Wendy Nelson*
Art Director: *Jeanne Schreiber*
Text Designer: *Glenda King*
Cover Designer: *Laurie Entringer*
Cover Image: © *Rubberball Productions/Getty Images*
Lead Production Supervisor: *Randy Hurst*
Composition: *10.5/12 Minion by Newgen*
Printing: *45# Pub Thinbulk, Quebecor*

Photo credits: The photo credits section for this book begins on page 627 and is considered an extension of the copyright page.

Library of Congress Cataloging-in-Publication Data

Payne, Wayne A.
    Understanding your health / Wayne A. Payne, Dale B. Hahn, Ellen B. Lucas—10th ed.
      p. cm.
    Includes index
    ISBN-13: 978-0-07-340464-6 (alk. paper)
    ISBN-10: 0-07-340464-0 (alk. paper)
    1. Health 2. College students—Health and hygiene. I. Hahn, Dale B. II. Lucas, Ellen B.
III. Title.

    RA777.3.P39 2009
    613—dc22

                2007020155

The Internet addresses listed in the text were accurate at the time of publication. The inclusion of a website does not indicate an endorsement by the authors or McGraw-Hill, and McGraw-Hill does not guarantee the accuracy of the information presented at these sites.

www.mhhe.com

Brief Contents

Contents

Part Four: Preventing Diseases 293

Part Six: Consumer and Safety Issues   503

Boxes in Text

Building Media Literacy Skills

Changing for the Better

Learning from Our Diversity

Discovering Your Spirituality

Considering Complementary Care

As We Go to Press

★ Star

Preface

As a health educator, you already know that personal health is one of the most exciting courses a college student will take. Today's media-oriented college students are aware of the critical health issues of the new millennium. They hear about environmental issues, substance abuse, sexually transmitted diseases, fitness, and nutrition virtually every day. The value of the personal health course is its potential to expand students' knowledge of these and other health topics. Students will then be able to examine their attitudes toward health issues and modify their behavior to improve their health and perhaps even prevent or delay the onset of certain health conditions.

Understanding Your Health accomplishes this task with a carefully composed, well-documented text that addresses the health issues most important to both instructors and students. As health educators, we understand the teaching issues you face daily in the classroom and have written this text with your concerns in mind.

Hallmarks of the Text

Several unique themes and features set *Understanding Your Health* apart from other personal health texts. These successful features continue to define *Understanding Your Health* in its tenth edition.

A Text for All Students

This book is written for college students in a wide variety of settings, from community colleges to large four-year universities. The content is carefully constructed to be meaningful to students of all ages. We have paid special attention to the increasing numbers of nontraditional-age students (those over age 25) who have decided to pursue a college education. *Understanding Your Health* continues to encourage students of all ages and backgrounds to achieve their goals.

Two Central Themes

Throughout the text, two central themes—the multiple dimensions of health and the developmental tasks—offer students a foundation for understanding their own health and achieving positive behavior change. The multiple dimensions of health are introduced in Chapter 1 and revisited in each part opener, where they are discussed in the context of the chapters that follow. The developmental tasks are also introduced in Chapter 1, where they are applied to young, middle, and older adulthood.

Flexible Organization

The tenth edition of *Understanding Your Health* has 21 chapters. The first stands alone as an introductory chapter that explains the focus of the book. The arrangement of the remaining chapters follows the recommendations of both the users of previous editions of the book and reviewers for this edition. Of course, professors can choose to cover the chapters in any sequence that suits the needs of their courses.

Wellness and Disease Prevention

Throughout this new edition, students are continually urged to be proactive in shaping their future health. Even the chapter titles invite students to take control of their health behavior.

Integrated Presentation of Aging

Topics of interest to midlife and older adults are integrated into appropriate chapters according to subject. This organization allows both traditional-age and non-traditional-age students to learn about the physical and emotional changes that take place as we age.

Separate Coverage of Cancer and Chronic Conditions

Rapid developments in cancer prevention, diagnosis, and treatment warrant a single comprehensive chapter on cancer, in which we present the latest research and information. In addition, *Understanding Your Health* features a separate chapter in which more than 20 of the most common chronic conditions are discussed.

Technology: The Key to Teaching and Learning

Just a quick glance through the pages of *Understanding Your Health* shows that technology is woven throughout every chapter, both in the content and in the chapter pedagogy. Similarly, the package of supplements that accompanies the text emphasizes technology. Together, the text and its supplements offer the ideal approach to teaching and learning—one that integrates the best tools that technology has to offer, challenging both instructors and students to reach higher.

Updated Coverage: New and Expanded Topics

As experienced health educators and authors, we know how important it is to provide students with the most current information available. The tenth edition of *Understanding Your Health* has been thoroughly updated with the latest information, statistics, and findings. Throughout each chapter, we have incorporated new examples and discussions, from information on newly available prescription drugs and medications (Chapters 2, 3, 11, and 12), to the latest information on dieting and supplements (Chapters 5, 6, and 16).

The following list gives a sample of some of the current concerns addressed in the tenth edition; visit the Online Learning Center (www.mhhe.com/payne10e) for a chapter-by-chapter list of changes to the new edition.

- Abuse of prescription drugs
- Avian influenza
- Global warming
- Food safety issues
- New contraceptive methods
- Body image
- Healthy weight loss strategies
- Complementary and alternative medicine
- Dietary supplements
- Sleep, time management, and other stress management strategies
- Food labeling
- Environmental carcinogens
- Stem cells and cloning
- Strategies for prevention of CVD and cancer
- Identity theft
- Guidelines for physical activity and exercise
- Depression and suicide
- Energy drinks and caffeine
- Metabolic syndrome
- Diabetes
- West Nile virus and other emerging infections
- Physician-assisted suicide
- Healthy relationship strategies

In addition to these topics, we have once again included chapter-ending "As We Go to Press" boxes in relevant chapters. These unique boxes allow us to comment on breaking news right up to press time, ensuring that the most current issues in health are addressed. For example, obesity vaccines are discussed in Chapter 6, warnings about drugs for attention deficit hyperactivity disorder are discussed in Chapter 7, and college binge drinking in Chapter 8.

Other changes to the tenth edition include streamlined chapter organization, new pedagogical features, and many new photos and illustrations; these changes are described in greater detail following.

Student-Friendly Chapter Pedagogy

Each chapter of *Understanding Your Health* is rich with pedagogical features that offer a variety of ways to address new and emerging health issues and to pique student interest in particular topics.

"What Do You Know?" Quizzes

New for the tenth edition, each chapter opens with a brief quiz to challenge students and help spark their interest in key topics. Quiz answers are found at the end of the chapter.

Building Media Literacy Skills

Face it—a student's world revolves around media of all types, especially the Web. Students get most of their health information not from instructors and textbooks but from television, self-help books, popular news magazines, the Web, and the radio. To meet students on this familiar ground, we've included Building Media Literacy Skills boxes, which take a critical look at these media sources of health information. For the tenth edition, the media boxes have been modified to focus on media literacy and critical thinking skills. More than half the media boxes are new or significantly updated—topics include evaluating websites and health news stories, media messages about body image, smoking in movies, product placement in grocery stores, alcohol ads directed at young people, and interpersonal relationships as portrayed in popular TV dramas and soap operas.

Discovering Your Spirituality

Spirituality has become an important focus in health courses. Discovering Your Spirituality boxes highlight the spiritual dimension of health and its effect on overall wellness. The boxes cover topics such as mindfulness, yoga, living well with cancer or a chronic infectious disease, making decisions about sex, and having an enjoyable social life without abusing alcohol or other drugs.

Considering Complementary Care

This feature highlights nontraditional approaches to health care. Topics include the use of herbal supplements, acupuncture, hypnotism, Ayurveda, and dietary aids. Students are encouraged to critique these approaches, weighing their possible advantages and disadvantages. Although methods that are known to be dangerous are clearly identified as such, students are invited to consider new approaches that are becoming more accepted because they show promising results. An underlying theme is patient responsibility coupled with a physician's advice.

 ### Changing for the Better

These unique question-and-answer boxes show students how to put health concepts into practice. Each box begins with a real-life question, followed by helpful tips and practical advice for initiating behavior change and staying motivated to follow a healthy lifestyle. Topics include enhancing self-esteem, choosing a diet plan, improving time management, eating more fruits and vegetables, dealing with an alcohol-related emergency, reducing risk of STDs, and performing self-exams for cancer.

Learning from Our Diversity

These boxes expose students to alternative viewpoints and highlight what we can learn from the differences that make us unique. Topics include women and alcohol, diverse food pyramids, gender and body image, violence against the disabled, smoking patterns around the world, and relationships among race, economic status, and exposure to pollution.

 ### Star Boxes

In each chapter, special material in Star boxes encourages students to delve into a particular topic or closely examine an important health issue. Topics covered in Star boxes include Internet addiction, food safety, cigar use, OxyContin abuse, and the risks of using a cell phone while driving.

Talking Points

Interspersed throughout each chapter, Talking Points offers students opportunities to explore how they might start a dialogue about specific health-related issues and situations.

 ### Personal Assessments

Each chapter ends with at least one Personal Assessment inventory. These self-assessment exercises serve three important functions: to capture students' attention, to serve as a basis for introspection and behavior change, and to provide suggestions for carrying the applications further.

 ### Taking Charge of Your Health

Located at the end of each chapter, these bulleted lists invite students to put the knowledge and information they've gleaned from the chapter to work in their everyday lives. Cross-referencing the text with Internet links and real-world situations allows students to see how what they've learned can be applied in their own lives.

Definition Boxes

Key terms are set in boldface type and defined in corresponding boxes. Pronunciation guides are provided where appropriate. Other important terms in the text are set in italics for emphasis. Both approaches facilitate student vocabulary comprehension.

Chapter Summaries

Each chapter concludes with a bulleted summary of key concepts and their significance or application. The student can then return to any topic in the chapter for clarification or study.

Review Questions

A set of questions appears at the end of each chapter to aid the student in review and analysis of chapter content.

Illustrations and Photos

The inviting look and bold colors of the tenth edition draw the reader into the book. Appealing photographs, attractive illustrations, and informative tables help support and clarify the chapter material. The tenth edition features more than 120 new photos and figures.

Comprehensive Health Assessment

The Comprehensive Health Assessment at the end of Chapter 1 allows students to take a close look at their current state of health, typical health behavior, and risk factors. Using this assessment, students can pinpoint trouble spots in their own health behavior and find out what they can do to reduce their risk of disease or other health conditions. At the end of the semester, they can take a look at their previous answers to see how their behavior changed as they learned more about health and wellness issues.

Health Reference Guide

The updated Health Reference Guide at the back of the book lists many commonly used health resources. Internet addresses, phone numbers, and mailing addresses of various organizations and government agencies are provided as available. The guide is perforated and laminated, making it durable enough for students to keep for later use.

Comprehensive Glossary

At the end of the text, all terms defined in boxes, as well as pertinent italicized terms, are merged into a comprehensive glossary.

First Aid Appendix

This updated appendix outlines important general first-aid measures, such as what to do when someone is choking, bleeding, or in shock. It includes a special section on recognition and first-aid treatment of epileptic seizures.

Supplements

An extensive supplements package is available to adopters to enhance the teaching-learning process. We have made a concerted effort to produce supplements of extraordinary utility and quality. This package has been carefully planned and developed to help instructors derive the greatest benefit from the text. We encourage instructors to examine them carefully. Many of the products can be packaged with the text at a discounted price. Beyond the following brief descriptions, additional information about these supplements is available from your McGraw-Hill sales representative.

Instructor's Media DVD

Organized by chapter, the Instructor's Media DVD includes resources to help you teach your course. The DVD will work in both Windows and Macintosh environments and includes the following elements:

- **Course Integrator Guide**. This guide includes all the useful features of an instructor's manual, such as learning objectives, suggested lecture outlines, suggested activities, media resources, and Web links. It also integrates the text with all the related resources McGraw-Hill offers, such as the Online Learning Center and the HealthQuest CD-ROM. The guide

also includes references to relevant print and broadcast media.

- **Test Bank.** This file includes more than 1,000 questions, including multiple-choice, true/false, and short essay. It has been rewritten to enhance clarity, and it now includes critical thinking questions and more applications questions.
- **Computerized Test Bank.** The test bank is available with **EZ Test** computerized testing software. EZ Test provides a powerful, easy-to-use test maker to create printed quizzes and exams. For secure online testing, exams created in EZ Test can be exported to WebCT, Blackboard, PageOut, and EZ Test online. EZ Test comes with a Quick Start Guide, and once the program is installed, users have access to a User's Manual and Flash tutorials. Additional help is available online at www.mhhe.com/eztest.
- **PowerPoint Slides.** A complete set of PowerPoint lecture slides for the course is included on the Instructor's Media DVD, as well as on the instructor's portion of the Online Learning Center. You can modify the presentations as much as you like to meet the needs of your course.
- **Image Bank.** This collection of illustrations from *Understanding Your Health* and other sources can be used to highlight lecture points or be incorporated into PowerPoint slides.
- **High-Definition Videos.** A collection of short video clips is included on the Instructor's Media DVD. These clips correlate with chapter topics and are designed to engage students in class discussions and promote critical thinking. The videos feature student interviews and historical health videos on body image, depression, alcohol and drug use, stress, intimate relationships, and many other topics. Videos can be downloaded to a computer or viewed directly from the DVD. Selected video clips include Instructor Video Guides with objectives and critical thinking and discussion questions. (Longer videos, including those from Films for the Humanities, are also available; check with your sales representative for more information.)

Online Learning Center

www.mhhe.com/payne10e

The Online Learning Center to accompany this text offers many additional resources for both students and instructors. Visit this website to find useful materials such as the following:

For the instructor

- PowerPoint presentations
- Course Integrator Guide

- Test Bank
- Image Bank
- Classroom Performance System (CPS) questions (see description below)
- Links to professional resources

For the student

- Self-scoring chapter quizzes
- Flash cards for learning key terms and their definitions
- Audio chapter summaries
- Learning objectives
- Interactive activities
- Web links for study and exploration of topics in the text
- Online self-assessments
- Articles on additional topics

HealthQuest CD-ROM, by Bob Gold and Nancy Atkinson

The HealthQuest CD-ROM (ISBN 0-07-295117-6) helps students explore their wellness behavior using state-of-the-art interactive technology. Students can assess their current health status, determine their risks, and explore options for positive lifestyle change. Tailored feedback gives students a meaningful and individualized learning experience without using valuable classroom time. Modules include the Wellboard (a health self-assessment); Stress Management and Mental Health; Fitness; Nutrition and Weight Control; Communicable Diseases; Cardiovascular Health; Cancer; Tobacco, Alcohol, and Other Drugs.

Fitness and Nutrition Log

This logbook (ISBN 0-07-332567-8) helps students track their diet and exercise programs. It serves as a diary to help students monitor their behaviors. It can be packaged with any McGraw-Hill textbook for a small additional fee.

NutritionCalc Plus

http://nutritioncalc.mhhe.com

NutritionCalc Plus is a dietary analysis program with an easy-to-use interface that allows users to track their nutrient and food group intakes, energy expenditures, and weight control goals. It generates a variety of reports and graphs for analysis, including comparisons with My-Pyramid and the latest Dietary Reference Intakes (DRIs). The database includes thousands of ethnic foods, supplements, fast foods, and convenience foods, and users can add their own foods to the food list. NutritionCalc Plus is available on CD-ROM or in an online version.

PageOut: The Course Website Development Center

www.pageout.net

PageOut, free to instructors who use a McGraw-Hill textbook, is an online program you can use to create your own course website. PageOut offers the following features:

- A course home page
- An instructor home page
- A syllabus (interactive and customizable, including quizzing, instructor notes, and links to the text's Online Learning Center)
- Web links
- Discussions (multiple discussion areas per class)
- An online gradebook
- Links to student Web pages

Contact your McGraw-Hill sales representative to obtain a password.

Course Management Systems

Now instructors can combine their McGraw-Hill Online Learning Center with today's most popular course management systems. Consult your McGraw-Hill sales representative to learn what other course management systems are easily used with McGraw-Hill online materials.

Classroom Performance System

Classroom Performance System (CPS) brings interactivity into the classroom/lecture hall. It is a wireless response system that gives instructors and students immediate feedback from the entire class. The wireless response pads are essentially remotes that are easy to use and that engage students. CPS is available for both IBM and Mac computers.

Primis Online

www.primisonline.com

Primis Online is a database-driven publishing system that allows instructors to create content-rich textbooks, lab manuals, or readers for their courses directly from the Primis website. The customized text can be delivered in print or electronic (eBook) form. A Primis eBook is a digital version of the customized text (sold directly to students as a file downloadable to their computer or accessed online by a password). *Understanding Your Health,* tenth edition, is included in the database.

Acknowledgments

The publisher's reviewers made excellent comments and suggestions that were very useful to us in writing and revising this book. Their contributions are present in every chapter. We would like to express our sincere appreciation for both their critical and comparative readings.

For the Tenth Edition

Norma Bowe, *Kean University*; Tyrone R. Burkett, *Penn State University Abington*; Dan Denson, *McNeese State University*; Joseph M. Flaherty, *Lehigh Carbon Community College*; Steve Gabany, *Indiana State University*; Bernard Griego, *University of California, Berkeley*; Charlene Gungil, *William Paterson University*; Will Stern, *University of Tennessee, Chattanooga*; Angela Willson, *Yuba College*; Lana Zinger, *Queensborough Community College*

For the Ninth Edition

Denise Colaianni, *Western Connecticut State University*; William Ebomoyi, *University of Northern Colorado*; Heidi Fuller, *Salem State College*; Kim Hyatt, *Weber State University*; John Kowalczyk, *University of Minnesota*; Janis McWayne, *Francis Marion University*; Dave Oster, *Jefferson College*; Lana Zinger, *Queensborough Community College*

For the Eighth Edition

Srijana Bajracharya, *Ithaca College*; Steve G. Gabany, *Indiana State University*; Rosann L. Poole, *Tallahassee Community College*; Kerry J. Redican, *Virginia Polytechnic Institute and State University*; Andrew L. Shim, *Southwestern College*; Lucille Talbot, *William Paterson University*

For the Seventh Edition

Charles R. Baffi, *Virginia Tech*; M. Basti, *Cuesta College*; Susan T. Burge, *Cuyahoga Community College*; Karen Camarata, *Eastern Kentucky University*; Kim Clark, *California State University, San Bernardino*; David P. Diaz, *Cuesta College*; Mark Doherty, *The University of Louisiana at Monroe*; Bridget Driscoll, *California State University, Fullerton*; Boyd Foster, *Eastern Washington University*; Sara Geist, *Ohio University*; Stephen Green, *Mississippi State University*; Kathryn Hilgenkamp, *Coastal Carolina University*; Kimberley Hyatt, *Weber State University*; Laurie Merges, *Kent State University*; Ron Murray, *University of Virginia*; Bill E. Pride, *Arizona State University*; DawnElla Rust, *Stephen F. Austin State University*; M. Ann Smith, *Chadron State College*;

Charles Tucker, *Valdosta State University*; Karen Vail-Smith, *East Carolina University*; Kathy Webster, *California State University, Fullerton*; Holly Willey, *Mississippi State University*

For the Sixth Edition

Srijana Bajracharya, *University of Maine-Presque Isle*; Gary Chandler, *Gardner-Webb University*; Patricia Cost, *Weber State University*; John Downey, *Long Beach City College*; Emogene Fox, *University of Central Arkansas*; Jolynn Gardner, *Anoka Ramsey Community College*; Ann Wertz Garvin, *University of Wisconsin-Whitewater*; Patricia Gordon, *Arkansas Tech University*; Rene Gratz, *University of Wisconsin-Milwaukee*; Loretta Herrin, *Benedict College*; Norm Hoffman, *Bakersfield College*; Carol Johnson, *University of Richmond*; Susan MacLaury, *Kean University*; Lori Marti, *Mankato State University*; Randy McGuire, *Eastern Kentucky University*; Phyllis Murray, *Eastern Kentucky University*; Carol Parker, *University of Central Oklahoma*; Alan Peterson, *Gordon College*; Kerry Redican, *Virginia Polytechnic Institute and State University*; McKay Rollins, *Brigham Young University*

For the Fifth Edition

Lori Dewald, *Shippensburg University*; Chester A. Halterman, *Northern Virginia Community College*; Richard Hurley, *Brigham Young University*; John Janowiak, *Appalachian State University*; Jacquelynn K. Lott, *Antelope Valley College*; Rosalie D. Marinelli, *University of Nevada*

For the Fourth Edition

Rosemary C. Clark, *City College of San Francisco*; Marianne Frauenknecht, *Western Michigan University*; Nancy Geha, *Eastern Kentucky University*; Jeffrey Hallam, *Ohio State University*; Dawn Larsen, *Mankato State University*; Loretta M. Liptak, *Youngstown State University*; Bruce M. Ragon, *Indiana University*

For the Third Edition

Charles A. Bish, *Slippery Rock University*; G. Robert Bowers, *Tallahassee Community College*; Donald L. Calitri, *Eastern Kentucky University*; Shae L. Donham, *Northeastern Oklahoma State University*; P. Tish K. Doyle, *University of Calgary*; Judy C. Drolet, *Southern Illinois University Carbondale*; Dalen Duitsman, *Iowa State University*; Mary A. Glascoff, *East Carolina University*; Sonja S. Glassmeyer, *California Polytechnic State University, San Luis Obispo*; Health Education Faculty, *Cerritos College*; Norm Hoffman, *Bakersfield College*;

C. Jessie Jones, *University of New Orleans;* Jean M. Kirsch, *Mankato State University;* Duane Knudson, *Baylor University;* Doris McLittle-Marino, *University of Akron;* Juli Lawrence Miller, *Ohio University;* Victor Schramske, *Normandale Community College;* Janet M. Sermon, *Florida A&M University;* Myra Sternlieb, *DeAnza College;* Mark G. Wilson, *University of Georgia*

Focus Group Participants

Danny Ballard, *Texas A&M University;* Robert C. Barnes, *East Carolina University;* Jacki Benedik, *University of Southwestern Louisiana;* Kathie C. Garbe, *Youngstown State University;* Virginia Peters, *University of Central Oklahoma;* Les Ramsdel, *Eastern Kentucky University;* James Robinson III, *University of Northern Colorado;* Linda Schiller-Moening, *North Hennepin Community College*

For the Second Edition

Dan Adame, *Emory University;* Judith Boone Alexander, *Evergreen Valley College;* Judy B. Baker, *East Carolina University;* Robert C. Barnes, *East Carolina University;* Loren Bensley, *Central Michigan University;* Ernst Bleichart, *Vanier College;* Shirley F. B. Carter, *Springfield College;* Vivien C. Carver, *Youngstown State University;* Cynthia Chubb, *University of Oregon;* Janine Cox, *University of Kansas;* Dick Dalton, *Lincoln University;* Sharron K. Deny, *East Los Angeles College;* Emogene Fox, *University of Central Arkansas;* George Gerrodette, *San Diego Mesa College;* Ray Johnson, *Central Michigan*

University; James W. Lochner, *Weber State College;* Linda S. Myers, *Slippery Rock University;* Virginia Peters, *University of Central Oklahoma;* James Robinson III, *University of Northern Colorado;* Merwin S. Roeder, *Kearney State College;* James H. Rothenberger, *University of Minnesota;* Ronald E. Sevier, *El Camino Community College;* Reza Shahrokh, *Montclair State College;* Albert Simon, *University of Southwestern Louisiana;* Dennis W. Smith, *University of North Carolina at Greensboro;* Loretta R. Taylor, *Southwestern College*

For the First Edition

Stephen E. Bohnenblust, *Mankato State University;* Neil Richard Boyd, Jr., *University of Southern Mississippi;* William B. Cissell, *East Tennessee State University;* Victor A. Corroll, *University of Manitoba;* Donna Kasari Ellison, *University of Oregon Umpqua, Community College;* Neil E. Gallagher, *Towson State University;* Susan C. Girratano, *California State University, Northridge;* Raymond Goldberg, *State University of New York College at Cortland;* Marsha Hoagland, *Modesto Junior College;* Carol Ann Holcomb, *Kansas State University;* Sharon S. Jones, *Orange Coast College;* Daniel Klein, *Northern Illinois University;* Susan Cross Lipnickey, *Miami University of Ohio;* Gerald W. Matheson, *University of Wisconsin La Crosse;* Hollis N. Matson, *San Francisco State University;* David E. Mills, *University of Waterloo;* Peggy Pederson, *Montana State University;* Valerie Pinhas, *Nassau Community College;* Jacy Showers, *Formerly of Ohio State University;* Parris Watts, *University of Missouri-Columbia;* Wayne E. Wylie, *Texas A&M University*

Special Acknowledgments

Authors do not exist in isolation. To publish successful textbooks, an entire team of professionals must work together for a significant amount of time. During the past three decades, we have worked with many talented people to publish more than 20 successful textbooks.

For this edition of *Understanding Your Health,* we used the professional expertise and writing talents of a team of three contributing authors. Leonard Kaminsky, Ph.D., Professor and Coordinator of Ball State University's Adult Fitness and Cardiac Rehabilitation Programs, took on the task of revising and updating Chapter 4 (Becoming Physically Fit) and Chapter 10 (Enhancing Your Cardiovascular Health). Robert Pinger, Ph.D., Professor in the Department of Physiology and Health Science at Ball State, revised Chapter 19 (Protecting Your Safety). And Chapter 20 (The Environment and Your Health) was written by David LeBlanc, Ph.D., Professor of Biology at

Ball State University. We thank these contributors for their professional dedication to this book and their personal commitment to the health of college students with whom they work on a daily basis.

This latest edition of *Understanding Your Health* bears the imprint of Joseph Diggins, Sponsoring Editor, Health and Human Performance. Joe's infectious excitement for *Understanding Your Health* and his positive vision for the future of our personal health texts have made us proud to be McGraw-Hill authors. We hope to work with Joe on many future editions.

New to this edition of *Understanding Your Health* is our Senior Developmental Editor, Kirstan Price. Among all the people who helped with this edition, Kirstan probably made the most critical impact. We believe her pedagogical perspectives combined with her vast knowledge about health topics helped to make this edition of *Under-*

standing Your Health especially meaningful to students and professors. Kirstan can turn chaos into clarity. For that we are so thankful.

On the production end of this edition, we interacted with many people for the first time. Wendy Nelson was our manuscript editor. She did a wonderful job juggling this book and its shorter version simultaneously. She did this with her own quiet enthusiasm, grace, and humor. We are certain that it was challenging for her to work on two books with three authors and three contributors. Thank you Wendy.

Finally, we would like to thank our families for their continued support and love. More than anyone else, they know the energy and dedication it takes to write and revise textbooks. To them we continue to offer our sincere admiration and loving appreciation.

Wayne A. Payne
Dale B. Hahn
Ellen B. Lucas

A Visual Guide to Understanding Your Health

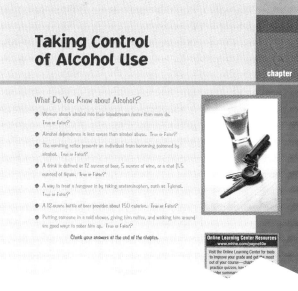

Whether you're trying to get in shape, looking for sound health advice, trying to interpret the health information you see in the media, or just working toward a good grade, *Understanding Your Health* is designed to help you succeed. Here's a brief guide to some of the useful and eye-opening features you'll find inside.

"What Do You Know?" Quiz

Each chapter opens with a brief quiz that highlights key points and allows you to check how much you know about chapter topics. Quiz answers are found at the end of the chapter.

Building Media Literacy Skills

Curious about all those ads you see for various drugs? Wondering about the reliability of the health information you find on the Internet? This feature investigates the way that written, broadcast, electronic, and personal media shape our perceptions about health, health care, and wellness. It also provides strategies that will help you be a more critical consumer of health information.

Changing for the Better

Learn to put health concepts into practice by following these useful tips. This feature provides practical advice for making positive changes and staying motivated to follow a healthy lifestyle.

Changing for the Better

Overcoming Barriers to Being Regularly Active

I've never really been active and can't seem to get started on an exercise program. What can I do?

Barriers to physical activity frequently listed by Americans are lack of time, motivation, and support and finding exercise inconvenient, boring, and unpleasant. Do you find it difficult to be regularly active? Take the quiz at the first InfoLink site listed below to find out your personal barriers. The same site also lists suggestions for overcoming common barriers, including the following strategies:

- *Lack of time.* Monitor your daily activities for a week to identify available time slots. Add physical activity to your daily routine, and select activities that require minimal time.
- *Lack of energy.* Sch ~tivity for times in the d~   ~ou f~   ~ your~

- *Fear of injury.* Choose activities involving minimum risk, and learn how to warm up, cool down, and work out in ways that are appropriate to your age, fitness level, and health status.
- *Lack of resources.* Select activities that require minimal facilities or equipment, such as walking or calisthenics. Investigate resources available on your campus.
- *Weather conditions.* Develop a set of regular activities that are always available regardless of weather. Look on outdoor activities that depend on weather conditions as extra bonus activities.
- *Family obligations.* Exercise with the kids or while the kids are bu~   ~leeping. Trade b~   ~ with a friend o~

Talking Points

Throughout each chapter, you'll find these tips for starting a dialogue about sensitive health topics.

TALKING POINTS A smoker says that she does not consider smoking to be a form of drug use. She becomes angry at the suggestion that cigarettes are part of a drug-delivery system. How would you respond to her position?

Discovering Your Spirituality

A healthy body and a healthy mind go hand in hand. This feature will help you tap into your spiritual side to improve your self-esteem, foster good relationships with others, and jump-start your physical health.

Discovering Your Spirituality

Mindfulness: Time to Pay Attention

Have you taken a moment today to be quiet and just be with yourself? Time alone can help you step away from a busy, fragmented world and draw inward for renewal. Having strengthened awareness of yourself in both mind and body allows you to experience the fullness of the moment, even to feel in sync with the universe. This is referred to as "mindfulness"—being aware of the present moment without judging, just accepting.

Mindfulness can also help you establish your identity, clarify what's important to you, and strengthen your independence. When we are observing ourselves in the present moment, we have the opportunity to fully emerge and become ourselves.

Any time you take for this meditation will be restorative. You may start with just five minutes every morning. You will need a place where you feel comfortable to be alone with your own thoughts, whether it be in bed, in the bath, at a coffee shop, in the library, or in the garden. Go for a walk, listen to music, do yoga, or just be still and concentrate on your breathing. All of these are ways to reconnect you to your life force. Pretty soon you may feel that your time of mindfulness is more energizing than sleep! When you are faced with a difficult project, a personal crisis, or something mo~ ~erious, such~ ~ sickness o~ ~ath, these re~ ~tive
~om~ ~ve y~ ~nd ~ ~wal~

Considering Complementary Care

Interested in nontraditional approaches to health care? What really works? What's really safe? This feature invites you to take a critical look at alternative approaches to health care and make up your own mind.

Considering Complementary Care

Alternatives for Stress Management

Complementary and alternative medicine are becoming increasingly popular in managing stress and alleviating insomnia. Herbal therapies, massage therapy, acupuncture, and ayurvedic medicine have been utilized to combat stress with good success. A national survey found that over 1.6 million Americans reported using some type of complementary care or alternative medicine for stress management or insomnia and thought it was helpful.

A majority of Americans reported taking a dietary supplement in the past month, and 40 percent of these people took them for insomnia or stress-related problems. The larger variety of herbal therapies include melatonin, kava kava, valerian, Siberian ginseng, lime blossom, catmint, skullcap, and chamomile, which are purported to have a calming effect and to help relieve stress and insomnia. Herbal supplements are made from extracts from plants and roots and can be taken in many different forms, such as pills or in teas or other beverages. Because they are considered dietary supplements, the FDA does not regulate them, and so there is no standardization for dosage nor anyone monitoring them for quality control. Little is known about their safety, side effects, or effectiveness. Melatonin is a natural hormone secreted by the pineal gland in the brain. Melatonin is one of on~ ~ hormones not reg~ ~ the FDA; it is sold
~r the c~ ~ orescri~ ~d a dietar~

of types of massage, including Swedish, deep-tissue, reflexology, and acupressure. Massage usually involves holding, pressing, and moving across particular stress points in the body to remove stress from these areas.

Acupuncture involves stimulation of anatomical points in the body by a variety of techniques using hair-thin, metallic needles. The goal of acupuncture is to release the energy flow that is blocked in your body and regain balance. This process stimulates endorphins, neurotransmitters, neurohormones, and immune cells.

Ayurvedic medicine is the "science of life" and is a holistic approach to stress management. It incorporates yoga, herbs, specific foods and diets, massage, and meditation to manage stress. It is based upon the belief that different body types require different diets, herbs, and regimes. Health and disease are seen to be related to the state of imbalance or balance of one's physical and mental states, as well as lifestyle factors.

More research needs to be conducted on how these therapies work and their rate of effectiveness, as well as any adverse side effects. If you want to try an alternative form of medicine, make ~hat the people you receive ~ ~ices from are certified
~ined, and k~ ~se alterna~

Learning from Our Diversity
Cardiovascular Disease Is Not Necessarily an Equal Opportunity Disease

Although cardiovascular disease is a significant problem for people of all races and ethnic backgrounds in the United States, there are distinct differences between some segments of our population. For example, did you know that African Americans have the highest rate of hypertension of any group of people throughout the world? Compared to white Americans, African Americans develop hypertension at an earlier age and have higher average blood pressure values. This is partly responsible for African Americans' higher death rates from stroke and heart disease and their higher rates of end-stage renal (kidney) disease.

two or more risk factors for coronary heart disease compared to other population groups.

What are the factors that contribute to these differences between different groups of people? The answers are not entirely clear, but it is likely that the differences result from a combination of factors. Certainly genetics could play a role. For example, it has been theorized that African Americans may have some nervous system differences that would cause their blood pressure to be higher. However, as with the population at large, cultural, environmental, and socioeconomic ... probably contribute to the ... rates of cardiovascular ... some ...

Personal Assessment
Risk Assessment for Marijuana Dependence or Abuse

You may wonder if your use or a friend's use of marijuana fits the criteria for being at risk for developing marijuana dependence or abuse. The following questions may help you determine if there is cause for you to be concerned.

1. Have you tried to cut down or stop smoking marijuana and not been able to do so?
2. Do you use daily?
3. Is it hard for you to imagine life without marijuana?
4. Do you find that who your friends is determined by your marijuana use?
5. Do you use marijuana to avoid dealing with your problems?
6. Do you use marijuana to cope with your feelings?
7. Has your marijuana use created conflict in your relationships?
8. Has your marijuana use created problems for you at work?
9. Has your marijuana use decreased your academic performance?
10. Has your use of marijuana caused problems with memory or concentration?
11. When your stash is nea~ ~ty, do you feel anxious or worried about ~
    you pl~   ~ana use

13. Have friends or relatives ever complained that your marijuana use is damaging your relationship with them?
14. Have you or others noticed a decrease in your overall motivation level?
15. Do you find that your marijuana use has increased over time?

Interpretation

Any yes answer could indicate problematic use of marijuana.

TO CARRY THIS FURTHER . . .

If you answered yes to any of these questions, you may want to reevaluate your marijuana use and talk to a medical or mental health care provider about a further assessment for drug abuse or dependence. If you are concerned about a friend's use, you might point to these specific behavioral criteria in sharing your concerns and encourage your friend to seek professional assistance.

~ from Ball State Uni~   ~ion~

Learning from Our Diversity

These unique boxes invite you to explore the rich diversity of your own campus and to gain perspective on the way such characteristics as age, racial/ethnic background, physical abilities, and sexual orientation can shape individuals' lives and well-being.

Personal Assessment

Do you eat too much fat? What's the best method of birth control for you if you are sexually active? Are you a perfectionist? Each chapter in *Understanding Your Health* includes an assessment to help you learn the answers to these and many other questions.

Shaping Your Health

What Do You Know about Health and Wellness?

◉ The label *Millennial Generation* encompasses all of today's traditional-age college students. True or False?

◉ Society holds developmentally oriented expectations for young adults, but not for middle-aged and older adults. True or False?

◉ Definitions of health derived from episodic and preventive medicine are strongly influenced by concerns related to morbidity and mortality. True or False?

◉ Persons with diagnosed disabilities, both visible and hidden, compose less than 5 percent of the current college student population. True or False?

◉ The loss of functionality is a reality for many older adults. True or False?

◉ Males' shorter life expectancy, compared to that of females, results almost completely from males' greater genetic weakness. True or False?

◉ A holistic perception of health is a perception totally focused on the structure and function of the body. True or False?

Check your answers at the end of the chapter.

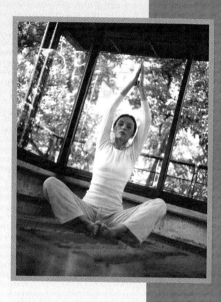

Online Learning Center Resources
www.mhhe.com/payne10e

Visit the Online Learning Center for tools to improve your grade and get the most out of your course—chapter objectives, practice quizzes, key terms flashcards, chapter summaries for your digital audio player, Web activities, self-assessments, and many other study aids.

"Take care of your health, because you'll miss it when it's gone," younger people hear often from their elders. This simple and heartfelt advice is given in the belief that young people take their health for granted and assume that they will always maintain the state of health and wellness they now enjoy. Observation and experience should, however, remind all of us that youth is relatively brief, and health is always changing.

How do you imagine your life in the future? Do you ever think about how your health allows you to participate in meaningful life activities—and what might happen if your health is compromised? Consider, for example, how your health affects the following activities:

• Your ability to pursue an education or a career
• Your opportunities to socialize with friends and family
• The chance to travel—for business, relaxation, or adventure

- The opportunity to meet and connect with new people
- The ability to conceive or the opportunity to parent children
- Your participation in hobbies and recreational activities
- Your enjoyment of a wide range of foods
- The opportunity to live independently

As you will learn in this chapter, quality of life is intertwined with activities such as these—indeed, your authors will present a new definition of health specifically related to accomplishing these important life tasks. But first, let's review the key growth and development tasks of adulthood and a few familiar perceptions about health. This chapter will provide you with a foundation for understanding your own health, as well as strategies to change problematic health behaviors.

The Millennial Generation

The general period of young adulthood (ages 18–39) is often divided into subperiods: early young adulthood (ages 18–24), middle young adulthood (25–33), and later young adulthood (34–39). Traditional-age college students are what we will call "early young adults" (ages 18–24). Non-traditional-age college students are students of all other age groups—middle young adults, later young adults, as well as older individuals in middle or older adulthood and the occasional teenager and even preteenager!

"Millennial generation" is the name given to today's early young adults, 18 to 24 years old.[1] If you are a nontraditional-age student reading this textbook, you will have your own generational "name." But if you are of traditional age (18–24), you are being placed in a larger group of persons, born between 1982 and 2000 and referred to collectively by sociologists as "millennials."

There have been some initial studies of the millennial generation's progress in mastering the developmental expectations for the transition from adolescence to early adulthood. (These expectations are discussed later in this chapter.) These studies have found that, compared to earlier generations, the millennials are:[2, 3, 4]

- More inclined to drop out of college for a period of time, and take longer to finish college even if they have not dropped out
- More likely to change colleges, and to change residence while at the same college
- More likely to return home to live after completing college—the "boomerang" phenomenon
- More likely to share a residence with friends from college than to live alone or to return home
- More likely to take less-substantive jobs, often in food services and retail sales, that pay relatively low wages

- Likely to leave a job rather than deal with job-related conflict, thus not experiencing advancement within the workplace, while protecting their self-concept
- More inclined to fill leisure time with technology-based media
- Less likely to have refined communications skills, due in large part to technology-based communication
- More likely to volunteer—not to pad their résumés, but for the well-being of others
- More likely to have a more diverse group of friends, in terms of both gender and race
- Less likely to marry, less likely to marry at a younger age, and more likely to delay parenting until older

Whether these generalizations about the millennial generation are compatible with our society's traditional developmental expectations will become clearer as time progresses. At this point, however, many experts believe that the millennials' growth and development are headed in a largely positive direction.[5]

If you are a nontraditional-age student (particularly if you were born before 1982), take an opportunity to look back to your early young adult years and assess, from the perspective of your current age, how you handled the developmental tasks just described. Also, speculate on how your soon-to-be-completed college education might have altered your initial progress through early young adulthood, if you had completed college at that younger age.

Developmental Tasks of Early Adulthood

Let's look next at some predictable areas of growth and development (defined as developmental expectations or tasks) that characterize the lives of young adults. Of course, society's expectations for the next generation of early young adults are always stated in the context of permissible "uniqueness," thus allowing you a fair measure of latitude so that you can do things "your way." Your textbook will provide a brief and general view of each early young adult developmental task—note that five of these tasks are more immediate in their completion, while two are traditionally brought to fruition a bit later. Making progress in these areas contributes to a sense of well-being and life satisfaction.

Forming an Initial Adult Identity

As emerging adults, most young people want to present a personally satisfying initial adult identity as they transition from adolescence into early young adulthood. Internally they are constructing perceptions of themselves as the adults they wish to be; externally they are formulating the behavioral patterns that will project this identity to others. Completion of this first developmental task is necessary for early young adults to establish a foundation on which to nurture their identity during the later stages of adulthood.

Establishing Independence

Society anticipates that, by the time their college education is completed, younger adults should be moving away from their earlier socialization and dependent relationships, particularly with their family and adolescent peer group. Travel, new relationships, military service, marriage, and, of course, college studies have been the traditional avenues for disengagement from the family.

Assuming Responsibility

Our society's third developmental expectation for traditional-age college students is that these early young adults will assume increasing levels of responsibility. Traditional-age students have a variety of opportunities, both on and off the college campus, to begin the process of becoming responsible for themselves and for other individuals, programs, and institutions. Central at this time is the need to assume increasing levels of responsibility in one's movement through the academic curriculum and for one's own and others' health (see the box "The Internet—Your Health Superstore").

 TALKING POINTS What does being an adult mean to you at this point? How would you explain this to your best friend?

Broadening Social Skills

The fourth developmental task for early young adults is to broaden their range of appropriate and dependable social skills. Adulthood ordinarily involves "membership" in a variety of groups that range in size from a marital pair to a multiple-member community group or a multinational corporation. These memberships require the ability to function in many different social settings, with an array of people, and in many roles. Accomplishing this task particularly requires that early young adults refine their skills in communication, listening, and conflict management.

Nurturing Intimacy

The task of nurturing intimacy usually begins in early young adulthood and continues, in various forms, through much of the remainder of life. Persons of traditional college age can experience intimacy in a more mature sense, centered on deep and caring relationships, than was true during adolescence. Dating relationships, close and trusting friendships, and mentoring relationships are the arenas in which mature intimacy will take root. From a developmental perspective, what matters is that we have quality relationships involving persons with whom we share our most deeply held thoughts, feelings,

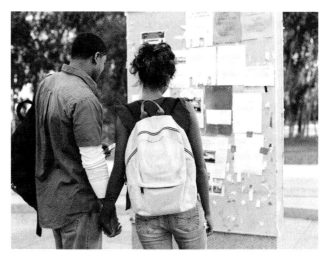

Developmental tasks for young adults include establishing independence from their families, assuming more responsibility for themselves and others, and nuturing intimate relationships.

and aspirations as we attempt to validate our own unique approach to life. Young adults who are unwilling or unable to create intimacy can develop a sense of emotional isolation.

Obtaining Entry-Level Employment and Developing Parenting Skills

In addition to the five developmental tasks just addressed, two additional areas of growth and development seem applicable to early young adults, but may come into "focus" more gradually. They include obtaining entry-level employment within the field of one's academic preparation and the development of parenting skills.

For nearly three-quarters of a century (thanks in part to the GI Bill after World War II) the majority of students have pursued a college education in anticipation that its completion would open doors (entry-level opportunities) in particular professions or fields of employment. In many respects these forms of employment meet needs beyond those associated purely with money. Employment of this nature provides opportunities to build new skills that expand upon those learned in academic majors, to undertake new forms of responsibility beyond those available on campus, and to play a more diverse set of roles, including colleague, supervisor, mentor, mentee, or partner. And today, more so than in the past, intimate relationships often have their origin in the workplace.

Although Americans today are having fewer children than in past generations, the fact remains that parenting-related decisions and skills are important components of the young adulthood years. Decisions regarding parenting (both biological and adoptive) involve important questions regarding age for the onset of parenting, number of children, and interval between subsequent children, as well as the manner in which parenting will be

The Internet—Your Health Superstore

Although the Pew Research Center (reporting 137 million Internet users) and TechWeb (reporting 172 million Internet users) do not agree on the number of Americans who have access to the World Wide Web, both reported numbers are, nevertheless, impressive. The TechWeb estimate suggests that approximately 70 percent of Americans have Web access from their homes. Access from work, school, and libraries greatly increases availability. As you might imagine, searches involving health-related information are high on the list of topical areas explored online.

Most frequently, online users seek information regarding specific medical problems, followed by information regarding aspects of treatment and longer term management of these problems. The use of the Internet for health-related purposes is, however, not a daily occurrence for most Americans with Internet access. When the Internet is used for this purpose, women are more likely to be seeking information than are men, and they most often do so for other persons (spouses, children, and friends). If you are not already, it is highly probable that you too will be an online consumer of health-related information, products, or services.

The biggest challenge for you as a health consumer is determining the credibility of the information you find on the Internet. How can you know that this information (and accompanying products or services) is trustworthy and that the persons responsible for the information, products, or services are motivated by concern for your health and well-being rather than just by profit? Recognized authorities offer these guidelines to help you:

- Who does the website belong to? Is it sponsored by an institution of higher education, a professional society, a government or not-for-profit agency, or a recognized pharmaceutical company? If not, who is responsible for the information? Remember, virtually anyone can develop a web page and begin disseminating information.

- Is the information carefully referenced, showing sources such as government reports, professional journal articles, or respected reference publications? Are the references clearly documented and current? Is the web page updated regularly? Does the information appear to agree with the titles of its own references?

- Does the content of the information seem to have a critical or negative bias toward a particular profession, institution, or treatment method? Does the information discredit others more than it supports its own position?

- Are "significant breakthroughs" promised in a way that suggests that only this source has the "ultimate answer" to certain problems? Does this answer involve throwing out your prescriptions, going against your physician's orders, or considering suicide as a way of escaping the pain and difficulties associated with your illness?

If you are skeptical about the credibility of any health care information you find online, submit the information to a respected health care professional or organization for assessment. If you and your physician find suspicious information or fraudulent health claims, report this to the Federal Trade Commission. Today, most health care practitioners feel comfortable with well-informed patients. In comparison to the public's ability to access health-related information prior to the World Wide Web, today's public is significantly more empowered (a term you will encounter later in the chapter) as they navigate the complex American health care system. Although one must be cautious about information found online, creditable sources can be instrumental in helping individuals enhance their own health.

---

undertaken and the role it will play relative to the overall aspirations of the adults involved. In today's complex society, young adults need to more clearly than ever understand the significant differences between reproduction and parenting; thus we assign the development of parenting skills as a socially anticipated developmental task.

Developmental Tasks of Middle and Older Adulthood

For students of traditional college age, help in more fully understanding the developmental tasks of middle and older adulthood can be supplied by the nontraditional-age students with whom you are in class with, as well as by your parents, family friends, older coworkers, and grandparents.

Midlife Developmental Tasks

If you are a traditional-age student, have you wondered what it would be like to be 20 or 30 years older than you are now? What would you be doing, feeling, and thinking if you were the age of your parents? What are your parents thinking about and trying to accomplish as they move through their midlife years?

One thought that probably recurs all too often is the reality of their eventual death (see the box "Why Men Die Young"). Their awareness that they will not live forever is a subtle but profoundly influential force that can cause them to be restless, to renew attention to their spirituality, and to be more highly motivated to master the developmental tasks of middle adulthood. This motivation and the awareness of the reality of death combine to produce the dynamic concept of being at "the prime of

Why Men Die Young

The extra longevity of women in our society is well established. In fact, the difference in life expectancy for infants born today is projected to be 80 years for females and only 75 for males. This 5-year difference has commonly been attributed to genetic factors. However, new evidence demonstrates that this discrepancy may be affected more by male behavior rather than genetic traits.

Men outrank women in all of the top 15 causes of death except for Alzheimer's disease. Men's death rates are twice as high for suicide, homicide, and cirrhosis of the liver. In every age group, American males have poorer health and higher risk of mortality than do females. Common increased risks include:

- More men smoke than women.
- Men are twice as likely to be heavy drinkers and to engage in other risky behaviors such as abusing drugs and driving without a seat belt.
- More men work in dangerous settings than women do, and men account for 90 percent of on-the-job fatalities.
- More men drive SUVs that are rollover prone and suffer fatalities in motorcycle accidents.

Perhaps some of these increased risks are associated with deep-seated cultural beliefs, which reward men for taking risks and facing danger head-on. This "macho" attitude seems to extend to the care that men take of their own physical and mental health. Women are twice as likely as men to visit their doctor on an annual basis and explore preventive medical treatments. Men are more likely to ignore symptoms and less likely to schedule checkups or seek follow-up treatment. Psychologically, men tend to internalize their feelings or stressors, or even self-medicate to deal with stress, while women tend to seek psychological help. Almost all stress-related diseases are more common in men.

In the final analysis, men and women alike must be responsible for their own health and well-being. By making sound choices regarding diet, exercise, medical care, and high-risk behaviors, both genders can attempt to maximize the full potential of their life expectancy.

---

life"—a time when there seems to be a great deal to accomplish and a diminishing amount of time in which to accomplish it.

Achieving Generativity   In a very real sense, people in middle adulthood are asked to do something they have not been expected to do previously. As a part of their development as unique people, they are expected to "pay back" society for the support it has given them. Most people in middle adulthood begin to realize that the collective society, through its institutions (families, schools, churches), has been generous in its support of their growth and development and that it is time to replenish these resources.[6, 7] Younger and older people may have needs that middle-aged people can best meet. By meeting the needs of others, people in middle adulthood can fulfill their own needs to grow and develop. *Generativity*, a term introduced into the field of adult emotional development by Erik Erikson,[8] reflects a process in which the emotional maturation needs of middle-aged people interact with society's need to support its most vulnerable members—its children and older adults, particularly the infirm and the frail.

The process of repaying society for its support is structured around familiar types of activities. Developmentally speaking, people in middle adulthood are able to select the activities that best use their abilities to contribute to the good of society.

The most traditional way in which people in middle adulthood repay society is through parenting. Children, with their potential for becoming valuable members of the next generation, need the support of people who recognize the contribution they can make. By supporting children, either directly through quality parenting or through institutions that function on behalf of children, middle-aged people repay society for the support they have themselves received. As they extend themselves outward on behalf of the next generation, they ensure their own growth and development. In a similar fashion, their support of aging parents and institutions that serve older adults provides another means to express generativity.

For people who possess artistic talent, generativity may be accomplished through the pleasure brought to others. Artists, craftspeople, and musicians have unique opportunities to speak directly to others through their talents. Volunteer work serves as another avenue for generativity. Most people in middle adulthood also express generativity through their jobs by providing quality products or services and thus contribute to the well-being of those who desire or need these goods and services.

Reassessing the Plans of Young Adulthood   People in middle adulthood must also begin coming to terms with the finality of their death. In conjunction with doing this, they often feel compelled to take time to think about their goals for adulthood they formulated 25 or more years previously. Their dreams are thus revisited. This reassessment constitutes a second developmental task of people in middle adulthood.

By carefully reviewing the aspirations they had as young adults, middle-aged people can more clearly study their short- and long-term goals. Specifically, strengths and limitations that were unrecognizable when they were young adults are now more clearly seen. The inexperience of youth is replaced by the insights gained through experience. A commitment to quality often replaces the

Accepting the physical changes of aging while maintaining a high level of functionality is a key developmental task for older adults.

desire for quantity during the second half of the life cycle. Time is valued more highly because it is now seen in a more realistic perspective. The dream for the future is more sharply focused, and the successes and failures of the past are more fully understood as this developmental task of reassessing earlier plans of young adulthood is accomplished.

Developmental Tasks of Older Adulthood

In this section, we focus on the developmental tasks confronted by older adults. Accepting the physical changes of aging, maintaining physical functionality, and reassessing one's sense of integrity are tasks of the older adulthood period.

Accepting the Changes of Aging   The general decline associated with the latter part of the life cycle is particularly serious between the seventh and ninth decades. Physically, emotionally, socially, intellectually, and occupationally, older adults must accept at least some decline. For example, a person may no longer be able to drive a car, which could in turn limit participation in social activities. Even a spiritual loss may be encountered at those times when life seems less humane. Clearly, a developmental task to be accomplished by the older adult is to accept the nature and extent of these changes.

Maintaining Functionality   Because each segment of the life cycle should be approached with the fullest level of involvement possible, the second developmental task

of the older adult is to maintain as much functionality as possible, particularly those aspects of physical functioning that support independence.

For areas of decline in which some measure of reversal is possible, older adults are afforded an opportunity to seek *rehabilitation*. Whether through a self-designed and individually implemented program or with the aid of a skilled professional, older adults can bring back some function to a previously higher level.

The second approach, often used in combination with rehabilitation, is *remediation*, whereby an alternative to the area of loss is introduced. Examples of remediation include the use of hearing aids, audiocassettes, and caregivers or home health aids. By using alternative resources, function can often be returned.

For a growing number of older adults, rehabilitation and remediation are rarely necessary because of the high level of health that they enjoy. For most, only minor modifications are necessary to enjoy full independence.

Reassessing a Sense of Integrity   The third major developmental task that awaits the older adult is to reassess their sense of integrity, or sense of wholeness, concerning the journey that may be nearly complete.[8] The elderly must look back over their lives to see the value in what they were able to accomplish. They must address the simple but critical questions: Would I do it over again? Am I satisfied with what I managed to accomplish? Can I accept the fact that others will have experiences to which I can never return?

If older adults can answer these questions positively, then they will feel a sense of wholeness, personal value, and worth. Having established this sense of integrity, they will believe that their lives have had meaning and that they have helped society.

Because they have already experienced so much, many older adults have no fear of death, even though they may fear the process of dying. Their ability to come to terms with death thus reinforces their sense of integrity.

Like all the other developmental tasks, this critical area of growth and development is a personal and, thus, a unique experience. Older adults must assume this last developmental task with the same sense of purpose they used for earlier tasks. When older adults can feel this sense of integrity, their reasons for having lived will be more fully understood.

Today's College Students

Readers of this textbook are college students, but they are also young adults, middle-aged adults, or even older adults. In some cases their decision to be a student has placed them in settings far different from those being experienced by other people their age. For many students, college classes are sandwiched in between other obligations—for example, full-time job, parenting, community involvement, even caring for older parents. Some might be the first members of their families to pursue higher education. Many students come from economic, racial, or ethnic backgrounds quite different from those of the majority of their classmates. Thus, today there is no one type of college student, but all students are progressing through life in predictable yet unique ways.

Traditional-Age Students

Projections issued by the National Center for Education Statistics[9] indicate that in the year 2015, more than 19 million persons will be enrolled in degree-granting U.S colleges and universities. Nearly 59 percent of these students will be women. Of course, much speculation exists as to why the discrepancy exists between male and female enrollment levels. Projected patterns of enrollment suggest that by 2015, nearly 37 percent of college student will be enrolled on a part-time basis.

Because today nearly 62 percent of all college students are traditional-age students, this book is directed first at these students. However, due to the significant growth in the percentage of older students, particularly those 30 or older, we also address a variety of life experiences that are appropriate to these students.

TALKING POINTS You are in charge of a campus event for students of various ages from several cultural groups. How would you go about finding out what would make the event attractive to students with backgrounds different from your own?

Nontraditional-Age Undergraduate College Students

In 2004, nearly 43.2 percent of U.S. undergraduate college students were classified as **nontraditional-age students.**[9] Included in this vast overlapping group are part-time students, military veterans, students returning to college, single parents, older adults, and evening students. These students enter the classroom with a wide assortment of life experiences and observations. Most of these students are 25 to 40 years old. (Read the box "Back to the Future" for a closer look at nontraditional-age students.)

Many nontraditional-age students are trying to juggle an extremely demanding schedule. The responsibilities of managing a job, a schedule of classes, and perhaps a family present formidable challenges. Performing these tasks on a limited budget compounds the difficulty. For many of these students, concerns over paying next month's rent, caring for aging parents, and finding affordable child care are among the challenges that confront them.

We want to make this textbook meaningful for both traditional-age and nontraditional-age students. Much of the information we present applies to both categories of students. We ask nontraditional-age students to do two things as you read this book: (1) reflect on your own young adult years and (2) examine your current lifestyle to see how the decisions you made as a younger adult are affecting the quality of your life now. Additionally, ask yourselves: (3) if you had taken this class as a traditional-age student on schedule to graduate, how would your overall younger adulthood have been different, and (4) how will the completion of college as a nontraditional-age student make the remainder of your life different from what you would otherwise have anticipated? Also, as a nontraditional-age student, you may have young adult children whose lives you can observe in light of the information you will find in this book.

Minority Students

Although enrollment patterns at colleges and universities vary, the overall number of minority students is increasing. In 2004, approximately 25 percent of all college students were minority students, with African Americans (13.8 percent), Hispanic Americans (12.9 percent), and Asian Americans (7.1 percent) representing the largest groups of minority students within the total college population.[10] These students bring a rich variety of cultural influences and traditions to today's college environment.

Students with Disabilities

People with reported disabilities are another rapidly growing student population, currently constituting 11 percent of all college students, with orthopedic conditions being the most prevalent (25 percent).[11] Improved diagnostic, medical, and rehabilitation procedures coupled with improved educational accommodations have opened up opportunities for these students at an increasing rate. In addition to students who have evident disabilities, such as blindness, deafness, or a physical disability requiring use of a wheelchair, an increasing number of students with "hidden" disabilities are on campus—students with learning disabilities (including attention deficit hyperactivity disorder), those with managed psychiatric and emotional problems, and those recovering from alcohol and substance abuse. Interestingly, many students with reported "hidden disabilities" often do not consider themselves to have a disability.

> **Key Terms**
>
> **nontraditional-age students** An administrative term used by colleges and universities for students who, for whatever reason, are pursuing undergraduate work at an age other than that associated with the traditional college years (18–24).

Learning from Our Diversity

Back to the Future: Nontraditional-Age Students Enrich the College Experience

To anyone who's visited a U.S. college campus in the last 15 years, it's abundantly clear that the once typical college student—White, middle class, between the ages of 18 and 24—is no longer in a majority on many campuses. In most institutions of higher learning, today's student body is a rich tapestry of color, culture, language, ability, and age. Wheelchair-accessible campuses roll out the welcome mat for students with disabilities; the air is filled with the sound of a dozen or more languages spoken by students from virtually every part of the world; students in their 60s chat animatedly with classmates young enough to be their grandchildren.

Of all the trends that are changing the face of college enrollment in the United States, perhaps the most significant is the increasing diversity in the age of students now on campus. Older students today are both a common and welcome sight in colleges and universities across the country. Many women cut short their undergraduate education—or defer graduate school—to marry and raise children. Divorcees, widows, and women whose children are grown often return to college, or enroll for the first time, to prepare for professional careers. And increasingly, both men and women are finding it desirable,

if not essential, to further their education as a means of either keeping their current job or qualifying for a higher position.

Just as children are enriched by the knowledge and experience of their grandparents and other older relatives, so too is today's college classroom a richer place when many of the seats are filled by students of nontraditional age. Without being didactic or preachy, older students can provide valuable guidance and direction to younger classmates who may be uncertain of their career path, or who may be wrestling with decisions about marriage and parenthood. In doing so, nontraditional-age students can gain helpful insights about young people's feelings, attitudes, challenges, and aspirations.

Among the many important benefits of today's increasingly diverse college campus, surely one of the most significant is the enhanced opportunity for intergenerational communication and understanding made possible by the growing numbers of students of nontraditional age.

In your classes, how would you characterize the interactions between traditional-age students and those of nontraditional age? In what ways are they enriching one another's college experience?

TALKING POINTS When controversial subjects are discussed in class, do you think that your opinions (or how you present them) are affected by the fact that students of different cultural backgrounds are involved in the discussion?

Sources of Our Traditional Definitions of Health

By the time they reach college age, most Americans are familiar with the many ways in which health care is provided. Following are some easily recognizable examples, all of which serve to reinforce our traditional definitions of health. Note that these examples involve the cure or management of illness and the extension of life, indicated by concerns about **morbidity** and **mortality.**

Episodic Health Care

The vast majority of Americans use the services of professional health care providers during periods (*episodes*) of illness and injury, that is, when we are "unhealthy." We consult providers, seeking a diagnosis that will explain why we are not feeling well. Once a problem is identified, we expect to receive effective treatment from the practitioners that will lead to our recovery (the absence of illness) and thus a return to health. If we are willing to comply with the care strategies prescribed by our practitioners, we should soon be able to define ourselves as "healthy" once again.

The familiarity of episodic health care is evident in the 911 million times that Americans visited physicians during 2004.[12] Although some of these visits were for preventive health care (see the discussion in the next section), the vast majority were in conjunction with illness. When viewed according to racial group, Whites averaged 3.3 visits, Blacks 2.7, Hispanic Americans 2.3, and Asian Americans 2.4 visits during that year.[12] A similar reporting in 2000 indicated that Native Americans made only 0.8 visit that year.

Differences in the number of office visits by race are most likely related to a combination of factors, including differences in the types and extent of illnesses within specific racial groups, health insurance or ability to pay for health care services, proximity to services, availability of dependable transportation, as well as personal and cultural practices related to illness.

Of the 911 million office visits in 2004, women were more likely to visit physicians than were men, and infants and persons over 65 were twice as likely to visit physicians than were older children, adolescents, and adults under age 65.[12] People living in metropolitan areas were one-third more likely to make physician visits than were people from nonmetropolitan areas. Again, no single factor accounts for these observed differences.

When office visits are viewed in terms of the types of physicians visited, primary care physicians accounted for the majority of visits (58.5 percent), while surgeons and other specialists accounted for the remainder. Usually surgeons and specialists become involved in a patient's care only after a referral from a primary care physician.[13]

What Is Complementary Medicine?

In addition to the episodic and preventive forms of medical care described earlier, a variety of other forms of health care, both curative and preventive, are moving more progressively into the medical care mainstream. Among these are chiropractic, reflexology, homeopathy, naturopathy, and herbalism (see Chapter 18), to mention but a few. Although the established medical community has long scoffed at these practices as being unscientific and ineffective, they are increasingly attractive to a growing segment of the population. Initially referred to collectively as *alternative* forms of health care, and more recently as *complementary* forms of care, today they are increasingly referred to as *integrative* forms of health care. This last term suggests a fusion (or integration) of various forms of care into traditional treatment/prevention approaches.

The increasing acceptance of integrative forms of health care is also seen in two relatively recent developments. The first is the formation in the mid-1990s of an Office of Complementary and Alternative Medicine within the National Institutes of Health. This office has been charged with the objective and systematic study of selected forms of nontraditional care. Clinical trials of various types are ongoing; they include *treatment trials, supportive care trials, prevention trials, screening trials* (early detection trials), and *diagnostic trials*, all employing forms of alternative or complementary treatments. Subsequent assessments will be released as they are completed.

A second expression of the growing popularity of integrative forms of health care is the increasing tendency of health insurance companies and HMOs (health maintenance organizations; see Chapter 18) to provide reimbursement of services from providers of nontraditional care. Today approximately 65 percent of all HMOs and several major insurance companies provide coverage for selective forms of integrative care.

As impressive as the "rush to coverage" described previously might appear, consumers of medical care services should remember that at this time relatively little carefully controlled research is available on the *efficacy* (effectiveness) of most forms of integrative care.

In spite of cautionary notes such as this, the *popularity* of alternative medical services for improving, maintaining, or restoring health is beyond dispute. A study conducted in 2002 by the Institute of Medicine found that prayer (for self and others), supplement use, relaxation breathing techniques, group prayer, meditation, chiropractic, yoga, and massage were all employed. Prayer, in various settings, was by far the most widely employed.

 TALKING POINTS Would you be hesitant to talk to your doctor about health advice you found on the Internet? How would you approach the subject?

Preventive or Prospective Medicine

Simple logic suggests that it makes more sense to prevent illness than to deal with it through episodic health (medical) care. This philosophy characterizes **preventive or prospective medicine.** Unfortunately, however, many physicians say they have little time to practice preventive medicine because of the large number of episodically sick people who fill their offices every day.

When physicians do practice preventive or prospective medicine, they first attempt to determine their patient's level of risk for developing particular conditions. They make this assessment by identifying **risk factors** (and **high-risk health behaviors**) with a variety of observational techniques and screening tests, some of which may be invasive (taking tissues from the body such as a biopsy or blood draw). Additionally, an important tool in assessing risk is an accurate family health history, something that over one-third of all adults cannot adequately provide to their health care providers.[14] So important is a health history that the federal government has established a website to assist us in becoming familiar with our family's health history (www.hhs.gov/familyhistory).[15] Certainly, if you identify any of the illness-related conditions shown in Table 1.1, share them with your primary care physician.[16, 17]

It is disconcerting to report that important medical information, including laboratory reports, comprehensive drug inventories, and family health histories, are often missing from medical files. A 2003 study involving primary care physician medical records suggests that perhaps one out of every seven patient files is missing information important to providing comprehensive health care.[18]

Once they have identified levels of risk in patients, health practitioners try to lower those risk levels through

---

Key Terms

morbidity Pertaining to illness and disease.

mortality Pertaining to death.

preventive or prospective medicine Physician-centered medical care in which areas of risk for chronic illnesses are identified so that they might be lowered.

risk factor A biomedical index such as serum cholesterol level or a behavioral pattern such as smoking, associated with a chronic illness.

high-risk health behavior A behavioral pattern, such as smoking, associated with a high risk of developing a chronic illness.

Table 1.1 Leading Causes of Adult Death, by Age, Sex, United States 2002

| 20–39 years | | 40–59 years | | 60–79 years | | 80+ | |
M	F	M	F	M	F	M	F
Accidents 21,627	Accidents 6,859	Heart 50,028	Cancer 49,570	Cancer 156,527	Cancer 129,694	Heart 136,941	Heart 231,969
Suicide 8,771	Cancer 5,403	Cancer 52,489	Heart 21,677	Heart 143,570	Heart 99,160	Cancer 73,839	Cancer 82,840
Homicide 7,827	Heart 2,640	Accidents 20,224	Accidents 8,076	Respiratory 31,438	Respiratory 29,905	Stroke 30,688	Stroke 67,702
Heart 5,590	Suicide 1,913	Suicide 9,325	Stroke 5,536	Stroke 24,573	Stroke 25,934	Respiratory 24,411	AD 35,225
Cancer 4,626	Homicide 1,723	Liver 9,082	Diabetes 4,675	Diabetes 16,886	Diabetes 17,038	Influenza 16,980	Respiratory 29,619
HIV 3,206	HIV 1,391	Diabetes 6,719	Respiratory 4,089	Accidents 10,825	Influenza 7,508	AD 12,384	Influenza 27,094
Diabetes 905	Stroke 740	HIV 6,450	Liver 3,617	Influenza 8,960	Kidney 7,357	Diabetes 9,737	Diabetes 16,556
Stroke 742	Liver 475	Respiratory 4,274	HIV 1,998	Septicemia 6,611	Septicemia 6,781	Accidents 8,236	Accidents 11,381
Congen 552	Congen 431	Homicide 2,875	Septicemia 1,983	Liver 6,313	AD 6,542	PD 5,805	Septicemia 9,614

Source: U.S. Mortality Public Use Data Tapes, National Centers for Health Statistics, Centers for Disease Control and Prevention, 2004

Note: Although first reported by Jemal A, et al. in Cancer Statistics, 2005 (*CA Cancer J Clin* 2005.55:10-30) deaths from cancer may have begun surpassing deaths from heart disease in adults between 19 and 79 years as early as 1999. Data reported above (for 2002) indicate that in this age group, cancer accounted for 393,688 deaths while heart disease accounted for 318,435. Underlying this reversal in the leading cause of death has been the significant reductions in heart disease mortality (52%), while cancer mortality has declined by considerably less (3%), as noted in Jemal A, et al. Trends in the leading causes of death in the United States, 1997–2002 (*JAMA*. Sept. 14, 2005. 294(10):1255-1259).

Abbreviations:

AD (Alzheimer's disease)—dementia (cognitive decline) resulting from deterioration of neural transmitter production in selected areas of the brain

Cong (congenital malformations)—structural errors formed during embryonic development that eventually prove incompatible with life

Kidney—usually end-stage renal failure associated with advanced diabetes mellitus and the decline of the body with advancing age

Liver (hepatic failure)—death resulting from the liver's inability to biotransform substances into nontoxic forms suitable for excretion from the body

PD (Parkinson's disease)—decline in fine muscular control resulting from the loss of dopamine production in selected areas of the brain

Septicemia (systemic blood poisoning)—widespread infection of the body associated with blood borne infectious agents

patient education, lifestyle modification, and, when necessary, medical intervention. Continued compliance on the part of the patients should result in a lower level of risk that will continue over the years. Note that preventive medicine is guided by practitioners, and patients are expected to be compliant with the directions they are given.

Although preventive medical care appears to be a much more sensible approach than episodic care in reducing morbidity and mortality, third-party payers (insurance plans) traditionally have not provided adequate coverage for preventive services. Managed health care plans that earn a profit by preventing sickness, such as health maintenance organizations, or HMOs (see Chapter 18), should be much more receptive to the concept and practice of preventive medicine.

In recent years the belief that preventive or prospective medical care can reduce the incidence of chronic illnesses, and thus reduce the likelihood of premature death, has been clouded by conflicting results from studies involving prevention-oriented changes in lifestyle, including, among others, dietary practices, exercise protocols, smoking cessation, weight management strategies, the use of hormone supplementation, and the inclusion of spiritual practices in daily routines. This inconsistency in effectiveness is seen by many experts as being largely a methodological problem in research study design. However, other health care experts suggest that factors not directly reachable by behavior change, such as age and genetic predispositions, make some people more successful than others in preventing illnesses and premature death. Regardless, when successful, this form of health care provides people with a personal sense of **empowerment** [19] that is always a useful resource for leading a healthy, productive, and satisfying life.

Key Terms

empowerment The nurturing of an individual's or group's ability to be responsible for their own health and well-being.

See the box "What Is Complementary Medicine?" on page 9 for more on broadening perspectives on health care.

Health Promotion—Personal and Collective Empowerment

High-level health is more likely to be obtained by people who have been exposed to the knowledge, behavioral patterns, and attitudinal stances required in adopting a health-enhancing approach to living. Whether these "tools" for better health are sought out by an individual person or developed by a group of people working

as a "learning community," they become the resources reflected in the term *empowerment*. Empowered persons, individually or collectively, are now active participants in their own health enhancement quest (see the box "The Importance of Risk Reduction"). Health promotion specialists have played an active role in leading people in this process.

Individually Oriented Health Promotion Throughout the United States, YMCA/YWCA-sponsored wellness programs, commercial fitness clubs, and corporate fitness centers offer risk-reduction programs under the direction of qualified instructors, many of whom are university graduates in disciplines such as exercise science, wellness management, and **health promotion.** Using approaches similar to those employed in preventive medicine, these nonphysician health professionals attempt to guide their clients toward activities and behaviors that will lower their risk of chronic illness. Unlike preventive medicine, with its sometimes invasive assessment procedures and medication-based therapies, health promotion programs are not legally defined as medical practices and thus do not require the involvement of physicians. In addition, the fitness focus, social interaction, and healthy lifestyle orientation these programs provide tend to mask the emphasis on preventing chronic illness that would be the selling point of such efforts if they were undertaken as preventive medicine. In fact, it is likely that people receiving health promotion in these settings do not recognize it as such. Rather, they are very often submitting to assessments and listening to health-related information only as incidental parts of personal goals, such as losing weight, preparing for their first marathon, or simply meeting friends for lunch-hour basketball.

Group-Oriented Health Promotion   In addition to the practices just described, a group-oriented form of health promotion is offered in many communities. This approach to improving health through risk reduction is directed at empowering community groups, such as church congregations or neighborhood associations, so that they can develop, operate, and financially sustain their own programs with little direct involvement of health promotion specialists.[20]

Empowerment programs have produced positive health consequences for groups that traditionally have been underserved by the health care system, such as minority populations. Once such people are given needed information, inroads into the political process, and skills for accessing funding sources, they become better able to plan, implement, and operate programs tailored to their unique health needs.

Perhaps no greater challenge in establishing health-related empowerment is that related to the devastating tsunami that occurred on December 26, 2004, in the Indian Ocean basin. In addition to coping with a death

Although not primarily interested in illness or premature death, wellness practitioners consider it essential to inform their clients about the role of elevated blood pressure in the development of cardiovascular disease.

toll approaching 200,000 and the displacement of entire communities, much of the effort and resources needed to rebuild viable communities will eventually need to be transitioned from professionally staffed international relief organizations into the hands of the local people. When successful, these empowerment programs stand as excellent examples of the fact that people can make a difference when they become empowered.

In virtually all areas of the country, small groups are engaged in the process of empowering people to eventually manage their own health and safety programs. These groups include neighborhood associations organizing Crime Watch programs and identifying "safe houses" for children to go to when they encounter situations they recognize as unsafe, churches sponsoring smoking abatement programs for members of their congregations, and locally organized groups of parents that petition the local school board to improve the healthfulness of the school lunch program.

Wellness

Expanded perceptions of health are the basis for **wellness.** Recall that episodic health care, preventive medicine, and group-oriented health promotion are directly aligned with concerns about morbidity and mortality, whereas health promotion at the individual level is focused on aspects of appearance, weight management, body composition, and physical performance capabilities. Wellness differs from these kinds of health care concerns because it has virtually no interest in morbidity and mortality.

Practitioners describe wellness as a process of extending information, counseling, assessment, and lifestyle-modification strategies leading to a desirable change in the recipients' overall lifestyle, or the adoption of a wellness lifestyle. Once adopted, the wellness lifestyle produces a

---

Key Terms

health promotion A movement in which knowledge, practices, and values are transmitted to people for use in lengthening their lives, reducing the incidence of illness, and feeling better.

wellness A process intended to aid individuals in unlocking their full potential through the development of an overall wellness lifestyle.

Which factors do today's adults associate with the ability to feel good about their lives? Check the following list for the answers given to this question. Note that virtually no respondent makes direct reference to being free of illness and disease or to living long into the future. Rather, respondents are more aligned with a personally defined sense of being adequately independent, self-sufficient, responsible, respected by other, and nurturing.

- A sense of *personal satisfaction* (82 percent) was identified as the most important feeling that should be experienced during adulthood.

- A sense of *being in control* of one's life (80 percent) was the second most identified index of adult well-being.

- A sense that one was a partner in a *good marriage* (78 percent) appeared as the third most important component of living well as an adult.

- A sense that one was *competent at one's job* (69 percent) placed employment in fourth position—important but clearly below the factors listed above. Also, note that *making a lot of money* was selected by only 25 percent as being of primary importance in defining adult life satisfaction.

- A sense that one's *children were (or would be) successful* was cited by 63 percent of the adults sampled as an important factor in feeling a sense of well-being.

Having studied these responses, you also may appreciate more fully the meaning we assign to having a sense of well-being and the role health plays in making it possible. In fact, the findings presented here might serve as a new and much-needed focus for the wellness movement, which currently replicates the morbidity- and mortality-reducing activities traditionally delivered by physicians practicing prospective medicine and health promotion professionals.

Source: Data from Yankelovich Monitor 1997, as reported in "What Is Success?" *USA Today* Jan 19: 1A.

sense of well-being that in turn enables recipients to unlock their full potential (see the box "Factors That Affect Well-Being").

This explanation of how wellness differs from episodic health care, preventive medicine, and health promotion does, on first hearing, seem progressive and clearly devoid of interest in morbidity and mortality concerns. But in practice, wellness programs are not all that different from other kinds of health care. We have consistently noted that wellness programs, as carried out on college campuses, in local hospital well centers, and in corporate settings, routinely transmit familiar health-related information and engage in the same risk-reduction activities that characterize preventive medicine and health promotion. It is in the final aspect of wellness, the "unlocking of full potential," that wellness might differ from other concepts of health.

Having learned about the sources of our familiar and traditional definitions of health, recall that a new and unique definition of health is presented later in the chapter.

Federal Programs to Improve the Health of People in the United States

To identify all the health-related concerns identified by members of the health community would be a monumental undertaking far beyond the scope of this book. However, in 2003 the Institute of Medicine released a list of priority health concerns that it believes need particular attention.[21] Among these priority concerns are

- Treatment of asthma
- Coordination of care for the 60 million or more persons with chronic health conditions
- Reduction in the development of diabetes
- Development of evidence-based cancer screening
- Enhanced rates of immunization, particularly for flu and pneumonia
- Improved detection of depression, which is now inadequately diagnosed and treated
- Aggressively promoted prevention of cardiovascular disease, presently the second leading killer of American adults under the age of 80
- Reduction of tobacco dependence through cessation and prevention of smoking
- Widened availability of prenatal care

While improvements in these areas are greatly needed, the Institute of Medicine has no specific programs in place at this time to address them. In comparison, well-established and ongoing programs, such as Healthy People 2000 and Healthy People 2010, have established specific goals and objectives to improve the health of Americans in many of these areas. A brief descripton of these ongoing programs follows.

In 1991 the U.S. Department of Health and Human Services document titled *Healthy People 2000: National Health Promotion and Disease Prevention Objectives*[22] outlined a strategic plan for promoting the health of the American public. The plan included 300 health objectives in 22 priority areas. Forty-seven of the 300 objectives were defined as "sentinel" ones, that is, particularly significant goals that could be used to measure the progress of the 1990s health promotion objectives.

Progress toward achieving the objectives was assessed near the middle of the decade and reported in a document titled *Healthy People 2000: Midcourse Review and 1995 Revisions.*[23] Although progress was reported in some areas, little or no progress was reported in many. Subsequently, a new plan, called *Healthy People 2010: Understanding and Improving Health,* Volume 1,[24] was formulated, refined, and is now being implemented.

Healthy People 2010: Understanding and Improving Health, Volume 2[25] is a health promotion program intended to be implemented at all levels, ranging from individual involvement through multinational cooperative efforts, including *Health for All in the 21st Century,* a World Health Organization health promotion initiative. Although the goals of *Healthy People 2000: National Health Promotion and Disease Prevention Objectives* and *Healthy People 2010: Understanding and Improving Health* are similar, the latter focuses on the projected needs of the United States during the first decade of the new century.

Central to the design of *Healthy People 2010: Understanding and Improving Health* are two paramount goals: (1) increasing quality and years of life and (2) eliminating health disparities in areas such as gender, race, and ethnicity, as well as income and education level. These goals in turn provide 28 more focused objectives. Progress in accomplishing these objectives is anticipated through the manipulation of the behavioral, biological, and environmental determinants of health as they relate to 10 of the leading health indicators: (1) physical activity, (2) weight management, (3) tobacco use, (4) substance abuse, (5) responsible sexual behavior, (6) mental health, (7) injury and violence, (8) environmental quality, (9) immunization, and (10) access to health care.

The success of *Healthy People 2010: Understanding and Improving Health*[25] will not be known for a few years. However, if its goals are ultimately reached, Americans can anticipate improved quantity and quality of life.

Improving Health through Planned Behavior Change

Although some health concerns can be successfully addressed through local, state, national, or international efforts, such as those just outlined, most are ultimately based on the willingness and ability of persons to change aspects of their own behavior. However, for many people health-related behavior change proves difficult or even impossible to make.

Why Behavior Change Is Often Difficult

Several factors can strongly influence a person's desire to change high-risk health behaviors, including these:

1. A person must know that a particular behavioral pattern is clearly associated with (or even causes) a particular health problem. For example: cigarette smoking is the primary cause of lung cancer.
2. A person must believe (accept) that a behavioral pattern will make (or has made) him susceptible to this particular health problem. For example: my cigarette smoking will significantly increase my risk of developing lung cancer.
3. A person must recognize that risk-reduction intervention strategies exist and that should she adopt these in a compliant manner she too will reduce her risk for a particular health condition. For example: smoking-cessation programs exist, and following such a program could help me quit smoking.
4. A person must believe that benefits of newly adopted health-enhancing behaviors will be more reinforcing than the behaviors being given up. For example: the improved health, lowered risk, and freedom from dependence resulting from no longer smoking are better than the temporary pleasures provided by smoking.
5. A person must feel that significant others in his life truly want him to alter his high-risk health behaviors and will support his efforts. For example: my friends who are cigarette smokers will make a concerted effort to not smoke in my presence and will help me avoid being around people who smoke.

When one or more of these conditions is not in place, the likelihood that persons will be successful in reducing health-risk behaviors is greatly diminished.

Transtheoretical Model of Health Behavior Change

The process of behavioral change unfolds over time and progresses through defined stages.[26, 27] James Prochaska, John Norcross, and Carol DiClemente outlined six predictable stages of change. They studied thousands of individuals who were changing long-standing problems such as alcohol abuse, smoking, and gambling. While these people used different strategies to change their behavior, they all proceeded through six consistent stages of change in the process referred to as **Prochaska's Transtheoretical Model of Health Behavior Change.**[28]

Key Terms

Prochaska's Transtheoretical Model of Health Behavior Change Six predictable stages—precontemplation, contemplation, preparation, action, maintenance, and termination—people go through in establishing new habits and patterns of behavior.

People can improve their health through planned behavior change. As part of a plan to improve his eating habits, this man shops for healthy food choices.

Precontemplation Stage   The first stage of change is called *precontemplation*, during which persons might think about making a change but ultimately find it too difficult and avoid making it. For example, during this phase a smoker might tell friends, "Eventually I will quit" but have no real intention of stopping within the next six months.

Contemplation Stage   For many, however, progress toward change begins as they move into a *contemplation* stage, during which they might develop the desire to change but have little understanding of how to go about it. Typically, they see themselves taking action within the next six months. For example: when the semester is finished and my stress level is lower, I'll start the stop smoking program that I have material about.

Preparation Stage   Following the contemplation stage, a *preparation* stage begins, during which change begins to appear to be not only desirable but possible as well. A smoker might begin making plans to quit during this stage, setting a quit date for the very near future (a few days to a month) and perhaps enrolling in a smoking-cessation program. For example: this is the last weekend of my "smoking career"—on Monday I plan to quit.

Action Stage   Plans for change are implemented during the *action* stage, during which changes are made and sustained for a period of about six months.

Maintenance Stage   The fifth stage is the *maintenance* stage, during which new habits are consolidated and practiced for an additional six months. For example: I think that I'm almost home, but I better continue paying attention to my maintenance plan for a bit longer—returning to the bar scene too soon could be my downfall.

Termination Stage   The sixth and final stage is called *termination*, which refers to the point at which new habits are well established, and so efforts to change are complete.

Today's Health Concerns

To this point in the chapter we have identified some health concerns and addressed the desirability of health-related behavior change. Earlier in the chapter we looked at those illnesses that are the major causes of death that afflict adults in the United States (see Table 1.1 on p. 10). However, in spite of astonishing progress on many fronts, we continue to face a number of serious health challenges from those and other illnesses. Heart disease, cancer, accidents, drug use, and mental illness all are important concerns for each of us, even if we are not directly affected by them. Also becoming increasingly troublesome are the complex problems of environmental pollution, violence, health care costs, a possible Avian flu epidemic, and the international scope of the HIV/AIDS epidemic, as well as other sexually transmitted diseases. World hunger, overpopulation, and the threat of domestic and international terrorism are other health-related issues that will affect us as well as the generations that follow.

The health concerns just mentioned are by no means unmanageable. Fortunately, we as individuals can reduce the likelihood of encountering many of these conditions by making choices in the way we live our lives (see the box "Keys to Longer Living"). On a personal level, we can decide to pursue a plan of healthful living to minimize the incidence of illness and disease and to extend life.

Taking Charge of Your Health

- Complete the Comprehensive Health Assessment on pages 22 to 31. Develop a plan to modify your behavior in the areas in which you need improvement.

- Take part in a new spiritual activity, such as meditating, creating art or music, or attending a religious service.

- To promote the social dimension of your health, try to meet one new person each week during the semester.

- Choose one developmental task you would like to focus on, such as assuming responsibility, and plan the steps you can follow to progress in this area.

- Volunteer to be an assistant in a community service program, such as a literacy project or a preschool program.

SUMMARY

- The Millennial generation encompasses persons born between 1982 and 2000.
- Each phase of the life cycle involves a set of personal developmental tasks that are common to all people yet may be undertaken differently by each individual. Young adulthood is characterized by five key developmental tasks: forming an initial adult identity, establishing independence, assuming responsibility, broadening social skills, and nurturing intimacy.
- Generativity and integrity are developmental tasks of midlife and older adulthood, respectively.
- Today's college campus is a dynamic blend of students of both traditional and nontraditional ages and of diverse backgrounds, cultures, and attributes.
- When we seek the services of health care practitioners because of symptoms of illness or disease, we are said to be seeking episodic health care.
- Preventive medical care attempts to minimize the incidence of illness and disease by identifying early indicators of risk to bring them under control.
- Individual-centered health promotion involves risk-reduction activities similar to those used in preventive medical care, except that the techniques cannot be invasive and are directed by professionals who are not physicians. Its most visible emphasis tends to be on fitness and body composition.
- Group-centered health promotion involves the empowerment of individuals so that they can organize collectively and participate in their own health promotion activities.

- Wellness contends a disinterest in morbidity and mortality, rather emphasizing living a wellness lifestyle that leads to a sense of well-being.
- A decision to change a health behavior is often difficult to make because of the multiplicity of factors underlying the maintenace of the high-risk behavior.
- Health behavior change requires movement through a multistaged process, including precontemplation, contemplation, preparation, action, maintenance, and termination.
- A wide array of health problems (for example, cancer, cardiovascular disease, HIV/AIDS) persist despite today's highly sophisticated health care technology.
- Complementary and integrative medicine involves the integration of alternative forms of care, such as acupuncture and therapeutic massage, into traditional medical practices.
- Current multidimensional definitions of health may include many or all of the following dimensions: physical, emotional, social, intellectual, spiritual, and occupational.
- Our new definition of health includes the role of health and the composition of health. The role of health is to enable individuals to participate in the activities that collectively constitute growth and development. The composition of health is the intrinsic and extrinsic resources on which individuals can draw to participate fully in their own growth and development.

REVIEW QUESTIONS

1. What birth years are encompassed within the label *Millennial generation*?
2. What are the five developmental tasks of young adulthood, and how can the accomplishing of one influence the accomplishing of any of the remaining four?
3. What is implied by the statement "growth and development are predictable yet unique"?
4. What is the most likely route that midlife adults will take in their quest for a sense of generativity?
5. In what ways is the current U.S. college student population more diverse than any that came before?

6. What are morbidity and mortality, and how are they involved in the more traditional definitions of health?
7. In preventive medical care, who determines a person's level of risk and decides what risk-reduction techniques should be implemented?
8. What does the term *empowerment* mean, and how would it appear as a component of a community-based health promotion program?
9. What is the main reason that proponents of wellness give for being uninterested in morbidity and mortality?

10. What factors could underlie the inability or unwillingness of persons to change their health behavior?
11. What are the six stages that persons pass through as they consider and then attempt to change their health behavior?
12. What are the most frequently included dimensions of a holistically centered definition of health?
13. How does your textbook define the role of health? Composition of health?
14. How does our definition of health differ from traditional definitions?
15. Why is it necessary to understand developmental expectations before we can answer the question "Are you healthy enough to . . . ?"

ANSWERS TO THE "WHAT DO YOU KNOW?" QUIZ

1. True   2. False   3. True   4. False   5. True   6. False   7. False

As We Go to Press

Church Attendance Attrition among Young Adults

The spiritual dimension of health, as described in the chapter is, for many people, inseparable from affiliation with an organized religious body. For the majority of Americans, affiliation is predominately in mainline and evangelical protestant churches. However, a recent study suggests these churches are having difficulty retaining young adults as members.

In a national survey of 1,023 young adults conducted by Lifeway Research, an affiliate of the Southern Baptist Church, it was found that attrition was unexpectedly high among adults who had themselves been regular attendees (twice a month or more) as high school students. In fact, 70 percent of those who had been regular attendees were not attending at all, or were only occasional attendees.

Underlying this attrition were a variety of factors that collectively suggested to experts that church youth programs were mainly functioning as "holding tanks held together with pizza." Factors underlying departure from membership following the end of high school Included "needing a break," "church members being too judgmental," "conflicts with college and employment," "relocation," and being "too busy."

Among the 30 percent of young adults who continued attendance following their teen years, two factors were pertinent: having had parents who were regular attendees and having had sermons that were relevant. Additionally, these young adults reported that it was vital for them to maintain "a personal relationship with God," that regular church attendance "provided guidance in making daily decisions in their lives," and as a consequence of attending, they were "better people for doing so." For the 40 percent who seem most disconnected, the churches appear to have few viable answers.

ENDNOTES

1. Strauss W and Howe N. *Generations: The History of America's Future: 1584–2069*. New York: William Morrow and Company. 1992.
2. Furstenberg FF, Kennedy S, McLoyd VC, et al. Growing Up Is Harder to Do. *Context*. 3(3), Summer 2004.
3. Diversity in Word and Deed: Most Teens Claim Multicultural Friends. *The TRU Study*. Teen Research Unlimited (TRU), November 2004.
4. Putman RD. *Bowling Alone: The Collapse and Revival of American Community*. New York: Simon & Schuster, 2000.
5. Verhaagen D. *Parenting the Millennial Generation: Guiding Our Children Born between 1982 and 2000*. Westport, CT: Praeger, 2005.
6. McAdams DP, St. Aubin ED (Eds.) *Generativity and Adult Development and Why We Care for the Next Generation*. Hoboken, NJ: American Psychological Association, 2001.
7. McAdams DP. Generativity in Midlife. In Lachman M (Ed.). *Handbook of Midlife Development*. Hoboken, NJ: Wiley, 2001.
8. Erikson EH. *Childhood and Society* (reissued ed.), New York: Norton, 1993.
9. U.S. Department of Education. National Center for Education Statistics: 2003–04. *National Postsecondary Student Aid Study*. NPSAS:04, August 2005.
10. U.S. Department of Education. National Center for Education Statistics. *Projection of Education Statistics to 2015*. NCES 2006–084. (Tables 10, 11, 19, 22.), November 2005.
11. U.S. Department of Education. National Center for Education Statistics. *Profile of Undergraduates in U.S. Postsecondary Education Institutions: 2003–04*. NCES 2006–184, September 2006.
12. Hing E, Cherry DA, Woodwell BA. *National Ambulatory Medical Care Survey: 2004 Summary*. Advanced Data from Vital and Health Statistics. Number 374. (Table 3.), June 23, 2006.
13. Hing E, Cherry DA, Woodwell BA. *National Ambulatory Medical Care Survey: 2004 Summary*. Advanced Data from Vital and Health Statistics. Number 374. (Table 10.), June 23, 2006.
14. Roper Center for Public Opinion Research (for Pfizer Women's Health), University of Connecticut. Adults Know Their Family History. *USA Today*, May 30, 2000. p. 5D.
15. *U.S. Surgeon General's Family History Initiative*. Washington, DC: U.S. Department of Health and Human Services, 2004, www.hss. gov/familyhistory/download.html.
16. Jermal A, et al. Cancer Statistics, 2005. *CA Cancer J Clin*. (55):10–30, 2005.
17. Jermal A, et al. Trends in the Leading Causes of Death in the United States, 1997–2002. *JAMA*. Sept. 14. 294(10):1255–1259, 2005.
18. Smith PC, et al. Missing Information During Primary Care Visits. 2005. *JAMA*, Feb 2; 293(5):567–571.
19. Cottrell RR, Girvan JT, McKenzie JF. *Principles and Foundations of Health Promotion and Education* (3rd ed.). San Francisco: Benjamin Cummings, 2005.

20. McKenzie JF, Neiger BL, Smeltzer JL. *Planning, Implementing and Evaluating Health Promotion Programs* (4th ed.). San Francisco: Benjamin Cummings, 2005.

21. *Priority Areas for National Action: Transforming Health Care Quality.* Washington, DC: National Academies Press, 2003.

22. *Healthy People 2000: National Health Promotion and Disease Prevention Objectives* (full report with commentary). Washington DC: U.S. Department of Health and Human Services. Public Health Services, 1991.

23. *Healthy People 2000: Midcourse Review and 1995 Revisions.* Washington, DC: U.S. Department of Health and Human Services. Public Health Services, 1995.

24. *Healthy People 2010: Understanding and Improving Health.* Volume 1 Washington, DC: U.S. Department of Health and Human Services, 2000.

25. *Healthy People 2010: Understanding and Improving Health.* Volume 2. Washington, DC: U.S. Department of Health and Human Services, 2000.

26. Prochaska JO, Velicer WF. The Transtheoretical Model of Health Behavior Change. *Am J of Health Promotion.* 12:38–48, 1994.

27. Norcross JC, Prochaska JO, Using the Stages of Change. *Harv Ment Health Lett.* 18(11):507, 2002.

28. Prochaska JO, Norcross JC, Clemente CC. *Changing for Good.* New York: William Morrow, 1994.

29. Smith-Lovin L, McPherson M, Brashears M. Social Isolation in America: Changes in Core Discussion Networks over Two Decades. *American Sociologica.* 353–375, June 2006.

30. *American Piety in the 21st Century: New Insights to the Depths and Complexity of Religion in the U.S.* Baylor Institute for Studies of Religion. Baylor University, September 2006. www.baylor .edu/isreligionj/index.[ip?id=40634.

31. Spirituality and the Professoriate: A National Study of Faculty Beliefs, Attitudes, and Information. *Spirituality in Higher Education.* Higher Education Research Institute. University of California, Los Angeles, March 2006.

Comprehensive Health Assessment

Now that you have read the first chapter, complete the following Comprehensive Health Assessment. We strongly suggest that you retake this assessment after you have completed your health course. Then compare your responses in each section of the assessment. Have your scores improved?

Social and Occupational Health

	Not true/ rarely	Somewhat true/ sometimes	Mostly true/ usually	Very true/ always
1. I feel loved and supported by my family.	1	2	3	4
2. I establish friendships with ease and enjoyment.	1	2	3	4
3. I establish friendships with people of both genders and all ages.	1	2	3	4
4. I sustain relationships by communicating with and caring about my family and friends.	1	2	3	4
5. I feel comfortable and confident when meeting people for the first time.	1	2	3	4
6. I practice social skills to facilitate the process of forming new relationships.	1	2	3	4
7. I seek opportunities to meet and interact with new people.	1	2	3	4
8. I talk with, rather than at, people.	1	2	3	4
9. I am open to developing or sustaining intimate relationships.	1	2	3	4
10. I appreciate the importance of parenting the next generation and am committed to supporting it in ways that reflect my own resources.	1	2	3	4
11. I recognize the strengths and weaknesses of my parents' childrearing skills and feel comfortable modifying them if I choose to become a parent.	1	2	3	4
12. I attempt to be tolerant of others whether or not I approve of their behavior or beliefs.	1	2	3	4
13. I understand and appreciate the contribution that cultural diversity makes to the quality of living.	1	2	3	4
14. I understand and appreciate the difference between being educated and being trained.	1	2	3	4
15. My work gives me a sense of self-sufficiency and an opportunity to contribute.	1	2	3	4
16. I have equal respect for the roles of leader and subordinate within the workplace.	1	2	3	4
17. I have chosen an occupation that suits my interests and temperament.	1	2	3	4
18. I have chosen an occupation that does not compromise my physical or psychological health.	1	2	3	4
19. I get along well with my coworkers most of the time.	1	2	3	4
20. When I have a disagreement with a coworker, I try to resolve it directly and constructively.	1	2	3	4

POINTS _____

Spiritual and Psychological Health

	Not true/ rarely	Somewhat true/ sometimes	Mostly true/ usually	Very true/ always
1. I have a deeply held belief system or personal theology.	1	2	3	4
2. I recognize the contribution that membership in a community of faith or spirituality can make to a person's overall quality of life.	1	2	3	4

3. I seek experiences with nature and reflect on nature's contribution to my quality of life.	1	2	3	4
4. My spirituality is a resource that helps me remain calm and strong during times of stress.	1	2	3	4
5. I have found appropriate ways to express my spirituality.	1	2	3	4
6. I respect the diversity of spiritual expression and am tolerant of those whose beliefs differ from my own.	1	2	3	4
7. I take adequate time to reflect on my own life and my relationships with others and the institutions of society.	1	2	3	4
8. I routinely undertake new experiences.	1	2	3	4
9. I receive adequate support from others.	1	2	3	4
10. I look for opportunities to support others, even occasionally at the expense of my own goals and aspirations.	1	2	3	4
11. I recognize that emotional and psychological health are as important as physical health.	1	2	3	4
12. I express my feelings and opinions comfortably, yet am capable of keeping them to myself when appropriate.	1	2	3	4
13. I see myself as a person of worth and feel comfortable with my own strengths and limitations.	1	2	3	4
14. I establish realistic goals and work to achieve them.	1	2	3	4
15. I understand the differences between the normal range of emotions and the signs of clinical depression.	1	2	3	4
16. I know how to recognize signs of suicidal thoughts and am willing to intervene.	1	2	3	4
17. I regularly assess my own behavior patterns and beliefs and would seek professional assistance for any emotional dysfunction.	1	2	3	4
18. I accept the reality of aging and view it as an opportunity for positive change.	1	2	3	4
19. I accept the reality of death and view it as a normal and inevitable part of life.	1	2	3	4
20. I have made decisions about my own death to ensure that I die with dignity when the time comes.	1	2	3	4

POINTS _____

Stress Management

	Not true/ rarely	Somewhat true/ sometimes	Mostly true/ usually	Very true/ always
1. I accept the reality of change while maintaining the necessary stability in my daily activities.	1	2	3	4
2. I seek change when it is necessary or desirable to do so.	1	2	3	4
3. I know what stress-management services are offered on campus, through my employer, or in my community.	1	2	3	4
4. When necessary, I use the stress-management services to which I have access.	1	2	3	4
5. I employ stress-reduction practices in anticipation of stressful events, such as job interviews and final examinations.	1	2	3	4
6. I reevaluate the ways in which I handled stressful events so that I can better cope with similar events in the future.	1	2	3	4
7. I turn to relatives and friends during periods of disruption in my life.	1	2	3	4
8. I avoid using alcohol or other drugs during periods of stress.	1	2	3	4
9. I refrain from behaving aggressively or abusively during periods of stress.	1	2	3	4

	Not true/ rarely	Somewhat true/ sometimes	Mostly true/ usually	Very true/ always
10. I sleep enough to maintain a high level of health and cope successfully with daily challenges.	1	2	3	4
11. I avoid sleeping excessively as a response to stressful change.	1	2	3	4
12. My diet is conducive to good health and stress management.	1	2	3	4
13. I participate in physical activity to relieve stress.	1	2	3	4
14. I practice stress-management skills, such as diaphragmatic breathing and yoga.	1	2	3	4
15. I manage my time effectively.	1	2	3	4

POINTS _____

Fitness

	Not true/ rarely	Somewhat true/ sometimes	Mostly true/ usually	Very true/ always
1. I participate in recreational and fitness activities both to minimize stress and to improve or maintain my level of physical fitness.	1	2	3	4
2. I select some recreational activities that are strenuous rather than sedentary in nature.	1	2	3	4
3. I include various types of aerobic conditioning activities among the wider array of recreational and fitness activities in which I engage.	1	2	3	4
4. I engage in aerobic activities with appropriate frequency, intensity, and duration to provide a training effect for my heart and lungs.	1	2	3	4
5. I routinely include strength-training activities among the wider array of fitness activities in which I engage.	1	2	3	4
6. I routinely vary the types of strength-training activities in which I participate in order to minimize injury and strengthen all of the important muscle groups.	1	2	3	4
7. I do exercises specifically designed to maintain joint range of motion.	1	2	3	4
8. I believe that recreational and fitness activities can help me improve my physical health and my emotional and social well-being.	1	2	3	4
9. I include a variety of fitness activities in my overall plan for physical fitness.	1	2	3	4
10. I take appropriate steps to avoid injuries when participating in recreational and fitness activities.	1	2	3	4
11. I seek appropriate treatment for all injuries that result from fitness activities.	1	2	3	4
12. I believe that older adults should undertake appropriately chosen fitness activities.	1	2	3	4
13. My body composition is consistent with a high level of health.	1	2	3	4
14. I warm up before beginning vigorous activity, and I cool down afterward.	1	2	3	4
15. I select properly designed and well-maintained equipment and clothing for each activity.	1	2	3	4
16. I avoid using performance-enhancing substances that are known to be dangerous and those whose influence on the body is not fully understood.	1	2	3	4
17. I sleep seven to eight hours daily.	1	2	3	4
18. I refrain from using over-the-counter sleep-inducing aids.	1	2	3	4

Comprehensive Health Assessment—*continued*

19. I follow sound dietary practices as an important adjunct to a health-enhancing physical activity program.	1	2	3	4
20. My current level of fitness allows me to participate fully and with reasonable comfort in my daily activities.	1	2	3	4

POINTS _____

Nutrition and Weight Management

	Not true/ rarely	Somewhat true/ sometimes	Mostly true/ usually	Very true/ always
1. I balance my caloric intake with my calorie expenditure.	1	2	3	4
2. I obtain the recommended number of servings from each of the food groups.	1	2	3	4
3. I select a wide variety of foods chosen from each of the food groups.	1	2	3	4
4. I understand the amount of a particular food that constitutes a single serving.	1	2	3	4
5. I often try new foods, particularly when I know them to be healthful.	1	2	3	4
6. I select breads, cereals, fresh fruits, and vegetables in preference to pastries, candies, sodas, and fruits canned in heavy syrup.	1	2	3	4
7. I limit the amount of sugar that I add to foods during preparation and at the table.	1	2	3	4
8. I examine food labels to determine the presence of trans-fats (trans-fatty acids) and select foods free of these fats.	1	2	3	4
9. I select primarily nonmeat sources of protein, such as peas, beans, and peanut butter, while limiting my consumption of red meat and high-fat dairy products.	1	2	3	4
10. I consume an appropriate percentage of my total daily calories from protein.	1	2	3	4
11. I select foods prepared with unsaturated vegetable oils while reducing consumption of red meat, high-fat dairy products, and foods prepared with lard (animal fat) or butter.	1	2	3	4
12. I carefully limit the amount of fast food that I consume during a typical week.	1	2	3	4
13. I consume an appropriate percentage of my total daily calories from fat.	1	2	3	4
14. I select nutritious foods when I snack.	1	2	3	4
15. I limit my use of salt during food preparation and at the table.	1	2	3	4
16. I consume adequate amounts of fiber.	1	2	3	4
17. I routinely consider the nutrient density of individual food items when choosing foods.	1	2	3	4
18. I maintain my weight without reliance on over-the-counter or prescription diet pills.	1	2	3	4
19. I maintain my weight without reliance on fad diets or liquid weight loss beverages.	1	2	3	4
20. I exercise regularly to help maintain my weight.	1	2	3	4

POINTS _____

Alcohol, Tobacco, and Other Drug Use

	Not true/ rarely	Somewhat true/ sometimes	Mostly true/ usually	Very true/ always
1. I abstain or drink in moderation when offered alcoholic beverages.	1	2	3	4
2. I abstain from using illegal psychoactive (mind-altering) drugs.	1	2	3	4
3. I do not consume alcoholic beverages or psychoactive drugs rapidly or in large quantities.	1	2	3	4
4. I do not use alcohol or psychoactive drugs in a way that causes me to behave inappropriately.	1	2	3	4
5. My use of alcohol or other drugs does not compromise my academic performance.	1	2	3	4
6. I refrain from drinking alcoholic beverages or using psychoactive drugs when engaging in recreational activities that require strength, speed, or coordination.	1	2	3	4
7. I refrain from drinking alcoholic beverages while participating in occupational activities, regardless of the nature of those activities.	1	2	3	4
8. My use of alcohol or other drugs does not generate financial concerns for myself or for others.	1	2	3	4
9. I refrain from drinking alcohol or using psychoactive drugs when driving a motor vehicle or operating heavy equipment.	1	2	3	4
10. I do not drink alcohol or use psychoactive drugs when I am alone.	1	2	3	4
11. I avoid riding with people who have been drinking alcohol or using psychoactive drugs.	1	2	3	4
12. My use of alcohol or other drugs does not cause family dysfunction.	1	2	3	4
13. I do not use marijuana.	1	2	3	4
14. I do not use hallucinogens.	1	2	3	4
15. I do not use heroin or other illegal intravenous drugs.	1	2	3	4
16. I do not experience blackouts when I drink alcohol.	1	2	3	4
17. I do not become abusive or violent when I drink alcohol or use psychoactive drugs.	1	2	3	4
18. I use potentially addictive prescription medication in complete compliance with my physician's directions.	1	2	3	4
19. I do not smoke cigarettes.	1	2	3	4
20. I do not use tobacco products in any other form.	1	2	3	4
21. I minimize my exposure to secondhand smoke.	1	2	3	4
22. I am concerned about the effect that alcohol, tobacco, and other drug use is known to have on developing fetuses.	1	2	3	4
23. I am concerned about the effect that alcohol, tobacco, and other drug use is known to have on the health of other people.	1	2	3	4
24. I seek natural, health-enhancing highs rather than relying on alcohol, tobacco, and illegal drugs.	1	2	3	4
25. I take prescription medication only as instructed, and I use over-the-counter medication in accordance with directions.	1	2	3	4

POINTS _____

Comprehensive Health Assessment—*continued*

Disease Prevention

	Not true/ rarely	Somewhat true/ sometimes	Mostly true/ usually	Very true/ always
1. My diet includes foods rich in phytochemicals.	1	2	3	4
2. My diet includes foods rich in folic acid.	1	2	3	4
3. My diet includes foods that are good sources of dietary fiber.	1	2	3	4
4. My diet is low in dietary cholesterol.	1	2	3	4
5. I follow food preparation practices that minimize the risk of foodborne illness.	1	2	3	4
6. I engage in regular physical activity and am able to control my weight effectively.	1	2	3	4
7. I do not use tobacco products.	1	2	3	4
8. I abstain from alcohol or drink only in moderation.	1	2	3	4
9. I do not use intravenously administered illegal drugs.	1	2	3	4
10. I use safer sex practices intended to minimize my risk of exposure to sexually transmitted diseases or infections, including HIV and HPV.	1	2	3	4
11. I take steps to limit my risk of exposure to the bacterium that causes Lyme disease and to the virus that causes hantavirus pulmonary syndrome.	1	2	3	4
12. I control my blood pressure with weight management and physical fitness activities.	1	2	3	4
13. I minimize my exposure to allergens, including those that trigger asthma attacks.	1	2	3	4
14. I wash my hands frequently and thoroughly.	1	2	3	4
15. I use preventive medical care services appropriately.	1	2	3	4
16. I use appropriate cancer self-screening practices, such as breast self-examination and testicular self-examination.	1	2	3	4
17. I know which chronic illnesses and diseases are part of my family history.	1	2	3	4
18. I know which inherited conditions are part of my family history and will seek preconceptional counseling regarding these conditions.	1	2	3	4
19. I am fully immunized against infectious diseases.	1	2	3	4
20. I take prescribed medications, particularly antibiotics, exactly as instructed by my physician.	1	2	3	4

POINTS _____

Sexual Health

	Not true/ rarely	Somewhat true/ sometimes	Mostly true/ usually	Very true/ always
1. I know how sexually transmitted diseases are spread.	1	2	3	4
2. I can recognize the symptoms of sexually transmitted diseases.	1	2	3	4
3. I know how sexually transmitted disease transmission can be prevented.	1	2	3	4
4. I know how safer sex practices reduce the risk of contracting sexually transmitted diseases.	1	2	3	4
5. I follow safer sex practices.	1	2	3	4
6. I recognize the symptoms of premenstrual syndrome and understand how it is prevented and treated.	1	2	3	4

Comprehensive Health Assessment—*continued*

	1	2	3	4
7. I recognize the symptoms of endometriosis and understand the relationship of its symptoms to hormonal cycles.	1	2	3	4
8. I understand the physiological basis of menopause and recognize that it is a normal part of the aging process in women.	1	2	3	4
9. I understand and accept the range of human sexual orientations.	1	2	3	4
10. I encourage the development of flexible sex roles (androgyny) in children.	1	2	3	4
11. I take a mature approach to dating and mate selection.	1	2	3	4
12. I recognize that marriage and other types of long-term relationships can be satisfying.	1	2	3	4
13. I recognize that a celibate lifestyle is appropriate and satisfying for some people.	1	2	3	4
14. I affirm the sexuality of older adults and am comfortable with its expression.	1	2	3	4
15. I am familiar with the advantages and disadvantages of a wide range of birth control methods.	1	2	3	4
16. I understand how each birth control method works and how effective it is.	1	2	3	4
17. I use my birth control method consistently and appropriately.	1	2	3	4
18. I am familiar with the wide range of procedures now available to treat infertility.	1	2	3	4
19. I accept that others may disagree with my feelings about pregnancy termination.	1	2	3	4
20. I am familiar with alternatives available to infertile couples, including adoption.	1	2	3	4

POINTS _____

Safety Practices and Violence Prevention	Not true/ rarely	Somewhat true/ sometimes	Mostly true/ usually	Very true/ always
1. I attempt to identify sources of risk or danger in each new setting or activity.	1	2	3	4
2. I learn proper procedures and precautions before undertaking new recreational or occupational activities.	1	2	3	4
3. I select appropriate clothing and equipment for all activities and maintain equipment in good working order.	1	2	3	4
4. I curtail my participation in activities when I am not feeling well or am distracted by other demands.	1	2	3	4
5. I repair dangerous conditions or report them to those responsible for maintenance.	1	2	3	4
6. I use common sense and observe the laws governing nonmotorized vehicles when I ride a bicycle.	1	2	3	4
7. I operate all motor vehicles as safely as possible, including using seat belts and other safety equipment.	1	2	3	4
8. I refrain from driving an automobile or boat when I have been drinking alcohol or taking drugs or medications.	1	2	3	4
9. I try to anticipate the risk of falling and maintain my environment to minimize this risk.	1	2	3	4
10. I maintain my environment to minimize the risk of fire, and I have a well-rehearsed plan to exit my residence in case of fire.	1	2	3	4

Comprehensive Health Assessment—*continued*

11. I am a competent swimmer and could save myself or rescue someone who was drowning.	1	2	3	4
12. I refrain from sexually aggressive behavior toward my partner or others.	1	2	3	4
13. I would report an incident of sexual harassment or date rape whether or not I was the victim.	1	2	3	4
14. I would seek help from others if I were the victim or perpetrator of domestic violence.	1	2	3	4
15. I practice gun safety and encourage other gun owners to do so.	1	2	3	4
16. I drive at all times in a way that will minimize my risk of being carjacked.	1	2	3	4
17. I have taken steps to protect my home from intruders.	1	2	3	4
18. I use campus security services as much as possible when they are available.	1	2	3	4
19. I know what to do if I am being stalked.	1	2	3	4
20. I have a well-rehearsed plan to protect myself from the aggressive behavior of other people in my place of residence.	1	2	3	4

POINTS _____

Health Care Consumerism

	Not true/ rarely	Somewhat true/ sometimes	Mostly true/ usually	Very true/ always
1. I know how to obtain valid health information.	1	2	3	4
2. I accept health information that has been deemed valid by the established scientific community.	1	2	3	4
3. I am skeptical of claims that guarantee the effectiveness of a particular health care service or product.	1	2	3	4
4. I am skeptical of practitioners or clinics who advertise or offer services at rates substantially lower than those charged by reputable providers.	1	2	3	4
5. I am not swayed by advertisements that present unhealthy behavior in an attractive manner.	1	2	3	4
6. I can afford proper medical care, including hospitalization.	1	2	3	4
7. I can afford adequate health insurance.	1	2	3	4
8. I understand the role of government health care plans in providing health care to people who qualify for coverage.	1	2	3	4
9. I know how to select health care providers who are highly qualified and appropriate for my current health care needs.	1	2	3	4
10. I seek a second or third opinion when surgery or other costly therapies are recommended.	1	2	3	4
11. I have told my physician which hospital I would prefer to use should the need arise.	1	2	3	4
12. I understand my rights and responsibilities as a patient when admitted to a hospital.	1	2	3	4
13. I practice adequate self-care to reduce my health care expenditures and my reliance on health care providers.	1	2	3	4
14. I am open-minded about alternative health care practices and support current efforts to determine their appropriate role in effective health care.	1	2	3	4
15. I have a well-established relationship with a pharmacist and have transmitted all necessary information regarding medication use.	1	2	3	4

Comprehensive Health Assessment—*continued*

16. I carefully follow labels and directions when using health care products, such as over-the-counter medications.	1	2	3	4
17. I finish all prescription medications as directed, rather than stopping use when symptoms subside.	1	2	3	4
18. I report to the appropriate agencies any providers of health care services, information, or products that use deceptive advertising or fraudulent methods of operation.	1	2	3	4
19. I pursue my rights as fully as possible in matters of misrepresentation or consumer dissatisfaction.	1	2	3	4
20. I follow current health care issues in the news and voice my opinion to my elected representatives.	1	2	3	4

POINTS _____

Environmental Health

	Not true/ rarely	Somewhat true/ sometimes	Mostly true/ usually	Very true/ always
1. I avoid use of and exposure to pesticides as much as possible.	1	2	3	4
2. I avoid use of and exposure to herbicides as much as possible.	1	2	3	4
3. I am willing to spend the extra money and time required to obtain organically grown produce.	1	2	3	4
4. I reduce environmental pollutants by minimizing my use of the automobile.	1	2	3	4
5. I avoid the use of products that contribute to indoor air pollution.	1	2	3	4
6. I limit my exposure to ultraviolet radiation by avoiding excessive sun exposure.	1	2	3	4
7. I limit my exposure to radon gas by using a radon gas detector.	1	2	3	4
8. I limit my exposure to radiation by promptly eliminating radon gas within my home.	1	2	3	4
9. I limit my exposure to radiation by agreeing to undergo medical radiation procedures only when absolutely necessary for the diagnosis and treatment of an illness or disease.	1	2	3	4
10. I avoid the use of potentially unsafe water, particularly when traveling in a foreign country or when a municipal water supply or bottled water is unavailable.	1	2	3	4
11. I avoid noise pollution by limiting my exposure to loud noise or by using ear protection.	1	2	3	4
12. I avoid air pollution by carefully selecting the environments in which I live, work, and recreate.	1	2	3	4
13. I do not knowingly use or improperly dispose of personal care products that can harm the environment.	1	2	3	4
14. I reuse as many products as possible so that they can avoid the recycling bins for as long as possible.	1	2	3	4
15. I participate fully in my community's recycling efforts.	1	2	3	4
16. I encourage the increased use of recycled materials in the design and manufacturing of new products.	1	2	3	4
17. I dispose of residential toxic substances safely and properly.	1	2	3	4
18. I follow environmental issues in the news and voice my opinion to my elected representatives.	1	2	3	4

19. I am aware of and involved in environmental issues in my local area.	1	2	3	4
20. I perceive myself as a steward of the environment for the generations to come, rather than as a person with a right to use (and misuse) the environment to meet my immediate needs.	1	2	3	4

POINTS _____

YOUR TOTAL POINTS _____

Interpretation

770 to 880 points—Congratulations! Your health behavior is very supportive of high-level health. Continue to practice your positive health habits, and look for areas in which you can become even stronger. Encourage others to follow your example, and support their efforts in any way you can.

550 to 769 points—Good job! Your health behavior is relatively supportive of high-level health. You scored well in several areas; however, you can improve in some ways. Identify your weak areas and chart a plan for behavior change, as explained at the end of Chapter 1. Then pay close attention as you learn more about health in the weeks ahead.

330 to 549 points—Caution! Your relatively low score indicates that your behavior may be compromising your health. Review your responses to this assessment carefully, noting the areas in which you scored poorly. Then chart a detailed plan for behavior change, as outlined at the end of Chapter 1. Be sure to set realistic goals that you can work toward steadily as you complete this course.

Below 330 points—Red flag! Your low score suggests that your health behavior is destructive. Immediate changes in your behavior are needed to put you back on track. Review your responses to this assessment carefully. Then begin to make changes in the most critical areas, such as harmful alcohol or other drug use patterns. Seek help promptly for any difficulties that you are not prepared to deal with alone, such as domestic violence or suicidal thoughts. The information you read in this textbook and learn in this course could have a significant effect on your future health. Remember, it's not too late to improve your health!

TO CARRY THIS FURTHER . . .

Most of us can improve our health behavior in a number of ways. We hope this assessment will help you identify areas in which you can make positive changes and serve as a motivator as you implement your plan for behavior change. If you scored well, give yourself a pat on the back. If your score was not as high as you would have liked, take heart. This textbook and your instructor can help you get started on the road to wellness. Good luck!

The Mind

Part One covers two topics that are closely linked to how we handle change in our lives. Chapter 2 discusses psychological health, and Chapter 3 deals with stress management. As explained below, your personal growth closely relates to each of the six health dimensions discussed in Chapter 1.

1. **Physical Dimension**
   The physical dimension of health concerns the structure and the function of all body systems. Many of the experiences that shape your feelings about yourself are made possible by good physical health. In addition, effective coping skills often require us to draw on the physical dimension of health.

2. **Psychological Dimension**
   Our responses to stress are primarily emotional. Feelings of uneasiness arising from the demands of college, relationships, parenting, or work are the hallmarks of stress. Fortunately, you can cope with change by using the resources of your psychological dimension of health. Your sense of humor, capacity for empathy, and attitude toward adversity will help you cope with demanding changes in your life.

3. **Social Dimension**
   Growth and development are influenced by the people with whom you interact. When things go well with roommates, coworkers, or your spouse or children, you begin to feel capable as a social person. Occasional failures in social relationships can produce stress but can also remind you that emotional growth and coping skills take time to develop.

4. **Intellectual Dimension**
   As you grow older, you will call on your intellectual resources with increasing frequency. These resources will help you enjoy life more fully and understand your emotional and spiritual growth. During difficult times, your mind may be your most dependable coping source. A book, a concert, or an art exhibit may be a refuge from the stress of the classroom, family, or office.

5. **Spiritual Dimension**
   Many of today's students are searching for a deeper understanding of the meaning of life. Some students feel pressured to accept the spiritual beliefs of the majority. The uncertainties of exploring what to believe and how to express those beliefs can create stress. Your spirituality can be a valuable resource during periods of stress. Meditation, introspection, and prayer can free people from some of the stress of living in a fast-paced, sometimes uncaring world. To believe deeply in something and to act on that belief by serving others leads to personal growth.

6. **Occupational Dimension**
   The vocation you choose will have a lasting effect on shaping the person you will become. Many people choose an occupation that allows them to serve others. However, work can be a primary source of life stress. Some of this stress is unwelcome and can be harmful. But occupational stress can also challenge you to perform at your peak, generating a sense of pride and accomplishment.

Achieving Psychological Health

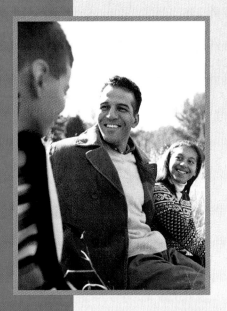

What Do You Know about Psychological Health?

◎ Psychological health has been associated with having a good sense of humor. True or False?

◎ Self-esteem is the highest level of psychological health on Maslow's hierarchy of needs. True or False?

◎ Pessimists tend to live longer than optimists do. True or False?

◎ It has been proven that personality is influenced more by heredity than by environment. True or False?

◎ Mental disorders are the leading cause of disability in the United States. True or False?

◎ You should always take seriously someone who talks about suicide. True or False?

◎ Schizophrenia is a mental disorder that involves having dissociative identity disorder. True or False?

Check your answers at the end of the chapter.

Defining Psychological Health

How many feelings are people capable of expressing? Happy, sad, fearful, and angry are the four primary emotions that humans universally feel. These emotions are considered to be hardwired into human neuroanatomy for survival. Permutations of these four primary emotions result in our capacity to express about 100 different emotions, such as feeling frustrated, although cultural differences do exist[1] (see the box "Cultural Differences in Emotional Expression" for more information). These feelings are all part of the psychological dimension of health. The terms *emotional wellness* and ***psychological health*** have been used interchangeably to describe how people function in the emotional and cognitive realms of their lives. Such functioning includes how people express their emotions; cope with stress, adversity, and success; and adapt to changes in themselves and their environment. Psychological health also addresses cognitive functioning—the ways people think and behave in conjunction with their emotions. There is

Learning from Our Diversity

Cultural Differences in Emotional Expression

Although humans share four primary emotions—happiness, fear, anger, and sadness—we do not all express them in the same way. For example, to express fear, Oriya women of Bhubansewar, India, extend their tongues out and downward, raise their eyebrows, and widen and cross thieir eyes,* whereas Europeans and Americans tend to open their eyes wide, raise their eyebrows, and open their mouths wide. There are also significant cultural differences in how acceptable it is to express feelings. Some cultures (such as Asian cultures) are more emotionally restrictive, while others (such as Italians) are more emotionally intense.

Expressing anger is rare for Tahitians and Utku Eskimos; in contrast, Americans and Western Europeans tend to frequently express this emotion.

Even though cultures share the same emotions, not all situations evoke the same emotional response in all cultures. For example, people from Bali laugh in response to grief and fall asleep in reaction to unfamiliar or frightening situations. Americans tend to see smiling at a stranger as a way to convey friendliness, but Japanese tend to interpret smiling at a stranger as being fake and shallow.*

Emotions communicate meaning and provide an interpretation of events through both nonverbal and verbal cues. Emotions are key in social interactions, as they influence behavior and elicit reactions from others. In addition, feelings convey social statements about you, others, and the situation.† Therefore, to avoid miscommunication, it is important to take into consideration the cultural context of emotional expression, as this can greatly change the meaning or interpretation of an event or an emotional expression.

*S. Planalp, *Communicating Emotion: Social, Moral, and Cultural Processes* (New York: Cambridge University Press, 1999).
†S. Kitayama and H. Markus, *Emotion and Culture* (Washington, DC: American Psychological Association, 1994).

---

some debate about whether thoughts influence feelings or feelings cause us to think and behave a certain way. However, the most accepted view is that the way we think can directly change how we feel about an event or a situation. Thus, you can change your feelings about something by changing your attitude and perspective about a situation. This ability has implications for how we can increase our self-esteem and confidence level, and enhance our interactions with others. You will learn more about psychological health in this chapter.

When you apply resources from the multiple dimensions of health (Chapter 1) in ways that allow you to direct your growth, assess deeply held values, deal effectively with change, and have satisfying relationships with others, you are psychologically healthy.

Research in the area of health psychology has shown that there is a mind-body connection in which biological, psychological, and social factors interact to influence health or illness. This is referred to as the **biopsychological model.**[2] We know that one's psychological state has a significant effect on physical health; stress, depression, and anxiety have been associated with how the immune system responds and can impair physical health. For example, studies have shown that terminally ill cancer patients who had good psychological health lived longer and reported having higher quality of life than did other cancer patients.[3]

Psychological health has also been associated with developing and maintaining a positive **self-concept,** positive **self-esteem,** and a higher level of **emotional intelligence.** However, as you will see, psychological health is much more than just the absence of mental illness.

Characteristics of Psychologically Healthy People

Your self-concept is the internal picture you have of yourself and is a reflection of your psychological health. Psychologically healthy people are not perfect. They have their share of stress, problems, and flaws, and they make their share of mistakes. However, it is how they perceive themselves and how they cope with their stress and

> ### Key Terms
>
> **psychological health** A broadly based concept pertaining to cognitive functioning in conjunction with the way people express their emotions; cope with stress, adversity, and success; and adapt to changes in themselves and their environment.
>
> **biopsychological model** A model that addresses how biological, psychological, and social factors interact and affect psychological health.
>
> **self-concept** An individual's internal picture of himself or herself; the way one sees oneself.
>
> **self-esteem** An individual's sense of pride, self-respect, value, and worth.
>
> **emotional intelligence** The ability to understand others and act wisely in human relations and measure how well one knows one's emotions, manages one's emotions, motivates oneself, recognizes emotions in others, and handles relationships.

problems that separate them from unhealthy individuals. Psychologically healthy people:

- Accept themselves and others
- Like themselves
- Appropriately express the full range of human emotions, both positive and negative
- Give and receive care, love, and support
- Accept life's disappointments
- Accept their mistakes
- Express empathy and concern for others
- Take care of themselves
- Trust others as well as themselves
- Establish goals, both short and long term
- Can function both independently and interdependently
- Lead a health-enhancing lifestyle that includes regular exercise, good nutrition, and adequate sleep

See the box "Fostering Your Psychological Health" for activities that may enhance your current level of psychological health.

Self-Esteem

What is self-esteem? How do you know when someone is lacking in self-esteem? Most people answer this question by saying that they define positive self-esteem as:

- Having pride in yourself
- Treating yourself with respect
- Considering yourself valuable, important, worthy
- Feeling good about yourself
- Having self-confidence, being self-assured
- Accepting yourself

People with low levels of self-esteem tend to allow others to mistreat them, don't take care of themselves, have difficulty being by themselves, and have little self-confidence. In addition, people with low self-esteem tend to take things personally and are sometimes seen as overly sensitive; they tend to be perfectionists who are highly critical of themselves and others. These individuals often have a pessimistic outlook on life and see themselves as undeserving of good fortune. We explore the concepts of optimism and pessimism as they relate to psychological health in a later section of this chapter.

Where do we get our self-esteem? Most people would say from their parents, teachers, peers, siblings, religious institutions, and the media. While these factors certainly can positively or negatively affect our self-concept and self-esteem, they are all *external* factors. Self-concept refers to our *internal* self-perception. People with low self-esteem tend to have a poor self-concept, meaning that their internal picture of themselves is very negative. Because of this poor self-concept, people with low self-esteem tend to allow others to mistreat or abuse them and fail to be assertive. Many psychological problems have their underpinnings in low self-esteem, including eating disorders, substance abuse problems, and depression.

People who suffer from low self-esteem tend to focus on outside factors. If our self-esteem and self-concept were based solely on external factors, then we would need to change only our environment and the people around us to raise our self-esteem. Thus, many people believe

I keep getting into unhealthy romantic relationships and have come to expect that the person I am dating will eventually find something wrong with me and leave me. What can I do to feel better about myself and change my attitude toward my chances of having a successful relationship?

As the saying goes, it is hard to allow others to love you when you don't love yourself. So the first step is to start accepting and liking yourself and develop a more positive self-concept. The following activities can help you start the process of enhancing your self-esteem.

Write down three things you like about yourself every day. Ask yourself what you did well today—not what you did wrong.

Share this list with a friend. It is generally more accepted to share your flaws and problems rather than your successes or positive qualities. We often hear people say, "That was a stupid thing for me to say" or "I'm having a bad hair day" rather than "I was proud of how I was able to answer a question in class today."

Accept compliments. Frequently, we deflect or laugh away compliments rather than accept them. One of the ways to test yourself to see if you took in a compliment is to see if you remember what that person said about you an hour later. Another way is to focus on how you are feeling—do you feel more positive, confident, happier with yourself?

Give compliments. Sometimes people with low self-esteem criticize others in order to feel better about themselves. To get out of this pattern, look for positives in other people and share your feedback, without belittling yourself. Instead of saying, "You do that so much better than I do" just say "You are really good at that."

Watch your body posture. Making eye contact with others, keeping your head up and shoulders back, and not folding your arms in front of you but keeping an open body posture help to build self-

esteem and confidence and project this image to others.

Take a risk, do something different. People with low levels of self-esteem tend to tell themselves "I can't do that" and so don't even try. Don't be afraid of making a mistake or looking foolish. Take a risk and do something new and different—you might surprise yourself and be more successful than you anticipated.

Disarm the critic. Don't listen to the critical voice in your head that tells you that you are stupid, lazy, or not good enough. Sometimes this critical voice is the voice of our parents, teachers, or someone else in our lives who told us these negative messages. Replace the negative statements with positive ones and tell the critic to ease up a bit.

Reward yourself and be good to yourself. We frequently do nice things for other people or wait for others to reward us. Do something fun or nice for yourself every day.

Signs and symbols of self-worth. Keep your list of positive qualities where you will see it—in your room or in your car. Have things around you that remind you that people care about you and that you are a worthwhile person, such as notes from friends, pictures of enjoyable times with others, or an item that is special to you in some way.

Set realistic goals and expectations for yourself. Changing patterns takes time and practice. You didn't develop your self-concept overnight, and it will take some time to change the way you talk to yourself and see yourself. Notice how much progress you have made rather than how much more you have to go.

InfoLinks

www.self-esteem-nase.org

---

that if they had more money, a nicer car, a better relationship, and so on they would feel better about themselves. This can become a vicious cycle, leaving these people always seeking more and being perpetually dissatisfied with themselves. This can also lead to perfectionism and not accepting yourself.

Although we don't have much control over other people, we do have control over what we internalize or accept as true and valid about ourselves (see the box "Enhancing Your Self-Esteem"). Self-esteem is not an all-or-none commodity. Most people have varying degrees of self-esteem, depending on their stage of development, events in their lives, and their environment.[4]

Emotional Intelligence

A third aspect of psychological health is the degree of emotional intelligence you possess. Emotional intelligence refers to "the ability to understand others and act wisely in

human relations."[5] Furthermore, emotional intelligence can be broken down into five primary domains:

- *Knowing your emotions.* This is considered to be the cornerstone of emotional intelligence and relates to how much self-awareness and insight you have. How quickly you are able to recognize and label your feelings as you feel them determines the level of your emotional intelligence.

- *Managing your emotions.* How well can you express your feelings appropriately and cope with your emotions? People who have trouble coping with anxiety, distress, and failures tend to have lower levels of emotional intelligence.

- *Motivating yourself.* People who can motivate themselves tend to be more highly productive and independent than are those who rely on external sources for motivation. The more you can self-motivate and engage in goal-directed activities, the higher your emotional intelligence.

- *Recognizing emotions in others.* Another aspect of emotional intelligence is the degree of empathy you have, or how sensitive you are to the feelings of others and how you relate to other people.

- *Handling relationships.* This refers to your level of social skills. The more interpersonally effective you are and the more you are able to negotiate conflict and build a social support network, the more emotional intelligence you possess.

Of course people have differing levels of emotional intelligence and may have higher levels in one domain than in another. People with overall high levels of emotional intelligence tend to take on leadership roles, are confident, are assertive, express their feelings directly and appropriately, feel good about themselves, are outgoing, and adapt well to stress.[5]

Personality

What is meant when someone says, "She has a good personality"? Is it possible to have no personality? **Personality** is generally defined as a specific set of consistent patterns of behaviors and traits that help to identify and characterize an individual. Personality includes thoughts, feelings, behaviors, motivation, instinct, and temperament.[6] Isn't it likely that you associate a "good" personality with the existence of psychological health?

There is some debate about how personality is formed and where we acquire our personality traits. A general consensus is that two factors, **nature** and **nurture,** influence the shaping of personality. Nature refers to the innate factors we are born with that genetically determine our personality traits. Nurture is the effect that the environment, people, and external factors have on our personality.[7] While it is agreed that both nature and nurture influence personality development, there is some debate about how much of a role each one plays in its formation. We all know people who are introverted or quiet or shy "by nature" or "naturally outgoing." We seem to be born with a predisposition toward certain personality traits that often resemble our parents'. "She is serious like her father" or "He is funny like his mother" are remarks people may make alluding to this genetic link. Environmental factors, such as social relationships, family harmony, financial resources, job and academic concerns, and living situations, can influence your personality.

Often assumptions are made about an individual's personality based largely on his or her appearance. Studies have shown that physically attractive people are seen as warm, friendly, and intelligent, and unattractive people are viewed as cold, humorless, and not as bright.[8] First impressions also play a major role in how we perceive other people's personalities. Research shows that we tend to make a decision about someone's personality within four minutes of meeting them. Once an impression is formed, it is difficult to change, regardless of how the person behaves or new information that you receive that might contradict what you initially perceived.[7] Thus, people can make errors in judgment because they have not taken the context into consideration or taken enough time to get to know someone over the course of several months and in a variety of settings.

The Normal Range of Emotions

You probably know people who seem happy all the time. Although some people like this may exist, they are truly the exceptions. For most people, emotions are more like a roller-coaster ride. At times, they feel happy, confident, and positive; other times, they feel sad, insecure, and negative. Once you know them better, these same people may show that they feel happy, sad, pleased, uncertain, confident, excited, and afraid all in the same day or week. To outsiders, they might even appear to be moody. To the mental health professional, however, these same people would probably seem to be normal, since the feeling states that they are demonstrating all fall within a normal range of emotions.

Experiencing a range of emotions is normal and healthy. You should not expect to remain calm and rational every minute of the day. You also should not expect to adjust effectively to every situation with which you are confronted. Life has its ups and downs, and the concept of the *normal range of emotions* reflects this. It is when emotions fluctuate to an extreme level (both up and down), aren't expressed appropriately, or are out of control and overwhelming that people can become psychologically unhealthy.

Maslow's Hierarchy of Needs

Abraham Maslow has been one of the most significant contributors to the understanding of personality and emotional growth. Central to Maslow's contribution to twentieth-century American psychological thought is his view of psychological health in terms of the individual's attempt to meet inner needs, what he called *the hierarchy of needs*[9] (see Figure 2-1).

Maslow's theory is a positive, optimistic theory of human behavior. He believed that people are motivated to grow and fulfill their potential, referring to this phenomenon as **self-actualization.** He described self-actualization as "the need to become more and more what one is, to become everything that one is capable of becoming."[10] Maslow differentiated between two different categories of needs: **basic needs** and **metaneeds.** Basic needs—physiological needs, safety and security, belonging and love, and esteem needs—are the deficiency

Figure 2-1 Maslow's Hierarchy of Needs Once basic needs are met, metaneeds such as creativity, spirituality, and justice come into play.

Source: Maslow AH. *Motivation and Personality* (2nd ed.). New York: Van Norstrand, 1970.

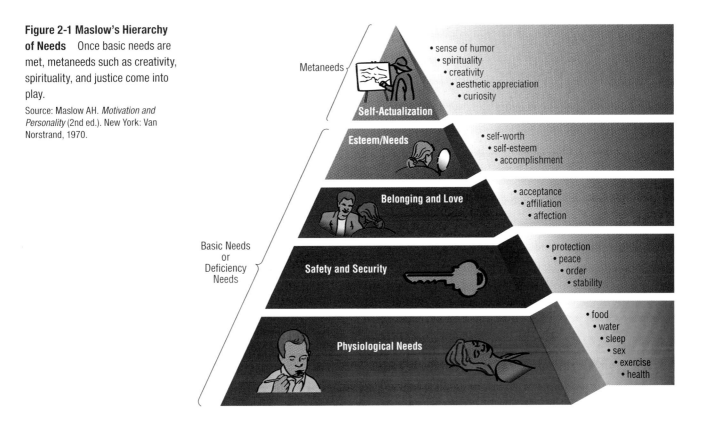

Metaneeds
- sense of humor
- spirituality
- creativity
- aesthetic appreciation
- curiosity

Self-Actualization

Esteem/Needs
- self-worth
- self-esteem
- accomplishment

Belonging and Love
- acceptance
- affiliation
- affection

Basic Needs or Deficiency Needs

Safety and Security
- protection
- peace
- order
- stability

Physiological Needs
- food
- water
- sleep
- sex
- exercise
- health

needs and are essential and urgent. Metaneeds come into play once the basic needs are met and include spirituality, creativity, curiosity, beauty, philosophy, and justice. Maslow's hierarchy of needs is arranged with the basic needs on the bottom, as they are the most fundamental and powerful needs. Lower-level needs must be met before the next level of needs can be satisfied. Maslow believed that people must fulfill their metaneeds in order to become completely developed human beings. Left unfulfilled, people can become cynical, apathetic, and lonely.[10]

Maslow arrived at this model by examining people whom he considered to be exceptionally healthy, people he defined as having developed to their fullest potentials. People whom Maslow identified as self-actualized included Albert Einstein, Albert Schweitzer, Eleanor Roosevelt, and Abraham Lincoln. He perceived these people to share similar personality characteristics, such as being self-assured, principled, innovative, compassionate, altruistic, goal-oriented, and internally motivated.[11]

Creative Expression

Another characteristic of people who have developed their psychological health is creativity. Allowing yourself to express your thoughts, feelings, and individuality in a creative manner entails having self-confidence, self-esteem, and flexibility. Confidence and self-esteem are essential so that you feel free to share your creative side

with others and don't feel embarrassed by your creativity. Children can easily do this when they draw a picture or make up a dance and say, "Look at me; look at what I made." However, as we age, some of us become inhibited

Key Terms

personality A specific set of consistent patterns of behavior and traits that helps to identify and characterize an individual; personality comprises thoughts, feelings, behaviors, motivation, instinct, and temperament.

nature The innate factors that genetically determine personality traits.

nurture The effect that the environment, people, and external factors have on personality.

self-actualization The highest level of psychological health at which one reaches his or her highest potential and values truth, beauty, goodness, faith, love, humor, and ingenuity.

basic needs Deficiency needs that are viewed as essential and fundamental, including physiological needs, safety and security, belonging and love, and esteem needs.

metaneeds Secondary concerns, such as spirituality, creativity, curiosity, beauty, philosophy, and justice, that can be addressed only after the basic needs are met.

and don't allow ourselves to be creative or to share this part of ourselves. If you don't exercise your creative side, it can atrophy, just as unexercised muscles do.

What are some resources that you might need to develop to foster your creativity?

- *Nonconformity.* Creative individuals aren't terribly concerned about what other people think of them. They are willing to risk looking foolish or proposing ideas that are divergent from others' ideas or traditional ways of thinking.

- *Independence.* Highly creative people tend to work well alone and sometimes prefer this to working in a group. As children, they often were encouraged to solve problems on their own rather than having someone else do so for them.

- *Motivation.* Creative people are motivated by intrinsic rather than external rewards, meaning they like to be creative for their own pleasure, not to please others or because it is expected of them. They enjoy creativity for creativity's sake alone, not to reap rewards or praise from others.

- *Curiosity.* Creative people have a wide range of interests and a broad base of knowledge. They are open to new experiences and question things that other people ignore or take for granted.

- *Persistence.* This is seen as one of the most important traits of a creative person. As Thomas Edison said, "Genius is one-tenth inspiration and nine-tenths perspiration." Persistence requires not giving up when your first efforts are not successful and thinking of new ways of doing something, problem solving, or thinking "outside the box."[12]

Some people reviewing the preceding list may recognize many of these characteristics as being already well developed in their own personalities. Others may not have demonstrated some of the traits listed, and the traits may appear far beyond their reach. Nevertheless, most people can increase their creativity by giving themselves permission to be creative. Some people state, "I'm not a creative person," and yet they haven't explored that part of their personality, perhaps since childhood. There are many avenues of creativity, and the first step is to experiment, to be open and spontaneous. In this way, you can gain greater psychological health from accessing your inner strengths and resources.

Spiritual Health

Having a sense of purpose, direction, and awareness is a dimension of spiritual health. This aspect of psychological health also refers to how well we integrate our beliefs and values with our behavior. People with spiritual health seek meaning and purpose in their lives and have a deep appreciation for a sense of unity and community

Discovering Your Spirituality

Mindfulness: Time to Pay Attention

Have you taken a moment today to be quiet and just be with yourself? Time alone can help you step away from a busy, fragmented world and draw inward for renewal. Having strengthened awareness of yourself in both mind and body allows you to experience the fullness of the moment, even to feel in sync with the universe. This is referred to as "mindfulness"—being aware of the present moment without judging, just accepting.

Mindfulness can also help you establish your identity, clarify what's important to you, and strengthen your independence. When we are observing ourselves in the present moment, we have the opportunity to fully emerge and become ourselves.

Any time you take for this meditation will be restorative. You may start with just five minutes every morning. You will need a place where you feel comfortable to be alone with your own thoughts, whether it be in bed, in the bath, at a coffee shop, in the library, or in the garden. Go for a walk, listen to music, do yoga, or just be still and concentrate on your breathing. All of these are ways to reconnect you to your life force. Pretty soon you may feel that your time of mindfulness is more energizing than sleep! When you are faced with a difficult project, a personal crisis, or something more serious, such as sickness or death, these reflective moments will give you mental and spiritual renewal.

It's not selfish to carve out whatever time you need alone to refresh yourself. By paying attention to your thoughts and feelings, you're reconnecting to your inner self. This nourished spirit is something you can share with others.

(see the box "Mindfulness"). Spiritual health also includes one's morals, ethics, intrinsic values, and beliefs. It also refers to an awareness and appreciation of the vastness of the universe, and recognition of a dimension beyond the natural and rational, involving, perhaps, a belief in a force greater than oneself.[13] Spirituality has been found to increase psychological health; people who incorporate it into their lives reported better psychological coping, increased well-being, increased satisfaction with life, lower anxiety and fewer depressive symptoms, less hostility and anger, and greater happiness in general.[14] Similarly, spirituality has also been related to better physical health. Studies have shown that no matter how *spirituality* was defined or measured, it has a positive effect on reducing coronary heart disease, high blood pressure, stroke, and cancer and increasing life expectancy.[15]

As a resource in the spiritual dimension of health, the existence of spirituality provides a basis on which your belief system can mature and your expanding awareness of life's meaning can be fostered. In addition, the existence of spirituality lends meaning to your career and assists you in better understanding the consequences of your vocational efforts. Further, spirituality can influence many of the experiences that you will seek throughout life and can temper the emotional relationships that you have with these experiences. In virtually all cultures, spirituality provides individuals and groups with rituals and practices that foster the development of a sense of community. In turn, the community provides the structure and guidance that nurtures the emotional stability, confidence, and sense of competence needed for living life fully.[16]

 TALKING POINTS How well do your actions reflect your beliefs and values? How much time and energy do you devote to what is most important to you?

Keys to Psychological Health

Cultivating a Sense of Humor

Perhaps the most prized emotion to be experienced is a feeling of happiness about life—a feeling that is more likely to occur when day-to-day events are entered into with an underlying sense of humor. Maintaining a sense of humor is now known to be a critically important component of the psychological dimension of health.[17] People who possess this ability understand that life is not meant to be taken too seriously.

Recognizing the humor in daily situations and occasionally being able to laugh at yourself will make you feel better not only about others but also, more importantly, about yourself. Others will enjoy being associated with you, and your ability to perform physically and to recover from injuries and illnesses will also be enhanced.[18] In addition, laughter reduces stress,[19] boosts the immune system,[20] alleviates pain,[21] stabilizes mood,[22] decreases anxiety,[23] enhances communication,[24] and inspires creativity.[25] The research suggests that we need to laugh 30 minutes total in a 24-hour period in order to attain these benefits. This is an easy task for children, who on average laugh 250 times a day, but more challenging for adults who tend to laugh only 15 times a day.[26] Employers have been putting the benefits of laughter to good use to increase productivity in factories. Factories in India have created "laughing clubs" in which people laugh together for 20 minutes a day, resulting in less absenteeism and better performance among the workers.[27]

 TALKING POINTS How would you describe your personality? How do you think your friends or family would describe you? Do you think the descriptions would be the same or different? Why?

Developing Communication Skills

When people find it difficult to initiate or even participate in conversations with others, it is likely, in part,

Laughing increases endorphin levels to help ease pain, decrease stress, and release tension from your body.

that they have not developed some of the communication skills with which others feel comfortable. In this section we investigate how speaking and listening can foster improved social relationships. We also look at the use of unspoken communication as an aid to social interaction.

Verbal Communication Communication between people can be viewed in terms of a particular person's role as sender or receiver. You can enhance your effectiveness as a sender of verbal information by implementing several important steps:[4]

- *Take the time to think before speaking.* Effective communication requires that you know what you want to say.

- *Focus your words on your most important thoughts and ideas.* Your main message may get lost in too many details or too long a story.

- *Speak clearly and concisely.* This will aid the listener, particularly when ideas are complex or new.

- *Talk with, rather than at, the listener.* Speaking with other people encourages listeners to share freely and comfortably with those speaking.

- *Start on a positive note.* Even when the message is negative, a more positive atmosphere is established when a conversation begins in this manner.

- *Seek feedback from listeners.* Provide frequent intervals between ideas to allow listeners to respond.

- *Use other forms of communication to transmit important ideas* when face-to-face conversation is not effective. Written communication or the use of a carefully selected third person is often highly effective.

Verbal communication requires that you function as skillfully as a listener, or receiver, as you do as a sender of spoken ideas. Certainly, there are skills for structuring the exchange of information. The following are a variety of listening approaches:

- *Focus on what is being said*, not on what you want to say next.
- *Ask for clarification* and summarize what you think you heard the speaker saying to ensure you have received the message accurately.
- On some occasions, *it may be necessary to guide the speaker* to ensure that excessive or confusing information is not being transmitted. This is accomplished by asking carefully worded questions intended to stay on the topic and not get off on a tangent.

Nonverbal Communication Nonverbal communication is what is communicated by your facial expressions, body posture, tone of voice, movements, and even the way you breathe, such as when you sigh or yawn. Nonverbal communication is a very powerful and sometimes more important aspect of the message than what is verbally communicated. Facial cues, particularly from the eyes, are attended to more than any other type of nonverbal communication, even when information from other sources, such as hand and body movements, may provide a more accurate picture of what the person is feeling. The following suggestions can enhance your nonverbal communication skills:

- *Facial expressions.* Facial expressions have been cited as one of the most important sources of nonverbal communication in terms of a person's emotional state.[28] When people speak with their eyebrows raised, they tend to be seen as more animated, excited, and happy. Flushing of one's face can indicate embarrassment, and crinkling one's nose can mean that you don't like something. Every part of your face can communicate some type of emotional reaction.
- *Eye contact.* Maintaining eye contact is an important component of positive nonverbal communication, while looking away or shifting your eyes can be read as seeming dishonest. But don't stare—five to seven seconds seems to be the maximum amount of time to look at someone's eyes before the person begins to feel scrutinized.
- *Personal space.* There are cultural differences in how much personal space or distance is comfortable and accepted when sitting or standing next to another person. For example, Americans' personal space—about 3 to 4 feet for a casual conversation—tends to be much greater than that of Arabs or Italians but less than for Japanese or Britons. Gender and age and degree of familiarity are other factors that can determine the amount of personal space you are comfortable having between you and another person.
- *Body posture.* Assertiveness is equated with people who carry themselves with their head up and shoulders back and maintain eye contact. Folding your arms, crossing your legs, and looking away from the speaker can indicate defensiveness and rejection.

As with verbal communication, when nonverbal components are recognized and well directed, communication is more effective.

Managing Conflict Communication can be especially challenging when there is a conflict or disagreement. Emotions such as anger, hurt, and fear might alter your ability to communicate as effectively as you would like. Some techniques for managing angry or upset people or conflictual situations are these:

- *Listen to and acknowledge the other person's point of view, even if it differs from your own.* To ensure that you have heard the person accurately and to let that person know you are listening, repeat back or summarize what you heard and ask if you misunderstood something that was said.
- *Use assertive communication.* Using "I" statements rather than "You" statements helps to avoid putting people on the defensive and is especially helpful when negotiating conflict or disagreements. Rather than saying "You are inconsiderate," you can say "I feel upset when you're late and don't call to let me know."
- *Focus not just on what you say but how you say it.* Pay attention to your tone of voice and speak in a conversational tone. People tend to talk louder because they think they will be better heard that way. This can result in a shouting match in which neither person hears the other.
- *Acknowledge the others person's feelings.* Use statements like "I can understand why this is so frustrating for you."
- *Watch your body posture.* Don't fold your arms in a closed, defensive posture, maintain eye contact, and be aware of your facial expression so that you are not conveying hostility nonverbally. Make sure your nonverbal communication matches your verbal communication.
- *Accept valid criticism.* If you made a mistake, admit to it and apologize for whatever you think you did to contribute to the misunderstanding or conflict (see the box "How to Say You Are Sorry and Mean

Some people avoid relationships because they don't want to get hurt. Of course they are also avoiding feeling cared about and sharing their lives with others. It is impossible not to hurt someone with whom you are in a relationship—you are going to forget something, inadvertently say the wrong thing, or have a grouchy moment—but it is possible to fix the damage you have done with little to no residual scarring. This is called "the art of effective apology."

There are some dos and don'ts that can make the difference between an effective, reparative apology and a lame, destructive one. In fact, an apology that is perceived as insincere, as blaming the other person, or as defensive can do more harm than good. Here are some important things to keep in mind as you consider an apology.

Apologize . . .

1. *As soon as you realize you have done something wrong.* Don't wait for the "right time," because it will probably never come. Remember that the right time is as soon as you have realized your error.

2. *When you have something truly to apologize for.* Don't apologize for everything and everyone, including the bad weather. When you overapologize, it dilutes the apology's meaning.

3. *By fully acknowledging what you did wrong.* Don't sugarcoat or minimize the error. For example, don't say "I didn't understand what you said" when really you understood but didn't agree with what she said.

4. And *include an explanation*, not an excuse, for your actions. Take responsibility for your actions, don't blame other people or the situation. Owning up to what you did and being willing to admit to it will increase trust in your relationship.

5. *With remorse.* Saying "I'm sorry that I hurt you" instead of "I'm sorry you feel that way" will make or break how an apology is received. Saying "I'm sorry I hurt you *but*" also diminishes the sincerity of an apology, because "but" tends to negate whatever comes before it. This doesn't mean you have to beat yourself up to show how badly you feel about the situation, but you do need to acknowledge that you hurt the other person's feelings.

6. *And fix what can be repaired.* Saying "I'm sorry" but not offering to resolve or repair the damage can cause further hurt. Ask the person what you can do to make things right. Don't say "I said I'm sorry, what else do you want from me?" or "Get over it and move on. It wasn't that big of a deal."

7. *And learn from your mistakes.* Saying you are sorry and then doing the same thing all over again destroys trust. You may be perceived as using an apology as a way of continuing the offensive behavior. The next time, do something different when that situation arises. Talk with the person about how you can handle that situation in a better way in the future.

With effective apologies can come forgiveness and rebuilding of trust and respect in relationships. An effective apology involves honesty, courage, humility, and a real commitment to the relationship. It means we admit to our imperfections and flaws, and it reinforces our commitment to improve ourselves and be acceptable as imperfect human beings.

Source: Martha Beck, "Love Means Never Having to Say You Are Sorry," *Oprah Magazine,* September 2004.

It!"). This will open the door for the other person to take responsibility for his or her part in the conflict as well.

- *Focus on the problem at hand.* If you try to resolve every disagreement you have ever had with this person, you will become overwhelmed and won't accomplish much. Stay on track by talking about the present situation.

- *Take a team approach by engaging in mutual problem solving.* Avoid the winner-versus-loser paradigm, and look for areas of compromise. Find a middle ground you can both live with.

- *Agree to disagree.* There is probably more than one right answer, and you can agree that you will not persuade the other person to change his or her point of view.

- *Agree to discuss this at a later time.* If the conversation becomes too volatile and heated, take some time to calm down and think about the situation. Some time and distance from the problem can be beneficial.

Taking an Optimistic Approach to Life

Is your happiness within your control? Are people born naturally happy or sad? One important key to psychological health is the way you think about and interpret events in your life. For example, if you say "hello" to someone and don't get a response, do you begin to wonder if that person is angry with you? Or do you surmise that he or she didn't hear you or perhaps was distracted? Research shows that having a positive interpretation of life's events, particularly how you cope with adversity, can make a significant difference in terms of your health, academic and work performance, as well as how long you will live.[29] Do you see the glass half empty, as pessimists do, or half full, as optimists do? Does it matter? Again studies overwhelmingly contend that your perspective

Optimists—those who see the glass as half full—interpret life's events positively and are better able to cope with setbacks and adversity.

makes a tremendous difference in your psychological health. Compared to pessimists, optimists tend to:

- Contract fewer infectious diseases
- Have better health habits
- Possess stronger immune systems
- Be more successful in their careers
- Perform better in sports, music, and academics

We do know that people can learn to be helpless and ultimately become depressed and even suicidal. Pavlov

---

---

demonstrated the concept of **learned helplessness** in his classic study in which he administered an electric shock to dogs that were harnessed and couldn't escape the shock. When he moved the dogs to another room and delivered the shocks, the dogs lay down and whimpered and didn't try to avoid the shocks. This time the dogs were not harnessed and could have easily escaped the shocks by moving to another side of the room. This reaction has been referred to as learned helplessness. The dogs learned that there was nothing they could do to affect their situation, and they lost hope and felt trapped and powerless.[30] We have seen this same phenomenon with humans. College students volunteered for an experiment in which they were subjected to an earsplitting noise and their efforts to stop the noise were unsuccessful. Later, when they were placed in another situation in which they could have easily pulled a control lever to turn off the noise, they made no effort to do so and just suffered with the noise until the experimenter stopped it.[31] Battered women have demonstrated this same sense of powerlessness and helplessness in their inability to escape the abuse they are subjected to by their partners.

So, if people can learn to be helpless and pessimistic, can they also learn to feel more optimistic, powerful, and in control? Martin Seligman, a prominent psychologist, conducted studies to prove that this is possible, and he called this concept **learned optimism.** Learned optimism refers to your explanatory style—in other words, if you describe the glass as being half full or half empty. Seligman identified three key factors that contribute to having an optimistic or pessimistic perspective: **permanence, pervasiveness,** and **personalization.**

Permanence   The first dimension is *permanence.* When something bad happens, pessimists tend to give up easily because they believe the causes of bad events are *permanent.* They say things like "Things never work out for me," "That won't ever work," or "He's always in a bad mood." They use permanence language—words like *never, always,* and *forever*—which implies that this negative situation is not temporary but will continue indefinitely. Optimists tend to use language of temporariness—such words as *sometimes, frequently,* and *often*—and they blame bad events on transient conditions. Examples of optimistic language are "It didn't work out this time," "Doing it that way didn't work," and "He's in a bad mood today." Optimists see failure as a small, transitory setback and are able to pick themselves up, brush themselves off, and persevere toward their goals.

Pervasiveness   The second factor that affects our outlook is *pervasiveness.* It refers to whether you perceive negative events as universal and generalize them to everything in your life, or if you can compartmentalize and

---

keep them defined to the specific situation. Pessimists tend to make universal explanations for their problems and when something goes wrong in one part of their lives, they give up on everything. While a pessimist would say that they are not good at math, an optimist would say that they didn't perform well in that particular class with that type of math: "I'm good at algebra but not as good with geometry." The last aspect of an optimistic or pessimistic explanatory style is determined by whether you blame bad things on yourself or on other people or circumstances.

Personalization   Pessimism and low self-esteem tend to come from personalizing events—blaming oneself and having an internal explanatory style for negative events. An optimist might say, "The professor wrote a very poor exam and that is the reason I received a lower score," whereas the pessimist would say, "I am stupid" or "I didn't study enough." This is different from not taking responsibility for one's actions and blaming other people for your problems or mistakes: the idea is to have a balanced perspective and outlook on life. Pessimists tend to give credit to other people or circumstances when good things happen and blame themselves when bad events occur. For example, a pessimist would say, "That was just dumb luck" rather than taking credit for a success. However, if pessimists fail, they readily blame themselves, saying, "I messed up." In contrast, optimists tend to give themselves credit for their accomplishments, saying "I worked hard and did a good job," and they don't belittle themselves when things go wrong.

Seligman conducted many studies to test how an optimistic explanatory style might be useful in daily living. For example, he worked with a swimming team from the University of California, Berkeley, to see how optimism or pessimism might affect their performance. He had the coaches tell the athletes that their times were slower than they actually were. The swimmers were then asked to swim the event again as fast as they could. The performance of the pessimists deteriorated in their 100-yard event by two seconds, the difference between winning the event and finishing dead last. The optimists got faster by two to five seconds, again enough to be the difference between losing and winning the race.[3] So how you interpret events, your attribution style, can make a tremendous difference in the eventual success or failure in your endeavors.

Building Optimism   How can you learn to be more optimistic? Albert Ellis developed a cognitive framework for positive thinking called the ABC method. When you encounter an event, the "A" part of the formula, you try to make sense out of it and explain what has happened. For example, if you receive a notice from the bank that you have overdrawn your checking account, you start to think, "How did this happen?" These thoughts are associated with your beliefs, the "B" in ABC. Your beliefs affect your feelings, and so you can control your emotions by changing your beliefs and thoughts.[32] So, if you think, "I'm irresponsible for letting this happen. I can't manage my money," then you will feel bad about yourself. But if you said, "The bank probably made a mistake" or "I might have added something incorrectly," you will most likely feel much better about yourself and the situation.

The "C" aspect is the consequence of the event, how you end up feeling about the situation. When someone feels depressed, he or she feels hopeless, trapped, and powerless. By adopting a more positive way of reframing or thinking about events, you create options, hope, and a strategy for solving problems rather than remaining stuck, like the whimpering dogs laying down and putting up with being shocked. In the previously described scenario with the overdraft, you can generate ideas such as "I need to check with the bank, go over my bank statement, be more careful in recording and calculating my balances, and request overdraft protection to prevent this from becoming a problem again."

Everyone encounters adversity sometime in his or her life. You can become discouraged by these events, blame yourself for these problems, and feel hopeless, worthless, and cynical about the world. Or you can be persistent and become stronger by overcoming these obstacles, by having positive beliefs, and by seeing these problems as short-lived, specific, and not a flaw in your character. When you embrace an optimistic perspective, you will feel more hopeful, stronger, and confident. You will be able to accept new challenges and take risks in your life. Take the Personal Assessment at the end of this chapter to find your level of optimism and pessimism.

TALKING POINTS Think about something bad that has happened in your life recently. What were your beliefs about this event? How did you feel? Using the concepts of permanence, pervasiveness, and personalization, how can you change your beliefs about this situation? How do you feel differently about the event?

Taking a Proactive Approach to Life

In addition to the approaches already discussed, the plan that follows is intended to give you other strategies for enhancing your psychological health. The following is a four-step process that continues throughout life: constructing perceptions of yourself, accepting these perceptions, undertaking new experiences, and reframing your perceptions based on new information.

Constructing Mental Pictures   Actively taking charge of your psychological health begins with constructing a mental picture of what you're like. Use the most recent and accurate information you have about yourself—what is important to you, your values, and your abilities. You may want to ask trusted friends and family members for their input.

To construct this mental picture, set aside a period of uninterrupted quiet time for reflection. Before proceeding to the second step, you also need to construct mental pictures about yourself in relation to *other people and material objects,* including your residence and college or work environment, to clarify these relationships.

Accepting Mental Pictures The second step of the plan involves an *acceptance* of these perceptions. This implies a willingness to honor the truthfulness of the perceptions you have formed about yourself and other people.

Psychological development is an active process. You must be willing to be *introspective* (inwardly reflective) about yourself and the world around you and to apply these new perceptions.

Undertaking New Experiences The next step of the plan is to test your newly formed perceptions. This *testing* is accomplished by *undertaking* a *new experience* or by reexperiencing something in a different way.

New experiences do not necessarily require high levels of risk, foreign travel, or money. They may be no more "new" than deciding to move from the dorm into an apartment, to change from one shift at work to another, or to pursue new friendships. The experience itself is not the goal; rather, it's a means of collecting information about yourself, others, and the objects that form your material world. The goal is to "try on" or test your perceptions to see what fits you.

Reframing Mental Pictures When you have completed the first three steps in the plan, the new information about yourself, others, and objects becomes the most current source of information. Regardless of the type of new experience you have undertaken and its outcome, you are now in a position to modify the initial perceptions constructed during the first step. Then you will have new insights, knowledge, and perspectives. This is a

continual process. As you grow and change, so will your perceptions.

Psychological Disorders

In the course of one year, an estimated 26 percent of Americans, about one in four, suffer from a diagnosable mental disorder. This translates to 57.7 million people being diagnosed with a mental disorder each year, with many people suffering from more than one mental disorder at a given time.[33] In addition, mental disorders are the leading cause of disability in the United States for Americans ages 15 to 44.[34] However, two-thirds of these people do not receive treatment owing to the stigma and cost associated with mental health treatment.[35] Overall, minorities and Caucasians share the same prevalence rate of mental disorders; however, there are great disparities in the rate of mental health care for minorities as compared to the nonminority population.

How common are these disorders? Quite common, as the figures just mentioned suggest. In addition, the lives of millions of other people who work, live, and have relationships with people with mental illness also suffer the effect of these disorders. While there are over 300 different types of mental illness that can be diagnosed, we will cover three major categories of mental disorder: mood disorders, including depression and bipolar disorder; anxiety disorders, including panic disorder, obsessive-compulsive disorder, and posttraumatic stress disorder; and schizophrenia.[36] We will also briefly discuss attention deficit hyperactivity disorder. Over 450 million people worldwide are affected by mental disorders at any given time, and these numbers are expected to increase in the future.[37]

In the sections that follow, we will investigate selected disorders, identify professionals who are trained to treat these conditions, and take a look at the techniques they employ to help those who are afflicted.

Mood Disorders

Mood disorders, such as depression, seasonal affective disorder, and bipolar disorder, refer to psychological problems in which the primary symptom is a disturbance in mood.[36] You might perceive someone as moody, unable to predict if the person will be in a good or bad mood from one day to the next.

Depression According to the World Health Organization (WHO), more than 340 million people worldwide, including 209 million of the U.S. adult population, are estimated to suffer from **clinical depression.**[37] WHO further contends that this will only worsen in the future, predicting that depression will become the second leading cause of disability worldwide by the year 2020, after heart disease, unless strides are made in prevention and

---

Key Terms

clinical depression A psychological disorder in which individuals experience a lack of motivation, decreased energy level, fatigue, social withdrawal, sleep disturbance, disturbance in appetite, diminished sex drive, feelings of worthlessness, and despair.

Figure 2-2 Rates of Major Depression by Age Percentage of American adults reporting a major depressive disorder episode in the year 2004, by age group.

Source: NSDUH Report, "Depression Among Adults." Office of Applied Studies, Substance Abuse and Mental Health Services Administration (SAMHSA), November 18, 2005.

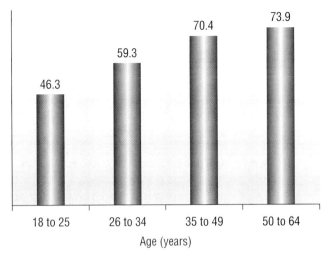

Figure 2-3 Rates of Treatment for Major Depression by Age Percentage of American adults reporting treatment for a major depressive episode in the year 2004, by age group.

Source: NSDUH Report, "Depression Among Adults." Office of Applied Studies, Substance Abuse and Mental Health Services Administration (SAMHSA), November 18, 2005.

treatment. We have already begun to see this trend, as the number of college students with depression has doubled over recent years.[38] About one in ten Americans suffers some form of depression, with women experiencing depression twice as often as men.[39] While depression can develop at any age, the average age of onset is the mid-20s. Figure 2-2 depicts the percentage of adult Americans who reported experiencing major depression in the past year, with the 35 to 49 age group and the 18 to 25 age group reporting the most, and the 65 and older group the least. However, Figure 2-3 shows that those who were 50 to 64 years old were the most likely to receive treatment for depression, and those who were 18 to 25 years old were the least likely.

Symptoms of Depression How can you tell the difference between having the blues and being clinically depressed? The symptoms of depression are as follows:

- Depressed mood most of the day, nearly every day
- Frequent crying
- Withdrawing, isolating yourself from others
- Lack of interest in activities that are typically enjoyable
- Increase or decrease in appetite resulting in significant weight loss or weight gain
- Insomnia, disturbed or restless sleep, or sleeping more than usual
- Feeling tired most of the time, regardless of how much sleep you have had
- Low self-esteem, feelings of hopelessness and worthlessness

- Difficulty concentrating, remembering things, and focusing on a task, and indecisiveness
- Frequent thoughts of suicide

Most people have experienced some of these symptoms at one point or another in their lives; however, clinically depressed individuals experience most of these symptoms every day and have felt this way for at least two weeks. Most people can find ways of pulling themselves out of feeling down, but for those suffering from clinical depression, the normal methods used to cope with the blues don't work. Clinical depression can range from mild to severe depression and can result in significant impairment in functioning, such as not being able to get out of bed to attend classes or go to work, or lacking the energy or motivation to take care of basic needs for food, hygiene, and rest. Some people tend to become irritable, negative, and uncommunicative, which can cause greater stress and conflict in their relationships. Depression has been described as constantly having a black cloud over your head, not being able to get out from underneath it no matter what you do. You might want to take the online self-assessment screening at www.mentalhealthscreening.org to assess your risk for clinical depression and to access more information on depression.

Causes of Depression There are several causes of or triggers for depression. Research suggests that if you have a family history of depression or any type of mood disorder, you are more prone to developing a depressive disorder. In fact, rates of depression for a child with a depressed parent are two to four times greater than for children without depressed parents.[40] While there is no single gene that causes depression, your genetic makeup can make you more vulnerable to depression. **Neurotransmitters** and hormone levels play a major role in the way your brain regulates your mood and emotions. Two neurotransmitters, serotonin and norepinephrine, are often found to be deficient in people with depression. (Chapter 7 includes a detailed discussion of neurotransmitters.)

However, biological processes are not the only explanation for depression. You may have a family history of depression and never develop depressive symptoms. Conversely, you may have no genetic predisposition and still become clinically depressed. Depression can be caused by many psychological factors, such as:

- Loss of a significant relationship
- Death of a family member or friend
- Physical or sexual abuse or assault
- Response to a serious illness or health problems
- Experiencing numerous setbacks and problems simultaneously

Key Terms

neurotransmitters Substances that transmit nerve signals; the chemical signals to activate or inhibit cell activity.

Having a support system, effective coping strategies, and a positive attributional style can make the difference between succumbing to depression or being protected during stressful and adverse times in our lives. Some people turn to the Internet to find increased social involvement and as a way to cope with depression. While it might seem that this would be a helpful way to build your support system and cope with depression, research shows that greater use of the Internet is associated with increasing depression, social isolation, and withdrawal. (See the box "A New Problem . . . Internet Addiction.")

Treatments for Depression There are many ways to treat depression, but the most effective treatment approach is a combination of counseling and medication (see the box "Taking the First Step in Fighting Depression"). Counseling can help people develop healthy coping skills, learn stress management strategies, focus on developing an optimistic explanatory style, and improve relationships and social skills. Medication, such as antidepressants, can be helpful in the treatment of depression because they act to increase the serotonin or norepinephrine levels to a normal and functional range. Antidepressants include fluoxetine (Prozac), paroxetine (Paxil), sertraline (Zoloft), mirtazapine (Remeron), venlafaxine (Effexor), escitalopram (Lexapro), citalopram (Celexa), and duloxetine (Cymbalta). It takes 4 to 6 weeks for an antidepressant to be fully effective, and there may be side effects such as dry mouth, decreased sexual drive, drowsiness, constipation, or diarrhea. Most of these side effects will disappear after 2 weeks of taking the medication. Interestingly, while the percentage of adults with depression taking antidepressants has increased from 37 percent to 75 percent, those receiving psychotherapy has declined from 71 percent to 60 percent.[41] Until 2003, the number of children and adolescents taking antidepressants had been skyrocketing. However, after the FDA issued warnings about the increased risk of suicide associated with this age group taking antidepressants, the trend reversed, decreasing by 20 percent.[42] Most people take an antidepressant for 6 months to a year and then are able to taper off the medication without a reoccurrence of symptoms. If you have had three separate episodes of depression, recovering from each episode and then relapsing, this can be a sign that your depression has a biological basis and an indication that you may need to continue taking an antidepressant medication long term.

Herbal supplements, such as St. John's Wort, have also been touted as a treatment for depression, although there is some debate as to how effective they truly are. Most clinicians agree that St. John's Wort can be somewhat effective in alleviating mild depression but not moderate or severe types of depression. As is the case with all herbal supplements, St. John's Wort is not subject to FDA approval, and it has not been put through the clinical trials that prescription medications have undergone to establish

The Internet has certainly changed the way we work, socialize, and educate ourselves. With a few key strokes, MySpace, Facebook, and blogging have opened up a new way of meeting and interacting with people. While the Internet has provided connections that otherwise could not be made very easily with people all around the world, it has also created unique psychological problems for some individuals. There is some question about the psychological implications the Internet may be having on our society as we are moving from a world in which we used to know our neighbors and interact with people face to face to developing serious and deep relationships with people from a distance. Marriages have broken up, affairs have taken place, and teenagers have been kidnapped by people they met over the Internet. In fact, one teenager was encouraged to overdose on drugs by his Internet friends and died while communicating over the net to this group.

There is a feeling of anonymity that is created by talking on the Web. You can be who you want to be, reveal as much or as little as you want, and not be judged by your appearance. Of course, this also means people can be deceitful and dishonest about who they are and what they want from you. In addition, there is a blending of home and work and increased solitude. Studies show that greater use of the Internet is associated with less communication among family members, decreased socializing with local friends, and increased depression and loneliness.* One study showed that using the Internet more than five hours a week resulted in less time with friends, family, and social activities.†

In fact, there is such concern about the potential adverse effects of spending too much time on the Internet that some mental health professionals propose adding "Internet addiction" as a diagnosable mental disorder. How can you tell if you are addicted? Here are some warning signs:

1. Preoccupation with the Internet—planning and thinking about the next time you can get online.
2. Increased use of the Internet over time.
3. Repeatedly making unsuccessful attempts to curtail your use of the Internet.
4. Feeling irritable, restless, and moody when you attempt to cut down your use of the Internet or are prevented from getting online when you would like.
5. Unaware of how much time you are spending on the Internet, staying online longer than you originally intended.
6. Lying to family members and friends about your use of the Internet.
7. Jeopardizing your job or risking losing a relationship because of the time you are spending on the Web.
8. Using the Internet as a way of escaping from problems and coping with depression.
9. Declining invitations to spend time with family and friends because you would rather be online.

Of course, answering "yes" to one of these statements does not indicate a concern. However, if you can answer "yes" to more than half of them, then you may want to examine your use of the Internet. Here are some ways you can avoid being an Internet addict:

- *Decide how much time you want to spend on the Internet before you get online* and set an alarm for that time. Stick to that time allotment.
- *Take frequent breaks.* Spend at least 5 minutes out of every hour or 15 to 20 minutes of every 3 hours on unwired activity. Take a walk, get up and eat a snack, or listen to music.
- *Visit the Net with a purpose and a strategy.* Surfing the Web aimlessly can lead to being online for longer than you anticipated.
- *Interact with people in a nonwired world.* Make a commitment to socially interact at least once a day with someone who is not online.
- *Don't let the Internet be the center of your existence* or the most important, enjoyable part of your day. Remind yourself of your life goals, values, and interests. What are other ways to achieve these goals besides via the Web?‡

*Kraut R, Patterson M, Lundmark V, Kiesler S, Mukopadyay T, Scherlis W. Internet paradox: A social technology that reduces social involvement and psychological well-being? *American Psychologist* 53(9), 1998;
†Streitfeld D. Study finds heavy Internet users are isolated. *Washington Post,* February 16, 2000;
‡Goldstein D Flory J. Best of the Net, *Online Guide Book Series.* New York: McGraw-Hill, Irwin Professional Publishing Inc., 1996.

therapeutic dose and efficacy. However, the National Institute of Mental Health, the National Center for Complementary and Alternative Medicine, and the Office of Dietary Supplements are currently conducting a $4 million collaborative four-year study to investigate the safety and the effectiveness of St. John's Wort, and so more definitive information will be available in the near future.

Exercise and activity level also play a significant role in alleviating and insulating people from depression. Again it seems that the endorphin levels and effects on brain chemistry and hormonal levels are part of the explanation for why this is a powerful antidote for depression.[43]

Electroconvulsive therapy (ECT) is another form of treatment for depression, with 100,000 Americans receiving this treatment each year. While ECT has fallen out of favor in recent years (owing in part to depictions of it in films such as *One Flew over the Cuckoo's Nest*), it has recently enjoyed a resurgence in popularity. This is due to improved technology. The procedure involves delivering a 90-volt burst of electricity, equal to the electricity in a 40-watt light bulb, for about a minute to the brain, causing a grand mal seizure. The patient is under anesthesia and receives muscle relaxants before receiving the shock, and heart rate and oxygen level are constantly monitored during the treatment. Most patients receive

Brightening Your Mood: Treating SAD with Light Therapy

Symptoms of seasonal affective disorder (SAD) often begin around October and subside in March or April, reflecting the hours of daylight in these months. With darker, colder, gloomier days, people find their moods become very similar—darker, distant, and gloomier. One form of treatment that has been increasing in popularity is light therapy.

With light therapy, you sit with your eyes open in front of a light box for anywhere from 15 minutes to 2 hours at a time, daily. It won't work to just turn on more lights around your house, as the amount of light required is between 2,500 and 10,000 lux (a bright sunny day may register 100,000 lux). The average household light intensity tends to be less than 400 lux. While exposing your eyes to the light, you can do other things, such as exercise or talk on the phone; however, you do need to have the light box positioned *above* your eyes, so that the light hits the bottom of your retina. This makes sense because this is the angle at which daytime sunlight usually enters the eyes. Light therapy is supported to mimic outdoor light, which in turn

decreases the amount of melatonin in your brain. Based on the idea that people with SAD are producing too much melatonin, the reduction of melatonin alleviates depressive symptoms. Light therapy was first used to treat SAD in the early 1980s and has become increasingly popular since then.

Light therapy boxes can be purchased over the counter without a prescription and range in price from $160 and up.

Some research has found that light therapy was more effective than taking an antidepressant in the treatment of seasonal affective disorder. However, more research needs to be done. Light therapy hasn't been approved by the FDA because there have not been enough clinical trials to provide evidence of its effectiveness.

Source: Mayo Foundation for Medical Education and Research (MFMER). Seasonal affective disorder: Treatment with light therapy, www.mayoclinic .com/health/seasonal-affective-disorder/MH00023, October 4, 2006.

---

3 ECT treatments each week, for a total of 6 to 12 sessions. Proponents of ECT claim that it is an effective treatment for depression when no other antidepressant or treatment regime has worked. Critics of ECT say that it causes brain damage and memory loss and that the decrease in depressive symptoms is only temporary.[44] Although ECT has been used for more than 60 years, no one knows exactly how it works or why it alleviates depression.

 TALKING POINTS Have you ever felt depressed? If so, what did you do to cope with these feelings? What did you do that worked and/or didn't help you to feel better?

Seasonal Affective Disorder In addition to the types of depression just described, some people may be especially vulnerable to depression on a seasonal basis. **Seasonal affective disorder (SAD)** is a form of depression that develops in relation to the changes in the seasons. While most people with SAD begin to feel increasingly depressed in October and report their depression lifts in March or April, about one in six SAD sufferers experience Summer SAD, beginning in May or June and ending in the fall months. Twice as many women as men are affected with SAD.[45]

SAD seems to be related to environmental factors such as amount of light, temperature, and situational stressors. Weight gain, fatigue, increased sleep, diminished sex drive, and mood swings are some of the symptoms of Winter SAD; agitation, loss of appetite, insomnia, and increased suicidal thoughts are characteristic of Summer SAD. Seasonal depression in the winter seems

linked to increases in the production of melatonin, a chemical that helps set the brain's daily rhythm, set off by the decrease in light. Antidepressants, counseling, and light therapy have been used to treat SAD (see the box "Brightening Your Mood"). Light therapy for Winter SAD involves sitting in front of a white fluorescent bulb, housed in a plastic diffusing screen, for 20 to 90 minutes each day so that the light is falling on the eyes.[45] For Summer SAD, which tends to occur in hotter locales, individuals are instructed to travel to cooler climates, to swim in cool water, and to stay in darkened, air-conditioned rooms.

Postpartum Depression Another unique form of depression is **postpartum depression,** a more severe kind of depression than is the commonly experienced "baby blues" that many women feel following childbirth. Postpartum depression occurs in one out of eight mothers who give birth and can last from a few days to over a year, but most commonly lasts for two weeks. Postpartum depression is characterized by fatigue, frequent crying, emotional withdrawal, anxiety, and other symptoms associated with depression. This should be differentiated from postpartum psychosis, which is marked by hallucinations and delusions. Sometimes people with postpartum depression have been associated with psychotic behavior, as was the situation with the much publicized case of Andrea Yates who in 2002 drowned her five children, ages 6 months to 7 years. Reportedly, Yates suffered from postpartum depression after the birth of her fourth child, and with the birth of her fifth child along with the death of her own father, became increasingly depressed and psychotic.

Do . . .

1. If possible, stay with the person until you can get further assistance.
2. Offer support and assistance. Tell them they are not alone.
3. Remain calm and talk about the person's feelings of sadness and helplessness.
4. Encourage problem solving and taking positive steps.
5. Emphasize the temporary nature of the problem. Suicide is a permanent solution to a temporary problem.
6. Seek help and don't try to handle this problem on your own. This might involve the person's family, religious advisor, friends, and teachers, or calling a mental health agency for consultation.

7. Ask the person to promise not to hurt or kill him or herself.

Don't . . .

1. Avoid talking about suicide or dancing around the topic. Talking about suicide doesn't upset people more. In fact, often people who are thinking about killing themselves say it is a relief to talk about it and it helps them to let go of this idea, not pursue it further.
2. Be judgmental or argumentative. Now is not the time to debate the morality of suicide—you will lose the debate and possibly the person.
3. Assume that the person is not serious. Saying "You're not serious" or "You don't mean that" may inadvertently encourage the person to show you how serious she or he truly is.
4. Argue that things aren't that bad or that other people have it worse and the person should be happy about his or her life. This approach can make people feel worse about themselves and guilty about their feelings of unhappiness.
5. Don't promise not to tell anyone. If you keep this promise and something happens to this person, how will you feel?

Suicide Suicide is the third leading cause of death for young adults 15 to 24 years old. It is the 11th leading cause of all deaths in the United States, but the second leading cause of death for college students. Men commit suicide four times more often than women do, and 72 percent of all suicides are committed by white men. Suicide occurs most often among Americans age 65 and older.[46] However, women are three times more likely than men to attempt suicide. Men tend to employ more violent methods such as firearms, hanging, or jumping from high places, whereas women tend to use methods such as overdosing with pills or cutting their wrists, which are slower methods and allow more time for medical intervention. An equal percentage of Caucasians and African Americans complete suicide. Asian Americans are one of the lowest-risk groups in terms of ethnicity. The suicide rate for the Hispanic American population is lower than for Caucasians and African Americans.

Why do people attempt or commit suicide? The majority of suicidal people have depressive disorders and feel helpless and powerless over their lives. They say things like "I just want the pain to stop" and don't see any other options available to them. There are some risk factors associated with suicidal behavior, such as:

- Little to no support system
- Previous suicide attempts
- Family history of mental illness, including substance abuse
- Family history of suicide
- Problems with drugs or alcohol
- Possession of a firearm

- Exposure to the suicidal behavior of others, including through the media

It is estimated that 300,000 suicide attempts occur each year in the United States, or one every 2 minutes. Eleven hundred of these suicides occur on college campuses. Some people say that suicidal gestures or threats are a "cry for attention" or a "cry for help" and think it is better to ignore the person. But left ignored, the person may go ahead and take the next step to attempt suicide because no one seems to care. It is always best to take any threats or talk about suicide seriously and act accordingly. What should you do if a friend or family member talks to you about thoughts of suicide? See the box "The Dos and Don'ts of Suicide Intervention" for suggestions.

Bipolar Disorder Another important mood disorder is **bipolar disorder,** a condition that was previously known as manic depression. The term *bipolar* refers to

---

Key Terms

seasonal affective disorder (SAD) A type of depression that develops in relation to the changes in the seasons.

postpartum depression A form of depression that affects women in the weeks and months following childbirth.

bipolar disorder A mood disorder characterized by alternating episodes of depression and mania.

the extreme mood swings individuals with this disorder experience, from feeling euphoric, energetic, and reckless to feeling depressed, powerless, and listless. An estimated 5.7 million American adults, or 2.6 percent, suffer from bipolar disorder, with men and women equally likely to develop this condition.[36] It is the least common of the mood disorders. The average age of onset for the first manic episode typically occurs in the early to mid-20s. This change in mood or "mood swing" can last for hours, days, weeks, or months. Bipolar disorder is found across all ages, races, ethnic groups, and social classes. When one parent has bipolar disorder, the risk to each child is estimated to be 15 to 30 percent; when both parents have bipolar disorder, the risk increases to 50 to 75 percent.[47] A recent study contended that a flawed gene appears to promote bipolar disorder. Further research is needed to examine this particular variant of the gene to better identify people at risk and develop more effective medications to treat this disorder.

We have already described depression in the previous section. Bipolar disorder involves having both depressive periods and manic episodes. Mania is characterized by:

- Excessive energy, needing little sleep, being highly excitable
- Racing thoughts, feeling as though your mind is going 50 mph
- Rapid speech, changing from topic to topic quickly in conversation
- Easily irritated and distracted
- Impulsive and reckless in behavior: for example, spending sprees, increased involvement in sexual activity, and drug and alcohol use
- Trying to do too much, feeling as though you can accomplish a great deal

Many people with bipolar disorder will tell you that they enjoy the "highs" but dread the lows. However, manic behavior can become very destructive because when people are in a manic phase, they can create enormous credit card debt, abuse drugs and alcohol, drive recklessly, and often feel invincible. They stay up all night and feel very little need for rest or food, and eventually their bodies can't function and they collapse. Mood stabilizers such as lithium carbonate (Lithobid) and anticonvulsant medications, such as valproic acid (Depakote), gabapentin (Neurontin), topiramate (Topomax), and lamotrigine (Lamictal), along with psychotherapy, have been used to treat bipolar disorder.

Anxiety Disorders

Bill, a very talented and bright 26-year-old, has a promising career as an executive in a large accounting firm. However, he is in jeopardy of losing his job because of his

Anxiety is one of the three most frequent problems students report experiencing during college.

absenteeism and tardiness. It can take him hours to get to work even though he lives 15 minutes away, and sometimes he doesn't go to work even though he is in the car and ready to go. Bill has a routine in the morning that involves checking the windows, doors, iron, stove, and garage door five times to ensure that things are secure and safe. Sometimes he drives away and then returns to the house to check again. He feels a need to turn the handles on doors five times, and if he loses track, he starts all over again.

Susan has been having such severe panic attacks in the car while driving to work that she has needed to pull over. Her heart races, her breathing is labored, and she sometimes feels as though she is having a heart attack and might die. She is frightened of being in the car alone and having an attack and not being able to get help or having a car accident. She is beginning to be afraid to leave her house and feels safer at home. She has declined invitations to go out with her friends and on vacations and goes out only when absolutely necessary. She feels as though she is losing control of her life.

John worries constantly about what other people think of him. When he passes a group of people who are laughing, he assumes that they are laughing at him. He has trouble having conversations with people because he believes whatever he says will sound "stupid" and people will not like him. He also plays conversations over and over in his head when he is trying to go to sleep, thinking about what he should have said and worrying about how people are judging him.

Bill, Susan, and John are all suffering from *anxiety disorders*. While everyone tends to feel nervous or worry about something at some point in their lives, people with anxiety disorders feel anxious most, if not all, of the time. They also feel powerless to alleviate their anxiety, and tend to worry about becoming anxious, so their anxiety causes them even greater anxiety. Anxiety is related to fear and is part of daily life. Some anxiety can even be helpful and motivating at times. Anxiety is a physiological, adaptive response to danger or potential threat and can enhance performance and keep us out of harm's way. In Chapter 3 we discuss the fight or flight response and how the stress response is related to anxiety. Anxiety disorders are differentiated from daily stress as being:

1. Intense, often debilitating, experiences during which people sometimes think they are going to die
2. Long lasting, persisting after the danger or stressful event has passed
3. Dysfunctional, causing significant interference in daily functioning

Anxiety disorders include generalized anxiety disorder, obsessive-compulsive disorder (such as Bill's problem), posttraumatic stress disorder, panic disorder (which describes Susan's symptoms), and phobias such as the social phobia John suffers from in his incessant worrying about what other people think about him. Approximately 40 million Americans, or 18 percent, have an anxiety disorder, and women are twice as likely as men to suffer from panic disorder, posttraumatic stress disorder, generalized anxiety disorder, agoraphobia, and specific phobias.[36] There are no gender differences with obsessive-compulsive disorder or social phobia.[47]

Generalized Anxiety Disorder (GAD)
Generalized anxiety disorder (GAD) involves experiencing anxiety for at least six months in which the intensity and frequency of the worry is excessive and out of proportion to the situation. GAD can be distinguished from specific phobias in which people feel worried about a particular situation or stimulus. An individual with GAD appears to worry all the time about everything, thinks the worst, and overreacts to situations. Restlessness, fatigue, irritability, difficulty concentrating, muscle tension, and trouble sleeping are some of the symptoms associated with GAD. Physical symptoms include excessive sweating, nausea, diarrhea, being easily startled, shortness of breath, racing heart, and feeling shaky.[36] Because people with GAD are tense and anxious much of the time, they experience impairment in their relationships, work performance, and general functioning. Most people with GAD say that they are afraid of losing control, of failing, of rejection or abandonment, and death or disease. In addition, they feel unable to cope with their fears and thus out of control in managing their anxiety.

Panic Disorder
Shortness of breath, pounding heart, dizziness, trembling, sweating, nausea, tingling in hands and feet, hot and cold flashes, chest pain, and a feeling of choking are the symptoms of **panic disorder,** exemplified by Susan's situation. Many panic disorder sufferers feel as though they are going to die, are losing control, or are going crazy, which of course makes them feel more anxious and panicked. Frequently, these individuals go to the emergency room thinking they are having a heart attack. This can seemingly occur out of the blue or because of some trigger, and can last for a few minutes or for hours. Because people become fearful of having a panic attack and don't know when the next attack might occur, they may develop **agoraphobia.** Agoraphobia is a fear of being in embarrassing situations or places in which you can't escape or get help if you need it.[48]

Panic disorder can be treated with antidepressant medications such as imipramine (Tofranil) and tranquilizers such as alprazolam (Xanax). Counseling can help individuals learn to recognize when a panic attack may be starting and to minimize and ward it off before it becomes a full-blown attack, using relaxation and stress-management exercises, as well as positive self statements such as "I'm not going to die. I can get through this."

Obsessive-Compulsive Disorder (OCD)
Obsessive-compulsive disorder, or OCD, affects 3 million Americans and symptoms often begin during childhood or adolescence.[36] OCD involves more than just being neat and orderly: symptoms include having recurring thoughts

---

Key Terms

mania An extremely excitable state characterized by excessive energy, racing thoughts, impulsive and/or reckless behavior, irritability, and being prone to distraction.

generalized anxiety disorder (GAD) An anxiety disorder that involves experiencing intense and non-specific anxiety for at least six months, in which the intensity and frequency of worry is excessive and out of proportion to the situation.

panic disorder An anxiety disorder characterized by panic attacks, in which individuals experience severe physical symptoms. These episodes can seemingly occur "out of the blue" or because of some trigger and can last for a few minutes or for hours.

agoraphobia A fear of being in embarrassing situations from which there is no escape or in which help would be unavailable should an emergency arise; often associated with panic disorder.

obsessive-compulsive disorder An anxiety disorder characterized by obsessions (intrusive thoughts, images, or impulses causing a great deal of distress) and compulsions (repetitive behaviors aimed at reducing anxiety or stress that is associated with the obsessive thoughts).

and behaviors that seem irrational and out of control, and which can be extremely time consuming. Obsessions are intrusive thoughts, images, or impulses causing a great deal of distress. Most people recognize that their obsessions are ungrounded and senseless but can't seem to push them out of their minds. Twenty-five percent of people with OCD have only obsessive thoughts without exhibiting any compulsive behavior.[48] Compulsions are repetitive behaviors aimed at reducing the anxiety and stress that are associated with the obsessive thoughts, such as checking that the iron is off or washing your hands a certain number of times. Some compulsions seem relevant to a particular fear (such as handwashing out of a fear of germs), but others might seem unrelated—for example, having to do something an odd number of times so that your parents will not come to any harm. The most common compulsions are washing, checking, and counting.[36]

Even though the goal of compulsive behavior is to alleviate distress brought about by obsessions, it is in itself a source of shame and anxiety. Individuals with OCD, like Bill in the earlier example, realize that their behavior is excessive and unreasonable but are unable to resist engaging in this behavior. This can cause great distress in their relationships, problems completing their work, and getting to places on time. In addition, once they have performed the compulsive behavior, their anxiety is only temporarily alleviated; the obsessive thoughts return and the cycle continues.

Treatment for OCD can include antidepressant medication such as fluoxetine (Prozac) and also counseling. Counseling might involve response prevention strategies such as exposing the individual to the situations that trigger the obsessive thoughts and then preventing the person from engaging in the compulsive behaviors to break this vicious cycle. For example, the individual might be exposed to a dirty environment and then allowed to wash his or her hands only once.

Phobias   John is suffering from one of the most common anxiety disorders, **social phobia,** previously called social anxiety disorder.[48] Social phobia involves feelings of extreme dread and embarrassment in situations in which public speaking or social interaction is involved, because the person worries she or he will be seen as stupid, clumsy, or lacking in some way. Social phobia is the third most common mental health problem in the United States, affecting 5.3 million each year. Twice as many women as men are afflicted, and the disorder typically begins in childhood or early adolescence and rarely develops after age 25. It is sometimes confused with shyness and is misdiagnosed much of the time. The most common social phobia is fear of public speaking. Commonly called stage fright, it is the most common of all phobias; many successful actors and performers suffer from this disorder, including actor Donny Osmond, gold

medalist swimmer Susie O'Neill, and actresses Kim Basinger and Barbra Streisand.

Social phobia differs from another disorder called **specific phobia** in which the person has a strong fear of and avoids one particular situation or object such as snakes, high places, or airplanes. Specific phobias affect 10 percent of the population and often begin as childhood fears that were never outgrown.[48] They are twice as common in women as in men. Sometimes a phobic reaction develops as a result of a traumatic event such as an accident or a particularly difficult visit to the doctor or dentist, or from an illness. Specific phobias tend to be easily treated with counseling in which the individual learns relaxation techniques and then is gradually exposed, first in imagery, then in real-life situations, to the feared situation.

Posttraumatic Stress Disorder (PTSD)   The essential feature of **posttraumatic stress disorder** is the development of symptoms following exposure to an extreme stressor involving threat of death or serious injury. This threat may be directly experienced or be the result of witnessing an event that is life threatening and dangerous.[36] This disorder was first identified during World War I when soldiers were observed to be suffering from anxiety, flashbacks, and nightmares. Posttraumatic stress can be the result of not only combat but any trauma that produces intense fear, horror, and feelings of helplessness, such as sexual assault, natural disasters like earth-quakes or tornados, a car accident, a life-threatening illness, or a mugging. The symptoms associated with PTSD are:

- Recurrent and distressing thoughts about the event
- Nightmares about the event
- Flashbacks—feeling as though one is reliving the event
- Emotional numbness, feeling detached from oneself and one's feelings
- Avoidance of anything that reminds one of the event
- Detachment from others
- Difficulty expressing one's feelings
- Sleep disturbance
- Irritability, angry outbursts
- Being easily startled
- Difficulty concentrating
- Hypervigilence—extreme awareness of one's environment

People with PTSD tend to be highly anxious and depressed, to have problems with their relationships, and to have difficulty trusting people, and they may restrict their activities because of their fearfulness. It is also not uncommon to experience panic attacks when exposed to something that triggers a memory of the trauma. Again, counseling to express and resolve the feelings, losses, and negative thoughts associated with the trauma, as well as antidepressant medications or tranquilizers, may be beneficial in treating PTSD.

Attention Deficit Hyperactivity Disorder (ADHD)

Once thought to be only a childhood disorder, **attention deficit hyperactivity disorder (ADHD)** is now being diagnosed in record numbers in adults. This increase might be the result of overlooking or misdiagnosing problems in childhood that later are accurately diagnosed in adults (see the box "Television Advertisements for Psychological Medications"). With symptoms that include being fidgety, disorganized, overactive, and easily distracted, a child may be seen as simply misbehaving rather than having a diagnosable disorder. It is often the child with ADHD who is seen as "disruptive" in the classroom and "lazy, stupid, a daydreamer" by friends and family. Actually, the truth about these individuals is often the opposite: they tend to be highly intelligent, motivated, creative, and energetic individuals.

It is currently estimated that over 15 million Americans suffer from this disorder, affecting males more than females, 3:1. There is strong evidence to support a genetic cause for ADHD, although environmental factors can certainly help or hinder the problem. One of the landmark studies in ADHD was conducted on adults and showed that there is a difference at the cellular level in energy consumption, between the parts of the brain that regulate attention, emotion, and impulse control in people with ADHD as compared to those without.[49]

Following are the symptoms often seen in adult ADHD:

- A sense of underachievement, not meeting one's goals
- Difficulty getting organized
- Chronic procrastination or trouble getting started
- Trouble with follow-through and completing tasks
- Having many tasks going on simultaneously, switching from one to another
- Easily bored and frequently searching for high stimulation
- Easily distracted, trouble focusing and sustaining attention
- Creative, intuitive, highly intelligent
- Impulsive, doesn't stop to think things through
- Impatient, low tolerance for frustration
- Tendency to worry needlessly and endlessly
- Insecure
- Moody

- Restless
- Tendency toward addictive behavior
- Low self-esteem
- Inaccurate self-concept, unaware of effect on others
- Childhood history of ADHD or presence of symptoms since childhood

Psychological tests such as the Test of Variability of Attention (TOVA) and an IQ test can help substantiate a diagnosis of ADHD. The TOVA tests the subject by flashing different shapes on a screen quantifying attention, distractibility, and impulsivity based on the subject's responses. The most effective treatment for ADHD involves a multimodal approach: counseling and coaching the individual to provide strategies, techniques, and structure for daily life; education; tools such as daily planners and organizers; goal setting and time management; and medication such as methylphenidate (Concerta, Ritalin), amphetamine-dextroamphetamine (Adderall), and atomoxetine (Strattera). (These medications are discussed in more detail in Chapter 7.)

Schizophrenia

Schizophrenia is one of the most severe mental disorders; it is characterized by profound distortions in one's

---

Key Terms

social phobia A phobia characterized by feelings of extreme dread and embarrassment in situations in which public speaking or social interaction is involved.

specific phobia An excessive and unreasonable fear about a particular situation or object that causes anxiety and distress and interferes with a person's functioning.

posttraumatic stress disorder An anxiety disorder that sometimes develops following exposure to an extreme stressor involving threat of death or serious injury. Symptoms include recurrent and distressing thoughts or nightmares about the event, emotional numbness, feelings of detachment, sleep disturbance, hypervigilance, and irritability.

attention deficit hyperactivity disorder (ADHD) An above-normal rate of physical movement; often accompanied by an inability to concentrate on a specified task. Also called *hyperactivity*.

schizophrenia One of the most severe mental disorders, characterized by profound distortions in one's thought processes, emotions, perceptions, and behavior. Symptoms may include hallucinations, delusions, disorganized thinking, and/or maintaining a rigid posture and not moving for hours.

Television Advertisements for Psychological Medications: Informative or Misleading?

"Trouble sleeping? Difficulty concentrating? Crying most of the time? You might want to talk to your physician about taking Paxil." We are barraged by these types of media message on a daily basis. In fact, a recent study showed that drug advertising increased from $800 million in 1996 to $9 billion in 2005, Does it work? Physicians report that an increasing number of patients are making appointments because of something they saw on television, and 70 percent of physicians write prescriptions for the specific medication the patient requests.

On the positive side, drug advertisements may assist in treating problems more quickly: people may feel less embarrassed, be more hopeful, and recognize problems sooner than they otherwise might have done. Research published in *Prevention Magazine* cited favorable responses to drug advertising on TV. It found that 84 percent of people felt better informed of new treatments. Seventy-eight percent said that the ads helped them to be more involved in their medical care, 34 percent reported talking to their physician about a drug they saw on TV, finding and 79 percent remembered hearing about risks and side effects. However, only 49 percent of these people said they paid attention to side effects, with the majority of people believing that they would not experience them. Understanding all the side effects and risks when they are rattled off at breakneck speed or displayed in the smallest print possible at the bottom of the TV screen can be difficult. Of course, some people may be scared off by the side effects and risks and, as a result, won't even talk to their doctors about their concerns.

Sometimes it is difficult to know from watching TV advertisements what condition or problem a drug is designed to treat. And some physicians may disagree with an advertisement's promises or suggest a different drug. The drugs typically being advertised are the newest ones on the market and so are often more expensive and haven't been used for very long. Some physicians are hesitant to prescribe these medications until more evidence exists to show that they work better than the older medications do. There is also a concern that there hasn't been enough time to reveal all the potential side effects or the long-term effects of these drugs. Often it is only after people have been taking them for some time that certain side effects become apparent, such as those associated with the antidepressant Serzone (nefazodone), which has recently been linked to an increased risk of liver failure, jaundice, and hepatitis.

Sometimes the advertisements make misleading or even fraudulent claims. For example, the Food and Drug Administration (FDA) recently sent a letter to GlaxoSmithKline requesting them to stop using a TV ad for Paxil. The letter stated that the ad was "false or misleading" because it suggested that the drug could be used by a broader range of patients than it was actually approved for and implied that it was safer than actually demonstrated. Pfizer Inc. was charged with illegal promotion of Neurontin, advertising it for use other than the one that the FDA approved. Also, the numbers of suicides and suicide attempts have increased with respect to individuals taking the drug. The FDA wanted the company to add suicide risk to its labeling, and Pfizer refused to do so, saying it remains "confident of the safety and effectiveness of this product."

A compromise might be to allow these ads to continue to air on television with more regulation. The FDA has announced a new proposal regarding consumer advertising and the health industry. The proposal would require ads for prescription drugs to contain language that consumers can better understand, to have possible adverse reactions displayed in larger type, and to include all warnings, contraindications, and major precautions.

Some strategies for being an informed consumer are to ask your doctor about:

- Side effects
- Length of time the medication has been on the market
- Realistic expectations regarding the medication's benefits and results
- Effectiveness compared to other similar medications
- Cost of the medication
- Interaction effects with other medications

Sources: "FDA Races to Keep Up with Drug Ads That Go Too Far" *USA Today*, May 30, 2005; "Plugged Into Prescription Drugs," *USA Today*, February 15, 2005; "Prescription Drugs and the Cost of Advertising," www.therubins.com, Allan Rubin, February 27, 2005; "Drug Advertising Skyrockets," CBS News, February 14, 2002; "Group Urges Ban of Antidepressant Serzone," www.intelihealth.com, March 6, 2003.

thought processes, emotions, perceptions, and behavior. People with schizophrenia experience hallucinations (seeing things that are not there, hearing voices), delusions (believing that they are Jesus, the CIA is after them, or radio waves are controlling their mind), and disorganized thinking (wearing multiple coats, scarves, and gloves on a warm day, shouting and swearing at passersby, maintaining a rigid posture and not moving for hours). The movie *A Beautiful Mind* gives a glimpse into the life of one schizophrenic, John Nash, and how he managed his symptoms.

There are several types of schizophrenia: paranoid, disorganized, catatonic, and undifferentiated. This disabling illness affects 1 percent of the U.S. population, and symptoms typically surface in people in their late teens and early 20s. Men and women are equally likely to develop schizophrenia, and it seems to run in families. Schizophrenia is often confused with dissociative identity disorder (formerly called "multiple personality disorder"), which is an entirely separate and distinct mental illness. People with dissociative identity disorder display two or more distinct identities or personalities that take control of the person's life; people with schizophrenia do not have multiple, separate, enduring personalities.

There are many theories to explain what causes schizophrenia. Some research suggests that heredity accounts for about 80 percent of the cause of schizophrenia and the other 20 percent is due to environmental stressors or situations. Researchers have also identified a number of abnormalities in the brains of diagnosed schizophrenics, including smaller temporal lobes, enlargement of the ventricles, and cerebral atrophy in the frontal lobes. Research is also being done on how the variations in chromosome-22 genes may be linked to schizophrenia. Individuals with schizophrenia also seem to have nearly double the number of dopamine receptors in their brains, leading to the theory that too much dopamine is being released into the brain pathways and causing schizophrenia symptoms. The antipsychotic medications act to block the receptors and prevent the transmission of dopamine, reducing the amount of dopamine in the system that is creating this chemical imbalance.[2]

Although there is no cure for schizophrenia, certain antipsychotic medications, such as quetiapine (Seroquel), risperidone (Risperdal), olanzapine (Zyprexa), aripiprazole (Abilify), and ziprasidone (Geodon), can effectively treat this illness and enable people to live functional, satisfying lives. Psychotherapy can be helpful in developing problem-solving approaches, in addition to identifying stressors and triggers, and early detection of a psychotic episode. Unfortunately, some people with schizophrenia are unable to recognize that they are delusional or irrational, and so do not get treatment or take their medications on a regular basis.

Health Providers Involved in the Treatment of Psychological Disorders

As in other areas of health care, a variety of practitioners, each of whom has unique training and uses specific therapies, treat and manage the mental health conditions just described.

Psychiatrists

A **psychiatrist** is a health care provider with a medical degree who has specialized in the field of psychiatry. Because psychiatrists are medical doctors, they may prescribe drugs and perform medical procedures such as electroshock therapy. Psychiatrists tend to treat psychological disorders through medical management and take a biological approach to addressing psychological disorders. They tend to give less focus to talking about one's problems and treat more severely and chronically ill patients.

Prescription medications are a common form of treatment for psychological disorders and may be used in combination with other therapies.

Psychologists

A **psychologist** is a mental health care provider whose educational background includes a doctoral-level degree in the field of counseling or clinical psychology. Psychologists practice general psychology, and their clients range from those with severe pathology to those with more temporary problems of living. There is a variety of subspecialties such as children and adolescents, neurological disorders and assessments, psychological evaluations and assessments, forensic psychology, industrial psychology, health psychology, career counseling, and marriage counseling. Until recently, one difference between psychiatrists and psychologists was that psychologists did not have prescription privileges and so couldn't use drug therapies in their treatment interventions. However, the lines are beginning to blur, as there has been a push in many states for legislation that would allow psychologists to prescribe psychiatric medicines; such legislation exists in New Mexico already. In general, psychologists treat psychological disorders using behavior therapy, problem-solving approaches, and talk therapy that focuses on changing the client's attitudes, behavior, affect, and cognitions. A psychologist must be licensed in the state in which he or she practices, and this typically requires passing a national certification examination and having

> ## Key Terms
>
> **psychiatrist** A medical doctor with specialized training in the diagnosis and treatment of psychological disorders through the use of biological and medical interventions.
>
> **psychologist** A doctoral-level practitioner with specialized training in the diagnosis and treatment of psychological disorders through the use of psychotherapy.

a specific number of hours practicing psychology under the supervision of a licensed psychologist.

Counselors

Counselors typically have a master's degree in counseling or clinical psychology. Individuals with master's degrees usually work in group counseling practices, clinics, and schools and may specialize in areas such as substance abuse, divorce recovery, vocational rehabilitation, school counseling, marriage and family therapy, sexual assault, domestic violence, and employee assistance programs. Master's-level counselors can be licensed as professional mental health counselors in all U.S. states except Nevada.

Social Workers

Social workers have a master's degree in social work and must be licensed to use the title *social worker*. Whereas psychologists, mental health counselors, and psychiatrists tend to focus on the individual's problems, social workers look at the bigger picture and take into consideration the environment, community, and system the individual is living in. Social workers provide both mental health and social services to the community and are the largest group of professionals to provide psychological services.

Social workers typically consult and counsel clients and arrange for services that can help them. Often, they refer clients to specialists in services such as debt counseling, childcare or eldercare, public assistance, or alcohol or drug rehabilitation. Social workers then follow through with the client to ensure that services are helpful and that clients make proper use of the services offered. Social workers may review eligibility requirements, visit clients on a regular basis, and provide support during crises.[50]

Approaches in Treating Psychological Disorders

There are over 200 approaches to treating psychological disorders and new variations and models are continuing to develop. Most approaches have their foundations based on a few basic therapeutic models, which we will look at in the section that follows. These therapies can be utilized with individuals, families, or couples.

Dynamic Therapy

Dynamic therapy is based on the belief that effective treatment must focus on the psychological forces underlying the individual's problems. These forces begin in early childhood and have great significance on later behavior and personality development. Because this type of therapy focuses on the person's childhood years to uncover the source of the current problem, it usually is a long-term, intensive, and expensive form of therapy that many insurance companies refuse to cover.

Humanistic Therapy

Humanistic treatment approaches are based on the belief that people, left to their own devices, will naturally grow in positive and constructive ways. The job of the therapist is to help clients unearth their natural potential and gain greater self-awareness and self-acceptance. Humanistic therapy has its roots in Carl Rogers's "client-centered therapy" and in Abraham Maslow's hierarchy of needs. In client-centered therapy, the client, not the therapist, is responsible for behavior change. The task of the therapist is to facilitate in a nondirective manner the process of helping individuals resolve their problems.[7] Rogers further believed that when people accept themselves, they will also accept other people.

Behavior Therapy

Behavior therapy focuses not on one's thoughts or feelings but on behavior modification. Thus the goal of treatment is not to uncover the reasons underlying the problems an individual is having but to eliminate the symptoms and change behavior. Insight, awareness, and past history are unimportant in behavior therapy. The idea is that behavior has been learned and so can be unlearned, and different, more adaptive behavior can be taught. This can be especially effective for the treatment of phobias, panic disorder, and anxiety.

Cognitive-Behavioral Therapy

Cognitive-behavioral therapy focuses on changing an individual's thoughts or cognitive patterns in order to change his or her behavior and emotional state. Pioneered by psychologists Aaron Beck and Albert Ellis in the 1960s, cognitive therapy assumes that maladaptive behaviors and disturbed mood or emotions are the result of inappropriate or irrational thinking patterns. As with behavior therapy, cognitive-behavioral therapy does not explore why someone is thinking or behaving in a particular way, nor does it look at the client's past history. Instead, cognitive therapists attempt to make the client aware of distorted thought patterns and change them through strategies such as cognitive restructuring, cognitive reframing, challenging irrational beliefs, and thought stopping. This type of treatment has been especially effective in treating obsessive-compulsive disorder, eating disorders, anxiety disorders, and mood disorders.

The learned optimism paradigm discussed earlier in this chapter was also based on cognitive-behavioral concepts.

Solution-Focused Therapy

Solution-focused therapy is a goal-oriented therapeutic approach that helps clients change by looking for solutions rather than dwelling on problems. Similar to cognitive-behavioral therapy, attention is directed to the present and the future, rather than to the past. Solution-focused therapists focus on the strength and resources within the individual. Clients are encouraged to envision a future in which their problems are no longer a dominant force in their lives, and in partnership with the therapist, treatment interventions are formulated in an effort to reach that goal.

Couples and Family Therapy

Couples counseling and family therapy includes premarital counseling, marital therapy, conflict mediation, and divorce counseling. Communication skills, assertiveness skills, sexual disorders, intimacy and commitment, anger management, step-parenting, and blended families are some of the psychological issues that are typically addressed by these therapies.

Group Therapy

Group therapy usually comprises five to eight people who meet regularly with a therapist to focus on the psychological problems with which they are struggling. Often the group members share common problems such as eating disorders, childhood sexual abuse, substance abuse, or divorce recovery, and so they can support one another and understand one another's experiences. The group members can help and learn from one another and don't feel so alone in their problems. Group therapy is very beneficial in breaking your sense of isolation and challenging the belief that you are the only one having this type of problem. The idea behind group therapy is that you can learn new ways of behaving and practice these skills and behaviors in a safe, supportive atmosphere. In fact, the research strongly suggests that group therapy can be superior to individual therapy or at least a necessary next step for particular psychological problems, such as sexual abuse, eating disorders, substance abuse, and interpersonal relationship problems.

 TALKING POINTS How do you think change occurs in people or yourself? What form of treatment might work best for you?

Psychological Health: A Final Thought

As you can see, psychological health involves how your emotions, thoughts, and behavior interplay with one another and with the world around you. There is an important mind-body connection in terms of your psychological health having a significant effect on your physical health and vice versa. Psychological health is not just the absence of mental illness, and there is a range or continuum of psychological health. Possessing a positive self-concept, developing high self-esteem, and cultivating an optimistic attitude toward life can promote psychological health and enhance relationships with others. While heredity plays a role in the development of personality and psychological health, environmental factors and stressors seem to have an equally important role. As people age and encounter developmental milestones, they also encounter new challenges, obstacles, and resources in continuing to maintain their psychological health.

Key Terms

social worker A professional with a master's degree in social work. Social workers provide both mental health and social services to the community and are the largest group of professional to provide psychological services.

dynamic therapy An intensive therapy based on the belief that effective treatment must focus on the psychological forces underlying the individual's problems.

humanistic therapy A treatment approach based on the belief that people, left to their own devices, will naturally grow in positive and constructive ways.

behavior therapy A behavior modification therapy based on the learning principles of reinforcement therapy, stimulus-response, and conditioning responses to change behavior.

cognitive-behavioral therapy An action-oriented form of therapy that assumes that maladaptive, or faulty, thinking patterns cause maladaptive behavior and negative emotions; treatment focuses on changing an individual's thoughts or cognitive patterns in order to change his or her behavior and emotional state.

solution-focused therapy A goal-oriented approach that helps clients change by looking for solutions rather than dwelling on problems.

- Take the Personal Assessment at the end of this chapter to assess your explanatory style.

- Apply the steps of a proactive approach to life to a situation in your life.

- Take the online screening assessment for depression, bipolar disorder, anxiety, or posttraumatic stress disorder at www.mentalhealthscreening.org.

- Keep a journal, and each day write down things you like about yourself or feel good about.

- Take a risk and do something you have been wanting to do, such as joining a club, trying a sport, or meeting new people.

SUMMARY

- Psychological health has also been associated with developing and maintaining a positive self-concept, positive self-esteem, and emotional intelligence.
- Personality is generally defined as a specific set of consistent patterns of behavior and traits that helps to identify and characterize an individual. Personality comprises thoughts, feelings, behaviors, motivation, instincts, and temperament.
- Two factors, nature and nurture, influence the shaping of personality. Nature refers to the innate factors we are born with that genetically determine our personality traits. Nurture is the effect that the environment, people, and external factors have on our personality.
- Nonverbal communication is what is communicated by your facial expression, body posture, tone of voice, and movements.
- Maslow's theory is a positive, optimistic theory of human behavior. He believed that people are motivated to grow and fulfill their potential, referring to this phenomenon as self-actualization.
- Having a positive interpretation of life's events, particularly how you cope with adversity, can make a significant difference in terms of your health and academic and work performance, as well as how long you will live.
- Anxiety disorders include generalized anxiety disorder, obsessive-compulsive disorder, posttraumatic stress disorder, panic disorder, and phobias.
- Schizophrenia is one of the most severe mental disorders, characterized by profound distortions in one's thought processes, emotions, perceptions, and behavior.
- A number of different health care professionals are trained to treat mental disorders, including psychiatrists, psychologists, social workers, and counselors.
- Treatments for psychological illnesses include dynamic, humanistic, behavioral, cognitive-behavioral, and solution-focused therapies, as well as drug therapies.

REVIEW QUESTIONS

1. What are three factors that have been associated with psychological health?
2. What are the characteristics commonly demonstrated by psychologically healthy people?
3. What is nonverbal communication?
4. Describe Maslow's theory of the hierarchy of needs.
5. How can having a positive interpretation of life's events make a significant difference in people's health?
6. How is clinical depression different from having the "blues"?
7. How should you respond to someone threatening or talking about committing suicide?
8. List five different types of anxiety disorders.
9. How does a psychiatrist differ from a psychologist?
10. What are five different types of therapy approaches to treat psychological disorders?

ANSWERS TO THE "WHAT DO YOU KNOW?" QUIZ

1. True   2. False   3. False   4. False   5. True   6. True   7. False

Antidepressant Use among Children and Teens

There has been a dramatic about-face in the number of children and teenagers taking antidepressants. This sudden retreat from prescribing antidepressants for kids and teens came as a result of the Food and Drug Administration's warning in 2003 that there is a higher risk of suicide associated with the use of antidepressants in these age groups. In fact, there has been a 20 percent decrease in the number of children and adolescents taking these medications, following a 20 percent increase just prior to the 2003 announcement. It was reported that 1 million children were taking antidepressants in early 2004. By March 2004, 18 percent fewer children were taking the drugs, and by June 2004 the number had dropped to 23 percent fewer.

There has been more focus on and concern about the use of medications to treat psychological disorders in children and adolescents because most clinical studies used to test these medications were performed with adults, not children.

In fact, only Prozac has been approved by the FDA to treat children and teens with depression; however, physicians routinely prescribe other antidepressants such as Paxil, Zoloft, Celexa, Effexor, and Remeron for this population. In October 2004, the FDA ordered "black box" labels, the most severe warning, on all antidepressants. Researchers suggest that antidepressants may be triggering "akathisia," a rapid increase in impulsivity and energy level that might contribute to already depressed kids taking the next step and attempting suicide. Often people with depression are so lethargic, unmotivated, and tired that they don't have the energy to act on suicidal thoughts. However, when the medication starts to work, the individual's energy level increases. If the level of hopelessness has not decreased or has stayed the same, the risk of suicidal behavior increases. Also, more is known about how these medications work for adults, and medications can work differently in children and teens. The medication can change teens from lovable, friendly, bright students to hateful, angry, unmotivated kids who seem like strangers to their friends and families.

GlaxoSmithKline, maker of Paxil, has been accused of withholding information and misleading doctors about the safety of treating kids with Paxil. The company has been accused of reporting only positive results from their clinical trials and not releasing information about any negative results.

There is also more concern over using antipsychotic drugs, such as Olanzapine, Quetipine, Ziprasidone, and Aripiprazol, with children and teenagers. The use of "atypical" or off-label drugs to treat aggressive behavior, schizophrenia, or bipolar disorder for children ages 2 to 18 jumped from half a million in 1995 to 2.5 million in 2002, a 500 percent increase. However, 45 deaths and 1,300 cases of dangerous side effects, such as convulsions and low white blood cell count, were also reported during this time period with this age group. Some physicians argue that antipsychotics are being overused in younger patients. They contend that antipsychotics should be used not as a first step but instead as a last resort after trying other treatment methods such as counseling, behavior management, and anger management.

It is no wonder that physicians are becoming more reluctant to prescribe these medications for children and teens. However, this reluctance may be putting our youth at risk because they may not be receiving appropriate treatment and medication that could alleviate their depression. While some physicians perhaps were writing these prescriptions too freely, we may now have a situation that has gone to the opposite extreme in which children and adolescents are suffering needlessly, not having the quality of life they could have, which may result in losing them to depression and suicide. The FDA has written a proposed medication guide about using antidepressants with children and teens.

Sources: "Fewer Kids Taking Anti-Depressants," *Web Md*, 22, 2004; "Spitzer Says Glaxo Withheld Paxil Info," *USA Today*, June 3, 2004; "Antidepressant Debate Takes a Delicate Turn," *USA Today*, October 18, 2004; "Questions, Answers on "Black Box" Labels," *USA Today*, October 18, 2004; "Warnings Slow Antidepressant Use," *USA Today*, February 1, 2005; "Suicide Alert Has Parents Rethinking Antidepressants," *USA Today*, February 1, 2005; "FDA Weighs Antidepressant Risk to Kids," www.intelihealth.com, January 27, 2004.

ENDNOTES

1. Turner I, Stels J. *The Sociology of Emotions*, New York: Cambridge University Press, 2005.
2. Papalia D, Olds S. *Psychology* (2nd ed.). New York: McGraw-Hill, 1988.
3. Seligman M. *Learned Optimism*. New York: Simon & Schuster., 1990.
4. McKay M, Fanning P. *Self-Esteem* (3rd ed.). Oakland, CA: New Harbinger, 1992.
5. Goleman D. *Emotional Intelligence*. New York: Bantam Books, 1997.
6. Wade C, Tavris C. *Psychology*. New York: Harper & Row, 1987.
7. Spear P, Penrod S, Baker T. *Psychology: Perspectives on Behavior*. New York: John Wiley, 1988.
8. Kagan J, Segal J. *Psychology: An Introduction* (6th ed.). Orlando, FL: Harcourt Brace Jovanovich., 1988.
9. Maslow AH. *The Farthest Reaches of Human Nature*. Peter Smith, 1983.
10. Maslow AH. *Motivation and Personality* (2nd ed.). New York: Van Nostrand, 1970.
11. Lindzey G, Thompson R, Spring B. *Psychology* (3rd ed.). New York: Worth, 1988.
12. Wade C., Tarns C. *Psychology*. New York: Harper & Row, 1987.
13. May R. Values, myths, and symbols. *American Journal of Psychiatry*, 132, 703–706, 1975.
14. Hemenway JE, et al. *Assessing Spiritual Needs: A Guide for Caregivers*. Minneapolis: Augsburg Press, 1993.
15. Ayele H, Mulligan T, Gheorghiu S, Reyes-Ortiz C. Religious activity improves life satisfaction for some physicians and older patients. *Journal of the American Geriatrics Society* 43, 453–455, 1999.
16. Levin JS. Religion and health: Is there an association, is it valid and is it causal? *Social Science Medicine* 38(11), 1475–1482, 1994.

17. Thorson JA, et al. Psychological health and sense of humor. *Journal of Clinical Psychology* 53(6), 605–619, 1997.
18. Yoshino S, Fujimori J, Kohda M. Effects of mirthful laughter on neuroendocrine and immune systems in patients with rheumatoid arthritis. *Journal Rheumatol* 23(4), 793–794, 1996.
19. Castro B, Eshleman J, Shearer R. Using humor to reduce stress and improve relationships. *Seminar Nurse Management* 7(2), 90–92, 1999.
20. Berk LS, et al. Immune system changes during humor-associated laughter. *Clinical Research* 39, 124a, 1991.
21. Cogan R, et al. Effects of laughter and relaxation on discomfort thresholds. *Journal of Behavioral Medicine,* 139–144, 1987.
22. Martin RA, Lefcourt HM. Sense of humor as a moderator between stressors and moods. *Journal of Personality and Social Psychology* 45, 1313–1324, 1983.
23. Nezu A, Nezu C, and Blissett S. Sense of humor as a moderator of the relationship between stressful events and psychological distress. *Journal of Personality and Social Psychology* 54, 520–525, 1988.
24. Miller J. Jokes and joking: A serious laughing matter, in Durant J and Miller J (Eds.) *Laughing Matters: A Serious Look at Humor.* Essex, England: Longman Scientific and Technical, 1988.
25. Lefcourt HM, Martin RA. *Humor and Life Stress: Antidote to Adversity.* New York: Springer-Verlag, 1986.
26. Kuhn C. *Humor Techniques for Health Care Professionals,* Presentation at Ball Memorial Hospital, April 22, 1998.
27. Nair M. A Documentary, *The Laughing Clubs of India,* 2001.
28. Collier G. *Emotional Expression.* Hillsdale, NJ: Erlbaum, 1985.
29. Peterson C, Seligman M, Vaillant G. Pessimistic explanatory style as a risk factor for physical illness: A thirty-five-year longitudinal study. *Journal of Personality and Social Psychology,* 55, 23–27, 1988.
30. Pavlov IP. *Conditioned Reflexes.* New York: Oxford University Press, 1927.
31. Hiroto D. Locus of control and learned helplessness. *Journal of Experiential Psychology* 102, 187–193, 1974.
32. Ellis A. *Reason and Emotion in Psychotherapy.* New York: Lyle Stuart, 1962.
33. Kessler RC, Chiu WT, Demler O, Walters EE. Prevalence, severity, and comorbidity of twelve-month DSM-IV disorders in the National Comorbidity Survey Replication (NCS-R). *Archives of General Psychiatry,* 62(6), 617–627, 2005.
34. U.S. Census Bureau population estimates by demographic characteristics. Table 2: Annual estimates of the population by selected age groups and sex for the United States: April 1, 2000 to July 1, 2004 (NC-EST2004–02). www.census.gov/popest/national/asrh/, Population Division, U.S. Census Bureau Release Data: June 9, 2005.
35. World Health Organization. *The World Health Report 2004: Changing History,* Annex table 3: Burden of disease in DALYs by cause, sex, and mortality stratum in WHO regions, estimates for 2002. Geneva: WHO, 2004.
36. American Psychiatric Association. *Diagnostic and Statistical Manual on Mental Disorders,* 4th ed. *(DSM-IV-TR).* Washington, DC: American Psychiatric Press, 2000.
37. World Health Organization. *Mental Health,* 2003.
38. Dramatic increases seen in college students' mental health problems over last 13 years. *Journal of Professional Psychology: Research and Practice,* February 2003.
39. National Institute of Mental Health, 2003.
40. Peterson K. Resilience, talking can help kids beat depression, *USA Today,* June 4, 2002.
41. Tanner L. With less stigma, more drugs, treatment for depression soars, *USA Today,* January 9, 2002.
42. Fewer kids taking antidepressants. WebMD Medical News, September 22, 2004.
43. Exercise better than drugs for depression. *British Journal of Sports Medicine* 35, 114–117, April 2001.
44. Study puts spotlight on electroshock therapy, *USA Today,* March 13, 2001.
45. Rosenthal NE. *Winter Blues.* New York: The Guilford Press, 1998.
46. Kochanek KD, Murphy SL, Anderson RN, Scott C. Deaths: Final data for 2002. *National Vital Statistics Reports.* 53 (5), 1–115, 2004.
47. Robins L, Regier D (Eds.). *Psychiatric Disorders in America: The Epidemiologic Catchment Area Study.* New York: The Free Press, 1991.
48. Bourne E. *The Anxiety and Phobia Workbook.* Oakland CA: New Harbinger, 1995.
49. Hallowell, E, Ratey, J. *Driven to Distraction.* New York: Simon & Schuster, 1995.
50. *Occupational Outlook Handout,* U.S. Department of Labor Bureau of Labor Statistics, 2002–2003.

Personal Assessment

What is your explanatory style?

Instructions: For each statement circle the response that best fits you.

1. The project you are in charge of is a great success.
   - A. I kept a close watch over everyone's work. 1
   - B. Everyone devoted a lot of time and energy to it. 0
2. You and your partner make up after a fight.
   - A. I forgave my partner. 0
   - B. I'm usually forgiving. 1
3. You get lost driving to a friend's house.
   - A. I missed a turn. 1
   - B. My friend gave me bad directions. 0
4. You were extremely healthy all year.
   - A. Few people around me were sick, so I wasn't exposed. 0
   - B. I made sure I ate well and got enough rest. 1
5. You forgot your friend's birthday.
   - A. I'm not good at remembering birthdays. 1
   - B. I was preoccupied with other things. 0
6. Your boss gives you too little time to finish a project, but you get it done anyway.
   - A. I am good at my job. 0
   - B. I am an efficient person. 1
7. They won't honor your credit card at a store.
   - A. I sometimes overestimate how much money I have. 1
   - B. I sometimes forget to pay my credit card bill. 0
8. Your car runs out of gas on a dark street late at night.
   - A. I didn't check to see how much gas was in the tank. 1
   - B. The gas gauge was broken. 0
9. You fail an important examination.
   - A. I wasn't as smart as the other people taking the test. 1
   - B. I didn't prepare for it well enough. 0
10. You lose your temper with a friend.
    - A. My friend is always nagging me. 1
    - B. My friend was in a hostile mood. 0
11. You win an athletic contest.
    - A. I was feeling unbeatable. 0
    - B. I trained hard. 1
12. A friend thanks you for helping her get through a bad time.
    - A. I enjoy helping her through tough times. 0
    - B. I am good at giving useful advice. 1

Scoring Key

Add together items 3, 5, 7, 8, 9, and 10 to get your B (bad event) score = _____

If you scored:

5 to 6—You tend to be very pessimistic and explain bad things as resulting from something you did or a personal characteristic that is lasting and extends to many areas in your life.

2 to 4—You have an average level of pessimism about negative events.

0 to 1—You tend to be very optimistic and explain bad things as resulting from something someone else did or a circumstance that is temporary and specific to only that situation.

Add together items 1, 2, 4, 6, 11, and 12 to get your G (good event) score = _____

If you scored:

5 to 6—You tend to be very optimistic and explain good things as resulting from something you did or a personal characteristic that is lasting and extends to many areas in your life.

2 to 4—You have an average level of optimism about positive events.

0 to 1—You tend to be very pessimistic and explain good things as resulting from something someone else did or a circumstance that is temporary and specific to only that situation.

TO CARRY THIS FURTHER . . .

How did you score? If your explanatory style tends to be pessimistic, try some of the strategies suggested in Chapter 2 for building optimism. When you encounter adversity, pay attention to your thinking patterns and consciously reframe them to be more positive and more focused on problem solving. Building a more optimistic approach to life can improve many dimensions of your health.

Source: Adapted from M. Seligman. *Learned Optimism.* New York: Pocket Books, 1990.

Managing Stress

What Do You Know about Managing Stress?

◉ Having stress is negative, and so stress should be eliminated from your life. True or False?

◉ Time management is the reason most college students cite for their academic success or failure. True or False?

◉ Laughing is important to managing stress. True or False?

◉ Different colors, sounds, and smells can affect your stress level. True or False?

◉ Breathing is the key to stress management. True or False?

◉ You can make up for not sleeping enough during the week by sleeping more or on the weekends, and it is the same as getting an average of seven to nine hours of sleep per night over a week's time. True or False?

◉ Exposing yourself to stressful situations can sometimes help you reduce your stress. True or False?

Check your answers at the end of the chapter.

What Is Stress?

How do you know when you are stressed? You might experience headaches, stomachaches, or back and neck aches, or you might feel irritable, tired, anxious, and depressed. Some people eat more, while others find eating difficult when they are stressed. **Stress** refers to physiological and psychological responses to a significant or unexpected change or disruption in one's life. It can be brought on by real or imagined factors or events.

Stress was first described in the 1930s by Hans Selye. During his second year of medical school, Selye observed that, although his patients suffered from a variety of illnesses, they all showed common symptoms, such as fatigue, appetite disturbance, sleep problems, mood swings, gastrointestinal problems, and diminished concentration and recall. He began developing his now-famous theory of the influence of stress on people's ability to cope with and adapt to the pressures of injury and disease. He discovered that patients with a variety of ailments manifested many similar symptoms, which he ultimately attributed to their bodies' efforts to respond to the stresses of being ill. He called this collection of symptoms—this stress disease—stress syndrome, or the **general adaptation syndrome (GAS).** He also described this as "the syndrome of being ill."[1] We will discuss Selye's discovery further later in the chapter.

Selye defines stress as "the nonspecific response of the body to any demand whether it is caused by or results in pleasant or unpleasant conditions." Stress can be both positive or negative. It is our response to stress—how we manage stress—that makes a difference in terms of how it affects us. Stress resulting from unpleasant events or conditions is called **distress** (from the Greek *dys,* meaning bad, as in displeasure). Stress resulting from pleasant events or conditions is called **eustress** (from the Greek *eu,* meaning good, as in euphoria). Both distress and eustress elicit the same physiological responses in the body, as noted in Selye's General Adaptation Syndrome model.

While stress may not always be negative, our responses to it can be problematic or unhealthy. Both positive and negative stressful situations place extra demands on the body—your body reacts to an unexpected change or a highly emotional experience, regardless of whether this change is good or bad. If the duration of stress is relatively short, the overall effect is minimal and your body will rest, renew itself, and return to normal. But, as you will learn in this chapter, long-lasting stress, experiencing multiple stressors simultaneously, and not managing your stress effectively can take a toll on your body.

Stress is actually normal and healthy at a certain level. With functional, healthy levels of stress, overall physiological equilibrium is maintained at a balanced level. However, you really don't want to eliminate all stress because stress is adaptive, functional, and can be beneficial. You need to understand how you uniquely deal with stress and what works and doesn't work well for you in coping with day-to-day pressures and problems (see the box "Different Cultures, Different Ways of Coping").

How We Respond to Stress

When we are stressed, we react in specific ways. The **stress response** is the result of learned and conditioned habits adopted early in life as a way of coping with problems, conflict, and disruptive events. But many of our responses to stress are innate, basic human survival mechanisms left over from our primordial roots. In prehistoric times, the best response to perceived danger, such as seeing a saber-toothed tiger about to attack, might be to either fight the animal or to run away. Stress in modern times remains the same except that we are responding to twenty-first century threats and dangers rather than to saber-toothed tigers. Again, it is not the events that determine how stressed we feel but our response to these stressors. We next discuss the way that this innate stress response affects our modern lives.

Fight or Flight Response

Our response to stress involves many physiological changes that are collectively called the **fight or flight response.** In situations in which you must react immediately to danger, it is advisable to either fight off the danger or flee. For example, you are walking back from class at night, thinking about all the studying you need to do and you begin to cross the street. Suddenly, out of nowhere, a car's headlights are coming right at you. Since your best response is probably not to fight the car, you run as fast as you can to the other side of the road. In that split second when you see the car careening quickly toward you, your muscles tense, your heart beats faster, your adrenaline pumps faster and is released at increased levels into your bloodstream, your breathing becomes more shallow and rapid, and your pupils dilate to see the car better.

This is the fight or flight response. Receiving alert signals from the brain, the sympathetic nerves signal most of the organs of the body, and the adrenal glands are activated. Within the brain itself, neural pathways, involved in increased attention and focus, are activated. In this way, performance and learning can be heightened. Again, all these changes are adaptive and helpful to your survival in getting out of harm's way. In the preceding example, when you get to the other side of the road and realize that you are okay, your body begins to relax and return to its

---

> ### Key Terms
>
> **stress** The physiological and psychological state of disruption caused by the presence of an unanticipated, disruptive, or stimulating event.
>
> **general adaptation syndrome (GAS)** Sequenced physiological responses to the presence of a stressor, involving the alarm, resistance, and exhaustion stages of the stress response.
>
> **distress** Stress that diminishes the quality of life; commonly associated with disease, illness, and maladaptation.
>
> **eustress** Stress that enhances the quality of life.
>
> **stress response** The physiological and psychological responses to positive or negative events that are disruptive, unexpected, or stimulating.
>
> **fight or flight response** The physiological response to a stressor that prepares the body for confrontation or avoidance.

Learning from Our Diversity

Different Cultures, Different Ways of Coping

While stressful situations can affect people differently, and we all have our unique ways of coping with stress, some important cultural differences exist in the types of stress and responses to stress that ethnic groups might experience. Clearly, being of minority status can cause a great deal of stress—for example, being the victim of hate crimes, having fewer opportunities for education and employment, earning less pay for the same work done by the majority population, experiencing higher mortality rates and illness and decreased access to health care, and suffering feelings of isolation and lack of support.

Latino/a Americans, for instance, are overrepresented among the poor, have a high unemployment rate, and often live in substandard housing. Many of those who do find employment hold semiskilled or unskilled jobs. Nearly one-third of Latino/a students drop out of high school, which is more than double the rate for African Americans and three times higher than the rate for Caucasians.

The rate of alcoholism is higher among Native Americans, with deaths owing to alcoholism being more than four times higher than those reported for the general population. The suicide rate among Native Americans is 77 percent higher than the national average. High school drop-out rates and unemployment rates are also higher for this group than for any other minority population.

Because different ethnic groups experience different stressors, the ways that groups effectivley manage their stress are important to consider. For example, Native Americans incorporate story telling, spirituality, dreams, and visions into their stress-management strategies. A "talking circle" may be employed to help alleviate stress. This involves sitting in a circle, connecting with others by shaking hands around the circle, sharing one's innermost feelings without interruption or response from others, burning incense and passing it around the circle, and passing a sacred object such as an eagle feather to the person who is speaking.

There are significant differences between the ways Asian and European cultures cope with stress. European cultures use social support in coping with stress; Asians tend to avoid drawing on social support for fear that they will disrupt group harmony, receive criticism about the problem, or feel ashamed. In Asian cultures people are taught to take responsibility for solving their own problems, and if they do go to others for support, they typically go to their own family. Yoga, meditation, and acupuncture are common methods for coping with stress in Asian cultures. Asian Americans focus more on logical, rational, and structured approaches, such as time management, relaxation techniques, and cognitive behavioral strategies.

African Americans tend to prefer to manage stress and problems using direct, active problem solving. In contrast to Asian cultures, African Americans tend to value social support—they tend to share their problems with others in times of stress and are more comfortable expressing feelings associated with the stress.

Hispanics tend to seek support from religion, family, and community in managing daily stressors. This culture values the present and emphasizes being rather than doing. Hispanic culture encourages accepting and enduring stress and problems rather than being assertive and provoking conflict.

Each of us needs to understand how we respond to stress and find strategies that work best to control stress levels. We should also consider issues of diversity in order to identify the unique stressors and stress-management techniques that might best fit us.

Sources: Dolph L. Hatfield, "The Stereotyping of Native Americans," *Humanist*, September 2000; "Native Americans of North America," Microsoft® Encarta® *Online Encyclopedia* 2005, http://encarta.msn.com © 1997–2005 Microsoft Corporation; D. Sue and D. Sue, *Counseling the Culturally Different* (New York: John Wiley and Sons, 1999).

normal state. You take a large, deep breath, expressing a big sigh of relief. Your muscles may feel even weaker than usual, your breathing may become deeper and heavier than is typical, and you may feel shaky as your body goes from extreme arousal to relaxing very quickly. Figure 3-1a depicts the changes from the normal state to an arousal state to a very relaxed state then back to normal.

Accompanying this fight or flight reaction is a slower response. During stressful events, the pituitary gland secretes a peptide called adrenocorticotrophin, or ACTH, into the blood. ACTH travels through the blood to the adrenal gland, where it signals the production of a hormone called cortisol.[2] Cortisol aids the body in recovering from stressful experiences by freeing up energy stores. The logic behind the slower stress response is that the quick fight or flight response uses up a lot of the body's available energy. The slower response helps to replenish that energy. The body usually has some small amount of cortisol circulating in the blood at all times. When the stress response lasts too long or is initiated too frequently, the cortisol level is increased. After enough of these small increases, the body soon resets its control mechanism to maintain a higher constant amount of cortisol in the body.

Chronic Stress

Now let's consider a different situation. You have a test in a week that you are very concerned about. It seems to be preoccupying your every waking thought, and you have trouble sleeping as well. You are worried that you won't perform well on the test, and you really need to do better than you did on your last test. Your parents have been putting a great deal of pressure on you to do better in school in general. Because our bodies respond similarly to perceived or anticipated threat, you can have the

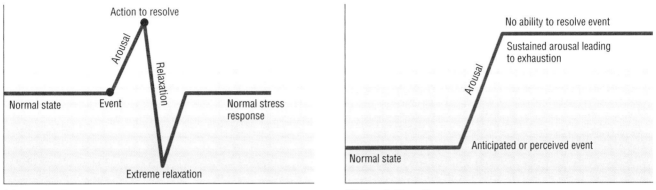

(A) Adaptive Stress Response

(B) Chronic Stress Response

Figure 3-1 Resolving Stress How quickly and effectively you act to resolve stress has a significant effect on how long your body remains at a high level of physiological arousal.

Source: H. Selye. "The Stress of Life," 1975.

same response to things that have and have not yet occurred. In other words, your heart races, breathing becomes labored, muscles are tense, the body sweats, and blood flow is constricted to the extremities and digestive organs and increases to the major muscles and brain. Your body is becoming ready to fight or flee the danger. However, you cannot take any action and make a fight or flight response, because nothing has happened yet. You haven't taken the test yet, and even once you have done so, you won't know your grade. So your body remains at this high level of arousal, as depicted in Figure 3-1b.

Remaining in a continued state of physiological arousal for an extended period of time is called **chronic stress.** This high level of arousal is similar to putting your foot on the accelerator of your car while it is in park and not letting up on the gas pedal. Since the fight or flight response is meant to be a very quick, short-acting response, your body begins to wear down if kept at this physiological state of arousal for too long; eventually, you will begin to feel exhausted. This is also the reason that people cope better with anxiety by taking some action, doing something about whatever they are worried about, rather than stewing about their problems. Thus the fight or flight response can be triggered inappropriately in response to phobias, irrational beliefs, an overactive imagination, or hallucinations or delusions.

The Three Stages of Stress

Once under the influence of a stressor, people's bodies respond in remarkably similar, predictable ways. For example, when asked to give a speech for a class, your heart rate may increase, your throat may become dry, your palms may sweat, and you may feel lightheaded, dizzy, and nauseous. If an individual lost her or his job or

discovered that her or his partner wanted to terminate their relationship, she or he might experience similar sensations. It is clear that different stressors are able to evoke common physical reactions.

Selye described the typical physical response to a stressor in his general adaptation syndrome model discussed earlier in the chapter.[3] Selye stated that the human body moves through three stages when confronted by stressors, as follows.

Alarm Stage

Once exposed to any event that is perceived as threatening or dangerous, the body immediately prepares for difficulty, entering what Selye called the **alarm stage.** These involuntary changes, shown in Figure 3-2, are controlled by the hormonal and the nervous systems, and they trigger the fight or flight response. For example, you realize that the final exam you thought was today was actually scheduled for yesterday. You may begin to experience fear, panic, anxiety, anger, depression, and restlessness.[4]

Key Terms

chronic stress Remaining at a high level of physiological arousal for an extended period of time; it can also occur when an individual is not able to immediately react to a real or a perceived threat.

alarm stage The first stage of the stress response, involving physiological, involuntary changes that are controlled by the hormonal and the nervous systems; the fight or flight response is activated in this stage.

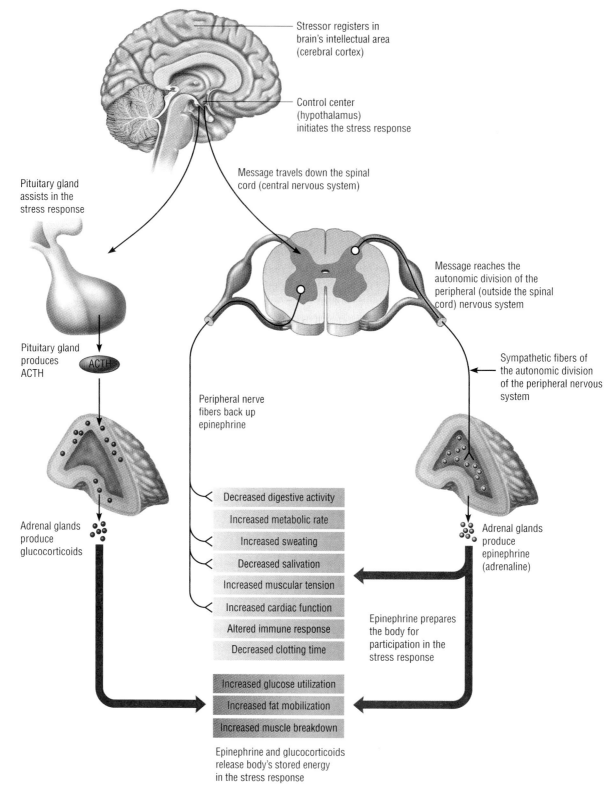

Stressor registers in brain's intellectual area (cerebral cortex)

Control center (hypothalamus) initiates the stress response

Pituitary gland assists in the stress response

Message travels down the spinal cord (central nervous system)

Message reaches the autonomic division of the peripheral (outside the spinal cord) nervous system

Pituitary gland produces ACTH

ACTH

Sympathetic fibers of the autonomic division of the peripheral nervous system

Peripheral nerve fibers back up epinephrine

Adrenal glands produce glucocorticoids

Decreased digestive activity

Increased metabolic rate

Increased sweating

Decreased salivation

Increased muscular tension

Increased cardiac function

Altered immune response

Decreased clotting time

Adrenal glands produce epinephrine (adrenaline)

Epinephrine prepares the body for participation in the stress response

Increased glucose utilization

Increased fat mobilization

Increased muscle breakdown

Epinephrine and glucocorticoids release body's stored energy in the stress response

Figure 3-2 The Stress Response Physiological reactions to a stressor are controlled by the hormonal and nervous systems.

Resistance Stage

The second stage of a response to a stressor is the **resistance stage,** during which the body attempts to reestablish its equilibrium or internal balance. The body is geared for survival, and because staying in the alarm stage for a prolonged amount of time is not conducive for the body's optimal functioning, it will resist the threat or attempt to resolve the problem and reduce the intensity of the response to a more manageable level. Specific organ systems, such as the cardiovascular and digestive systems, become the focus of the body's response.[5] During this phase, you might take steps to calm yourself down and relieve the stress on your body: you might deny the situation, withdraw and isolate yourself from others, and shut down your emotions. Thus, in the previous example, you may not tell anyone about missing the exam, may tell yourself that you don't care about that class anyway, and go back to bed.

Exhaustion Stage

Your ability to move from the alarm stage to a less damaging resistance stage determines the effect that the stressor has on your physical and psychological health. As you gain more control and balance is reestablished, you can begin to recover from the stress.

The length of time, the energy, and the effort required to accomplish recovery determines how exhausted your body becomes as a result of the stressor. Of course, the longer the body is under stress and out of balance, the more negative the effect will be on your body. Long-term exposure to a stressor or coping with multiple stressors at the same time often results in overloading your system. Specific organs and body systems that were called on during the resistance stage may not be able to resist a stressor indefinitely. When all the psychological and physical resources we rely on to deal with stress are used up, an **exhaustion stage** results, and the stress-producing hormones such as adrenaline increase again. This is when chronic and serious illnesses can begin to develop, and the individual may even develop clinical depression.

The Effects of Stress

If not managed well, stress can affect us in a variety of negative ways. For instance, stress can give us medical problems, interpersonal and relationship conflicts, and academic and work difficulties. However, a moderate level of stress can be beneficial.

The Physical Toll of Stress

Constant arousal and increased levels of adrenaline in your system will eventually wear down your body's

Chronic stress can contribute to headaches, anxiety, insomnia, and many other health problems.

immunological system. As this occurs, you will be less able to cope with stress, and so it takes less and less to cause a stress reaction. When you are chronically stressed, it takes very little to frustrate you, and you can feel easily irritated and stressed at the littlest thing. Your body is both psychologically as well as physically less able to cope with stress. This can compromise your immune system, and you may become ill more easily. It may also take longer for you to recover from illness.

The following medical problems have been associated with stress[6] (to examine stress indicators for your personal stress, complete the rating scale at the end of this chapter):

- Cardiovascular problems (heart attacks, strokes, hypertension)
- Gastrointestinal problems (ulcers, irritable bowel syndrome, diarrhea, constipation, diverticulitis)

Key Terms

resistance stage The second stage of a response to a stressor, during which the body attempts to reestablish its equilibrium or internal balance.

exhaustion stage The point at which the physical and the psychological resources used to deal with stress have been depleted.

The newly emerging field of psychoneuro-immunology addresses the apparent interplay of the mind, the nervous system (the hypothalamus and the autonomic nervous system), and the immune system (see Chapter 13).

On the basis of clinical observation and laboratory studies, it is recognized that feelings associated with stress (depression and anxiety) and the disruption of social support systems relate to the weakening of the immune response and the development of some illnesses. For example, a study showed that happy, relaxed people are more resistant to illness than are those who tend to be unhappy and tense. In addition, work-related or personal stress experienced for at least one month increases a person's chances of catching a cold. In other words, the longer you live in a stressful state, the more likely you are to catch a cold. People in unhappy marriages, particularly wives, also have higher incidences of colds. Extroverts are less likely to catch a cold, as are those with diverse social roles such as spouse, parent, worker, friend, community member, student. This situation makes sense, since we know that incorporating positive social interactions into our lives helps to alleviate stress, which in turn minimizes the risk of catching a cold. In another study, immunizations were less effective in producing an immune response in students stressed by upcoming examinations than in those not scheduled to take exams.

Stress triggers the release of inflammatory particles, cytokines and histamines, that fight off infection but can also cause cold symptoms. Researchers suspect that a sense of well-being decreases the release of cytokines and eases symptoms. This phenomenon may also explain why people can get through a state of acute stress and then become ill after the crisis is over, since stress produces adrenaline, which stimulates the immune system, releasing cortisol. This is the hormone that battles inflammation but weakens immunity.

Our growing understanding of the relationship between our thoughts, the nervous system, and the functional status of the immune system enhances our insight into illnesses and their relationship to stress. As this understanding continues to mature, we will develop more effective coping strategies that enhance the connection between our feelings and their effect on nervous system and endocrine system function and the maintenance of immune system capabilities.

Sources: Masek K et al. Past, present and future of psychoneuroimmunology. *Toxicology* 2000; 142(3): 179–188; Marilyn Elias, "In the War on Colds Personality Counts," *USA Today*, December 1, 2003; Cohen S et al. Types of stressors that increase susceptibility to the common cold in healthy adults. *Health Psychol* 1998; 17(3): 214–223.

- Rheumatoid arthritis
- Lupus
- Headaches and migraines
- Muscle spasms and cramps
- Sleep disorders
- Anxiety
- Jaw problems (temporomandibular joint [TMJ] syndrome)
- Allergies
- Cancer
- Back pain
- Asthma
- Kidney disease
- Sexual dysfunction
- Infertility
- Alcoholism and drug abuse

The Immune System and Stress

Corticosteroids are produced in the adrenal cortex as part of the stress response. Cortisol increases the body's fuel supply of carbohydrates, glucose, and fat, which are needed to respond to stress. It is important not to keep these levels elevated for very long, though, as too much cortisol in the system can also act to suppress the immune system. Remember that the stress response is meant to be a rapid, temporary response. Individuals who are chronically stressed are constantly pumping out a high level of corticosteroids. Over time, this can result in a breakdown of muscle, a decreased number of immune cells, and a decreased inflammatory response. This can render the body less able to defend against bacteria and viruses—a stressed person is more likely to become ill. Hypertension and fluid retention are also associated with constant high levels of corticosteroids. On the other hand, if the level of corticosteroids in your system is too low, you can have an overactive immune system—this can harm healthy cells, resulting in autoimmune diseases such as lupus and rheumatoid arthritis. Therefore it is important to maintain a healthy level of corticosteroids (in other words, a moderate level of stress) to keep the body in balance. See the box "Psychoneuroimmunology" for more on the links between stress and health.

Cardiovascular Disease and Stress

Your level of stress also contributes to your risk for developing cardiovascular disease. Chronic stress exposes your body to unhealthy, persistently elevated levels of stress hormones like adrenaline and cortisol. Studies also link stress to changes in the way blood clots, which increases the risk of heart attack. Job stress, personality factors, and social isolation have all been suggested as factors contributing to cardiovascular disease. For example, one study found that people who worked more than 60 hours a week were twice as likely to have a heart attack as those working 40 hours a week.[7] High levels of stress can make other risk factors (such as high cholesterol or high blood pressure) worse, which in turn increases the chances of developing cardiovascular disease.

Type A and Type B Personalities   Cardiologists Meyer Friedman and Roy Rosenman identified two basic types of personalities when they interviewed individuals in order to identify people who may be susceptible to stress-related heart disease.[8] In the interview, they asked individuals the following questions:

1. Does your job carry heavy responsibility?
2. Is there any time when you feel particularly rushed or under pressure?
3. When you are under pressure, does it bother you?
4. Would you describe yourself as a hard-driving ambitious type of person in accomplishing the things you want, or would you describe yourself as a relatively relaxed and easy-going person?

From the responses to these questions, Friedman and Rosenman were able to distinguish two types of personalities with respect to stress: type A and type B personalities. Type A individuals often feel pressured, are ambitious, impatient, competitive, walk and talk rapidly, and can be easily annoyed by delays. Type B individuals tend to be calm, relaxed, easy-going, and patient. They also found that many cases of heart disease couldn't be attributed to other cardiac risk factors such as smoking or dietary habits but could be linked to stress. Type A personalities tend to share qualities of workaholism and perfectionism, such as having high expectations and feeling out of control, irritable and overwhelmed, stressed and pressured most of the time. There is a constant sense of needing to go faster and hurry through activities to get onto the next task. Thus type A people tend not to enjoy what they are doing because they are thinking about the next activity rather than enjoying the present.[9] This can of course cause tension in their relationships as well. Type A people tend to drive themselves to exhaustion and stop only when they collapse or become ill.

While Friedman and Rosenman didn't describe type A personalities as an illness but more as a personality type, they did find correlations with stress. Type A people sometimes need to slow down, lower their expectations of themselves, delegate responsibilities to others, and prioritize their tasks. Type A individuals often complain that they have trouble relaxing and don't know how to relax. They also don't allow themselves to have fun until all of the work is done, which rarely occurs. Scheduling social activities and time to relax is one important component in alleviating the stress that accompanies type A personalities. Exercising, meditation, massage, spiritual activities, and yoga are other ways to relax.

The Stress-Hardy Individual   While some people are chronically stressed, which leads to exhaustion, other people seem to have a high stress tolerance. These "stress-hardy" individuals have a lower frequency of illness and absenteeism.[8] They view stressors as challenges and chances for new opportunities and seem to thrive with increased stress. They feel more in control of their lives and perceive themselves as having options and the power to make choices and influence situations. So it is not just the level of stress that an individual experiences that determines how he or she will respond but also the individual's ability to manage varying degrees of stress. Stress-hardy individuals who have a good social support system, exercise regularly, and maintain a healthy diet have fewer stress-related illnesses than do those who have less healthy lifestyles.

Benefits of Stress

As we have said, while too much stress can have a negative effect and cause some serious health problems, a moderate level of stress is positive and beneficial. Stress can be motivating and energizing. Without some stress, many of us may not get much accomplished in our day or even get out of bed! Look at the diagram in Figure 3-3. What do you notice? Too little and too much stress are not helpful. When you are not stressed at all, you can be apathetic and lethargic. When you are too stressed, you are paralyzed with fear, like deer in the headlights. This is referred to as the **Yerkes-Dodson Law,** which uses a bell-shaped curve to demonstrate that there is an optimal level of stress for peak performance. This fact holds true for any type of performance, from academic or work

---

Key Terms

type A personality A personality type that tends to be competitive, ambitious, and impatient; often associated with heart attacks and other stress-related conditions.

type B personality A personality type that tends to be more relaxed and patient.

Yerkes-Dodson Law A bell-shaped curve demonstrating that there is an optimal level of stress for peak performance; this law states that too little or too much stress is not helpful, whereas a moderate level of stress is positive and beneficial.

Figure 3-3 The Yerkes-Dodson Law Too little or too much stress is not helpful, but a moderate level of stress encourages peak performance.

Source: Hebb DO. Drive and the CNS (conceptual nervous system). *Psychological Review* 62(4), 243–254, 1955.

activities to music or athletics.[9] Recognizing the appropriate level of stress for your ideal performance level is important in reaching your potential.

The Sources of Stress

There are other causes of stress besides experiencing positive or negative events in life.[10] What events or situations trigger stress for you? For some it is financial worries, for others it might be relationship conflict, and for still others it is work-related stress. Even positive events, such as getting married, starting a new job, or moving to a new place, can be **stressors.** Going on vacation can be stressful as you get things done ahead of time to prepare for being away, pack your belongings, spend money on the trip, and completely change your routine. Any type of change in your life has the potential to trigger a stressful response.

Because stress involves a physiological response, it has a direct link to your physical and psychological health. The work of Thomas Holmes and Richard Rahe

> ### Key Terms
>
> **stressors** Factors or events, real or imagined, that elicit a state of stress.

has found direct connections between changes in people's lives and physical illness. They developed a widely used inventory, called the Social Readjustment Rating Scale, to assess the degree of stress people experience in connection with particular life events. While one of these events alone might be tolerable, a combination of too many life changes within a short period of time may lead to illness.[10] To effectively manage your stress, you need to understand what specific sources trigger stress for you. Students experience some specific types of stress that other people do not necessarily encounter. In this next section, we will discuss stressors unique to students and how to manage them.

To assess your level of stress and potential vulnerability to illness, complete the Personal Assessment inventory at the end of this chapter.

Student Stressors

Going to college has been likened to "crossing into a new culture" where students face unique challenges and stressors.[11] Similar to going to live in another country, students must learn new customs and traditions, new ways of doing things, a new language, and must leave comfortable and familiar surroundings. This can cause a high level of stress for students, many of whom have left their support system behind to live in a place where they know few people. In the sections that follow, we cover some of the specific stressors college students face and offer ways to manage these situations.

Interpersonal Stressors

Homesickness Homesickness is one of the most common problems facing college students—which is understandable given that they are separated from friends and family and learning to live in an entirely new environment. When you are undergoing a great deal of change in your life, it is helpful to have the comfort and security of knowing that your home base remains stable and consistent. Moving from home to college can disrupt this sense of safety. While the college years can be an exciting and challenging time in your life, you may be missing your friends and family at home with whom you normally share these events. You may have also lost your sense of belonging while you struggle with finding a way to fit in with and navigate your new surroundings.

Often homesickness doesn't hit until a few weeks or maybe a month after you have moved, since the first few weeks are filled with meeting new people, social activities, and unpacking. After the dust settles, some people begin to feel lonely and alone. See the box "Overcoming Homesickness" for advice on how to deal with homesickness.

Overcoming Homesickness

I just started college, and my family and friends are five hours away from me. I tend to be on the shy side and don't know anyone at my college. I miss my friends and family and don't feel like I belong here. I am thinking about withdrawing from school and going home. What should I do?

The following are some strategies to combat these feelings:

- *Get involved!* Become active in extracurricular social activities such as special interest clubs, student government, religious clubs, fraternities, and sororities. Clubs associated with your major are a great way to meet people, further your academic and career interests, and keep you from feeling homesick.
- *Call, e-mail, or text message* your family and friends regularly and let them know you would like to hear from them.
- *Be open to meeting new people.* Introduce yourself to people in your classes, and exchange e-mail addresses and phone numbers. This is also an excellent way to get a study partner or study group together. Keep your door open when you are in your

room, and spend time in public, common areas—not just hiding away in your room when you have spare time. Strike up a conversation while doing your laundry in the common laundry room area.

- *Don't eat alone.* Ask someone to join you to eat, or ask people at a table if you can eat with them.
- *Don't go home on the weekends.* Even though it may be tempting to visit your family and friends, the weekends are the best time to meet people and participate in the activities going on around campus.
- *Be patient with yourself.* Accept that loneliness and longing for home are normal, and it will take some time for you to adjust to all the changes you are experiencing. Don't decide to throw in the towel after the first few days! It may take a month or more before you begin to feel more comfortable in your new home. Give yourself some time to face this new challenge.

Relationship Problems Along with homesickness, another very common stressor for students is relationship problems. Often students are separated by long distances from their best friends and romantic partners. While it can be difficult to maintain long-distance relationships, it is not impossible. Studies show that the key to effective long-distance relationships is communication. The quality of a long-distance relationship is improved if you both are committed to each other, you can talk openly about your concerns, feelings, and fears, and you can agree on the rules of the relationship, such as dating other people. In addition, there needs to be a strong level of trust between the partners, since trust is often tested in long-distance relationships. Both of you will change, and you must share these changes so that you can grow together, not apart. Agree on how often you will see each other, call or e-mail, and focus on spending high-quality time together.

It can be beneficial to have your friends visit you at college (rather than you going home) so that they can interact with you in your new environment and meet your new friends. Often students feel as though they live in two worlds, home and school, and it can be stressful to negotiate going from one to the other. The more you can connect these two worlds, the less stress you will experience. So it can be helpful to share what you are doing in your day—activities around campus, details of your classes, even who you ate lunch with—with your friends and family back home, and ask them what they have been doing.

Balancing Work, Home, and School It is estimated that about two-thirds of students work while going to college, and more students are working full-time to pay for the costs of tuition (see Figure 3-4). In addition, it is estimated that between 5 and 10 percent of college students also have children. This, of course, adds stress to a student's life in balancing time for school, children, work, and household responsibilities. The increase in the number of students who have children is partly a result of a nationwide trend of more women in their mid-20s or older starting or returning to college. In fact, a national study by the University of Michigan showed that the number of full-time female students over 25 years old grew by 500 percent over recent years.[12]

Percentages of college students who also work at paying jobs

Figure 3-4 Balancing Work and School Almost two-thirds of the nation's 1.8 million college students under age 25 worked at paying jobs in recent years.

Source: Data from the U.S. Department of Labor, Bureau of Labor Statistics, March 25, 2005.

While some campuses offer child care, many do not, which leaves students having to coordinate schedules and juggle responsibilities, causing even more stress. Also, the cost of child care can be exorbitant for some and can certainly add to financial worries. Managing time well and having a strong support system are essential for students with children, particularly single parents. Often there is little to no time available for relaxation, socializing, or exercising, and so employing stress relief strategies can be challenging.

Academic Stressors

Stress and Learning How does stress affect learning? Research suggests that people who are highly anxious tend to perform better than others do at simple learning tasks but less well than others do at difficult tasks, particularly those involving reasoning activities and time-limited tests. One interesting study showed that college students with average scholastic ability earned significantly better grades when they had low levels of anxiety as compared to highly anxious average students.[13] When you are more stressed or anxious, you have a diminished ability to concentrate, to recall information, and to master problem-solving activities. You may find yourself reading the same page in your textbook over and over again, not knowing what you read.[13]

Test Anxiety You have studied for the test you are about to take and are well prepared. You look at the first test question and suddenly your mind goes blank. The harder you try to think, the more nervous and distressed you feel. You just can't think clearly and feel as though you have some type of mental block—what is happening? One-fifth of students experience these feelings, referred to as **test anxiety.** Exams are one of the greatest sources of stress for college students. The physical sensations associated with test anxiety are similar to those of general anxiety, such as fidgeting; having the feeling of butterflies in your stomach; rapid heart rate; difficulty breathing; nausea; tension in your neck, back, jaw, and shoulders; headaches; sweaty palms; and feeling shaky. People suffering from test anxiety make more mistakes on their tests, don't read the test accurately, and tend to make simple mistakes, such as spelling errors or adding something incorrectly. Many don't pace themselves well and have a hard time finishing exams. Test anxiety is a form of performance anxiety—people anticipate that they will perform poorly on the test.[13] To help determine if test

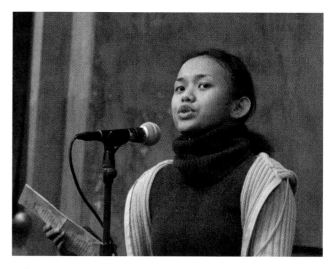

Effective behavioral and psychological interventions exist to treat speech anxiety.

anxiety is a problem for you—and what to do about it—refer to the box "Do You Suffer from Test Anxiety?"

 TALKING POINTS What are some problems with stress described in this chapter that you have experienced?

Speech Anxiety As we have mentioned, speech anxiety, or fear of public speaking, is one of the most common anxiety disorders. Since students are frequently required to give oral presentations, expected to engage in class discussion, and graded on class-participation points, this can present a problem for some.

In addition to the basic stress-management techniques outlined in this chapter, the following strategies can be used to cope with speech anxiety:

- *Volunteer to go first.* Anxiety is dealt with best by taking action. Pressure and expectations tend to mount with each person who takes a turn so you can lessen your stress level by being the first to present. Another advantage is that your performance is judged on its own merit without being compared to anyone else's.

- *Practice in front of a mirror and for your friends.* Solicit feedback: Do you need to slow down or speak louder? Practice will also help you to remember your talk so that you don't read it word for word, which can seem less interesting to your audience.

- *Engage in positive visualization.* Take deep, comfortable breaths and imagine yourself giving your speech with confidence and receiving positive feedback and compliments about your performance.

- *Vary your presentation style and format.* Use visuals such as slides, and engage your audience

Do You Suffer from Test Anxiety?

Test anxiety is a commonly experienced problem and can significantly impair your academic performance. Here are some questions you can ask yourself to help analyze if you might be suffering from test anxiety.

1. Are you aware of being really nervous on a test, maybe so nervous that you don't do your best, even though you know you've studied well and are prepared?
2. Does your stomach ever get tight or upset before or during a test? Hands cold and sweaty? Headaches? Do you have trouble sleeping the night before a test?
3. Do you ever find your mind racing or seeming dull or cloudy so that you can't think clearly while taking a test?
4. During a test, do you ever forget material you studied and learned, only to remember it again after the test is over?
5. Do you overanalyze questions, see too many possibilities, choose the complex answer, and overlook the simple, correct one?
6. Do you make many careless errors?
7. Have you had some bad experiences with tests and made poor grades when you didn't expect them?

8. Do you spend a lot of time and energy preparing for tests, yet fail to make grades that represent what you know?
9. Are tests and finals a particularly miserable time for you?

If you answered yes to more than half these questions, you might want to consider getting some help in managing the anxiety associated with test taking. College counseling centers frequently offer stress-management programs and can teach you techniques to manage your anxiety. Similar to managing other types of stress and anxiety, test anxiety can be coped with by using the following suggestions:

- Prepare well in advance. Don't cram at the last minute for the test. Rehearsal and repetition are the best ways of remembering information.
- Improve your odds by getting a good night's sleep before the test and eating a nutritious meal to give your brain needed energy.
- Watch your test talk. Don't talk about the test beforehand with friends, since this tends to increase anxiety.

- Go into the test with a confident attitude, reminding yourself that you are well prepared and have taken many tests and performed satisfactorily in the past.
- Activity reduces anxiety. If you stumble on a question, don't linger over it; go on to the next question and return to that one later.
- Ask for clarification if you don't understand a question or something on the test.
- Don't pay attention to the people around you. Focus on the test and don't allow yourself to get distracted.
- Take deep breaths, allow your breathing to help you to relax, and bring more oxygen to the brain so you can think more clearly.
- Pace yourself and be aware of your time. Know when you need to be halfway through the test according to the time allotted for the exam.

Source: Newman E. *No More Test Anxiety*. Los Angeles, CA: Learning Skills Publications, 1996. Used with permission by E. Newman.

---

in discussion so that they are an active not a passive part of your presentation. This takes some of the focus and pressure away from you.

Math Anxiety   Another common stressor for college students is math anxiety. Math anxiety is an intense emotional feeling of anxiety that some people have about their ability to understand mathematics. People who suffer from math anxiety feel that they are incapable of performing well in activities and classes that involve math. The incidence of math anxiety among college students has risen significantly over the last decade. Many students have even chosen their college major on the basis of how little math is required for the degree. Math anxiety has become so prevalent on college campuses that many schools have designed classes and special counseling programs to help math-anxious students.

Typically, people with math anxiety have the potential to perform well in math; the anxiety is more of a psychological, rather than an intellectual, problem. However, since math anxiety interferes with a person's ability to learn math, it can create an intellectual problem. Often math anxiety is the result of a student's negative

or embarrassing experience with math or a math teacher in previous years. Or perhaps the student was repeatedly told that he or she would not be able to perform well in math by a parent or a teacher. Such an experience can leave a student believing him- or herself deficient in math ability. This belief can actually result in poor performance, which serves as confirming evidence to the student. This phenomenon is known as a self-fulfilling prophecy; it is described more fully later in this chapter.[14]

Students who fear math often avoid asking questions to save embarrassment, sit in the back of the classroom, fail to seek help from the instructor, and usually put off studying math until the last moment. All these negative behaviors are intended to reduce the student's anxiety but actually result in more intense anxiety. However, there are a number of strategies to overcome math anxiety:

1. *Be sure to have developed a solid arithmetic foundation.* Since complex concepts build cumulatively on more simplistic ones, a remedial course or short course in arithmetic is often a significant first step in reducing the anxiety response to math.

2. *Take an easier, slower math course* as opposed to a faster-paced, more challenging one. It is better to stack the odds in your favor than to risk reinforcing your negative experiences with math.

3. *Be aware of thoughts, feelings, and actions* as they are related to math. Develop a positive perspective toward math.

4. *There is safety in numbers!* Math anxiety is learned and reinforced over a long period of time and may take time to eliminate. You can reduce your anxiety with the help of a tutor, studying with a friend, and talking with your instructor.

5. *Sit near the front of the class* where you will experience fewer distractions and feel more a part of what is being discussed.

6. If you have questions or can't keep up with the instructor, *ask for clarification and repetition* of whatever you missed.[15]

7. *Review the material.* As with most things, skill in math comes from practice. Make sure you review the material covered in the class, and identify questions you need to ask the instructor as soon as possible after the class. Research shows that you will remember 50 percent of what you heard in class if you review it immediately after class, but only 20 percent is retained 24 hours later if you didn't review the material right away.[16]

Internal Stressors

We can also generate stress within ourselves by putting too much pressure on ourselves, procrastinating, expecting too much of ourselves, and being self-critical. These intrapsychic stressors refer to our internal worries, criticisms, and negative self-talk, which were discussed in Chapter 2. Students say that procrastination, perfectionism, and poor goal setting are common sources of stress in their lives.

Procrastination   Procrastination means postponing something that is necessary to do to reach a goal.[17] Putting things off is a common problem that plagues students and can cause stress. A survey of college students found that approximately 23 percent of students said they procrastinated about half the time, and 27 percent of students said

they procrastinated most of the time.[17] Procrastination has been viewed as a time-management problem, but it is really more than that, and so time-management strategies tend to be ineffective in resolving this problem. Procrastination is also different from indecision, because people can make a decision but still have trouble implementing it.

Typically there is a psychological aspect to procrastination because we tend to delay doing those things that we don't want to do. Emotions such as anxiety, guilt, and dread often accompany thinking about the task. By putting the dreaded activity off, you can temporarily alleviate your anxiety and discomfort, which is a reinforcing aspect of procrastination. In the short term, procrastination seems to be a good solution and helps you to feel better. However, in the long run, procrastination usually leads to bigger problems and more work. For example putting off paying your bills may feel good at the moment, but when your electricity is turned off and you have to pay late fees, and your roommates are upset with you because they thought you had paid the bill, your pleasurable feelings soon turn sour.

Men and women procrastinate equally often, but more people in the mid- to late 20s and 60-year-olds procrastinate more than people in any other age group do.[18] Individuals who procrastinate are frequently referred to as "lazy" or "stupid," but actually there are no differences in levels of intelligence between procrastinators and non-procrastinators. However, students who procrastinate tend to perform less well and retain less than students who do not. You might want to take the survey at the end of this chapter to assess your risk for procrastination.

Many people who procrastinate report feeling overwhelmed and highly anxious. They have difficulty tuning out external stimulation and concentrating on the task at hand. They also worry about how their performance will be judged by others and have perfectionistic standards for themselves. We discuss perfectionism and setting unrealistic goals in the next section.

Perfectionism   Perfectionism leads to undue stress because perfection is an unattainable goal. By setting the standard at perfect, you will set yourself up to fail. Perfectionists tend to be their own worst critic; they are harder on themselves than anyone else is on them, and they are also critical of others. These individuals are described as neat and organized, seeming to "have it all together" and to be able to do more than most people and do it exceptionally well. Often people envy perfectionistic people because they seem very confident and competent; however, individuals who are perfectionistic never feel good enough and often feel out of control in their lives.[19] People who are perfectionists focus on what they haven't accomplished or haven't done right rather than on what they have completed or have done well. Making mistakes feels especially humiliating to persons

---

┌─ **Key Terms** ─────────────────────────────┐

intrapsychic stressors Our internal worries, self-criticisms, and negative self-talk.

procrastination Putting off completing tasks until some later time, sometimes resulting in increased stress.

perfectionism A tendency to expect perfection in everything one does, with little tolerance for mistakes.

└───┘

who are perfectionistic, and they tend to feel a strong sense of shame and low self-esteem when someone catches them in error. They have difficulty with criticism or any negative feedback because much of their self-esteem is based on being accurate, competent, and being the best. While striving to do your best is an admirable quality, expecting to be perfect in everything you do and never making a mistake places a great deal of stress and pressure on yourself.

People with perfectionistic behavior tend to be rigid in their thinking, saying "I must be perfect or else I am a failure" and tend to put 100 percent of their effort into something or don't want to attempt it at all, which can lead to procrastination. In expecting perfection, there seems, to these individuals, to be a right and wrong way to do things. Thus, perfectionism can create a great deal of anxiety and distress.

Problems with Goal Setting and Time Management

With the rising cost of education, many students feel pressured to earn their degrees as quickly as possible, and this adds another layer of stress for them. Learning for the sake of learning can sometimes seem like a luxury, because earning top grades to get into graduate programs and land well-paying jobs tend to take priority. Research shows that many students drop out of college because they don't know why they are in school, haven't found a direction or major, and feel pressured to either declare a major or quit. In addition, an overwhelming number of students identify time management as the reason for their academic success or failure. Setting priorities and goals, balancing academic life with your social life, and finding time for sleeping, eating, exercising, and working along with studying are essential aspects of managing your stress effectively; strategies will be discussed later in this chapter.

Job Stressors

Americans are spending more time at work than ever. In fact, the United States has overtaken Japan as the industrialized country with the longest working hours. Americans work 350 more hours per year than European workers.[7] What is the cost of these increased work hours? Less leisure time; less time for family, exercise, and sleep; less time for anything else but work! Seventy-five percent of workers stated that they experience job stress or burnout at work. Conflict with coworkers was the number one source of job stress, followed by unrealistic work loads, tight deadlines, last-minute projects, and difficult bosses. What are the signs of job burnout?

- Coming in late for work and leaving early
- Frequently calling in sick to work
- Feeling unmotivated and apathetic at work
- Withdrawing from coworkers
- Watching the clock during work hours
- Doing other things at the job instead of work, such as surfing the Net and chatting online

What are some strategies for overcoming job stress? First, you need to identify what is causing you the most stress and focus on resolving that issue. If it is conflict with your boss or a coworker, talk it out (see the tips on conflict negotiation and communication strategies in Chapter 2). Set a goal of finding one thing you are looking forward to or like about your job. Are there ways you can make your job more enjoyable? Take a walk—get out of the office and take a break—when you notice you are feeling frustrated or unmotivated. Organize and prioritize your workload, and start with the most urgent tasks first. Ask for assistance if you need help with something and set reasonable goals for your workday. Getting enough rest, relaxation time, and good nutrition also go a long way in decreasing job stress.

Technological Stressors

We are having to learn how to deal with a whole new type of stress—technological stress. Destructive computer viruses; hundreds of junk mail ads sent through e-mail, instant messages, cell phones, and voicemail; and increasing worry about identity theft have brought new meaning to stress management. Over 450 new viruses are discovered each month and 82,000 hacking attacks are made each year.[20] Seventy-six colleges reported security breaches in the past year. Hacking costs companies over $17 billion a year and creates paranoia, extreme stress, and frustration in victims of these attacks. Computer attacks have become increasingly wider in scope, automated, and harder to trace.[20]

If you are swamped by the catalogs, junk mail, and credit card applications you receive through the U.S. mail, your stress level will probably only intensify with the deluge of junk mail received via e-mail, voicemail, and instant messaging. And Internet telephony spam, called "spit," is predicted to become a bigger problem in the future as more people make phone calls over the Internet rather than use the regular phone lines.[21] Marketers can program their computers to send 1,000 voice messages a minute over Internet telephony. "Spim" is spam sent out as an instant message, and it has increased to 2 billion messages in 2004, four times more than were sent in 2003.[22]

Even personal Web logs, or blogs, are not immune from these invasive advertisements. Spam messages masquerade as comments from readers, with some bloggers receiving 20 spam messages on their Web journals each day.

Phishing is the practice of sending e-mails and using fake websites to lure unsuspecting customers into

Protecting Yourself from Spim, Spam, Phish, and Viruses

How much "junk" do you receive via e-mail and instant messages every day? E-mail offers marketers a new way to reach many potential customers—and scammers a new way to reach potential victims. Although new technologies offer many advantages, they also create new types of stressful challenges in our lives, and you may need to develop new skills to meet those challenges. Be aware of the potential risks in the e-mail you receive, and learn to protect yourself from the hassles and stress that come with our increasingly technological society:

- Don't reply to e-mail or pop-up messages that ask for personal or financial information, and don't click on or cut and paste links in a message. Scammers can send an e-mail that appears to be from a legitimate business and ask you to click on a link or call a number to verify or update your account information. Do not follow these instructions. Legitimate companies don't ask for this information via e-mail.
- If you need to reach an organization you do business with, call the number on your financial statements or on the back of your credit card—not the number shown in a potentially fraudulent e-mail. Or type in the Web address yourself; phishers can make links look like they go to one place but actually send you to a different site.
- Cure-all products, weight-loss claims, and work-at-home schemes are among the most prevalent spam scams. If you are considering an offer you receive via e-mail, use the same caution you would in evaluating any type of ad for a product or service. Read the small print, and get all promises in writing. Resist any urge to "act now," despite an attractive offer and terms. And don't do business with any company that doesn't provide its name, street address, and telephone number.
- Don't start or forward chain letters that involve money or valuable items and promise big returns; these are illegal, and if you start a chain e-mail or letter or send one on, you are breaking the law.
- Don't e-mail personal or financial information. E-mail is not a secure method of transmitting personal information. Don't give our your Social Security number unless you absolutely have to, and don't give out your credit card or bank account information online unless you are certain you are using a legitimate and secure site.
- Review credit card and bank account statements as soon as you receive them to check for unauthorized charges.
- Install antivirus and antispyware software, and make sure you update it regularly.
- Install updated software and filters to block spam and spim. Almost all e-mail software includes some type of antispam program.
- Be cautious in opening e-mail attachments, particularly from senders you don't recognize. However, be wary even of attachments sent by accounts you recognize, because viruses can send e-mails from infected computers owned by people known to you. Use the same precaution when downloading files from the Internet.
- Use hard-to-guess passwords, and change them frequently. (Don't use names of pets or family members, significant dates, or similar data.)
- Back up key documents frequently using removable media.
- Consider installing a firewall security program to further protect your computer. If needed, consult with your university's computing services staff about security issues.
- When you receive spam that is phishing for information, forward it to spam@uce.gov and to the company, bank, or organization impersonated in the phishing e-mail.

Sources: "Phishing," OnGuard Online, www.onguardonline.gov/phishing.html, October 2006; "Spam Scams," OnGuard Online, www.onguardonline.gov/spam.html, September 2005; "All Email Users: What You Need to Know About Chain Emails & Letters," Federal Trade Commission, www.ftc.gov/bcp/conline/pubs/online/emailusers.htm, November 2002.

sharing personal and financial data such as credit card account numbers, checking account numbers, and Paypal account numbers. Phishers create websites that look almost identical to the real ones, such as those of financial institutions like Citibank, and then ask their customers to verify their account information, which allows phishers easy access to people's financial data. An estimated 57 million people received phish e-mails in 2004 alone.[23] E-mails received from phishers are convincing because phishers copy the "from" line from the real company to make them look authentic. Banks, eBay, and even some government agencies, including the IRS and the FBI, have been spoofed by phishers.

Spending an inordinate amount of time deleting these messages or losing hours of work on one's computer because of a virus or a worm can create a sense of powerlessness and hopelessness. When word spreads that a new virus is circulating, people become increasingly anxious. They can become angry with friends, coworkers, and family members for inadvertently spreading a virus to their computers.

For tips on reducing the technological stressors in your life, refer to the box "Protecting Yourself from Spim, Spam, Phish, and Viruses."

Environmental Stressors

Light, sounds, smells, air quality, and temperature can all affect your stress level. Some people feel more stressed if their environment is disorganized or messy, and feel a

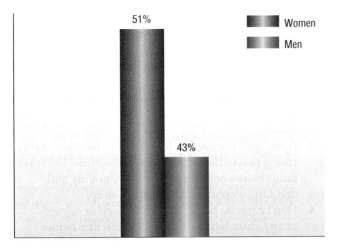

Figure 3-5 Stress and Gender   43 percent of men and 51 percent of women feel concerned about their level of stress.

Source: "Only Half of Worried Americans Try to Manage Their Stress," *USA Today*, February 23, 2006.

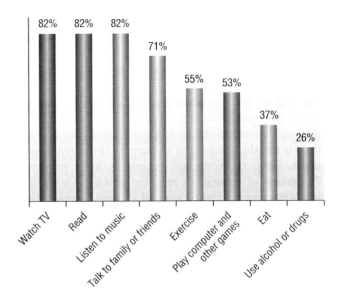

Figure 3-6 How Americans Cope with Stress   People have different ways of coping with stress, such as watching TV, reading, listening to music, or playing video games. How do you cope with stress?

Source: "Research Reveals Casual Games Provide Mental Balance, Stress Relief and Relaxation," www.realnetworks.com, August 14, 2006; "Americans Reveal Top Stressors, How They Cope," Mental Health America, www.nmha.org, November 16, 2006.

need to clean it up before they can concentrate or relax. As you read in Chapter 2, the amount of light and type of lighting you are exposed to can affect your levels of stress and depression. Artificial light, as well as certain colors, can increase one's stress level. People tend to associate the color red with anger and hostility and blue with depression.[24] Stress has also been linked to being exposed to prolonged, daily noise such as in a factory, at a construction site, or in a crowded room.[25] Air that is too cold or too warm, or that contains mold or pollutants, can be a source of stress. Higher temperatures have been associated with an increase in violence and aggression and decreased concentration and productivity. Situations in which one does not have control over one's environment—such as being stuck in a traffic jam, in line, or in an elevator—can also be stressful. Your stress level might also increase if you don't have control over the noise, temperature level, or appearance of your environment.

Approaches to Stress Management

The research on how people cope with crisis and stress in their lives has shown that people tend to resolve problems within two weeks of experiencing a crisis. Because stress involves a disruption in equilibrium, and the body does not function well in a chronic state of unbalance, it is human nature to seek a way to alleviate the stress the body is experiencing and return to a steady state. As we discussed previously, our bodies cannot function for very long in a sustained fight or flight response without serious damage, and so a person will naturally strive to make changes to resolve the stress for survival (Figure 3-5).

However, the way that people resolve their problems and alleviate stress may be positive or negative.

A number of negative ways of dealing with stress are quite common and often quite harmful. As indicated in Figure 3-6, some people turn to alcohol and drugs to avoid their problems and numb their feelings, and cigarettes are also cited as a way of relieving stress. Many people use food to comfort themselves. Putting off distasteful tasks and avoiding stressful situations is another negative way of coping with stress. Some people use sleep as a way of escaping their problems, and certainly depression has been associated with not having the ability to effectively manage stress. In the next section, we discuss ways of effectively managing stress.

What are some positive, effective methods to cope with stress? Different strategies and methods for stress management involve the physical, social, environmental, and psychological aspects of stress. We will review techniques and strategies within each of these dimensions, and you will need to practice and experiment to find the stress-management techniques that are right for you.

Physical Aspects of Stress Management

The physical aspects of stress management involve meeting your basic needs of sleep, exercise, and nutrition as was discussed in Chapter 2 under Maslow's hierarchy of needs.[26]

Our culture has developed an increasing need for speed. We are a fast-paced society, encouraged to eat, work, play, and move faster and faster. Our addiction to speed makes us a slave to time. What is the first thing you do in the morning when you wake up? Look at the clock, of course. Time tells us what to do when, and how long we have to engage in that activity. We have a need for speed that feeds our thirst for excitement and pumps out more adrenaline.

However, this pressure to do more in less time also causes stress in our lives. We can never be fast enough; there is never enough time. As Carrie Fisher once said, "Instant gratification takes too long." In order to beat the clock, we are consuming more caffeine and amphetamines and sleeping less. We are eating more fast food and gaining weight. We are working longer hours and taking less time to exercise, socialize, and enjoy leisure activities. The increase of road rage, relationship conflicts, and general lack of civility in our society has also been linked to our obsession with saving time. Time management and finding ways to do things more efficiently were originally intended to give us more leisure time and reduce the level of stress in our lives, but the opposite has occurred and we now pay a high price for speed.

However, there is a new, growing trend in the media called the "Slow movement." Books such as *In Praise of Slowness* discuss the merits of finding a balance in our lives and becoming more calm, careful, patient, and reflective and developing real, meaningful connections with people. In fact, the author contends that slower can be better, as we can develop healthier relationships, work, and family life. We can have higher quality in our food, exercise, and other aspects of our lives if we take the time to do things well. Sometimes doing something more slowly can yield faster results, because doing things quickly can result in making mistakes and having to redo things. The comedian Lily Tomlin once said, "For fast-acting relief from stress, try slowing down."

We are beginning to see this trend in many facets of life. Yoga and meditation have become increasingly popular, as has the Slow Food movement. In the United States and around the world, some cities are becoming "slow cities"—which means these communities have made a commitment to create an environment that helps people slow down. The slow philosophy translates into city ordinances such as banning motorized vehicles from some streets, banning fast-food chains and neon signs, and lowering speed limits. These communities have speed bumps that read "Ready, Set, Relax," and they set aside days for "family focus night" with no school practices, no homework, and no meetings. October 24 has been designated "Take Back Your Time Day" in the United States, because by October 24 each year, Americans have worked as much as Europeans do all year.

How can you begin to break away from the cult of speediness? Here are some tips:

1. Don't overschedule yourself.
2. Don't multitask. Focus on one thing only.
3. Take time to play.
4. Do nothing. Just sit there.
5. Meditate or do yoga.
6. Make a meal from scratch.
7. Eat without watching television, reading, or doing anything else.
8. Walk and talk slower than you normally do.
9. Don't wear a watch.
10. Let someone else go before you in line.
11. Don't drink caffeinated beverages.
12. Sleep eight hours a night.

Test yourself to see how difficult it is for you to do these things. Do you have trouble relaxing and doing nothing? Are you suffering from time sickness? It is important to note that the Slow movement doesn't necessarily mean that we do everything at a snail's pace. Instead, it means finding a balance in our lives. There may be times when it is appropriate to act quickly, to be time oriented, or to multitask. The Slow movement suggests only that we take back control of our time and go at our own pace, instead of rushing around because that is what we are supposed to do.

Sources: C. Honore, *In Praise of Slowness* (New York: HarperCollins, 2004); "Worldwide, We Seem to Have Lost the Art of Doing Nothing," *USA Today*, May 16, 2006.

produces calming effects such as lowered blood pressure and decreased heart rate. Cardiac patients who own pets tend to live much longer than those who have no pets.[33]

Environmental Aspects of Stress Management

To effectively manage your stress, you need to take into consideration environmental stressors such as noise level, amount of light, and aesthetic quality of the space you inhabit. Natural light tends to elevate your mood.[24] Having plants or photos of friends and family around your living and workspace can also alleviate stress.

Smell can also play a significant role in managing stress. As the saying goes, "Stop and smell the roses." Studies have shown that aromatherapy, using different aromas or odors therapeutically, can lower stress levels. When you breathe in the oils, they send a direct message to your brain via your olfactory nerves, where they can then affect the endocrine and the hormonal systems via the hypothalamus. Odors have an amazing effect on our emotional states because they hook into the emotional or primitive parts of our brains. Aromatherapy has been used to relieve pain, enhance relaxation and stress relief, unknot tense muscles, soften dry skin, and enhance immunity. So it is wise to pay attention to your aromatic surroundings, because they may affect you much more than you may realize.

While social interaction has been shown to have positive results on lessening the effects of stress, this beneficial effect depends on the type of friends with whom you surround yourself. Spending time with negative, pessimistic people can increase your stress level rather than decrease it. It is obviously more advantageous to surround yourself with positive, optimistic friends.[34] Feeling crowded in a room and not having enough personal space can also lead to an increase in stress.[35] Interestingly, it is not being in crowds itself but how familiar you are with the people, the activity that is taking place, and how much control you feel over your personal space that makes the difference. In other words, being in a crowded room filled with your friends during a party feels subjectively different than feeling trapped in a crowded restaurant filled with strangers.

Other important aspects of managing stress in your environment include having meaningful work and challenging and interesting classes. Having work that is stimulating but not beyond your abilities helps to keep your stress response at a moderate, optimal level for performance.

Psychological Aspects of Stress Management

Last, you can effectively cope with stress by using a variety of cognitive and psychological strategies. There are several different techniques, but as you will see, many are focused on deep breathing, which is the key to managing stress.

Relaxation and Deep Breathing The relaxation response, developed by Herbert Benson, M.D., is an effective way to ensure that you do not remain in the stress response too long. It is effective because it entails the opposite of the stress response. Rather than taking shallow breaths, you are required to breathe deeply, inhaling to a count of four and exhaling to a count of four while sitting in a comfortable position. As you breathe deeply, your muscles unwind and relax, again the opposite of the stress response. It is generally advised not to cross your legs or arms so that your muscles can relax easily. Blood flows to the extremities, and your heart rate slows. In fact, experienced users of this technique can temporarily lower their breathing rate from a typical rate of 14 to 18 breaths per minute to as few as 4 breaths per minute. Body temperature decreases, and blood pressure is lowered as well. The entire nervous system is slowed, in direct opposition to its role in the stress response. You are instructed to focus on your breathing and inner experience and become less aware of your external environment.

To help to tune out the outside world, you are instructed to close your eyes and let go of the worries and concerns of the day.[36]

To try this technique, take a moment to focus on your breathing and breathe in for a count of four and out for four. After doing so a few times, tighten your body, clench your hands, teeth, and jaw, close your eyes tightly, and pull your shoulders up while you are still breathing deeply. Are you able to do so? It is virtually impossible to tense your body and breathe deeply because they are mutually exclusive activities. Thus, the relaxation response is the foundation of most of the stress-management techniques described in this chapter. Deep breathing is the fundamental aspect of stress management, and it can also be used to alleviate anger; see the box "The Antidote for Anger . . . Relaxation."

Progressive Muscle Relaxation (PMR) In 1929 Edmund Jacobson, M.D., published a book describing a simple procedure of deliberately tensing and releasing major muscle groups in sequence from head to toe to achieve total relaxation of the body. His technique, called Progressive Muscle Relaxation, still enjoys popularity.[37] By learning to recognize the difference between contracted and relaxed muscles, Jacobson believed that people would be able to have more of a sense of control over their bodies and the stress response. Progressive muscle relaxation enables you to intentionally put certain muscles into a controlled state of relaxation and reduce your overall stress level.

PMR is based on the use of positioning your body in a comfortable position, sitting or lying down, and concentrating on certain muscle groups. As you inhale, breathing in for a count of four, you contract your muscles starting with your forehead and count to four as you exhale and relax your muscles. Continue to clench and relax the muscles, using your breathing to help you to tighten and release, working your way down your body all the way to your feet and toes. Concentrate on the sensations of relaxation and how different they are from the feelings of tension and stress. Fifteen minutes, twice a day, is the recommended schedule. In one to two weeks, you will have mastered the basics and will be aware of which muscles need more attention in order to relax. You will also be more sensitive to the buildup of tension in your body so that you will be able to decrease your stress level before it becomes overwhelming.[38]

Guided Imagery and Visualization In the early 1900s, Emil Coué, a French pharmacist, first suggested using human suggestibility to overcome the stress syndrome, to enhance recovery from illness, and to facilitate the accomplishment of positive goals.[39] By forming an image of a peaceful, serene place or seeing yourself being successful in accomplishing a task, you can use guided imagery or

The Antidote for Anger . . . Relaxation

When we are angry, our muscles tense, we breathe shallowly, and our adrenaline level increases, similarly to how we feel when we are stressed. Tension tends to build with the stress of increasing frustration, worry, discomfort, or unmet needs. The greater the stress, the more tension you feel. Expressing your anger can help to get rid of this tension, but only temporarily. You may have noticed that right after you get angry, maybe even blow up, you feel more relaxed and calm. Your muscles relax, the tension leaves your body, and you breathe more easily—but only briefly. Anger can create more anger because of the reinforcing effect that blowing up has in temporarily helping you feel better. Blowing up makes it easier to react the same way the next time, and the outbursts are usually stronger and harder to control each time.

As with the stress response, the key to managing anger is to change how we respond to events and express our anger. So, instead of blowing up, should you just keep your anger inside? No; this can eventually result in an explosion similar to that caused by pressure that builds in a pressure cooker or a shaken soda can. This is the "last straw" kind of anger response. To an observer, you may seem to be overreacting to a particular situation when you are really responding to a *multitude* of situations and frustrating events. You may take your anger out on an innocent bystander, or the dog.

Here are some tips on effective, respectful anger management:

1. *Relax,* take a deep breath, count to 10.
2. *Take a time-out if needed.* Don't continue to engage in a discussion if it is getting too heated.

3. *Avoid name calling.* Use "I" language, as was discussed in the previous chapter.
4. *Stay connected to the individual with whom you are speaking.* Don't withdraw physically or psychologically unless you need a time out, and then say this directly.
5. *Ask yourself what underlies your anger.* Hurt, guilt, feelings of rejection and shame, and fear of abandonment may be feelings that you need to express but that come out as anger. Especially for men, anger tends to be a more comfortable emotion to express.
6. *Is there a hidden agenda to your anger?* Are you using your anger to control, change, or punish someone? If so, use assertive language instead, and share your thoughts and feelings directly.
7. *Speak in a quieter, calmer voice than you typically do.* People tend to yell, speaking more loudly than normal in order to get the other person's attention. You may feel that you don't have power or people's attention unless you yell. While anger can be attention grabbing, this kind of attention is probably not what you want. People may tend to yell back, tune you out, or agree with you without meaning it, just to stop the yelling.
8. *Choose your battles wisely.* Don't argue every point. Ask yourself "Is this something that is really important to me and will be as meaningful tomorrow as it is right now?"

9. *Express your anger in a timely fashion.* Don't wait a week or a month to bring up issues when you have accumulated a bunch of things that have been bothering you over time. However, it may be more productive to wait until morning to express your anger if you are tired and irritable in the evenings. Another option is to wait and arrange a specific time to talk to avoid rushing through a conversation as you get ready to leave for work or class.
10. *It might feel easier or safer to redirect the anger you feel* toward your boss at your best friend or partner, but that doesn't solve your conflict with your boss and might create conflict with your friend or partner.

After you have respectfully expressed your anger, make sure you allow time and opportunity for the other person to express his or her feelings. Tell the person you appreciate how he or she listened to you and responded to you. Share other feelings besides the primary ones of hurt and anger, so that the person knows you can be angry with him or her and still care about him or her. Remember that your way of expressing anger and resolving conflict can either be destructive or be a way of connecting with people and improving relationships.

Sources: M. McKay, and P. Rogers, *The Anger Control Workbook* (Oakland: CA: New Harbinger, 2000): K. Paleg, and M. McKay, *When Anger Hurts Your Relationship* (Oakland: CA: New Harbinger, 2001).

---

visualization to manage your stress. Guided imagery involves having someone describe a beautiful, relaxing scene while you focus on taking deep, comfortable breaths. While in a comfortable position, in an environment free from interruptions and distractions, you breathe deeply, relax your muscles, and imagine a pleasant scene. The imagery includes all the senses, not just what you see but pleasant smells, sounds, touch, and even taste. Guided imagery can be self-taught, or you can listen to recordings of narrated scripts.

Visualization is similar to guided imagery with the scene being more specifically focused on something

you are about to do or want to accomplish, or on some performance or activity that may be causing you distress. Guided imagery and visualization techniques help you to change through positive mental images. For example, you might imagine yourself auditioning for a part in a play, seeing yourself go through your lines effortlessly and flawlessly, and feeling confident and proud of yourself. You are probably already skilled at visualization; unfortunately, we frequently engage in negative visualization and are unaware of doing so. For example, we imagine ourselves making fools of ourselves or making mistakes.

Yoga: The Union of Mind and Body

Yoga is often associated with Indian philosophy, such as Buddhism, but it has recently gained in popularity as a form of stress management. *Yoga* is a Sanskrit word meaning "union" of the individual soul with the universal soul. The practice of yoga directs and channels energy in a specific manner in the body. Individuals who practice yoga say they experience greater clarity in thinking and improved balance in their lives.

The reported benefits of regular yoga relaxation are numerous. They include:

- Better overall physical and mental health
- Increased energy and a feeling of restfulness
- "Spiritual unfoldment," which refers to an improved mind-body integration and an increased sense of harmony and peacefulness
- Enhanced concentration and focus
- A greater ability to cope with anxiety and daily stressors

Yoga has been shown to reduce heart rate and blood pressure, increase lung capacity, improve muscle relaxation, assist with weight management, and increase overall physical endurance. Yoga may affect levels of brain or blood chemicals, including monoamines, melatonin, dopamine, stress hormones (cortisol), and GABA (gamma-aminobutyric acid). Changes in mental functions, such as improved attention, cognition, processing of sensory information, and visual perception, have been described in some research studies in humans.

There are many different types of yoga, involving varying levels of meditation, posing, and activity. If you are interested in taking a yoga class, ask what type of yoga they teach:

- *Hatha yoga* is the most commonly known type of yoga. It focuses on simple poses that flow from one to the other at a very comfortable pace, while also focusing on breathing and meditation.

- *Kundalini yoga* is designed to activate the kundalini energy in the spine through poses, breath control, chanting, and meditation. It incorporates mantras (chanting), meditations, visualizations, and guided relaxation.
- *Kripalu yoga* starts with meditation and centering, breathing, warm-up movements, yoga postures, and relaxation.
- *Lyengar yoga* uses props such as chairs, straps, blocks, and pillows to help people do the poses more comfortably.
- *Ashtanga*, or *power yoga*, is the preferred yoga for athletes. Ashtanga yoga is light on meditation but heavy on developing strength and stamina. The poses are more difficult than those performed in other styles, and one moves quickly from one pose to another in an effort to build strength and flexibility.
- *Bikram yoga* is performed in a room that is at a temperature of 38 degrees C (100.4 degrees F) or higher to replicate the temperature of yoga's birthplace in India. The exercises are physically demanding and intense, with 26 postures that are performed in a certain order to warm up and stretch muscle, ligaments, and tendons.
- *Sivananda yoga* has a series of 12 poses, with the Sun Salutation, breathing exercises, relaxation, and mantra chanting as the basis.
- *Viniyoga yoga* is a slower, more individualized form of yoga that focuses on developing strength, balance, and healing.

To learn more about yoga, find a yoga class at your college or in the community.

Sources: www.yoga.about.com; "Complementary & Alternative Medicine," *Alternative Modalities for Health and Well-Being*, www.inteliheath.com, July 8, 2005; Kimbrough, J. Yoga for Better Health and Living, www.stress.about.com.

Athletes are trained in using positive visualization to improve their performance and visualize their goals.[38] Positive visualization has also been used in managing pain, especially in chronic pain management. This technique has also been effective in weight management, smoking cessation, insomnia, and for almost any type of behavior change. Some images commonly used to decrease stress are to visualize tightly twisted rope as uncoiling; hard, cold wax melting and softening; creaky hinges being oiled and becoming silent and gliding smoothly; or the feeling of sandpaper turning into silk. Again, guided imagery and visualization exercises have optimal benefit when practiced at least once a day, every day for 15 to 20 minutes.

Meditation Meditation allows the mind to transcend thought effortlessly when the person concentrates on a focal point. In transcendental meditation, a widely recognized approach to meditation, people repeat a mantra, or a personal word, while using deep-breathing and relaxation techniques. In other meditation approaches, alternative focal points are used to establish the depth of concentration needed to free the mind from conscious thought. Physical objects, music, and relaxing environmental sounds or breathing can be used as focal points. Meditation is also used in yoga; see the box "Yoga" for more information. Students who meditated twice a day for 15 minutes reported lowered blood pressure, better class attendance rates, and felt less stressed during their classes.

Hypnosis Hypnosis is an artificially induced state, resembling, but physiologically distinct from, sleep. It involves a heightened state of suggestibility that creates flexible and intensified attention and receptiveness, and an increased responsiveness to an idea or to a set of

Meditation can reduce blood pressure and lower stress level.

Use of a daily planner is a strategy that can help you manage your time more effectively as well as reduce your stress level.

ideas. The focus is on the unconscious rather than on the conscious state of mind, using deep-breathing and relaxation techniques. Hypnosis is perhaps the oldest and most misunderstood type of relaxation technique. It has been given a bad reputation by stage entertainers who use hypnosis to have unsuspecting audience members engage in embarrassing behavior.

Hypnosis is a natural state of mind that occurs spontaneously in nearly every person. It is a trancelike state, similar to those that you experience upon awakening, before falling asleep, or when you are engrossed in thought while performing other tasks—such as driving down a highway—on autopilot. It is possible to learn self-hypnosis from a trained professional or participate in hypnosis sessions with a qualified hypnotherapist.

Biofeedback The word *biofeedback* was coined in 1969 to describe procedures to teach people to alter brain activity, blood pressure, muscle tension, heart rate, and other bodily functions that are not normally controlled voluntarily. Biofeedback is a training technique in which people are taught to improve their health and performance by using signals from their own bodies. It operates on the premise that individuals can alter their involuntary responses by being "fed back" information either visually or audibly about what was occurring in their bodies. In addition, studies have shown that we have more control over so-called involuntary bodily functions than we once thought possible.

One commonly used device, for example, picks up electrical signals from the muscles and translates the signals into a form that people can detect. This device triggers a flashing light or activates a beeper every time muscles become more tense. To slow down the flashing or beeping, you need to relax tense muscles by breathing more slowly and deeply. People learn to associate sensations from the muscle with actual levels of tension and develop a new, healthy habit of keeping muscles only as tense as is necessary for as long as necessary. After

treatment, individuals are then able to repeat this response at will without being attached to the sensors. Other biological functions that are commonly measured and used in a similar way to help people gain control are skin temperature, heart rate, sweat gland activity, and brainwave activity. People can manage stress by decreasing the physiological components of the stress response.

Cognitive Aspects of Stress Management

Time Management Managing your time effectively can help you cope with your stress by feeling more in control, having a sense of accomplishment, and having a sense of purpose in your life. Establishing good time management habits can take two to three weeks. By using specific systems, even the most disorganized persons can make their lives less chaotic and stressful.

Assess Your Habits The first step is to analyze how you are spending your time. What are your most productive and least productive times of day and night? Do you tend to underestimate how long something will take you to complete? Do you waste time or allow interruptions to take you off task? Carrying a notebook with you for a week and writing down how you spend your time might provide you with some insight into the answers to these questions and how you spend your time. You might find that you've been devoting most of your time to less important tasks. Perhaps it is tempting to do your laundry rather than to start writing that term paper, but this is probably not the best use of your time.

Use a Planner Keeping a daily planner to schedule your time is the next step in managing your time more effectively. First block off all of the activities that are consistent,

I am always running from one thing to another and never get everything done that I plan to do. I am constantly late, doing things at the last moment, and this is causing me a great deal of stress and my friends are also getting aggravated with me. What can I do to better manage my time?

- Make a list of the things you need to accomplish, and then go back and prioritize the list using the A B C method to signify their urgency. Focus on getting the A tasks done first. Start on the Bs and Cs only if you have extra time.
- Break large tasks into smaller, more manageable pieces so that they don't seem so overwhelming.
- Set deadlines that are realistic, and give yourself a cushion of extra time in case things don't go according to plan.
- Check off items on your to-do list and consult it regularly.
- Do tasks that fit your time schedule and energy level.

- Ask yourself, "What is the best use of my time right now?"
- Do it now and don't procrastinate.
- Handle each piece of paper only once.
- Delegate.
- Say no to overcommitment. Be selective about what you volunteer to do, and give yourself permission to say no to your friends if necessary.
- Reward yourself when you finish a task.
- Vary your tasks so that you don't become bored.
- Set your goal at getting things done well enough and not perfectly.

Source: McGee-Cooper A. *Time Management for Unmanageable People*. New York: Bantam Books, 1994.

---

regular, weekly activities, such as attending classes, eating meals, sleeping, going to meetings, exercising, and working. Then look at the open, available time remaining. Schedule regular study time, relaxation time, and free time. Remember to schedule your study time during the more productive part of your waking hours. When you have a one-hour block of time, what can you realistically get done in that time? This could be a good time to review your notes from class, pay bills, or get some reading done.

Set Goals and Prioritize Set goals for the week as well as for each day. If something unexpected interferes with your time schedule, modify your plans but don't throw out the entire schedule.

Making a to-do list can be helpful, but it is only the first step (see the box "Tips for Better Time Management"). Breaking the large tasks into smaller, more manageable pieces and then prioritizing them is the key to effective time management. When you prioritize your tasks, try the ABC method of task management. The A tasks are those items that are most urgent and must be done today. Then the B tasks are those things that are important but, if need be, could wait 24 hours. The C tasks are activities that can easily wait a few days to a week. Don't fall into the C trap, which is when you do the less important tasks because they are quick and can be checked off your list with ease. This can lead to putting off the more important A activities, leaving them until you feel stressed and overwhelmed.

Stress Inoculation Working in a manner similar to a flu shot, stress inoculation involves exposing an individual to specific stressful situations, a little at a time, under controlled, safe conditions. Stress inoculation teaches

individuals to relax using deep breathing and progressive muscle relaxation while they are being exposed to stressful situations.

The first step is to construct your personal list of stressful situations and arrange the list from the least to the most stressful items, and learn how to evoke each of these situations in your mind while at the same time focusing on your breathing and relaxing your muscles. The second step is to create an arsenal of stress-coping thoughts, such as "I'm going to be all right," "I've succeeded with this before," and "Getting started is the hardest part, then it will get easier for me." The third step is to practice this *in vivo*, meaning in real-life situations, while using the relaxation and cognitive techniques to minimize the stress response.[39] In addition to stress management, stress inoculation has also been helpful in anger management.

Cognitive Self-Talk What we tell ourselves, our self-talk, has a tremendous effect on how well we manage our stress. Stress can be generated from faulty conclusions, misinterpretations, and expecting the worst. Some people claim that if they expect the worst, they won't feel disappointed or hurt, but in reality, they still feel the pain from their disappointment. We need to be careful about what we expect because we may inadvertently make it happen, a phenomenon referred to as a **self-fulfilling prophecy.**[40]

> ### Key Terms
>
> **self-fulfilling prophecy** The tendency to make something more likely to happen as a result of one's own expectations and attitudes.

Self-fulfilling prophecies can work for you or against you. If you expect that work will be boring and uninteresting, you will tend to portray a negative, unmotivated attitude and will probably have a miserable time. However, if you expect to enjoy yourself at work, you are more likely to go looking for challenge and to have fun.

If we look more closely at how we make faulty conclusions and misinterpretations, we recognize a number of cognitive distortions that lead to a more stress-filled life, such as:

1. *Filtering.* Selectively paying attention to the negative and disregarding the positive.
2. *Polarized thinking.* Putting things into absolute, all-or-nothing categories with no middle ground. For example, you have to be right or else you are wrong.
3. *Overgeneralization.* From one isolated event, you make a general, universal rule. For example, if you have failed once, you will always fail.
4. *Mind reading.* Without people saying so, you believe you know what people are feeling and the reasons they behave the way they do. For example, if your friend seems tired, you think she doesn't really want to go out to the movies tonight as you had planned and so you cancel the plans thinking that is what she really wants.
5. *Catastrophizing.* Expecting disaster or the worst-case scenario.
6. *Personalization.* Thinking that things people do or say is in reaction to you and comparing yourself with others. For example, you walk past a group of people laughing and assume that they are laughing at you.
7. *Fallacy of fairness.* Feeling resentful when situations don't seem fair or just. Believing that good things happen to good people and bad things happen to bad people.
8. *Shoulds.* Telling yourself what you are supposed to do, what is expected of you, or what you feel obligated to do rather than what you want to do. This is often something we don't want to do but think we should do and feel somewhat pressured or forced to do.

To change these cognitive distortions, you need to generate some rebuttals to your negative self-statements. This entails finding middle ground between all-or-nothing thinking by asking yourself what evidence proves that a statement is true and identifying some exceptions to this statement. Look for balance by asking yourself what is the opposite of this negative self-statement. Rather than telling yourself what you "should" do ask yourself what you "want" to do. Be specific instead of overgeneralizing, and avoid labeling yourself and others. Instead of telling yourself "I'm lazy," you might say, "I wish I would have studied a few more hours for that test." Stick

to the facts without blaming yourself or others. Question yourself as to how you know something is true and if you might be making an assumption or "mind reading." Be mindful of your self-fulfilling prophecies. It may be wiser to acknowledge that you don't know or consider many different possible outcomes rather than to expect the worst.

Changing negative self-talk requires time, practice, and patience. We develop these patterns of thinking over years, and they become almost automatic. It takes concentrated effort to be aware of and change negative thinking. Remember that your rebuttals need to be strong, nonjudgmental, and specific. Practice developing more flexible and balanced thinking about people, behavior, and situations.

Conquering Procrastination   Some techniques for combating procrastination involve time management, stress management, assertiveness training, and increasing self-esteem and self-acceptance. Specifically with regard to time management, procrastinators tend to both over- and underestimate how much time a task will take. When they underestimate the time, they feel justified in procrastinating because they erroneously believe they have plenty of time to complete the task. When they overestimate the time needed, they feel intimidated by the magnitude of the job, feel anxious, and so have trouble getting started. So it is important to give yourself more time than you think you might need for a project and start earlier than needed in case of unforeseen delays. Breaking the task down into manageable pieces can also help it seem less daunting.

People also report procrastinating when they feel forced or pressured to do something they don't want to do. Rather than communicating assertively, they rebel by agreeing to do something but constantly put it off, which can be a passive-aggressive way of behaving. They fear the consequences of saying no or not fulfilling their obligations but are also angry about what they perceive as unfair expectations and demands on them. This is when some assertiveness training may be helpful. Finally, increasing self-esteem can solve problems with procrastination because feeling better about yourself relieves you of worrying about what others think of you and having constantly to prove yourself to them. Some people procrastinate because they think they need to do everything perfectly or not at all. With increased self-esteem, you are more accepting of mistakes and don't expect yourself to perform perfectly.

Combating Perfectionism   Perfectionism is often associated with obsessive-compulsive disorder as well as with eating disorders. Having perfectionistic tendencies can also create stress and conflict in relationships because people who interact with perfectionists feel as

Combating Perfectionism

My girlfriend is a perfectionist and she is driving me crazy. Nothing I do seems good enough for her as much as I try to please her. Her unrealistic expectations are causing a great deal of stress in our relationship and our friends are beginning to stay away from us because they don't like to hear us argue. What can I do?

Sometimes people who are perfectionists tend to blame others for their own sense of failure or rejection. Here are some ways to respond better to your girlfriend:

1. Communicate how you feel when she is critical of you or shows her disapproval. Suggest more positive ways that she can give you feedback or share her disappointments.
2. Give specific examples of how she may be expecting too much, and find a compromise between all or nothing.
3. Don't retaliate. It is tempting to point out her flaws when she is doing the same to you. Instead, reassure her that you think highly of her and point out her successes and accomplishments, since she is probably focusing on her failures.
4. Communicate your confidence in her abilities and ask her to have the same trust in you.
5. Model acceptance of imperfection in yourself and others. Show her that everybody is flawed, no one is perfect, and this makes us human.
6. Don't focus on her mistakes or tease her when she makes an error. Instead give positive reinforcement when she doesn't do something well.
7. Help her to relax and have fun even if all the work is not yet done.
8. Talk about how she is feeling rather than the content of her message, such as saying "You sound very stressed and overwhelmed."
9. Don't fall into the perfectionist trap yourself. It is easy to think, "If I just try harder, she will be happy with me." Perfectionism is an impossible goal to reach, and so you are setting yourself up for failure and rejection.
10. Help her to see the forest rather than the trees. It is easy for perfectionists to get lost in the details and lose sight of the overall goal. It may help to alleviate her stress if you can help her to refocus on what is really important and what the overall goal is, such as having fun at the party you are throwing and not having the house perfectly clean.

though nothing they do is good enough or will please that person.

To help alleviate the stress of perfectionism, base your self-esteem on who you are rather than on what you do. This involves accepting yourself and others unconditionally, including imperfections (see the box "Combating Perfectionism"). Lowering your expectations of yourself and others and aiming for 80 percent rather than 100 percent is another strategy in battling perfectionism. Note what you are doing well and have accomplished rather than what is still left to do. Push yourself to take risks and allow yourself to make mistakes. It can be useful to make mistakes on purpose in order to get accustomed to this experience and realize that people still like and accept you and nothing bad will happen. Relaxation and stress-management techniques such as the ones described at the end of this chapter can also help alleviate the stress that comes with perfectionism. You might want to take the survey at the end of this chapter to assess your level of perfectionism.

As you can see, there are many different aspects to consider in managing stress, as well as its physical, social, environmental, and psychological components. As you think about how you can more effectively manage your stress level, you will need to practice and experiment to find the stress-management techniques most beneficial for you.

TALKING POINTS Think back to stressful times in your life. What were some positive ways you coped, and what were some negative things you did to cope?

A Realistic Perspective on Stress and Life

The development of a realistic approach to today's fast-paced demanding lifestyle may best be achieved by fostering many of the following perspectives:[41]

Anticipate problems and see yourself as a problem solver. Although each specific problem is unique, it is most likely similar to past ones. Use these past experiences to quickly recognize ways of resolving new problems.

Search for solutions. Act on a partial solution, even when a complete solution seems distant. By resolving some aspects of a problem, you can gain time for more focused consideration of the remaining difficulties. In addition, some progress is a confidence builder that can help you remain committed to finding a complete solution.

Take control of your own future. Set out to accomplish your goals. Do not view yourself as a victim.

Also, recall from Chapter 2 that being proactive and optimistic is an excellent way to take charge of your life and recognize capabilities that you were previously unaware of.

Be aware of self-fulfilling prophecies. Do not extend or generalize difficulties from one area into another. Further, negativity about yourself, in the form of self-doubt and self-blame, is certain to erode your feelings of success.

Visualize success. Focus on those things that are necessary and possible to ensure success. The very act of "imaging," seeing oneself performing skillfully, has proven beneficial in a variety of performance-oriented activities.

Accept the unchangeable. Focus on taking control of what you can and letting go of the rest. The direction your life takes is only in part the result of your own doing. Cope as effectively as possible with those events over which you have no direct control; beyond a certain point, however, you must let go of those things over which you have little control.

Live each day well. Combine activity, contemplation, and a positive attitude approaching the many things that must be done each day. Celebrate special occasions. Undertake new experiences. Learn from your mistakes. Recognize your accomplishments. Most importantly, however, remember that the fabric of our lives is far more heavily influenced by day-to-day events than it is by the occasional milestones of life.

Act on your capacity for growth. Undertake new experiences and then extract from them new information about your own interests and capacities. The multiple dimensions of health identified in Chapter 1 will, over the course of your lifetime, provide a wide array of resources that will allow growth to occur throughout your entire life.

Allow for renewal. Make time for yourself, and take advantage of opportunities to pursue new and fulfilling relationships. Foster growth in each of the multiple dimensions of health—physical, psychological, social, intellectual, spiritual, and occupational. Initial renewal in one dimension may serve as a springboard for renewal in others.

Accept mistakes. Both you and others will make mistakes. Recognize that these can cause anger, and learn to avoid feelings of hostility. Mistakes, carefully evaluated, can serve as the basis for even greater knowledge and more likely success in those activities not yet undertaken.

Keep life simple. Keep the demands of life as orderly and manageable as you can. Just as adding too many appliances to an electrical circuit will quickly overload it and cause a power outage, excess demands and commitments added to our daily schedule can quickly burn out our psyches. Learning to prioritize and postpone activities is key to building a productive and enjoyable life.

Taking Charge of Your Health

- Complete the Student Stress Checklist at the end of this chapter.

- Determine if you suffer from perfectionism by completing the Perfectionism assessment at the end of this chapter.

- Join a yoga, meditation, or exercise class on campus or in the community.

- Assess your sleep hygiene and incorporate into your sleep habits some of the tips recommended in this chapter.

- Prioritize your daily goals in a list that you can accomplish, allowing time for recreational activities.

- Counteract a tendency to procrastinate by setting up imaginary (early) deadlines for assignments and rewarding yourself when you meet those dates.

- Replace a negative coping technique that you currently use, such as smoking, with an effective alternative, such as deep breathing, relaxation exercises, yoga, or exercise.

- List the positive aspects of your life, and make them the focus of your everyday thoughts.

SUMMARY

- Stress refers to physiological changes and responses your body makes in response to a situation, a real or a perceived threat.
- The fight or flight response is a physiological response to perceived, anticipated, or real threat; it causes the heart to race, breathing becomes labored, muscles are tense, the body sweats, and blood flow is decreased to the extremities and digestive organs and increased to the major muscles and brain.
- Chronic stress refers to remaining at a high level of physiological arousal too long and not being able to take immediate, effective action to alleviate the perceived or real threat.

- While too much stress can have a negative effect and cause some serious health problems, a moderate level of stress is positive and beneficial.
- Constant arousal and increased levels of adrenaline in your system will eventually wear down your body's immunological system. You will be less able to cope with stress, and so it takes less and less stress to cause a stress reaction.
- General Adaptation Syndrome is a sequenced physiological response to the presence of a stressor, involving the alarm, resistance, and exhaustion stages of the stress response.
- An overwhelming number of students identify time management as the reason for their academic success or failure. Setting priorities and goals and balancing academic life are essential aspects of managing your stress effectively.

- To effectively manage your stress, you need to take into consideration environmental stressors such as the noise level, amount of light, and aesthetic quality of the space you inhabit. It is also important to get adequate amounts of sleep, excercise, and nutrition.
- The relaxation response is effective because it entails the opposite of the stress response. Rather than taking shallow breaths, breathe deeply, inhaling to a count of four and exhaling to a count of four while sitting in a comfortable position.
- Effective psychological tools for stress management include progressive muscle relaxation, visualization, guided imagery, meditation, hypnosis, biofeedback, stress inoculation, cognitive self-talk, conquering procrastination, combating perfectionism, and setting realistic goals.

REVIEW QUESTIONS

1. What is stress?
2. How does stress relate to your physical and psychological health?
3. What is the fight or flight response?
4. What are some long-term physiological effects of chronic stress?
5. Describe the Yerkes-Dodson Law.
6. Explain the three stages of the General Adaptation Syndrome.
7. List at least five types of stressors students can experience.
8. List some environmental stressors, and explain how high levels of stress have been linked to environmental factors.
9. Describe the relaxation response and how it is effective for stress management.
10. Name seven cognitive and psychological stress-management techniques, and explain how they work.

ANSWERS TO THE "WHAT DO YOU KNOW?" QUIZ

1. False   2. True   3. True   4. True   5. True   6. False   7. True

As We Go to Press

Stress Elimination: Just Take a Pill to Forget Your Stress?

Taking a pill to erase your memory sounds like something out of the movie *X-Men*. In the case of propranolol, life imitates art. Propranolol (Inderol) is a beta blocker historically used in the treatment of hypertension. Its controversial proposed new use is to erase traumatic memories and stress. When people are stressed, adrenaline is released. Adrenaline can enhance performance when produced at a moderate level. Increased adrenaline can also enhance memory. However, propranolol acts to block adrenaline, and in doing so it weakens memory or stops memories from becoming stronger. It has been suggested that propranolol be used for victims of trauma, such as rape victims, soldiers, and accident victims, to weaken the intensity of their psychological trauma and help them go on with their lives. There is currently an experimental study underway using propranolol to weaken or alter memories.

Although alleviating the anxiety, depression, and stress associated with a trauma may seem to be effective treatment for people with posttraumatic stress disorder, the Council on Bioethics has questioned the ethics of changing people's memories. They contend that our memories are part of who we are, and that changing people's memories of the past is paramount to rewriting people's lives and can fundamentally alter our identities.

Proponents for propranolol defend the use of this drug by comparing it to giving morphine to someone in severe pain. They contend that since we prescribe medications to take away physical pain, why not also prescribe them for psychological pain?

The bioethicists want to know where the line will be drawn—in other words, what experiences will be considered traumatic enough to warrant administering propranolol to erase the person's memories of them? If you had a relationship breakup, were fired from your job, or just had a bad day, would you want to take a pill to forget it?

Sources: "A Pill to Forget" Leslie Stahl, CBS, *60 Minutes*, November 26, 2006; "Unmaking Memories: Interview with James McGaugh," http://scientificamerican.com, December 13, 2003.

ENDNOTES

1. Selye H. Stress *Without Distress*. New York: New American Library, 1975.
2. Scott LV, Dinan T. Vasopressin and the regulation of hypothalamic-pituitary-adrenal functions: Implications for the pathophysiology of depression. *Life Sci* 1998; 62(22): 1985–1998.
3. Selye, H. *The Stress of Life. New York*: McGraw-Hill, 1984.
4. Girdano DA, Everly GS, Dusek DE. *Controlling Stress and Tension.* Boston: Allyn & Bacon, 1996.
5. Raber M, Dyck G. *Managing Stress for Mental Fitness.* Menlo Park, CA: Crisp, 1993.
6. Baucum D, Smith C, Kagan J. *Psychology: An Introduction.* 9th ed. Orlando, FL: Harcourt Brace Jovanovich, 2003.
7. Honore C. *In Praise of Slowness.* New York: HarperCollins, 2004.
8. Davis M, Eshelmar E, McKay M. *The Relaxation and Stress Reduction Workbook.* Oakland, CA: New Harbinger, 2000.
9. Robinson B. *Overdoing It. How to Slow Down and Take Care of Yourself.* Deerfield Beach, FL: Health Communications, 1992.
10. Holmes T, Rahe R. Social Readjustment Rating Scale. *Journal of Psychosomatic Research,* 11, 1967.
11. Rowh M. *Coping with Stress in College.* New York: College Board Publications, 1989.
12. Affordable care for kids squeezes college students. *Detroit News,* November 23, 2001.
13. Newman E. *No More Test Anxiety.* Los Angeles, CA: Learning Skills, 1996.
14. Lindzey G, *Thompson R, Spring B. Psychology* (3rd ed.). New York: Worth, 1988.
15. Arem C. *Conquering Math Anxiety: A Self-Help Workbook.* Pacific Grove: CA: Brooks/Cole, 1993.
16. Kahn N. *More Learning in Less Time.* Berkeley, CA: Ten Speed Press, 1992.
17. Roberts M. *Living Without Procrastination.* Oakland, CA: New Harbinger, 1995.
18. Ferrari J, Johnson J, McGown W. *Procrastination and Task Avoidance: Theory, Research and Treatment.* New York: Plenum, 1995.
19. Basco M. *Never Good Enough.* New York: Simon & Schuster, 1999.
20. Tech pros get to know their enemy. *USA Today,* Septmber 23, 2003.
21. Irritated by spam? Get ready for spit. *USA Today,* November 10, 2004.
22. Spam's irritating cousin, spim, on the loose. *USA Today,* March 1, 2004.
23. Fighting phish, fakes, and frauds. *E. commerce Security,* September 1, 2004.
24. Rosenthal NE. *Winter Blues.* New York: Guilford Press, 1998.
25. Goliszek AG. *Breaking the Stress Habit.* Winston-Salem, NC: Carolina Press, 1987.
26. Maslow AH. *Motivation and Personality* (2nd ed.). New York: Van Nostrand, 1970.
27. Ferber R. *Solve Your Child's Sleep Problems.* New York: Simon & Schuster, 1985.
28. Sleep treatments rise to the occasion *USA Today,* February 27, 2006.
29. Saladin KS. *Anatomy & Physiology: The Unity of Form and Function.* New York: McGraw-Hill, 2001.
30. Lefcourt HM, Martin RA. *Humor and Life Stress: Antidote to Adversity.* New York: Spring-Verlag, 1986.
31. Asterita MF. *The Physiology of Stress.* 4–5. New York: Human Sciences Press, 1985.
32. Hugging warms the heart and also may protect it. USA *Today,* March 10, 2003.
33. Allen K, Shykoff BE, Izzo JL, Jr. Pet ownership but not ACE inhibitor therapy blunts home blood pressure responses to mental stress. *Hypertension 2001,* October, 38(4), 815–820.
34. Seligman M. *Learned Optimism.* New York: Simon & Schuster, 1990.
35. Wade C, Tavris C. *Psychology.* New York: Harper & Row, 1987.
36. Benson H. *The Relaxation Response.* New York: Avon, 1976.
37. Jacobson E. *Progressive Relaxation.* Chicago: University of Chicago Press, 1942.
38. Fanning P. *Visualization for Change.* Oakland, CA: New Harbinger, 1988.
39. McKay M, Davis M, and Fanning P. *Thoughts and Feelings: The Art of Cognitive Stress Intervention.* Oakland, CA: New Harbinger, 1981.
40. Jones RA. *Self-Fulfilling Prophecies.* Hillsdale, NJ: John Wiley, 1977.
41. McGinnis L. *The Power of Optimism.* New York: Harper & Row, 1990.

Personal Assessment

Student Stress Checklist

Put a check next to those stressors that apply to you.

Academic

_____ Difficulty managing time

_____ Deadlines

_____ Poor grades

_____ Competition

_____ Exams

_____ Pressure to do well (parents', own, and/or others' expectations)

_____ Study skills deficit

_____ Earned academic awards

_____ Completion of a big project

_____ Keeping scholarships

_____ Other

Interpersonal Relationships

_____ Too much or too little social activity

_____ Dating

_____ Conflict with others

_____ Few or no supportive relationships

_____ Long-distance relationship issues

_____ Sexual difficulties

_____ Beginning a new romantic relationship

_____ Negotiating relationships with professors

_____ Joining an organization

_____ Other

Personal

_____ Poor physical or psychological health

_____ Family difficulties

_____ Lack of social support

_____ Death of a loved one

_____ Financial problems

_____ Having a gay/lesbian/bisexual/transgendered identity

_____ Homesickness

_____ Change in eating or sleeping pattern

_____ Conflict in values

_____ Recent life changes (moved to a new location, new job, marriage, etc.)

_____ Becoming more independent

_____ Not belonging/fitting in

_____ Having a pet

_____ Holiday/semester breaks

_____ Dissatisfaction with appearance

_____ Peer pressure

_____ Difficulty controlling alcohol and/or drug use

_____ Other

Career

_____ Lack of career direction

_____ Unhappy with major

_____ Declaring a major

_____ Internship placement (e.g., student teaching)

_____ Graduation

_____ Other

Employment

_____ Difficulty with boss

_____ Unstable work hours

_____ Change in working conditions

_____ Job offer

_____ Promotion (more responsibility)

_____ Possible military deployment of self/friends/family

_____ Other

Environment

_____ Discrimination

_____ Unsatisfactory living environment

_____ Transportation difficulties

_____ Commuting

_____ Parking

_____ Other

_____ **Total Stressors Checked**

TO CARRY THIS FURTHER . . .

How well do you think you are managing your stress? (Make a mark on the continuum where you think you fit.)

0 . . . . 1 . . . . 2 . . . . 3 . . . . 4 . . . . 5 6
Not at   Very
all   well

Keep in mind that two people with the same number of stressors may experience their stress differently. A person with a small number of stressors may feel overwhelmed by them, while a person with many stressors may feel they are manageable. As you consider the number of stressors in your life, it is important to recognize how well you manage them. Regardless of the number of stressors, if you are not managing your stress well, we encourage you to seek help in developing positive coping skills.

Personal Assessment

Am I a perfectionist?

Below are some ideas that are held by perfectionists. Which of these do you see in yourself? To help you decide, rate how strongly you agree with each of the statements below on a scale from 0 to 4.

0	1	2	3	4
I do not agree		I agree somewhat		I agree completely

_____ 1. I have an eye for details that others can miss.

_____ 2. I can get lost in details and forget the real purpose of the task.

_____ 3. I can get overwhelmed by too many details.

_____ 4. It stresses me when people do not want to do things the right way.

_____ 5. There is a right way and a wrong way to do most things.

_____ 6. I do not like my routine to be interrupted.

_____ 7. I expect a great deal from myself.

_____ 8. I expect no less of others than I expect of myself.

_____ 9. People should always do their best.

_____ 10. I am neat in my appearance.

_____ 11. Good grooming is important to me.

_____ 12. I do not like being seen before I have showered and dressed.

_____ 13. I do not like making mistakes.

_____ 14. Receiving criticism is horrible.

_____ 15. It is embarrassing to make mistakes in front of others.

_____ 16. Sharing my new ideas with others makes me anxious.

_____ 17. I worry that my ideas are not good enough.

_____ 18. I do not have a great deal of confidence in myself.

_____ 19. I'm uncomfortable when my environment is untidy or disorganized.

_____ 20. When things are disorganized it is hard for me to concentrate.

_____ 21. What others think about my home is important to me.

_____ 22. I have trouble making difficult decisions.

_____ 23. I worry that I may make the wrong decision.

_____ 24. Making a bad decision can be disastrous.

_____ 25. I often do not trust others to do the job right.

_____ 26. I check the work of others to make certain it was done correctly.

_____ 27. If I can control the process it will turn out fine.

_____ 28. I am a perfectionist.

_____ 29. I care more about doing a quality job than others do.

_____ 30. It's important to make a good impression.

_____ **TOTAL SCORE**

Scoring

Add all 30 items together to get your total score. If your score was less than 30, then you are probably not a perfectionist, although you may have a few of the traits. Scores from 31 to 60 suggest mild perfectionism. When you are stressed your score may be higher. Scores of 61 to 90 suggest moderate perfectionism. This probably means that perfectionism is causing you trouble in some specific areas, but is not out of control. Scores higher than 91 suggest a level of perfectionism that could cause you serious problems.

TO CARRY THIS FURTHER . . .

If you or a friend of family member scored in the moderate to high range for perfectionism, consider taking some of the steps described in this chapter for combating perfectionism. Allow yourself to take risks and make mistakes. General relaxation strategies can also be helpful in overcoming an unhealthy degree of perfectionism.

Source: Adapted with the permission of The Free Press, a Division of Simon & Schuster Adult Publishing Group, from *Never Good Enough: Freeing Yourself from the Chains of Perfection* by Monica Ramirez Basco, Ph.D. Copyright © 1999 by Monica Ramirez Basco. All rights reserved.

The Body

Part Two contains three chapters whose content is especially relevant to college students: fitness, nutrition, and weight management. This part will help you learn how to improve your health in these areas.

1. **Physical Dimension**
   Health experts believe that fitness, nutrition, and weight management are interrelated. How well our bodies work depends on what we eat and how we exercise. Healthy bodies allow us to participate in daily activities and recover more quickly from illness and injury.

2. **Psychological Dimension**
   When you start a fitness program or begin to pay attention to your diet, you learn about your level of motivation and commitment. You will be challenged, but the psychological rewards for your efforts, such as an improved self-concept and greater confidence, can be substantial.

3. **Social Dimension**
   The social dimension of health is closely related to fitness, nutrition, and weight management. Exercising with friends offers an opportunity for social interaction. Participation in most group fitness activities involves listening, sharing, and counseling. Food, like alcohol, can function as a "social lubricant" by bringing and holding people together. However, excessive food intake and lack of exercise can hinder social relationships when a person is significantly above his or her desirable weight.

4. **Intellectual Dimension**
   Some evidence suggests that people feel mentally sharper after they exercise. Many students report that they can study more efficiently after a workout. People deprived of adequate exercise and proper nutrition may suffer intellectual impairment. Regular physical activity, a sound diet, and effective weight management will allow you to enjoy a wide range of new experiences that can lead to improved intellectual functioning.

5. **Spiritual Dimension**
   Throughout this text we emphasize that an important part of your spiritual growth is serving others. Staying physically fit, following a healthful diet, and managing your weight can enhance your ability to serve others. You can express your own spirituality and help others find meaning in their lives when you take proper care of your health.

6. **Occupational Dimension**
   Just as you can better serve others when you feel your best, you can also pursue a career and carry out daily occupational tasks when you take care of your body. Some job functions, such as traveling and heavy lifting, require that you be in good physical condition. In addition, being fit can help you deal more effectively with the stress that inevitably accompanies employment. Taking care of your body can increase your self-esteem and improve your confidence—a definite plus when you are trying to land a job or earn a promotion.

Becoming Physically Fit

What Do You Know about Exercise and Physical Activity?

- One of the benefits of endurance (aerobic) exercise training is that it improves both your good (HDL) and bad (LDL) cholesterol. True or False?

- The old saying "Use It or Lose It" is correct when applied to exercise training. True or False?

- You can estimate your maximal heart rate by subtracting your age from 200. True or False?

- You will burn more calories in a typical aerobic exercise training session than you will in a typical resistance training session. True or False?

- Exercise is a subcategory (that is, a specific type) of physical activity. True or False?

- A person will obtain a greater improvement in aerobic fitness by exercising at higher intensity for a shorter duration compared with a more moderate intensity performed for a longer duration. True or False?

- Ballistic stretching, which involves repetitive, forceful movements, is the recommended type for flexibility training. True or False?

Check your answers at the end of the chapter.

Online Learning Center Resources
www.mhhe.com/payne10e

Visit the Online Learning Center for tools to improve your grade and get the most out of your course—chapter objectives, practice quizzes, key terms flashcards, chapter summaries for your digital audio player, Web activities, self-assessments, and many other study aids.

For many people, the day begins early in the morning; continues with classes, assignments, study, a job, and/or recreational activities; and does not end until after midnight. This kind of pace demands that one be physically fit. Even a highly motivated college student must have a conditioned, rested body to maintain such a schedule.

Of course, many college students do not look at **physical fitness** as a means to a more satisfying, exciting life. Instead, many students look for the cosmetic benefits of fitness. They want to look in the mirror and see the kind of body they see in the media: one with well-toned muscles, a trim waistline, and an absence of flabby tissue, especially on the arms, legs, abdomen, and hips. Thus, many students become motivated to start exercise programs because they hope that they can build a better body. Through their efforts to do so, students usually start to feel better, physically and mentally. They realize that physical fitness can improve every aspect of their lives, because they see it happening with each passing week.

Fortunately, you need not become a full-time athlete to enjoy the health benefits of fitness (see the box "What Is Your Goal: Health or Fitness?"). Indeed, the Surgeon General has reported that significant

Have you received mixed messages about how much exercise is necessary? Some reports tout that all you need to do is more general types of activities (raking leaves, walking the dog.) Others suggest that you can get benefits with multiple short walks throughout the day. And of course, you can go to the gym and hear that you have to feel the burn to make it worthwhile. So which message is correct? Surprisingly, all of them! It just depends on what your goal is.

Prior to the 1990s, fitness professionals recommended that you needed to exercise above certain minimal (of time, intensity, and frequency) levels to obtain fitness benefits. Their message was correct; however, many people believed that if they could not meet the minimums, they were obtaining no benefits. Thus, it was viewed as an all-or-none proposition.

In 1995 the American College of Sports Medicine and the Centers for Disease Control and Prevention issued a public health statement on Physical Activity and Health. This report documented that there are clear benefits to 30 minutes a day of moderate-intensity physical activity and suggested that activities such as gardening and housework could be beneficial to health. Another important aspect of this report was that the health benefits could be obtained by accumulating activity throughout the day (for example: three 10-minute bouts of activity; one in the morning, one in the afternoon, and one in the evening). Unfortunately, many individuals misunderstood this message and started suggesting that more vigorous forms of activity (exercise) were not really necessary and the term exercise lite was born.

What got confused was the difference between health benefits and fitness benefits. The Surgeon General's Report on Physical Activity and Health was issued in 1996 and helped clarify the message from the ACSM/CDC report. Clearly there are numerous health benefits to regular physical activity. Among these benefits are control of body weight, blood pressure, blood sugar, and cholesterol. The Surgeon General also operationalized the amount of activity required to obtain health benefits as 150 kilocalories per day. The Report suggested that this could be achieved in a variety of ways (15 minutes of jogging, 30 minutes of walking, or 45 minutes of playing volleyball). Additionally, they clarified that doing more than this amount would result in additional benefits. In other words the more activity (dose), the greater the benefits (response).

The publication *Dietary Guidelines for Americans,* published in 2005, concurred with these recommendations and advised additional physical activity to help control body weight. Specifically, they recommend 60 minutes of moderate-to-vigorous intensity activity to prevent weight gain, and 60–90 minutes of daily moderate intensity activity to sustain weight loss in adulthood.

Because exercise is a form of physical activity, when one exercises regularly, one gets the same (or greater) health benefits as those who choose to just maintain a regularly active lifestyle. Of course the bonus for those who exercise is that they will also derive physical fitness benefits from their program.

So, the choice is yours. If your principle goal is to maintain good health, accumulating a moderate amount of physical activity on most days will work. However, if your goal is health and physical fitness, then exercise is required.

---

health benefits can be achieved if you accumulate a moderate amount of physical activity on most, preferably all, days of each week.[1]

Four Components of Physical Fitness

People who engage in regular exercise often choose physical activities that fit their lifestyles and individual preferences. These activities have the potential for helping them achieve a state of physical fitness. Physical fitness is characterized by the ability to perform occupational and recreational activities without becoming unduly fatigued and to have the capacity to handle unforeseen emergencies.

In the following sections, we discuss cardiorespiratory endurance, muscular fitness, flexibility, and body composition. These characteristics of physical fitness can be categorized as health-related physical fitness. Other characteristics, such as speed, power, agility, balance, and reaction time are associated with what would be called performance-related physical fitness. Although the latter type is most important for competitive athletes, it is the former type that has the most relevance to general population. Thus, this chapter focuses on health-related physical fitness.

Cardiorespiratory Endurance

If you were limited to improving only one area of your physical fitness, which would you choose—muscular

---

Key Terms

physical fitness A set of attributes that people have or achieve that relates to the ability to perform physical activity.[2]

physical activity Any bodily movement produced by skeletal muscles that results in energy expenditure.[2]

exercise A subcategory of physical activity; it is planned, structured, repetitive, and purposive in the sense that an improvement or maintenance of physical fitness is an objective.[2]

strength, muscular endurance, or flexibility? Which would a dancer choose? Which would a marathon runner select? Which would an expert recommend?

The experts, exercise physiologists, would probably say that another fitness dimension is of even greater importance than those just listed. These research scientists regard improvement of heart, lung, and blood vessel function as the key focal point of a physical fitness program.

Cardiorespiratory endurance forms the foundation for whole-body fitness. Cardiorespiratory endurance increases your capacity to sustain a given level of energy production for a prolonged period. Development of cardiorespiratory endurance helps your body to work longer and at greater levels of intensity.

Aerobic vs. Anaerobic Exercise Occasionally your body cannot produce the energy it needs for long-term activity. Certain activities require performance at a level of intensity that outstrips your cardiorespiratory system's ability to transport oxygen efficiently to contracting muscle fibers.

This oxygen-deprived form of energy production is called **anaerobic** (without oxygen) **energy production,** the type that fuels many intense, short-duration activities. For example, rope climbing, weight lifting for strength, and sprinting are short-duration activities that quickly cause muscle fatigue; they are generally considered anaerobic activities. The key factor is if the energy demand of the activity exceeds the aerobic energy production capability. Thus, even activities that typically are considered to be aerobic (walking or cycling) can require anaerobic energy if the intensity is high.

If you usually work or play at low intensity but for a long duration, you have developed an ability to maintain **aerobic** (with oxygen) **energy production.** As long as your body can meet its energy demands in this oxygen-rich mode, it will not convert to anaerobic energy production. Thus fatigue will not be an important factor in determining whether you can continue to participate. Marathon runners, serious joggers, distance swimmers, bicyclists, and aerobic dancers can perform because of their highly developed aerobic fitness. The cardiorespiratory systems of these aerobically fit people have developed a large capacity to take in, transport, and use oxygen.

Benefits of Cardiorespiratory Endurance Following a program of regular aerobic exercise improves the capacity of your cardiovascular and muscular systems. More specifically, regular aerobic exercise strengthens the muscles of your heart, enabling your heart to pump more blood with fewer strokes to meet the demands you place on it. As a result, your resting heart rate may become slower than in the past, indicating that you have become more physi-

cally fit. At the same time, your skeletal muscles develop improved metabolic machinery to allow them to use more oxygen and thus produce more energy. This cardiorespiratory endurance (also called cardiorespiratory fitness or aerobic fitness) enables you to deal more easily with the routine and extraordinary demands of your daily life.

In addition, improving your cardiorespiratory (aerobic) fitness has a variety of benefits that can improve nearly all parts of your life.[3] Aerobic fitness can help you gain the following physical benefits:

- Control of your weight
- Greater ability to perform a wide variety of activities throughout your life
- Ability to ward off infections
- Increased efficiency of your other body systems
- Reduced concentration of triglycerides and increased concentration of high-density lipoproteins ("good cholesterol") in your blood
- Reduced risk of heart disease and certain types of cancer (breast and colon)
- Increased capillary network
- Prevention of hypertension, type 2 diabetes, and osteoporosis
- Increased longevity
- Improved psychological health
- For women, reduced number and severity of symptoms associated with premenstrual syndrome (PMS); see Chapter 14 for more information.

Aerobic fitness also offers a variety of other benefits that, although not immediately obvious, are no less important. For example, the increased stamina that comes with cardiorespiratory fitness enables you to complete and better enjoy your daily activities. In addition, your improved fitness level may reduce the severity and shorten the duration of common illnesses. Likewise, you will find your ability to cope with stressors to be increased with your fitness level. As a result, you may find your sense of well-being and confidence to be improved (see the box "Harnessing the Spirit").

Older adults will find that improving their cardiorespiratory fitness enables them to enjoy their later years to a greater extent, giving them the energy and ability to participate in activities that they might have delayed for many years, such as traveling, or even activities they might never have considered, such as joining a square dance club or learning how to line dance.

When you become aerobically fit, you may be able to achieve a long-held goal, such as hiking part of the Appalachian Trail, climbing Mt. Rainier, or bicycling through Europe. Others might find that becoming physically fit reduces their dependence on substances such as

Harnessing the Spirit: The Saga of Lance Armstrong

In the summer of 1999, American cyclist Lance Armstrong made one of the most amazing sports comebacks in history. Armstrong won the Tour de France, the most grueling cycling event in the world. In October 1996, Armstrong had been diagnosed with advanced testicular cancer and was given less than a 50 percent chance of survival. At the time of the diagnosis, the cancer had already spread to Armstrong's abdomen, lungs, and brain.

After being diagnosed with cancer, but before starting aggressive therapy, Armstrong declared himself "a cancer survivor, not a cancer victim." He convinced himself, his family, and his medical support team that he could beat the long odds facing him. He even established the Lance Armstrong Foundation (www.laf.org) before he had surgery and chemotherapy. He battled through his therapy without giving up the hope that the cancer would be defeated.

Miraculously, Armstrong's cancer disappeared. He then stunned the cycling world by returning to active training and planning a comeback that included competing for the 1999 Tour de France title. As Armstrong's physical condition improved and his training regimen became more demanding, cycling enthusiasts believed that Armstrong might be able to compete in—but certainly not win—the world's most famous bike race.

Armstrong proved his doubters wrong by winning the 1999 Tour de France. Perhaps even more amazingly, he has won the Tour de France *again* in the years 2000, 2001, 2002, 2003, 2004, and 2005, and he participated on the U.S. Olympic Cycling Team at the Sydney Olympics in 2000, winning a bronze medal in the Men's Individual Time Trial event. Armstrong chronicled his battle with testicular cancer in his best-selling book *It's Not About the Bike* (Putnam) and followed this with a cycling training book called *The Lance Armstrong Performance Program* (Rodale Press). Clearly, his powers of the mind and spirit worked to help him overcome his physical barriers. His success story has undoubtedly inspired others to take charge of their lives by doing their best to rise above mental and physical barriers to pursue the dreams that sometimes seem impossible.

---

alcohol, cigarettes, or other drugs and that they sleep more soundly.

Finally, while you are pursuing your physical fitness activities, you probably will meet other healthy, active people and find that you are expanding your circle of friends. The box "A Different Kind of Fitness" takes a look at the physical and social benefits for persons with disabilities who participate in the Special Olympics.

Muscular Fitness

Muscular fitness is the term used to represent the capabilities of the skeletal muscles to perform contractions. The capacity of the muscles have two distinct yet integrated characteristics: **muscular strength** and **muscular endurance.** The strength of the muscle is related to its ability to perform at or near its maximum for a short period of time. The endurance of the muscle is related to its ability to perform at submaximal levels for a long period of time.

Muscular fitness is essential for your body to accomplish work. Your ability to maintain good posture, walk, lift, push, and pull are familiar examples of the constant demands you make on your muscles to maintain or increase their level of contraction. The stronger you are, the greater your ability to contract muscles and maintain a level of contraction sufficient to complete tasks.

Benefits of Muscular Fitness Training People who regularly perform muscular fitness exercises obtain a variety of benefits. Strength training will improve

Key Terms

cardiorespiratory endurance The ability of the heart, lungs, and blood vessels to process and transport oxygen required by muscle cells so that they can contract over a period of time; cardiorespiratory endurance is produced by exercise that requires continuous, repetitive movements.

anaerobic energy production The body's alternative means of energy production, used when the available oxygen is insufficient for aerobic energy production; anaerobic energy production is a much less efficient use of stored energy.

aerobic energy production The body's primary means of energy production, used when the respiratory and the circulatory systems can process and transport sufficient oxygen to muscle cells to convert fuel to energy.

muscular fitness The ability of skeletal muscles to perform contractions; includes muscular strength and muscular endurance.

muscular strength The component of physical fitness that deals with the ability to contract skeletal muscles to a maximal level; the maximal force that a muscle can exert.

muscular endurance The aspect of muscular fitness that deals with the ability of a muscle or muscle group to repeatedly contract over a long period of time.

body composition, both by maintaining or increasing muscle mass and possibly by lowering body fat. Muscular fitness exercises reduce body fat largely by raising the person's resting metabolic rate, which is directly related to the amount of muscle mass a person has. Such exercises also promote improved clearance of glucose from the blood. Impaired glucose clearance can lead to diabetes.

It is also well known that people with good levels of muscular fitness can perform a variety of activities of daily living (ADLs), such as carrying a bag of groceries with more ease. These functional benefits of muscular fitness become even more important as people age. Regular resistance training can help improve balance and may increase bone mass. Thus, it may help prevent falls in the elderly, which often result in bone fractures leading to disability.

Key Terms

flexibility The ability of joints to function through an intended range of motion.

Flexibility

The ability of your joints to move through their natural range of motion is a measure of your **flexibility.** This fitness trait, like so many other aspects of structure and function, differs from point to point within your body and among different people. Not every joint in your body is equally flexible (by design), and, over the course of time, use or disuse will alter the flexibility of a given joint. Certainly gender, age, genetically determined body build, and current level of physical fitness affect your flexibility.

One's inability to move easily during physical activity can be a constant reminder that aging and inactivity are the foes of flexibility. Failure to use joints regularly will quickly result in a loss of elasticity in the connective tissue and shortening of muscles associated with the joints. Benefits of flexibility include improved balance, posture, and athletic performance and reduced risk of low-back pain and injury.

Body Composition

Body composition refers to what the body is made up of (muscle, bone, fat, water, minerals).[4] Of particular inter-

Muscular fitness training has both functional and health benefits. People with good muscular fitness can perform daily tasks more easily and enjoy more recreational activities. Muscular fitness training can also improve body composition.

est to fitness experts are percentages of body fat and fat-free weight. Health experts are especially concerned about the large number of people in American society who are overweight and obese. Cardiorespiratory fitness trainers increasingly are recognizing the importance of body composition and are including strength-training exercises to help reduce body fat. (See Chapter 6 for further information about body composition, health effects of obesity, and weight management.)

 TALKING POINTS Which benefits of exercise are most important to you? What would motivate you to become and stay active?

Developing a Personalized Fitness Program

Principles of Training

A personalized exercise program should meet both the needs and the preferences of the individual. The best exercise program is the one that the person will perform regularly. However, there are a number of principles of training that need to be followed for the program to be successful.

The most basic of all the principles of exercise training is *overload*. The objective of exercise is to improve something in the body (such as heart function). To obtain this improvement, the body must be placed under a stress to make it work harder than it is usually accustomed to. When a body part or system is overloaded in an appropriate manner, that body part undergoes adaptation, increasing the capability of that body part.

A second important principle of training is *specificity*. To produce an adaptation, the exercise must be specific to the outcome that is targeted for improvement. A good example of this can be seen by considering two different types of strength training, isometric and isotonic. Over time, persons who regularly perform isometric exercises will increase their capacity to perform an isometric contraction (they will be able to generate more muscular force without lengthening their muscle); however, their ability to perform muscular contractions throughout the full range of motion will not be improved significantly.

A third important principle of training is *reversibility* (sometimes referred to as regression). This is basically what is meant by the old saying "Use It or Lose It." In order for people to maintain the benefits of exercise, they must perform the exercise on a regular basis. See the box "Sticking to Your Exercise Program" for advice on keeping your program on track. Specific details of how to train will be discussed in the following sections.

Cardiorespiratory Endurance

For people of all ages, cardiorespiratory conditioning can be achieved through many activities. As long as the activity you choose places sufficient demand on the heart and lungs, improved fitness is possible. In addition to engaging in the familiar activities of swimming, running, cycling, and aerobic dance, many people today participate in brisk walking, rollerblading, cross-country skiing, swimnastics, skating, rowing, and even weight training (often combined with some form of aerobic activity). Regardless of age or physical limitations, you can select from a variety of enjoyable activities that will condition the cardiorespiratory system. (Complete the Personal Assessment at the end of this chapter to determine your level of fitness.)

Many people think that any kind of physical activity will produce cardiorespiratory fitness. Often people consider golf, bowling, hunting, fishing, and archery to be forms of exercise. If performed regularly and for sufficient periods of time, they may enhance your health. However, they do not meet the requirements to be called exercise and would not necessarily improve physical fitness. The American College of Sports Medicine (ACSM), the nation's premier professional organization of exercise physiologists and sport physicians,[5] has well-accepted guidelines for exercise training.

The ACSM's most recent recommendations for cardiorespiratory conditioning were published in 2005.[6] The four major factors that are important for cardiorespiratory training are (1) mode of activity, (2) frequency, (3) intensity, and (4) duration. ACSM has also made recommendations for muscular fitness and flexibility training. We summarize these recommendations. You may wish to compare your existing fitness program with these standards.

Mode of Activity The ACSM recommends that the mode of activity be any continuous physical activity that uses large muscle groups and can be rhythmic and aerobic in nature. Among the activities that generally meet this requirement are continuous swimming, cycling, aerobics, basketball, cross-country skiing, rollerblading, step training (bench aerobics), hiking, walking, rowing, stair climbing, dancing, and running. Water exercise (water or aqua aerobics) has become a popular fitness mode, because it is especially effective for pregnant women and older, injured, or disabled people.[7]

Endurance games and activities, such as tennis, basketball, racquetball, and handball, are fine as long as you and your partner are skilled enough to keep the ball in play; walking after the ball will do very little for you. Softball and football are generally less than sufficient continuous activities—especially the way they are played by weekend athletes. An old coaching adage applies here: You get in shape to play the game, you do not play the game to get in shape. In other words, using recreational sports is not an effective method to develop physical fitness; however, it may be a useful (and enjoyable) way to maintain fitness.

Regardless of which continuous activity you select, it should also be enjoyable. Running, for example, is not for everyone—despite what some accomplished runners say! Find an activity you enjoy. If you need others around you to have a good time, corral a group of friends to join you.

Cross-training is the use of more than one aerobic activity to achieve cardiorespiratory fitness. For example, runners may use swimming, cycling, or rowing periodically to replace running in their training routines. Cross-training allows certain muscle groups to rest and injuries to heal. In addition, cross-training provides a refreshing change of pace for the participant.

Vary your activities to keep from becoming bored. You might cycle in the summer, run in the fall, swim in the winter, and play racquetball in the spring. The box "Exercising in an Urban Environment" has suggestions for meeting the special challenges posed by urban environments.

Frequency of Training Frequency of training refers to the number of times per week a person should exercise. The ACSM recommends three to five times per week. For most people, participation in fitness activities more than five times each week does not significantly further improve their level of conditioning. Likewise, an average of only two workouts each week does not seem to produce a measurable improvement in cardiorespiratory conditioning. Thus, although you may have a lot of fun cycling twice each week, do not expect to see a significant improvement in your cardiorespiratory fitness level.

Intensity of Training How much effort should you put into an activity? Should you run quickly, jog slowly, or swim at a comfortable pace? Must a person sweat profusely to become fit? These questions all refer to **intensity** of effort.

The ACSM recommends that healthy adults exercise at an intensity level of between 65 percent and 90 percent of their maximum heart rate, which is estimated by subtracting one's age from 220. However, be aware that there could be a considerable difference between estimated maximal heart rate and actual maximal heart rate (measured during a maximal exercise test). Or, one should exercise at an intensity level between 50 percent and 85 percent of one's heart rate range. This level of intensity is called the **target heart rate** (THR) (see the box "How

---

Key Terms

frequency The number of exercise sessions per week; for aerobic fitness three to five days are recommended.

intensity The level of effort put into an activity; for aerobic fitness 50 percent to 85 percent of heart rate range is recommended.

target heart rate (THR) The number of times per minute the heart must contract to produce a cardiorespiratory training effect.

duration The length of exercise time of each training session; for aerobic fitness, 20–60 minutes per session is recommended.

People who live in large cities face special challenges as they pursue fitness activities. Some of these challenges are just annoying, but some challenges can be life-threatening. News reports occasionally tell of someone who was seriously injured or killed (accidentally or intentionally) while trying to exercise in an urban environment. Visitors to cities can also be confronted with these difficulties, and visitors may be less experienced adjusting to these challenges than those who live year-round in the city.

Among the obstacles are pollution, heavy vehicular and pedestrian traffic, and the possibility of criminal activity. These problems may also exist in small towns, but they likely exist to a lesser degree. Resist the temptation to use "the city" as an excuse not to exercise. Fortunately, you can tailor a fitness program to fit the urban environment in numerous ways. Consider these strategies as you plan your fitness activities in the city.

- *If you are unfamiliar with the environment, exercise indoors.* It can be dangerous to jog, rollerblade, or cycle in a place where you could become lost. Exercise inside your home or apartment, a local health club or YMCA, or in your hotel. Many indoor exercise machines provide a good cardiorespiratory and strength-training workout. Some facilities also have swimming pools, indoor tracks, handball courts, and special fitness classes.

- *If you plan to exercise outdoors, always do so with a partner.* There is, indeed, safety in numbers. Exercising with a friend or two (or jogging with a large, leashed dog) can provide a measure of protection. If you become injured, friends can help summon medical assistance.

- *Try to avoid heavily congested areas.* Cycling or jogging in heavy traffic is dangerous not only for you but also for other pedestrians and motorists. This is especially true during rush hours (7–9 a.m., noon, and 4–6 p.m.). Try to locate a relatively quiet place that also seems secure. If you are a visitor to an area, make certain you know whether a particular area is safe for walking, cycling, or jogging. Don't assume that every urban park is a safe haven for exercisers.

- *Do not exercise outside at night.* A city can take on an entirely different mood during the night. It is foolish to place yourself at risk by exercising outside when it is dark. Stick to the daylight hours.

- *Be aware of pollution levels before you exercise.* If there is a pollution warning, consider exercising indoors until the alert is over. If you are one who must exercise outside, you might wish to use a pollution mask; the mask will filter a significant amount of large particles. However, it may also serve to attract unnecessary attention.

- *Consider carrying an alarm or protective spray device when exercising outdoors.* This suggestion has both proponents and opponents. Carrying a protective spray device or alarm can be helpful, if you know how to use it in an emergency. Remember, some devices can be used against you, especially if an assailant surprises and overpowers you.

to Calculate Your Target Heart Rate"). This rate refers to the minimum number of times your heart needs to contract (beat) each minute to have a positive effect on your heart, muscles, and blood vessels. This intensity produces a *training effect*. Activity at an intensity below the THR will be insufficient to make a significant improvement in your fitness level. Although intensity below the THR will still help you expend calories and thus lose weight, it will probably do little to make you more aerobically fit. However, intensity that is significantly above your THR will probably cause you to become so fatigued that you will be forced to stop the activity before the training effect can be achieved.

Choosing a particular THR depends on your initial level of cardiorespiratory fitness. If you are already in relatively good physical shape, you might feel comfortable starting exercise at 70 percent of your heart rate range. A well-conditioned person needs to select a higher THR for his or her intensity level, whereas a person with a low cardiorespiratory fitness level will still be able to achieve a training effect at a lower THR of 50 percent of heart rate range.

In the example in the box, the younger person would need to participate in a continuous activity for an extended period while working at a THR of 158 beats per minute. The older person would need to function at a THR of 150 beats per minute to achieve a positive training effect.

Determining your heart rate is not a complicated procedure. Find a location on your body where an artery passes near the surface of the skin. Pulse rates are difficult to determine by touching veins; the blood pressure is lower in veins than in arteries, making it more difficult to feel a pulse. Two easily accessible sites for determining heart rate are the carotid artery (one on each side of the windpipe at the front of your neck) and the radial artery (on the inside of your wrist, just above the base of the thumb).

Practice placing the front surface of your index and middle fingertips at one of these locations and feeling for a pulse. Once you have found a regular pulse, look at the second hand of a watch. Count the number of beats you feel in a 15-second period. Multiply this number by 4. This number is your heart rate. With a little practice, you can become proficient at determining heart rate.

Duration of Training The ACSM recommends that the **duration** of training be between 20 and 60 minutes of continuous aerobic activity. Generally speaking, the duration can be on the shorter end of this range for people whose activities use a high intensity of training (75 percent to 85 percent of heart rate range). Those who choose activities with a low range of intensity (50 percent to 60 percent of heart rate range) should

Key Terms

overload principle The principle whereby a person increases the resistance load to levels above which they are normally accustomed to; this principle also applies to other types of fitness training.

isometric exercises (**eye** so **met** rick) Muscular strength-training exercises in which the resistance is so great that the object cannot be moved.

isotonic resistance exercises Muscular strength-training exercises in which traditional barbells and dumbbells with fixed resistances are used.

isokinetic exercises (**eye** so kin e tick) Muscular strength-training exercises in which machines are used to provide variable resistances throughout the full range of motion at a fixed speed.

maintain that activity for a longer time. Thus a fast jog and a moderate walk require different amounts of time to accomplish the training effect. The fast jog might be maintained for 25 minutes, whereas the brisk walk should be kept up longer—perhaps for 50 minutes. The bottom line is to achieve what ACSM calls an adequate volume (total amount) of exercise. ACSM recommends that individuals should expend between 1,000–2,000 kilocalories per week in aerobic exercises to obtain a cardiorespiratory training effect. This total volume can be achieved in a variety of ways. For example, some people may choose to exercise at a moderate intensity (50 percent to 60 percent of heart rate range) for a longer duration (40 minutes per session) and higher frequency (5 days per week), whereas others can get similar benefits by choosing higher intensity (75 percent to 80 percent of heart rate range) with a shorter duration (30 minutes per session) and lower frequency (4 days per week).

Muscular Fitness

Recognizing that overall body fitness includes muscular fitness, the ACSM now recommends resistance training in its current standards. The ACSM suggests participation in resistance training two or three times a week. This training should help develop and maintain a healthy body composition—one with an emphasis on lean body mass. The goal of resistance training is not to improve cardiorespiratory endurance but to improve overall muscle strength and muscular endurance. For some people (individuals with hypertension or type 2 diabetes), resistance training with heavy weights is not recommended because it can induce a sudden and dangerous increase in blood pressure.

Muscular strength can best be improved by training activities that use the **overload principle.** By overloading, or gradually increasing the resistance (load, object, or weight) your muscles must move, you can increase your muscular strength. The following three types of training exercises are based on the overload principle.

Types of Muscular Fitness Exercises Muscular endurance can be improved by performing repeated contractions of a less than maximal level. This aspect of muscular fitness is most related to common physical activities (leaf raking, pushing a lawn mower). Although it is not as glamorous as muscular strength, muscular endurance is an important part of muscular fitness.

In **isometric** (meaning "same length") **exercises,** the resistance is so great that the contracting muscles cannot move the resistant object at all. For example, you could contract your muscles against an immovable object such as a wall. Because of the difficulty of precisely evaluating the training effects, isometric exercises

Many types of inexpensive accessory equipment are available for muscular fitness training, including resistance bands (left), stability balls (center), and weighted "medicine" balls (right).

are not usually used as a primary means of developing muscular strength and can be dangerous for people with hypertension.

Isotonic resistance exercises, also called *same-tension exercises,* are currently the most popular type of strength-building exercises and include the use of traditional free weights (dumbbells and barbells), as well as many resistance exercise machines. People who perform progressive resistance exercises use various muscle groups to move (or lift) specific fixed resistances or weights. Although during a given repetitive exercise the weight remains the same, the muscular contraction effort required varies according to the joint angles in the range of motion.[4] The greatest effort is required at one angle (sticking point) in the range of motion of the movement.

Isokinetic (meaning "same motion") **exercises** use mechanical devices that provide resistances that consistently overload muscles throughout the entire range of motion. The resistance moves only at a preset speed regardless of the force applied to it. For the exercise to be effective, a user must apply maximal force. Isokinetic training requires elaborate, expensive equipment. Thus the use of isokinetic equipment may be limited to certain athletic teams, diagnostic centers, or rehabilitation clinics. The most common isokinetic machines are Cybex, Mini-Gym, ExerGenie, KinCom, and Biodex.

Free Weights or Machines? Which type of strength-building exercise (machines or free weights) is most effective? Take your choice, since all will help develop muscular strength. Some people prefer machines because they are simple to use, do not require stacking the weights, and are already balanced and less likely to drop and cause injury. Other people prefer free weights because they encourage the user to work harder to maintain balance during the lift. In addition, free weights can be used in a greater variety of exercises than can weight machines.

Accessory Equipment What about other types of equipment? There are many types of equipment that can be used for strength training. Some types may focus on one part of the body (such as the abdominal muscles), while others also train additional skills, such as balance. Here are just a few of the many available types of accessory equipment:

- *Resistance tubes and bands* come in different levels of resistance and are useful for training a variety of muscle groups in movement patterns that mimic everyday activities. They are small and lightweight, making them easy to store and ideal for taking along on a trip.

- *Stability balls* come in different sizes and are useful for training the core muscle groups (principally the abdominal and back muscles).

- *Inflatable exercise discs* can be used to train both strength and balance.

- *Weighted exercise ("medicine") balls* come in different weights and are useful both for training the upper body muscles and as an added source of resistance when doing abdominal exercises. Throwing and catching the balls can also assist in balance training.

- *Abdominal isolation devices* comes in variety of different styles and are useful for training the abdominal muscles.

- *Hard foam rollers* come in different sizes and are useful for training the core muscle groups, for balance, and for therapeutic relief for some forms of muscular tension.

Talk with an exercise professional to learn what pieces of equipment might work best for you and how to properly use the equipment. The good news is that many of these exercise accessories are inexpensive enough to purchase for use at home.

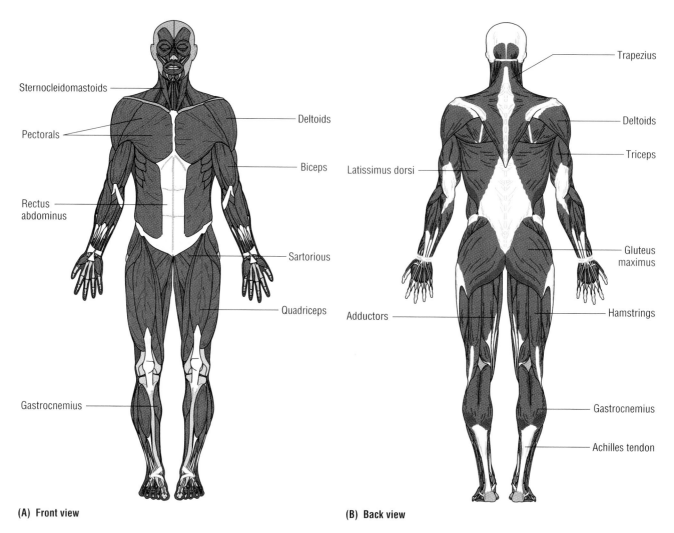

(A) Front view

(B) Back view

Figure 4-1 Major Muscle Groups

Frequency, Intensity, and Duration The resistance training recommended by the ACSM includes one set of 8 to 12 repetitions (10 to 15 repetitions for individuals over age 50) of 8 to 10 different exercises performed twice per week. Although any weight that produces an overload will result in improvement, the greatest muscular fitness gains will be achieved if the weight lifting results in fatigue of the muscle (that is, more than 12 repetitions cannot be performed). These exercises should be geared to the body's major muscle groups (for example, legs, arms, shoulders, trunk, and back) and should not focus on just one or two body areas (Figure 4-1). Isotonic (progressive resistance) or isokinetic exercises are recommended. For the average person, resistance training activities should be done at a moderate-to-slow speed, use the full range of motion, and not impair normal breathing. With just one set recommended for each exercise, resistance training is not very time consuming. See the box "Considering Strength Training? Think Safety . . ." for additional guidelines for a safe and effective program.

Changing for the Better

Considering Strength Training? Think Safety . . .

I'm a 22-year-old college student thinking about starting a strength training program. What kinds of safety precautions should I take?

- Warm up appropriately.
- Use proper lifting techniques.
- Always have a spotter if you are using free weights.
- Do not hold your breath during a lift.
- Avoid single lifts of very heavy weights.
- Before using a machine (such as Nautilus, Paramount, or Cybex), be certain you know how to use it correctly.
- Seek advice for training programs from experts (individuals with academic training and fitness training certification).
- Understand your current strength level; avoid exercises that are beyond your capacity.

Flexibility Training

To develop and maintain a healthy range of motion for the body's joints, the ACSM suggests that flexibility exercises be included in one's overall fitness program. Stretching can be done in conjunction with other (cardiorespiratory or muscular fitness) training or can be performed separately. Note that if flexibility training is done separately, a general warm-up should be performed before stretching so that the muscles are warm before they are stretched.

Types of Stretching Exercises   Flexibility can be developed through **static stretching,** which involves the slow lengthening of a muscle group, or through **ballistic stretching,** which involves repetitive and forceful bouncing movements. Athletic trainers generally prefer static stretching for people who wish to improve their range of motion, because ballistic stretching carries a higher risk of soft-tissue tears and injury. For most people, static stretching is the best type.

Frequency, Intensity, and Duration   The ACSM recommends that a flexibility program include stretches for all the major muscle and/or tendon groups. Stretching exercises should be performed at least three days per week, but stretching is an activity that can be safely performed daily. Each stretch should extend to a position where you feel mild discomfort in the muscle. Slowly extend each stretch and then hold the extended position for 10–30 seconds. Repeat each stretch three to four times per training session. See the box "Guidelines for Static Stretching" for additional advice on safe and effective stretching.

Training Considerations for Body Composition

When training to improve body composition, the goal is to increase muscle (and possibly bone) mass, decrease body fat, or a combination of both. Training to maintain or increase muscle mass was covered earlier in this chapter in the discussion of muscular fitness. It is important to recognize that muscle mass declines with age, beginning sometime after age 35. This loss of muscle mass is called **sarcopenia.** Thus, strength training to maintain the amount and the quality of muscle is a recommended component of adult exercise programs.

The most common exercise goal related to body composition is to lose body fat. To achieve this, the exercise program should seek to maximize the caloric expenditure. Aerobic exercise activities are the best to produce relatively high rates of energy expenditure for a prolonged period of time. The ACSM recommends that an exercise session should produce an energy expenditure of 300–400 kilocalories. Any combination of duration and intensity in suitable, as long as the total caloric

---

★ Guidelines for Static Stretching

Take the following precautions to reduce the possibility of injury during stretching:

- Warm up using a slow jog or fast walk before stretching.
- Stretch only to the point at which you feel tightness or resistance to your stretching. Stretching should not be painful.
- Be sure to continue normal breathing during a stretch. Do not hold your breath.
- Use caution when stretching muscles that surround painful joints. Pain is an indication that something is wrong—it should not be ignored.

---

expenditure target is achieved. Frequency should be most, if not all, days of the week.

Overtraining

The human body is an amazing piece of equipment. It functions well regardless of whether you are conscious of its processes. It also delivers clear signals when something goes wrong. You should monitor any sign that seems abnormal during or after your exercise. "Listen to your body" is a good rule for self-awareness. The box "Exercise Danger Signs" lists some common warning signs to monitor.

However, such occurrences are extremely unusual. Fear of developing these difficulties should not deter you from starting a fitness program. These risks are minimal—and the benefits far outweigh the risks. Sports injuries are discussed later in this chapter.

The Workout Routine

A training session consists of three basic parts: the warm-up, the conditioning phase, and the cooldown.[6]

Warm-Up   The warm-up should last 5–10 minutes. During this period, you should begin slow, gradual,

---

Key Terms

static stretching   The slow lengthening of a muscle group to an extended stretch, followed by a holding of the extended position for 10–30 seconds.

ballistic stretching   A "bouncing" form of stretching in which a muscle group is lengthened repetitively to produce multiple quick, forceful stretches.

sarcopenia   A reduction in the size of the muscle fibers, related to the aging process.

---

comfortable movements related to the upcoming activity, such as walking or slow jogging. If the upcoming activity requires specific types of movement, some range of motion exercises mimicking those movements are beneficial. All body segments and muscle groups should be exercised as you gradually increase your heart rate. Near the end of the warm-up period, the major muscle groups should be stretched. This preparation helps protect you from muscle strains and joint sprains.

The warm-up is a fine time to socialize. Furthermore, you can mentally prepare yourself for your activity or think about the beauty of the morning sky, the changing colors of the leaves, or the friends you will meet later in the day. Mental warm-ups can be as beneficial for you psychologically as physical warm-ups are physiologically.

Conditioning The second part of the training session is the conditioning phase, the part of the session that involves improving muscular fitness, cardiorespiratory endurance, and flexibility. Workouts can be tailor-made, but they should follow the ACSM guidelines discussed previously in this chapter (Table 4.1).

Cooldown The third important part of each fitness session is the cooldown. Ideally, one should not abruptly stop exercise as this could cause circulatory problems (insufficient blood returning to the heart). The cooldown consists of a 5- to 10-minute session of relaxing exercises, such as slow jogging, walking, and stretching. Note, this is the ideal time for flexibility training, since the muscles and joints are warmed from the conditioning phase. This activity allows your body to cool and return to a resting state. A cooldown period helps reduce muscle soreness.

Exercise over the Life Span

Regardless of age, exercise provides health and fitness benefits. However, there are modifications to the exercise recommendations that are age-specific.

Children's Physical Activity

Major research studies published during the last 10 years have indicated that U.S. children and teenagers lead very

Table 4.1 Summary of Exercise Training Recommendations for Each Component of Physical Fitness

	Cardiorespiratory Endurance	Muscular Strength	Muscular Endurance	Flexibility	Body Composition
Mode	Any using large muscle groups in a rhythmic pattern	Free weights, machines, resistive devices	Free weights, machines, resistive devices	Static is recommended	Aerobic for fat loss and strength for muscle mass gains
Intensity	65–90% HR_{max} or 50–85% HRR	Amount of weight that can be moved only 12–15 times without rest	Less than maximal	To point of mild to moderate discomfort	Specific to mode of training
Duration	20–60 minutes per day	1 set of 8–10 using major muscle groups	1 set of 8–10 using major muscle groups	3–4 repetitions of 10–30 seconds each, for all major joints	200–300 minutes per week
Frequency	3–5 days per week	2–3 days per week	3–5 days per week	3–5 days per week	5–7 days per week

Note: HR_{max} = maximum heart rate; HRR = heart rate range.

Source: Adapted from American College of Sports Medicine.

sedentary lives. Children ages 6 to 17 score extremely poorly in the areas of strength, flexibility, and cardiorespiratory endurance. In many cases, parents are in better shape than their children are. A major consequence of these sedentary habits in children is obesity. The 1999–2000 National Health and Nutrition Examination Survey (NHANES) indicates that 15 percent of children and adolescents ages 6 to 19 years are overweight. Indeed, from NHANES II (1976–80) to NHANES III (1988–1994), the prevalence of overweight nearly doubled among children and adolescents and has continued to rise. The seriousness of these data is revealed by the fact that most obese children become obese adults.

This situation presents a challenge to educators and parents to emphasize the need for strenuous play activity. Television watching and parental inactivity were implicated as major factors in these studies. The National Center for Chronic Disease Prevention and Health Promotion recommends that children and teenagers get at least 60 minutes per day of moderate-intensity physical activity.[8] Furthermore, they advise that part of this should be of moderate-to-vigorous intensity, 20 or more minutes per session, on 3 or more days per week.

Exercise and Aging

With aging, physical decline occurs and the components of physical fitness become more difficult to maintain. From the fourth decade onward, a gradual decline in vigor and resistance eventually gives way to various types of illnesses. In the opinion of many authorities, people do not die of old age. Rather, old age worsens specific conditions responsible for death. However, physical decline can be slowed, and the onset of illness delayed, by staying physically active. The process of aging can be described on the basis of predictable occurrences,[9] as follows:

- *Change is gradual.* In aging, gradual changes occur in body structure or function before specific health problems are identified.
- *Individual differences occur.* When two people of the same age are compared for the type and the extent of change that has occurred with age, important differences can be noted. Even within the same person, different systems decline at differing rates and to varying extents.
- *Greatest change is noted in areas of complex function.* In physiological processes involving two or more major body systems, the most profound effects of physiological aging can be noted.
- *Homeostatic decline occurs with age.* Becoming older is associated with a growing difficulty in maintaining homeostasis (the dynamic balance among body systems). In the face of stressors, the older adult's

Choosing activities that are safe, convenient, and enjoyable can help people maintain an exercise program throughout the life span.

system takes longer to respond, does not respond with the same magnitude, and may take longer to return to baseline.

Like growth and development, aging is predictable yet unique for each person.

Exercise for "30-Somethings"

People who are in their 30s need to make few, if any, significant adjustments in their fitness programs. Men and women can continue physical activities they have used since their 20s—the key word being *continue*. Unfortunately, many "30-somethings" have developed sedentary habits and have suffered the consequences of gaining excess body fat and acquiring cardiac risk factors (such as high blood pressure). It is important for these individuals to either increase their activity gradually, say by walking more each day, or to seek the assistance of an exercise professional to guide them through the first 1 to 3 months of a new exercise program. See the box "Overcoming Barriers to Being Regularly Active" for ideas on how to get started on an exercise program.

Those 30-somethings who feel mired in activities that now seem boring might try a new activity. However, any new activity (or increase in the intensity of a current activity) should be undertaken gradually.

Exercise for Older Adults

Health Concerns   The body experiences a number of changes as a person ages. Some of these changes are accelerated or magnified for those whose lifestyle does not include regular physical activity.

Changes in Midlife Adults   The period between 45 and 64 years of age brings with it a variety of subtle changes in the body's structure and function. When life is busy and the mind is active, these changes are generally not evident. Even when they become evident, they are not usually the source of profound concern. Nevertheless, older students in your class and people with whom you work could be experiencing these changes:[9]

- Decrease in bone mass and density
- Increase in vertebral compression
- Degenerative changes in joint cartilage
- Increase in adipose tissue; loss of lean body mass
- Decrease in capacity to engage in physical work
- Decrease in visual acuity
- Decrease in resting energy requirements
- Decrease in fertility
- Decrease in sexual function

For some midlife adults these health concerns can be quite threatening, especially for those who view aging with apprehension and fear. Some middle-aged people reject these physical changes and convince themselves they are sick. Indeed, hypochondriasis is much more common among midlife people than among young people.

Changes in Older Adults   In older people, it is frequently difficult to distinguish between changes caused by aging and those caused by disease. For virtually every body system, biomedical indexes for the old and young can overlap. In the respiratory system, for example, the cardiorespiratory endurance of a man of 70 may be no different from that of a man of 55 who has a history of heavy cigarette smoking. Is the level in the older man to be considered an indicator of a disease, or should it be considered a reflection of normal old age? In dealing with older adults, physicians frequently must make this kind of distinction.

In older people, as in midlife people, structural and physiological changes are routinely seen. In some cases, these are closely related to disease processes, but in most cases they reflect the gradual decline that is thought to be a result of the normal aging process. The most frequently seen changes include the following:

- Further decrease in bone mass, resulting in changes in the structure of bone
- Decrease in muscle bulk and strength
- Decrease in cardiorespiratory endurance
- Loss of nonreproducing cells in the nervous system
- Decrease in hearing and vision abilities

- Decrease in all other sensory modalities, including the sense of body positioning
- Slower reaction time
- Gait and posture changes resulting from a weakening of the muscles of the trunk and legs

In addition to these changes, the most likely change seen in older adults is the increased sensitivity of the body's homeostatic mechanism. Because of this sensitivity, a minor infection or superficial injury can be traumatic enough to decrease the body's ability to maintain its internal balance. An illness that would be easily controlled in a young person could even prove fatal to a seemingly healthy 75-year-old person.

Continuing to follow a physical fitness plan throughout midlife and older adulthood is essential to minimizing age-related health problems. The plan should be modified as necessary to accommodate changes in physical functioning.

Safe Exercise Programs An exercise program designed for younger adults may be inappropriate for older people, particularly those over age 50. Special attention must be paid to matching the program to the interests and abilities of the participants. Often, this is best achieved by having older individuals begin their exercise program under the supervision of a certified exercise professional. The goals of the program should include both social interaction and physical conditioning.

Older adults, especially those with a personal or family history of heart problems, should have a physical examination before starting a fitness program. This examination should include an evaluation of all the physiological systems of the body, especially the cardiovascular, respiratory, and musculoskeletal. Ideally, the evaluation should also include a maximal exercise test (a "stress" test). Participants should learn how to monitor their own cardiorespiratory status during exercise.

Well-designed fitness programs for older adults will include activities that begin slowly, are monitored frequently, and are geared to the enjoyment of the participants (see the box "Older Adults and Tai Chi Chuan").[10] The professional staff coordinating the program should be familiar with the signs of distress (excessively elevated heart rate, nausea, breathing difficulty, pallor, and pain) and must be able to perform CPR. Warm-up and cooldown periods should be included. Activities to increase flexibility are beneficial in the beginning and ending segments of the program. Participants should wear comfortable clothing and appropriate shoes, and they should be mentally prepared to enjoy the activities.

A program designed for older adults will largely conform to the ACSM criteria specified previously in this chapter, including both cardiorespiratory and muscular fitness training. Certainly, specific modifications or restrictions to the exercise program may be required due to

Older Adults and Tai Chi Chuan

Continuing to follow a program of physical fitness is vital throughout midlife and older age. However, which types of exercise are most appropriate for older adults?

Many older adults choose gentle aerobic activities that put less stress and strain on joints, such as walking or water aerobics. Another option is the Chinese discipline tai chi chuan. Practitioners say that the slow, gentle movements of tai chi provide a variety of health benefits, such as improving physical strength and balance. Research supports these beliefs, reporting that geriatric practitioners of tai chi enjoy greater flexibility, improved balance, and lower blood pressure. Thus tai chi may be prescribed as a suitable conditioning exercise for older adults.

Source: J. Cheng, "Tai Chi Chuan: A Slow Dance for Health," *Physician and Sports Medicine*, June 1999.

health concerns of the individual. For example, because of possible joint, muscular, or skeletal problems, certain activities may have to be done in a sitting position. Pain or discomfort should be reported immediately to the fitness instructor.

Fortunately, properly screened older adults will rarely have health emergencies during a well-monitored fitness program. Many fit older adults can also safely exercise alone.

 TALKING POINTS If your screening tests indicate that you cannot start a vigorous fitness program, are you prepared to ask your doctor about alternative activities?

Special Health Concerns
Low-Back Pain

A common occurrence among adults is the sudden onset of low-back pain. Four out of five adults develop this condition at least once in their lifetime, which can be so uncomfortable that they miss work, lose sleep, and generally feel incapable of engaging in daily activities. Many of the adults who have this condition will experience these effects two to three times per year.

Although low-back pain can reflect serious health problems, most low-back pain is caused by mechanical (postural) problems. As unpleasant as low-back pain is, the symptoms and functional limitations usually subside within a week or two. The services of a physician, physical therapist, or chiropractor are generally not required.

By engaging in regular exercise, such as swimming, walking, and bicycling, and by paying attention to your back during bending, lifting, and sitting, you can minimize the occurrence of this uncomfortable and incapacitating condition. Many commercial fitness centers and campus recreational programs are starting to offer specific exercises geared to muscular improvement in the lower back and abdominal areas.

Female Athlete Triad

In the early 1990s, the ACSM identified a three-part syndrome of disordered eating, **amenorrhea** (lack of menstruation), and osteoporosis as the female athlete triad.[11] The conditions of this syndrome appear independently in many women, but among female athletes they appear together. The female athlete triad is most likely to be found in athletes whose sport activities emphasize appearance (for example, diving, ice skating, or gymnastics) and can also be observed in women who become compulsive exercisers.

Parents, coaches, athletic trainers, teammates, and friends should be watchful for signs of the female athlete triad. This syndrome has associated medical risks, including inadequate fuel supply for activities, inadequate iron intake, reduced cognitive function, altered hormone levels, reduced mental health, early onset of menopause, increased likelihood of skeletal trauma, altered blood fat profiles, and increased vulnerability to heart disease.[11] Vitally important is an early referral to a physician who is knowledgeable about the female athlete triad. The physician will likely coordinate efforts with a psychologist, a nutritionist, and an athletic trainer to improve the health of the athlete and prevent recurrences.

Pregnancy

Pregnant women should continue to exercise.[12] During pregnancy a woman's entire body undergoes many physical changes. Muscles are stretched, joints are loosened, and tissues are subjected to stress. If a woman is in good physiological condition, she is more likely to handle these changes with few complications. The baby

may also benefit. Studies have shown that women who exercise moderately during pregnancy tend to give birth to healthier babies.[13]

Some reports suggest that exercise during pregnancy can make delivery of the baby easier and faster. Exercise can also help control her weight gain and improve her balance during pregnancy, and make it easier to get back to normal weight after delivery.

The types of exercises a woman should perform during pregnancy depend on the individual and the stage of pregnancy.[6] Most pregnant women should perform general exercises that increase overall fitness and stamina, as well as exercises that strengthen specific muscle groups. Muscles of the pelvic floor, for example, should be exercised regularly, because these muscles will be supporting most of the extra weight of the baby.

A variety of exercises are appropriate, including walking, swimming, stretching, and strengthening exercises. Yoga and tai chi are also good forms of exercise for pregnant women. The muscles of the pelvic floor, abdomen, and back are especially subject to stress and strain during pregnancy and delivery, so certain exercises can also be performed to strengthen these muscles. Exercises can also be performed to speed up recovery after delivery. Such postpartum exercises can be started in some cases within 24 hours after delivery. Exercises can even be started before conception if a pregnancy is anticipated.

Some types of exercise can put the fetus at risk. A pregnant woman should avoid any activity in which she becomes overheated, because her elevated body temperature will warm up the fetal environment. Thus pregnant women should not use saunas or hot tubs, nor should they exercise in a hot, humid environment. During the last trimester of pregnancy, women should also avoid any strenuous or high-impact exercise that involves bouncing, jumping, or jarring motions. Obviously, pregnant women should first consult with their obstetricians to develop a safe, productive exercise routine.

Osteoporosis

Osteoporosis is a condition frequently seen in older middle-aged women. However, it is not fully understood why menopausal women are so susceptible to the increase in calcium loss that leads to fractures of the hip, wrist, and vertebral column. Approximately 80 percent of the 10 million people with osteoporosis are women. Estimates from the National Osteoporosis Foundation are that half of women and one in four men over age 50 will have an osteoporosis-related fracture in their lifetime.[14]

The endocrine system plays a large role in the development of osteoporosis. At the time of menopause, a woman's ovaries begin a rapid decrease in the production of estrogen, one of two main hormones associated with the menstrual cycle. This lower level of estrogen

> ### Key Terms
>
> **amenorrhea** The absence of menstruation.
>
> **osteoporosis** Decrease in bone mass that leads to increased incidence of fractures, primarily in postmenopausal women.
>
> **osteoarthritis** Arthritis that develops with age; largely caused by weight bearing and deterioration of the joints.

may decrease the conversion of the precursors of vitamin D into the active form of vitamin D, the form necessary for absorbing calcium from the digestive tract. As a result, calcium may be drawn from the bones for use elsewhere in the body.

Additional explanations of osteoporosis focus on two other possibilities—hyperparathyroidism (another endocrine dysfunction) and the below-average degree of muscle development seen in osteoporotic women. In the latter case the reduced muscle mass is associated with decreased activity, which in turn deprives the body of the mechanical stimulation needed to facilitate bone growth.

Premenopausal women have the opportunity to build and maintain a healthy skeleton through an appropriate intake of calcium. Depending on age, current recommendations are for an intake of 1,000–1,300 mg of calcium per day. Three to four daily servings of low-fat dairy products should provide sufficient calcium. The diet also must contain adequate vitamin D because it aids in the absorption of calcium.

Many women do not consume an adequate amount of calcium. Calcium supplements, again in combination with vitamin D, can be used to achieve recommended calcium levels. It is now known that calcium carbonate, a much-advertised form of calcium, is no more easily absorbed by the body than are other forms of calcium salts. Consumers of calcium supplements should compare brands to determine which, if any, they should buy.

In premenopausal women, calcium deposition in bone is facilitated by exercise, particularly exercise that involves movement of the extremities. Today, women are encouraged to consume at least the recommended servings from the milk group and engage in regular physical activity that involves the weight-bearing muscles of the legs, such as aerobics, jogging, and walking.

Postmenopausal women who are not elderly can markedly slow the resorption of calcium from their bones through the use of estrogen-replacement therapy. When combined with a daily intake of 1,500 mg of calcium, vitamin D, and regular exercise, estrogen therapy almost eliminates calcium loss. Of course, women need to work closely with their physicians to monitor the use of estrogen because of continuing concern over the role of estrogen-replacement therapy in the development of breast cancer and the increased risk of coronary heart disease events and stroke.

Osteoarthritis

Arthritis is an umbrella term for more than 100 forms of joint inflammation. The most common form is osteoarthritis. It is likely that as we age, all of us will develop osteoarthritis to some degree. Often called "wear and tear" arthritis, osteoarthritis occurs primarily in the weight-bearing joints of the knee, hip, and spine. In this form of arthritis, joint damage can occur to bone ends, cartilaginous cushions, and related structures as the years of constant friction and stress accumulate.

The object of current management of osteoarthritis (and other forms) is not to cure the disease but rather to reduce discomfort, slow the progression of the disease, and maintain or improve function in daily activities.[15] Analgesics and nonsteroidal anti-inflammatory agents are the medications most frequently used to treat osteoarthritis.

It is now believed that osteoarthritis develops most commonly in people with a genetic predisposition for excessive damage to the weight-bearing joints. Thus the condition seems to run in families. Further, studies comparing the occurrence of osteoarthritis in those who exercise and those who do not demonstrate that regular movement may decrease the likelihood of developing this form of arthritis.

Fitness Questions and Answers

Along with the major components of your fitness program, you should think about many additional issues when you start a fitness program.

Should I See My Doctor before I Get Started?

First of all, it is highly desirable to have regular checkups as part of your overall health plan. However, the Surgeon General has suggested that most adults can safely increase their activity level to a moderate amount without the need for a comprehensive medical evaluation.[1] Individuals with chronic diseases should consult with their physician before increasing their activity level.

If vigorous forms of exercise are desired, then a medical exam is recommended for men over 40 and women over 50. It is also recommended for individuals with more than one risk factor for coronary artery disease or with any other notable health problems. The American College of Sports Medicine also recommends an exercise ("stress") test for these individuals.[6]

What Causes a "Runner's High"?

During or after exercise, a person occasionally experiences feelings of euphoria. Runners and joggers call these feelings the "runner's high." However, these positive feelings of relaxation, high self-esteem, and reduced stress are not limited to runners. Almost any fitness activity can leave participants with these intense positive feelings. Swimmers, aerobic exercisers, hikers, and cyclists all have reported exercise-induced highs.

Although these pleasurable feelings can be attributed in part to psychological causes, there is plenty of scientific evidence to suggest a physiological cause. During physical activity, the brain releases its own morphinelike (opiate-like) substances called *endorphins*. These chemicals are released by brain neurons and produce sensations that are pleasurable, and sometimes even numbing. Exercisers report that these episodes of euphoria are unpredictable. Sometimes they experience highs and sometimes they do not. However, endorphin highs are more likely to occur during or after a strenuous, challenging workout.

How Beneficial Is Aerobic Dance Exercise?

One of the most popular fitness approaches is aerobic exercise, including aerobic dancing. Many organizations sponsor classes in this form of continuous dancing and movement. The rise in popularity of aerobic exercise video programs reflects the enthusiasm for this form of exercise. Because extravagant claims are often made about the value of these programs, the wise consumer should observe at least one session of the activity before enrolling. Discover for yourself whether the program meets the criteria outlined earlier in this chapter in terms of mode of activity, frequency, intensity, duration, resistance training, and flexibility training.

Street dancing, swing dancing, and Latin dancing have become some of the most popular aerobic exercises. Popularized by rap music, hip-hop music, and the growth of vigorous dancing in music videos, these forms of dancing provide an excellent way of having fun and maintaining cardiorespiratory fitness. Have you experienced the exhilaration that results from an hour or two of dancing?

What Are Low-Impact Aerobic Activities?

Because long-term participation in some aerobic activities (for example, jogging, running, aerobic dancing, and rope skipping) may lead to injury of the hip, knee, and ankle joints, many fitness experts promote low-impact aerobic activities. Low-impact aerobic dancing, water aerobics, bench aerobics, and brisk walking are examples of this kind of fitness activity. Participants still conform to the principal components of a cardiorespiratory fitness program. THR levels are the same as in high-impact aerobic activities.

The main difference between low-impact and high-impact aerobic activities is the use of the legs. Low-impact aerobics require having one foot on the ground at all times. Thus, weight transfer does not occur with the forcefulness seen in traditional, high-impact aerobic activities. In addition, low-impact activities may include exaggerated arm movements and the use of hand or wrist weights. All these variations are designed to increase the

Wearing appropriate clothing and safety equipment and drinking adequate amounts of fluid are good strategies for any type of exercise.

heart rate to the THR without undue strain on the joints of the lower extremities. Low-impact aerobics are excellent for people of all ages, and they may be especially beneficial to older adults.

In-line skating (rollerblading) is one of the fastest-growing fitness activities. This low-impact activity has cardiorespiratory and muscular benefits similar to those of running without the pounding effect that running can produce. However, it should be recognized that it requires both skill and balance. Rollerblading requires important safety equipment: sturdy skates, knee and elbow pads, wrist supports, and a helmet. Obviously, the potential for falling makes this a higher-risk activity.

What Is the Most Effective Way to Replace Fluids during Exercise?

Despite all the advertising hype associated with commercial fluid-replacement products, for an average person involved in typical fitness activities, water is still the best fluid replacement. The availability and cost are unbeatable. However, when activity is prolonged and intense, commercial sports drinks may be preferred over water because they contain electrolytes (which replace lost sodium and potassium) and carbohydrates (which replace depleted energy stores). However, the carbohydrates in sports drinks are actually simple forms of sugar. Thus, sports drinks tend to be high in calories just like regular soft drinks. Regardless of the drink you choose, exercise physiologists recommend that you drink fluids before and at frequent intervals throughout the activity, particularly in warm, humid environments.

What Clothing Should I Wear for Exercise?

The two points of emphasis for exercise clothing are to wear clothing that is comfortable, more than stylish, and that promotes temperature regulation. Generally, loose-fitting attire that does not restrict movement is desirable. However, new materials have been developed that are more form-fitting, yet are comfortable, do not restrict movement, and do not impede temperature regulation.

In warmer temperatures the goal is to prevent the body from overheating. Generally, in a warm or hot environment, less clothing should be worn and the materials should allow for the transfer of moisture from the skin so that it can evaporate. Evaporation is what results in heat loss. Sweat that drips off or is wiped off the body does not produce any cooling. Also, for outdoor exercising, light-colored clothing should be worn to diminish radiant heat transfer to the body.

In cooler temperatures the goal is to prevent losing too much heat, which can result in hypothermia. In cold environments, a layered approach to dressing is recommended. When you exercise, even in the cold, you will produce body heat. Layering enables you to remove the outermost layer of clothing during exercise. (Note: You might need to put this layer back on if you perform your cooldown routine outdoors.) The innermost layer should be made of a material that will transfer moisture away from your skin. Cotton is not recommended, because it tends to absorb and retain moisture from sweat, which can increase the amount of heat loss in cold temperatures. The outermost layer should be of a material that will shield the body from the wind but allow for moisture to be transferred away from the body. Material such as Gore-Tex is ideal for this. Additionally, you should protect your extremities by wearing a hat that covers your ears and using gloves or mittens as dictated by the outdoor temperature.

Where Can I Find Out about Proper Equipment?

College students are generally in an excellent setting to locate people who have the resources to provide helpful information about sports equipment. Contacting physical education, exercise science, or health education faculty members who have an interest in your chosen activity might be a good start. Most colleges also have a number of clubs that specialize in fitness interests—cycling, hiking, and jogging clubs, for example. Attend one of their upcoming meetings. For many activities, the only equipment you'll need is a good pair of athletic shoes; see

the box "Choosing an Athletic Shoe" for advice on finding shoes that are right for you.

Many types of cardiorespiratory fitness equipment are now available for home use. Home fitness equipment can be especially helpful for those who do not have access to a health or fitness club, who prefer to exercise alone and at home, or who must exercise at irregular hours. Some of the most popular devices are described following.

Stationary bicycles come in models ranging in price from about $150 to $3,500. Some upright bikes can also be used for an upper body workout because the user can pump the handlebars. Recumbent bikes, so named because the user sits back while pedaling, take the pressure off the lower back and permit the rider to exercise the hamstring muscles to a greater degree than on an upright bike. Also available are stands that allows the user to convert a regular bicycle into a stationary bike.

Treadmills consist of a moving belt stretched over rollers. Less expensive varieties, starting at a few hundred dollars, are driven manually by the walking or running action of the user. More expensive treadmills are driven by an electric motor and typically allow the user to change speeds and the incline angle of the platform to increase the intensity of the workout; top-of-the-line models can cost thousands of dollars. If you are a first-time user of a motorized treadmill, start slowly so you can become familiar with the motion. Also take special care getting on and off the moving belt.

Stair climbers simulate climbing up a series of stair steps while saving the knees from much of the pressure normally associated with stair climbing. Prices vary from about $200 for a simple level model to $5,000 for a programmable model that varies the speed and amount of resistance. Some models come with an upper-body component that allows the user to pump the arms while climbing.

Rowing machines have a sliding seat and movable handles that are similar to oars and allow the user to simulate the movements of rowing a racing scull. Users push their feet against footplates while pulling back on the handles and sliding the seat. Rowing machines can range in cost from about $300 to more than $3,000.

Elliptical trainers provide a low-impact simulation of the action of walking or running. The feet describe an ellipse, which is roughly the same pattern that we move in when we walk or run. These trainers can require more involvement of the gluteal and thigh muscles than do treadmills or stationary cycles. Prices range from several hundred to several thousand dollars.

Most forms of equipment can provide a good cardiorespiratory workout, but you may have to add strength training to your fitness program in order to obtain a complete workout. In terms of effectiveness, a *Journal of the American Medical Association* study found that treadmill users walking or running "somewhat hard" burned more calories per hour than users of five other common home exercise machines; in this study, people using regular and dual-action stationary cycles burned the fewest calories per hour.[16]

The machine that is best for you is the one that you enjoy using and that lasts. Unfortunately, many people purchase a machine and seldom use it. Using just one piece of equipment can become monotonous, and you may find yourself avoiding exercise due to boredom. It is advisable to thoroughly test out equipment before purchase. Check the quality of the equipment and its appropriateness for you. See the box "Infomercials and Advertisements for Fitness Equipment" for consumer guidelines.

How Worthwhile Are Commercial Health and Fitness Clubs?

The health and fitness club business is booming. Fitness clubs offer activities ranging from free weights to weight machines to step walking to general aerobics. Some clubs have saunas and whirlpools and lots of frills. Others have course offerings that include wellness, smoking cessation, stress management, time management, dance, and yoga. The atmosphere at most clubs is friendly, and people are encouraged to have a good time while working out.

If your purpose in joining a fitness club is to improve your cardiorespiratory fitness, measure the program offered by the club against the ACSM standards.[17] If your primary purpose in joining is to meet people and have fun, request a trial membership for a month or so to see whether you like the environment.

Before signing a contract at a health club or spa, do some careful questioning. Find out when the business was established, ask about the qualifications of the employees, contact some members for their observations, and request a thorough tour of the facilities. You might even consult your local Better Business Bureau for additional information. Finally, make certain that you read and understand every word of the contract.

What Are Steroids, and Why Do Some Athletes Use Them?

Steroids are drugs that physicians can legally prescribe for a variety of health conditions, including certain forms of anemia, inadequate growth patterns, and chronic debilitating diseases. Steroids can also be prescribed to aid recovery from surgery or burns. **Anabolic steroids** are drugs that function like the male sex hormone testosterone. They can be taken orally or by injection.

 TALKING POINTS If you suspected a young person you know was using steroids, what strategies would you use to encourage the person to change his or her behavior?

Anabolic steroids are used by athletes who hope to gain weight, muscular size and strength, power, endurance, and aggressiveness. Over the last few decades, many bodybuilders, weightlifters, track athletes, and football players have chosen to ignore the serious health risks posed by illegal steroid use. More recently, steroid use among high school and college campuses has reached epidemic levels. The mass media has begun to focus attention on the dangers of steroid use, but many young athletes choose to ignore these warnings.

The use of steroids is highly dangerous because of serious, life-threatening side effects and adverse reactions. These effects include heart problems, certain forms of cancer, liver complications, and even psychological disturbances. The side effects on female steroid users are as dangerous as those on men. Figure 4-2 shows the adverse effects of steroid use.

Steroid users have developed a terminology of their own. Anabolic steroids are called "roids" or "juice." "Roid rage" is an aggressive, psychotic response to chronic steroid use. "Stacking" means using multiple steroids at the same time.

Many organizations that control athletic competition (such as the National Collegiate Athletic Association or the NCAA, The Athletics Congress, the National Football League, and the International Olympic Committee) have banned steroids and are testing athletes for

> **Key Terms**
>
> **anabolic steroids** (ann uh **bol** ick) Drugs that function like testosterone to produce increases in muscle mass, strength, endurance, and aggressiveness.

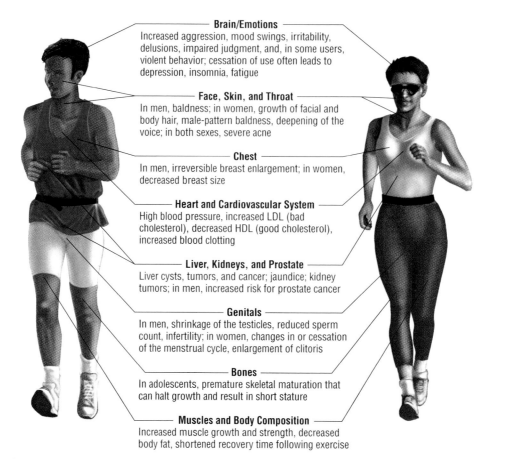

Brain/Emotions
Increased aggression, mood swings, irritability, delusions, impaired judgment, and, in some users, violent behavior; cessation of use often leads to depression, insomnia, fatigue

Face, Skin, and Throat
In men, baldness; in women, growth of facial and body hair, male-pattern baldness, deepening of the voice; in both sexes, severe acne

Chest
In men, irreversible breast enlargement; in women, decreased breast size

Heart and Cardiovascular System
High blood pressure, increased LDL (bad cholesterol), decreased HDL (good cholesterol), increased blood clotting

Liver, Kidneys, and Prostate
Liver cysts, tumors, and cancer; jaundice; kidney tumors; in men, increased risk for prostate cancer

Genitals
In men, shrinkage of the testicles, reduced sperm count, infertility; in women, changes in or cessation of the menstrual cycle, enlargement of clitoris

Bones
In adolescents, premature skeletal maturation that can halt growth and result in short stature

Muscles and Body Composition
Increased muscle growth and strength, decreased body fat, shortened recovery time following exercise

Figure 4-2 Effects of Steroids In addition to the effects listed above, people who inject steroids run the added risk of contracting or transmitting HIV infection or hepatitis.

Sources: "Steroids (Anabolic-Androgenic)," *NIDA InfoFacts*, National Institute on Drug Abuse, March 2007; "Anabolic Steroids," *NIDA Community Drug Alert Bulletin*, National Institute on Drug Abuse, April 2000.

illegal use. Fortunately, some athletes finally seem to be getting the message and are steering clear of steroids. For more information on the potential health hazards of using anabolic steroids, see the National Institute on Drug Abuse's Info Facts, found on the Web (www.nida.nih.gov/infofacts/steroids.htm). For more on other supplements taken by athletes, see the box "Evaluating Nutritional Supplements Promoted to Enhance Exercise."

Why Has Bodybuilding Become So Popular?

The popularity of bodybuilding has increased significantly in recent years for many reasons. Bodybuilders often start lifting weights to get into better shape—to improve muscle tone. They may just want to look healthier and feel stronger. When they realize that they can alter the shape of their bodies, they find that bodybuilding offers challenges that, through hard work, are attainable. Bodybuilders also report enjoying the physical sensations (the "pump") that result from a good workout. The results of their efforts are clearly visible and measurable.

Some bodybuilders become involved in competitive events to test their advancements.

Perhaps we should dispel a few myths about bodybuilding. Are bodybuilders strong? The answer is emphatically—yes! Will muscle cells turn into fat cells if weight-lifting programs are discontinued? No, muscle cells are physiologically incapable of turning into fat cells. Will women develop bulky muscles through weight training? No, they can improve muscle size, strength, and tone, but unless they take steroids, their muscle mass cannot increase to the same degree as men's muscle mass. Is bodybuilding socially acceptable? Yes, for many people. Just observe all the health clubs and campus exercise rooms that cater to weightlifters and bodybuilders.

Exercise Injuries

At any time during your participation in fitness or sport activities, it is possible that you will become injured, even if you carefully warm up before your exercise and cool down after your exercise. If you are lucky, the injury will be only a minor one and after a short period of rest you will be able to resume your fitness interests. Sometimes, however, an injury can be significant and require you to seek medical care and undergo extensive rehabilitation.

It is beyond the scope of this textbook to provide a comprehensive discussion of the prevention, care, and treatment of sports injuries. (You can find this information in an athletic training textbook, a fitness textbook, or a sports medicine book.) However, here we provide you with some general principles related to the prevention and care of sports injuries and a table that lists many common fitness injuries.[18] (See Table 4.2.)

1. *A well-planned fitness program starts at a low level and progresses gradually and consistently.* This principle supports the concept of starting at a level of activity that can be handled comfortably. If the activity is a walking program, an unfit person should not begin with walks of five or six miles a day but should start with a shorter distance and gradually add additional distance in a consistent manner to avoid muscle, skeletal, or joint injuries.
2. *If you stop exercising for an extended time, do not restart the activity at the level at which you stopped.* Do not plan on returning to a high level of activity if you have been inactive for an extended time. Rather, reduce your activity significantly and gradually return to your earlier levels of activity.
3. *"Listen to your body."* Always be aware of the nature of your body as you are exercising. If you sense that something is wrong, stop the activity and assess the situation. For example, if you think you might be hurting your back or that a joint or muscle is being strained, stop and evaluate the situation. If you think something is wrong, by all means don't test your body by returning to the activity. (Have you ever seen a person with a suspected ankle injury "test" the ankle by hopping up and down on the injured leg? This makes no sense at all.) Pain indicates that something is wrong. If this is the case, seek a professional evaluation, perhaps from an athletic trainer or a physical therapist. A physician, especially one trained in sports medicine, can make an accurate diagnosis of the injury.
4. *Follow rehabilitation instructions carefully.* Athletic trainers and physical therapists are trained to design effective rehabilitation programs. If you are injured, it is very important that you follow the

Table 4.2 Common Injuries Associated with Physical Activity

Injury	Condition
Achilles tendinitis	A chronic tendinitis of the "heel cord" or muscle tendon, located on the back of the lower leg just above the heel. It may result from any activity that involves forcefully pushing off with the foot and ankle, such as in running and jumping. This inflammation involves swelling, warmth, tenderness to touch, and pain during walking and especially running.
Ankle sprains	Stretching or tearing of one or several ligaments that provide stability to the ankle joint. Ligaments on the outside or lateral side of the ankle are more commonly injured by rolling the sole of the foot downward and toward the inside. Pain is intense immediately after injury, followed by considerable swelling, tenderness, loss of joint motion, and some discoloration over a 24- to 48-hour period.
Groin pull	A muscle strain that occurs in the muscles located on the inside of the upper thigh just below the pubic area and that results from either an overstretch of the muscle or from a contraction of the muscle that meets excessive resistance. Pain will be produced by flexing the hip and leg across the body or by stretching the muscles in a groin-stretch position.
Hamstring pull	A strain of the muscles on the back of the upper thigh that most often occurs while sprinting. In most cases, severe pain is caused simply by walking or in any movement that involves knee flexion or stretch of the hamstring muscle. Some swelling, tenderness to touch, and possibly some discoloration extending down the back of the leg may occur in severe strains.
Patellofemoral knee pain	Nonspecific pain occurring around the knee, particularly the front part of the knee, or in the kneecap (patella). Pain can result from many causes, including improper movement of the kneecap in knee flexion and extension; tendinitis of the tendon just below the kneecap, which is caused by repetitive jumping; bursitis (swelling) either above or below the kneecap; and osteoarthritis (joint surface degeneration) between the kneecap and thigh bone. It may involve inflammation with swelling, tenderness, warmth, and pain associated with movement.
Quadriceps contusion, "charley horse"	A deep bruise of the muscles in the front part of the thigh caused by a forceful impact or by some object that results in severe pain, swelling, discoloration, and difficulty flexing the knee or extending the hip. Without adequate rest and protection from additional trauma, small calcium deposits may develop in the muscle.
Shin splints	A catch-all term used to refer to any pain that occurs in the front part of the lower leg or shin, most often caused by excessive running on hard surfaces. Pain is usually caused by strain of the muscles that move the ankle and foot at their attachment points in the shin. It is usually worse during activity. In more severe cases it may be caused by stress fractures of the long bones in the lower leg, with the pain being worse after activity is stopped.
Shoulder impingement	Chronic irritation and inflammation of muscle tendons and a bursa underneath the tip of the shoulder, which results from repeated forceful overhead motions of the shoulder, such as in swimming, throwing, spiking a volleyball, or serving a tennis ball. Pain is felt when the arm is extended across the body above shoulder level.
Tennis elbow	Chronic irritation and inflammation of the lateral or outside surface of the arm just above the elbow at the attachment of the muscles that extend the wrist and fingers. It results from any activity that requires forceful extension of the wrist. Typically occurs in tennis players who are using faulty techniques hitting backhand ground strokes. Pain is felt above the elbow after forcefully extending the wrist against resistance or applying pressure over the muscle attachment above the elbow.

Source: WE Prentice, *Get Fit, Stay Fit*, 4th ed., McGraw-Hill, 2007. Reproduced with permission of The McGraw-Hill Companies.

advice of these professionals. This is especially true in cases where you start to feel better before the rehabilitation program is finished. Even though you feel better, your body may not be fully recovered. A return to activity too quickly may result in an even more serious injury than your original one. (This is especially true for adults over the age of 40.) The best advice is to resist the urge to return to your activity until you are given full clearance from your trainer or therapist.

5. *Develop a prevention approach.* After you recover from an injury, try to discover ways to prevent that injury from happening again. Learn about proper stretching exercises, effective strength-training activities, appropriate equipment, and the proper mechanics for your selected sports/fitness activities. Use this collective knowledge to prevent the injury from recurring.

For example, if you have injured your hamstring muscles while running, you will need to learn how to effectively stretch these muscles in the future. You will also need to learn how to strengthen these muscles through resistance training. If your running shoes are old and worn, they may have to be replaced. Finally, don't run too fast before warming up; start slowly and gradually increase your speed after the muscles are fully warmed up. Preventive actions such as these will allow you to have a fitness program that is not regularly interrupted by a nagging injury.

Taking Charge of Your Health

- Assess your level of fitness by completing the National Fitness Test on pages 125–126.

- Implement or maintain a cardiorespiratory fitness program that uses the most recent American College of Sports Medicine recommendations.

- Start a daily stretching program based on the guidelines in this chapter.

- Recognize that a comprehensive physical fitness program includes performing muscular fitness exercises at least twice a week.

- Monitor your physical activities for potential danger signs indicating that you should consult an athletic trainer, physical therapist, or physician.

- Make sure that you always include a warm-up and a cooldown with each exercise session.

SUMMARY

- Physical fitness allows one to avoid illness, perform routine activities, and respond to emergencies.
- The health benefits of exercise can be achieved through regular, moderate exercise.
- Fitness comprises four components: cardiorespiratory endurance, muscular fitness, flexibility, and body composition.
- The American College of Sports Medicine's program for cardiorespiratory fitness has four components: (1) mode of activity, (2) frequency of training, (3) intensity of training, and (4) duration of training. Additionally, ACSM now recommends that everyone also include (5) resistance training and (6) flexibility training.
- The target heart rate (THR) refers to the number of times per minute the heart must contract to produce a training effect.

- Training sessions should take place in three phases: warm-up, conditioning, and cooldown.
- Static stretching is the recommended type of stretching.
- Fitness experts are concerned about the lack of fitness in today's youth.
- Street dancing, swing dancing, step aerobics, and rollerblading are currently popular aerobic activities.
- Low-impact aerobic activities have a lower risk of muscle and joint injuries than do high-impact activities.
- College students who are interested in fitness should be as knowledgeable as possible about the important topics of supplement use, cross-training, fluid replacement, and bodybuilding.
- Following a few simple principles can help prevent many common sports injuries.

REVIEW QUESTIONS

1. Identify the four components of fitness described in this chapter. How does each component relate to health?
2. What is the difference between anaerobic and aerobic energy production? What types of activities are associated with anaerobic energy production? With aerobic energy production?
3. List some of the benefits of fitness.
4. Describe the various methods used to promote muscular fitness.
5. What does the principle of overload mean in regard to fitness training programs?
6. Identify the ACSM's components of an effective cardiorespiratory conditioning program. Explain the important aspects of each component.

7. Under what circumstances should you see a physician before starting a physical fitness program?
8. Identify and describe the three parts of a training session.
9. Describe some of the negative consequences of anabolic steroid use.
10. Name three common types of nutritional supplements used related to exercise programs.
11. Describe the three-part female athlete triad.
12. Discuss the five basic principles important in avoiding sports injuries.

ANSWERS TO THE "WHAT DO YOU KNOW?" QUIZ

1. False   2. True   3. False   4. True   5. True   6. False   7. False

Scoring standards (hanging time)

Age	18–29		30–39		40–49		50–59		60+	
Gender	F	M	F	M	F	M	F	M	F	M
Excellent	>1:30	>2:00	>1:20	>1:50	>1:10	>1:35	>1:00	>1:20	>:50	>1:10
Good	:46–1:30	1:00–2:00	:40–1:20	:50–1:50	:30–1:10	:45–1:35	:30–1:00	:35–1:20	:21–:50	:30–1:10
Average	<:46	<1:00	<:40	<:50	<:30	<:45	<:30	<:35	<:21	<:30

Curl-Ups

Abdominal and low back strength. Equipment: stopwatch. Procedure: Lie flat on upper back, knees bent, shoulders touching the floor, arms extended above your thighs or by your sides, palms down. Bend knees so that feet are flat and 12 inches from the buttocks. Curl up by lifting head and shoulders off the floor, sliding hands forward above your thighs or the floor. Curl down and repeat. Your score is the number of curl-ups in 1 minute.

Scoring standards (number in 1 minute)

Age	18–29		30–39		40–49		50–59		60+	
Gender	F	M	F	M	F	M	F	M	F	M
Excellent	>45	>50	>40	>45	>35	>40	>30	>35	>25	>30
Good	25–45	30–50	20–40	22–45	16–35	21–40	12–30	18–35	11–25	15–30
Average	<25	<30	<20	<22	<16	<21	<12	<18	<11	<15

Push-Ups (Men)

Upper body strength. Equipment: stopwatch. Assume a front-leaning position. Lower your body until chest touches the floor. Raise and repeat for 1 minute. Your score is the number of push-ups completed in 1 minute.

Modified Push-Ups (Women)

Upper body strength. Equipment: stopwatch. Assume a front-leaning position with knees bent up, hands under shoulders. Lower your chest to the floor, raise, and repeat. Your score is the number of push-ups completed in 1 minute.

Scoring standards (number in 1 minute)

Age	18–29	30–39	40–49	50–59	60+
Excellent	>50	>45	>40	>35	>30
Good	25–50	22–45	19–40	15–35	10–30
Average	<25	<22	<19	<15	<10

Scoring standards (number in 1 minute)

Age	18–29	30–39	40–49	50–59	60+
Excellent	>45	>40	>35	>30	>25
Good	17–45	12–40	8–35	6–30	5–25
Average	<17	<12	<8	<6	<5

TO CARRY THIS FURTHER . . .

Note your areas of strengths and weaknesses. To improve your fitness, become involved in a fitness program that reflects the concepts discussed in this chapter. Talking with fitness experts on your campus might be a good first step.

Source: Data from the National Fitness Foundation.

Understanding Nutrition and Your Diet

What Do You Know about Nutrition?

- Coffee is Americans' number one source of antioxidants. True or False?

- Whole-grain bread does not have the same nutritional benefits as wheat bread. True or False?

- It is better to eat foods that are labeled "low carb." True or False?

- Saturated fats are the same thing as trans fats. True or False?

- The new dietary guidelines do not make recommendations for how much water you should drink each day. True or False?

- Foods with phytochemicals are bad for you and should be avoided. True or False?

- Fruit juice is a good way to meet the dietary recommendations for the fruit group. True or False?

Check your answers at the end of the chapter.

Online Learning Center Resources
www.mhhe.com/payne10e

Visit the Online Learning Center for tools to improve your grade and get the most out of your course—chapter objectives, practice quizzes, key terms flashcards, chapter summaries for your digital audio player, Web activities, self-assessments, and many other study aids.

Healthy eating is important from the prenatal period throughout life, in order to prevent malnourishment and minimize the development of illnesses. Food supports growth and development by providing the body with the nutrients needed for energy, repair of damaged tissue, growth of new tissue, and regulation of physiological processes. Our food selections also reflect personal, familial, and cultural traditions. The preparation and serving of food at regular mealtimes and during holiday gatherings and other special occasions enhance all of the dimensions of health (see the box "Mealtime—A Chance to Share and Bond"). For example, sharing a meal with fellow parishioners after a religious service supports the spiritual dimension of health; sharing popcorn at the movies with your friends can enhance the social dimension of health; and learning about the cuisine of another culture develops the cultural dimension of health. As you read this chapter, keep in mind this balanced view of food as sustenance and food as a resource for the dimensions of health.

Mealtime—A Chance to Share and Bond

Food is important to your physical well-being—for energy, growth, repair, and regulation of your body and its functions. But it's also important to the well-being of your spirit. The sharing of food nourishes our spiritual sense of community. This happens through the type of foods selected, the method of preparation, the uniqueness of presentation, and the people involved. From a spiritual perspective, the sharing of food can be a highly satisfying activity.

When food is shared in the company of those who care about us, we experience a sense of community and well-being. The simple act of being together and engaging in a familiar and comfortable practice is reassuring. Meals that involve family or friends, especially for special occasions or important holidays, can provide a chance to reconnect and build relationships.

Food is often at the center of the celebration of special occasions. Weddings, birthdays, anniversaries, graduations, promotions, retirements, and funerals take on a special meaning when people come together to share food and drink. From the first birthday cake through the retirement dinner to the lunch provided by neighbors after the funeral of a loved one, food can help to symbolize and acknowledge these events in our lives.

Food has been part of many religious practices and customs for centuries. Some foods have symbolic meanings related to major life experiences, and ceremonies and religious rites. Food can take on symbolic and spiritual meaning, such as bread representing the body of Christ in the Christian religion. The use of food in spirituality helps to bring groups together to build a stronger sense of community. For example, Ramadan, the ninth month of the Islamic Calendar, is considered one of the holiest months of the year in Islam, and from dawn to sunset Muslims abstain from food. The fast is broken at sunset when families and friends come together and enjoy traditional dishes such as fattoush, a salad. For Jews, the Seder is the most important event in the Passover celebration. Gathering family and friends together, the Seder maintains long-held traditions and customs involving food. The home is cleaned and cleared of all leavened food (foods containing yeast) and grains, and only foods that are kosher are consumed. In the Christian religion, family and friends celebrate Easter by having a meal together on Easter Sunday, usually including lamb, which represents Christ and is seen as a good omen.

Finally, food connects people on a spiritual level by allowing them to share traditions, religious practices, and beliefs. These customs help people build a sense of fellowship and can unify them in times of joy and sorrow.

Types and Sources of Nutrients

Your body relies on seven **nutrients** to carry out its physiological functions: carbohydrates, fats, protein, vitamins, minerals, dietary fiber, and water.* The first three—carbohydrates, fats, and protein—will be discussed together because they provide **calories.** These calories are either used quickly by our bodies in energy metabolism or are stored in the form of glycogen or fat for delayed use as energy sources. The other nutrients—vitamins, minerals, dietary fiber, and water—are not sources of calories for the body. However, regardless of their relationship to calories, all nutrients are essential to human health. The function of each is discussed later in the chapter.

Carbohydrates

Carbohydrates are various combinations of sugar units, or saccharides, and are the major energy source for the body.

Types and Sources of Carbohydrates Carbohydrates occur in three forms, depending on the number of saccharide (sugar) units that make up the molecule. Carbohydrates are divided into two categories: simple (monosaccharides and disaccharides) and complex carbohydrates (polysaccharides).

- *Monosaccharides—carbohydrates with one saccharide unit.* These are the primary source of the body's energy. Examples include glucose, found in vegetables, honey, fruits, and syrup; and fructose, found in fruits and berries.

- *Disaccharides—carbohydrates with two saccharide units, one of which is always a glucose unit.* Examples include sucrose, or table sugar; maltose, which is

---

> **Key Terms**
>
> **nutrients** Elements in foods that are required for the growth, repair, and regulation of body processes.
>
> **calories** Units of heat (energy); specifically, 1 calorie is the amount of energy needed to raise the temperature of 1 gram of water by 1 degree C. In common usage, on food labels, and in this chapter, the term *calorie* is used to refer to a larger energy unit, *kilocalorie* (1,000 calories).
>
> **carbohydrates** The body's primary source of energy for all body functioning; carbohydrates are chemical compounds including sugar, starches, and dietary fibers.

---

*Since most of our water intake comes from beverages rather than from food, some nutritionists do not consider water a nutrient, even though it is essential for life.

Are There Really Good and Bad Carbs?

I have heard there are good and bad carbohydrates and that this makes a difference in terms of weight gain or loss. What is the difference between good and bad carbs?

Carbohydrates are the energy food. All carbohydrates are broken down into glucose, a simple sugar, to be used for energy by the body. The difference between "good" and "bad" carbs is that "good" carbs are high in fiber and bran, which are removed from "bad carbs" in the refining process. This is why the USDA's new dietary guidelines recommend eating more whole grains, which are the good carbs. Bad carbs also include the simple carbohydrates—refined sugars such as table sugar and honey.

Because of their fiber and bran, good carbs are absorbed more slowly and you tend to feel more full and eat less. Because the fiber and bran have been removed from bad carbs, these foods are easier to digest and are absorbed very quickly. Simple carbs or sugars, the bad carbs, cause your blood sugar to spike and you typically feel a quick rush of energy. This, in turn, stimulates your pancreas to make more insulin to remove the excess sugar from your system. Insulin then lowers your blood sugar and transports excess glucose to be stored in fat cells. Your lower blood sugar levels then can cause you

to feel tired, and then you feel hungry again very quickly. In this cycle of spiking and plummeting blood sugar levels, bad carbs can cause you to eat too many calories without your getting full, and these extra calories become converted into fat. Bad carbs include white bread, white rice, white pasta, and anything else labeled *enriched, refined bleached,* or *processed,* as well as foods high in sugar, such as ice cream, donuts, and soda.

While we are on the subject of carbohydrates, the phrases "net carbs" and "low carbs" have also been used in advertising. Actually, there is no such thing as a low carb or net carb: that is just a gimmick to make a product sound healthier so you will buy it. The FDA has not defined or approved these terms—so this type of advertising is misleading and illegal.

You want to get your carbohydrate needs met by eating more good carbs—foods that are high in fiber, such as whole-grain breads, oatmeal, vegetables, brown rice, whole-wheat pasta, and fruit. This will give you a more constant feeling of energy throughout the day and will reduce your blood sugar swings.

---

derived from germinating cereals; and lactose, found in human and animal milk.

- *Polysaccharides—carbohydrates with more than two saccharide units.* Polysaccharides include starches and dietary fiber. Examples are vegetables, breads, cereals, legumes, and pasta.

Both simple and complex carbohydrates contain 4 calories per gram, and both are digested into glucose. Simple carbohydrates are digested more quickly because they are composed of fewer saccharide units than complex carbohydrates. Complex carbohydrates also take longer to digest because they have more fiber, vitamins, and minerals. (See the box "Are There Really Good and Bad Carbs?" for more information.)

How Much Carbohydrate Is Recommended? Each gram of carbohydrate contains 4 calories. Since the average person requires approximately 2,000 calories per day and about 45–65 percent of our calories come from carbohydrates, it is recommended that approximately 1,200 of our daily calories come from carbohydrates.[1] However, age, gender, and activity level affect the number of calories an individual requires each day; individual energy needs are discussed later in this chapter.

Simple Sugars: The American Sweet Tooth The average adult American consumes approximately 140 pounds of sweeteners (sugar, corn sweetener, syrup, and honey)

each year,[2] an increase of 19 percent in the past 30 years (Table 5.1). These sugars are usually found in sodas, candy, and bakery items, which have little nutritional value. Corn sweetener consumption increased to 79

Table 5.1 Per Capita Consumption of Food and Calories

Commodity Group	Per Capita Consumption			
	1970	2003	Increase in Pounds, 1970–2003	Increase in Daily Calories, 1970–2003
	Pounds		*Percentage*	*Number*
Fats and oils	53	86	63	216
Grains	136	194	43	188
Sugar and sweeteners	119	142	19	76
Meat, eggs, and nuts	226	242	7	24
Vegetables	337	418	24	16
Fruits	242	275	12	14
Dairy	564	594	5	−11
Total	1,675	1,950	16	523

Source: USDA, "U.S. Food Consumption Up 16% Since 1970," Economic Research Service, December 2005.

The Economic Research Service per capita data represent the amount of food and calories available for consumption after adjusting for spoilage, plate waste, and other losses in the home or marketing system.

pounds in 2003, up 400 percent from 1970, largely due to the high-fructose corn syrup found in many beverages. This increase in sugar consumption is a major contributor to the more than 500-calorie-per-day increase in overall energy consumption since 1970 (see Table 5.1).

Much of the sugar we consume is hidden; that is, sugar is a principal product we may overlook in a large number of food items. Foods such as ketchup, salad dressings, cured meat products, and canned vegetables and fruits can contain much hidden sugar. Corn syrup, frequently found in these items, is a highly concentrated sucrose solution. Whether the sugar is overt or hidden, the USDA has suggested a limit of 8 teaspoons of sugar per day for a 2,000 calorie diet.

Sugar Substitutes For a number of years, sugar substitutes have been used in a wide array of beverages, candy, baked goods, chewing gum, frozen desserts, gelatins and puddings, jams, toppings, and syrups. Among the most familiar of these are saccharin and aspartame (Nutrasweet), both of which are several hundred times sweeter than sucrose. Since 1977, saccharin has been linked to cancer, particularly bladder cancer, and warnings were given about its use until 2000, when Congress removed this requirement.[3] Some of the newer artificial sweeteners are: sorbitol, found in ice cream; acesulfame potassium (ace K), used in Pepsi ONE; xylitol, found in some brands of chewing gum; neotame, found in candy and soft drinks; sucralose (Splenda); and tagatose, found in Slurpees. These sweeteners can be more than 600 times sweeter than sugar; neotame is 7,000 to 13,000 times sweeter than sugar. Stevia is an herbal sweetener made from the leaves of the South American shrub by this name. It is 200 to 300 times sweeter than table sugar and is sold as a dietary supplement in the United States. There has been concern that consumption of stevia could cause infertility.

Fats

Fats (lipids, fatty acids) have been given a bad name but are an important nutrient in our diets. Fats provide a concentrated form of energy (over double that of carbohydrates—there are 9 calories per gram consumed versus 4 for carbohydrates and protein). Fats provide a sense of **satiety** and keep us from feeling hungry. Because fats take longer to leave the stomach than either carbohydrates or proteins do, our stomachs feel full for a longer period of time, decreasing our appetite. Fats also help to give our food its pleasing taste, and they serve as carriers of fat-soluble vitamins A, D, E, and K. Without fat, these vitamins would quickly pass through the body. Fat insulates the body and helps it retain heat.

Sources of Fat Dietary sources of fat are often difficult to identify. The visible fats in our diet, such as butter, salad oils, and the layer of fat on some cuts of meat, represent only about 40 percent of the fat we consume. Most of the fat we eat is "hidden" in food because it is incorporated into the food during preparation or used to fry the food, or it is in food that we have not learned to recognize as being high in fat, such as a candy bar.

Parents of infants and toddlers need to know that current medical opinion advises strongly against any limiting of fats in the diets of children younger than two years of age.[4] This recommendation is, of course, based on the demands for energy and the nutritional requirements that accompany the rapid growth that occurs during this formative stage of life.

Types of Fat Every type of dietary fat is made up of a combination of three forms of fat (saturated, monounsaturated, and polyunsaturated), based on its chemical composition (Figure 5-1). In each of the three forms of fat, the absence of double bonds (saturated fats) or the presence of double bonds (monounsaturated and polyunsaturated fats) and the location of the double bonds within the molecule determine the nature and degree of restructuring that the body can do in changing dietary fat into physiology-friendly forms. Today, consumers need to pay attention to the amount of each type of fat in dietary fat because of the role that each form plays in heart disease (see Chapter 10).

Saturated and Trans Fats Not all fats are created equal. **Saturated fats,** including those found in animal sources and in vegetable oils to which hydrogen has been added (hydrogenated), becoming **trans-fatty acids,** need to be carefully limited in a modern healthy diet. The presence of trans-fatty acids (an altered form of normal vegetable oil molecule or from meat and dairy products, having formed naturally by fermentation in the intestinal tract of animals)[5] is associated with changes in the cell membrane, including those cells lining the artery wall. This possibly prevents these vessel wall cells from freeing cholesterol from their surfaces.[6] Processing can change the structure of fat, making it more saturated. As a result, the oils become semisolid and more stable at room temperature. The term *trans* describes the chemical makeup of a fatty

---

> **Key Terms**
>
> **satiety** (suh **tie** uh tee) The feeling of no longer being hungry; a diminished desire to eat.
>
> **saturated fats** Fats in solid form at room temperature; primarily animal fats.
>
> **trans-fatty acids** An altered form of an unsaturated fat molecule in which the hydrogen atoms on each side of the double bond(s) are on opposite sides; also called *trans fats.*

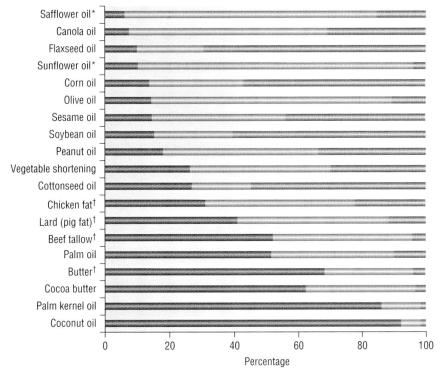

Figure 5-1 Composition of Dietary Fats

* Safflower and sunflower oil come in several forms; those given here are high oleic (monounsaturated) forms.
† Only animal fats contain cholesterol; per tablespoon, chicken fat has 11 mg; lard, 12 mg; beef tallow, 14 mg; and butter, 31 mg.

Source: Data from USDA Nutrient Database for Standard Reference (Release 19), April 2007.

acid. Most trans-fatty acids come from hydrogenated oil, which is found in foods such as stick margarine, peanut butter, and crackers. They are popular in food manufacturing because they can extend the shelf life of the food: the oil stays mixed in the food and doesn't rise to the top, and the food doesn't become too soft at room temperature. The fast-food industry uses these fats to fry many foods.[7] Additionally, trans-fatty acids are associated with increases in low-density lipoprotein (LDL) the "bad" cholesterol, without corresponding increases in high-density lipoprotein (HDL), the "good" cholesterol[8] (see Chapter 10). The amount of trans-fatty acids in the diet should be limited.

Trans fats can act like saturated fat, potentially raising LDL blood cholesterol levels and decreasing HDL cholesterol. This is the reason nutritionists encourage us to use butter rather than stick margarine. To reduce your intake of trans fat, make sure you check the labels on foods to see if they list "partially hydrogenated vegetable oil" as one of the ingredients. Foods such as cakes, cookies, crackers, snack foods, stick margarine, vegetable shortening, and fried foods are most likely to contain hydrogenated vegetable oil.

Trans fat is seen as being so unhealthy it has been called a "dangerous and unnecessary ingredient" and

has been banned for use in restaurants in New York City. The Cheescake Factory chain announced it is trying out a trans-fat-free menu in Los Angeles, and Kentucky Fried Chicken and Wendy's have pledged not to use trans fat in their cooking oil. The FDA now requires food manufacturers to list trans fat on any product that contains at least 0.5 grams of trans fat. Many food producers are jumping on the no-trans-fat bandwagon, and you will see more cereals, chips, crackers, and other foods labeled "No trans fat."

Monounsaturated Fats Fortunately, the replacement of saturated fats with monounsaturated and polyunsaturated fats and oils appears to lower blood cholesterol levels and reduce the risk of heart disease. Vegetable oils tend to be low in saturated fats, with the exception of the tropical oils (coconut, palm, and palm kernel oils). Monounsaturated fats are found in high quantities in olive oil, peanut oil, and sesame oil.

Polyunsaturated Fats Polyunsaturated fats are especially prevalent in soybean oil and corn oil. Monounsaturated fats can reduce the harmful low-density lipoproteins (LDLs). Polyunsaturated fats both reduce LDLs and total cholesterol. However, polyunsaturated fats also *lower* the healthful high-density lipoproteins (HDLs), which is not a desirable outcome. Omega-3 fatty acids, found in most varieties of fish, are a type of polyunsaturated fat and have received a great deal of attention lately in being associated with decreased risk of heart disease. Our bodies require omega-3 fatty acids, but we can't produce them on our own, and therefore we must get them from the foods we eat. You can also consume omega-3 fish oil as a dietary supplement. Flax seed, walnuts, and olive oil are also good sources for omega-3 fatty acids.

Tropical Oils   Although all cooking oils (and fats such as butter, lard, margarine, and shortening) have the same number of calories by weight (9 calories per gram), some oils contain high percentages of saturated fats. All oils and fats contain varying percentages of saturated, monounsaturated, and polyunsaturated fats. The tropical oils—coconut, palm, and palm kernel—contain much higher percentages of saturated fats than do other cooking oils. Coconut oil is 92 percent saturated fat. Tropical oils can still be found in some brands of snack foods, crackers, cookies, nondairy creamers, and breakfast cereals, although they have been removed from most national brands. Do you check for tropical oils on the ingredients labels of the food you select?

How Much Fat, and What Type, Is Recommended?   The new dietary guidelines recommend that no more than 20–35 percent of our calories come from fat. In addition it is suggested that people:

- Consume less than 10 percent of calories from saturated fatty acids and less than 300 mg/day of cholesterol, and keep trans-fatty acid consumption as low as possible.
- Get most fats from sources of polyunsaturated and monounsaturated fatty acids, such as fish, nuts, and vegetable oils.
- Make choices that are lean, low-fat, or fat-free when selecting and preparing meat, poultry, dry beans, and milk or milk products.

Cholesterol   **Cholesterol** is a white, fatlike substance found in cells of animal origin. It is not found in any vegetable product, so products such as peanut butter and margarine that claim they are cholesterol-free never had it in the first place. Cholesterol is used to synthesize cell membranes and also serves as the starting material for the synthesis of bile acids and sex hormones. Although we consume cholesterol in our diet, in such foods as shrimp and other shellfish, animal fat, and milk, we don't need to obtain cholesterol from external sources—the human liver can synthesize enough of the substance to meet the body's needs.

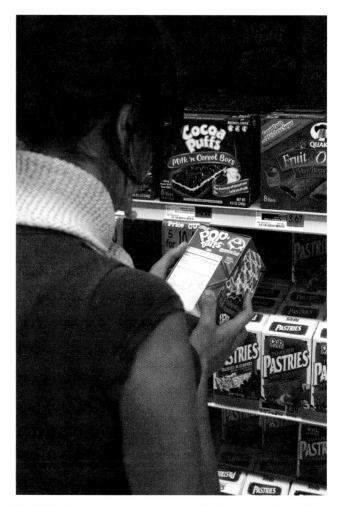

Food labels are an important source of information about the type and amount of fats, carbohydrates, and other nutrients contained in a food.

Cholesterol is essential for many of the body's functions. However, if you have too much cholesterol, it builds up in your bloodstream and clogs arteries, putting you at risk for heart disease, heart attack, and stroke. There are different kinds of cholesterol. LDL is often referred to as "bad" cholesterol. LDL cholesterol builds up on the walls of arteries to form artery-clogging "plaques" that contribute to the development of heart disease and stroke. HDL, or good cholesterol, helps remove excess LDL cholesterol from the blood and transports it back to the liver, where it can be eliminated from the body. You want to have lower LDL (under 130) and higher HDL (higher than 60), with total cholesterol under 200 (see Chapter 10). Almonds, oatmeal, fish, soy, and red wine (a limit of one glass daily) help lower overall cholesterol levels. Whole milk, processed meats, and foods with trans fats and tropical oils, such as fast foods and baked goods, can increase overall cholesterol levels and should be avoided.

A number of medical conditions can give rise to high blood cholesterol, such as liver disease, kidney failure, hypothyroidism, and diabetes. Certain medications, (some diuretics, for example) can also raise blood cholesterol, irrespective of diet.

Nutritionists recommend that people restrict their dietary intake of cholesterol to 300 mg or less per day. In addition, no more than 20–35 percent of your total caloric intake should come from fat, with most fats being monounsaturated and polyunsaturated.

Low-Fat Foods   *Low-fat* and *low-calorie* do not mean the same thing, but often people confuse the two. Fat-free, low-fat, and reduced-fat foods have been popular for many years, with people thinking they can eat as much as they want of these foods. This is far from true; a fat-free or reduced-fat product may have as many if not more calories per serving than regular products do. For example, 2 tablespoons of fat-free caramel topping have 103 calories, the same amount as homemade-with-butter caramel topping; 2 tablespoons of Skippy peanut butter have the same number of calories as 2 tablespoons of Skippy reduced-fat peanut butter, 190 calories; and 2 tablespoons of Cool Whip are equal to lite Cool Whip, 25 calories.[9]

Fatty foods make people feel fuller longer than do fat-free foods; thus people tend to eat more of the fat-free foods and so consume more calories. In general, the lower the fat, the higher the price tag, because the food industry recognizes that Americans are willing to pay more for products labeled *reduced-fat* and *fat-free*. However, food such as low-fat sour cream, yogurt, or salad dressings are healthier choices, because they have less saturated fat.

Fat-Free Substitutes   Newly developed fat-free products containing fat substitutes (Simplesse, Simple Pleasures, Olestra, and Trailblazer) are available or soon to be available in the marketplace. These products contain no cholesterol and have 80 percent fewer calories than do similar products made with fat. Although fat-free substitutes first appeared only in snack foods, today they are found in ice cream, salad dressing, cheese spreads, yogurt, cakes, pies, and French fries.

The development of Olestra (marketed as Olean) as an example, required more than 25 years and $200 million on the part of Procter & Gamble, as an array of new technologies were required. In general, fat-free substitutes are made through processes called *microparticulation*, in which several fatty acids are bonded to a sugar molecule to create a triglyceride-like molecule that imparts all the characteristics of fats but is incapable of being enzymatically broken down by the body as are the triglycerides.

In spite of the apparent desirability of the fat-free technology, concerns have been voiced regarding the inability of these "nouveau fats" to carry fat-soluble vitamins (vitamins A, D, E, and K). Additional concern was raised over side effects in some people, such as abdominal cramping, loose stools, anal leakage, and an unpleasant aftertaste.[10]

 TALKING POINTS What would you say to a friend who is following a low-carbohydrate, high-fat weight-loss diet to help that person see the potential pitfalls of the diet?

Proteins

The word *protein* derives from the ancient Greek word *proteios*, meaning "first importance." Protein serves primarily to promote growth and maintenance of body tissue. However, when calorie intake falls, protein is broken down for glucose. This loss of protein can impede growth and repair of tissue. From this, it can be seen that adequate carbohydrate intake prevents protein from serving as an energy source.[11] Protein also is a primary component of enzyme and hormone structure; it helps maintain the *acid-base balance* of our bodies and serves as a source of energy (4 calories per gram consumed).

Sources and Types of Proteins   Proteins are manufactured in every living cell; they are composed of chains of amino acids. Amino acids are the "bricks" from which the body constructs its own protein. Twenty amino acids are used in various combinations to build the protein required for physiological processes to continue in a healthy manner.

The human body obtains amino acids from two sources—by breaking down protein from food (as if to take a brick wall apart for its bricks) or by manufacturing its own bricks (amino acids) within its cells. The latter process is less than fully successful because only 11 of the necessary 20 amino acids can be built by the body. The 9 amino acids that *cannot* be built by the body are called *essential amino acids* (indispensable amino acids), because they must be obtained from outside the body through the protein in food. The 11 amino acids that the body itself can make are called *nonessential amino*

Key Terms

cholesterol A primary form of fat found in the blood; lipid material manufactured within the body, as well as derived from dietary sources.

proteins Compounds composed of chains of amino acids; primary components of muscle and connective tissue.

amino acids The building blocks of protein; manufactured by the body or obtained from dietary sources.

The Dietary Reference Intakes (DRIs) replaced the Recommended Daily Allowances (RDAs) in 1997. The RDA recommendations were based upon the levels that might prevent nutrition-related diseases; the **Dietary Reference Intakes (DRIs)** are much more comprehensive and based on health promotion and prevention. The DRI refers to three types of reference values: **Estimated Average Requirement (EAR), Recommended Dietary Allowance (RDA),** and **Tolerable Upper Intake Level (UL).** The Estimated Average Requirement (EAR) is the intake value that is estimated to meet the requirement in 50 percent of an age- and gender-specific group. At this level of intake, the remaining 50 percent of the specified group would not have its needs met. The Recommended Dietary Allowance (RDA) is the dietary intake level that is sufficient to meet the nutrient requirements of nearly all individuals in the group. The Tolerable Upper Intake Level (UL) is the maximum level of daily nutrient intake that is unlikely to pose risks of adverse health effects for almost all of the individuals in the group for whom it is designed. The specific DRIs for vitamins and minerals are discussed later in this chapter.

The Food and Nutrition Board sets an additional standard for the energy nutrients known as **Acceptable Macronutrient Distribution Ranges (AMDRs).** These values are the range of intakes for energy sources that are associated with adequate nutrient intake and reduced risk of chronic disease; the AMDRs for adults are as follows:

Carbohydrate: 45–65 percent of total calories
Fat: 20–35 percent of total calories
Protein: 10–35 percent of total calories

Source: Food and Nutrition Board, Institute of Medicine of the National Academies. Dietary Reference Intake Tables, 2004.

---

acids (dispensable amino acids), because the body does not have to rely solely on food protein to obtain these bricks.[11]

In terms of food sources of amino acids, foods can be classified into one of two types, depending on whether they can supply the body with the essential amino acids or not. Complete protein foods contain all nine essential amino acids and are of animal origin (milk, meat, cheese, and eggs). The incomplete protein foods do not contain all the essential amino acids and are of plant origin (vegetables, grains, and legumes [peas or beans, including chickpeas and butter beans]). Vegan vegetarians (see page 151), people with limited access to animal-based food sources, and those who have significantly limited their meat, egg, and dairy product consumption, need to understand how essential amino acids can be obtained from incomplete protein sources. When even one essential amino acid is missing from the diet, deficiency can develop.

Soybeans are a good source of protein for vegetarians. Soybeans provide the same high-quality protein as animal protein.[12] Furthermore, soybeans contain no cholesterol or saturated fat. In 1999 the FDA stated, "Diets low in saturated fat and cholesterol that include 25 grams of soy protein a day may reduce the risk of heart disease." The sale of soy foods doubled since that proclamation. However, the research on which that claim was based has not been replicated, and in February 2006 the American Heart Association concluded that soy doesn't lower cholesterol as much as was originally suggested. Three long-term government-funded studies currently are investigating the effects of soy on cholesterol levels and its role, if any, in the prevention of cancer and heart disease.[12]

How Much Protein Is Recommended? The latest recommendations for protein intake are part of a set of standards known as the Dietary Reference Intakes, or DRIs (see the box "Dietary Reference Intakes" for more information). Protein intake recommendations are based on body weight and activity level. The current DRI for protein is 0.36 grams per pound of body weight per day, based upon a sedentary lifestyle, and is higher for athletes and those who are more active. In terms of overall energy intake, nutritionists recommend that 10–35 percent of our total caloric intake come from protein.[13]

Vitamins

Vitamins are organic compounds that are required in small amounts for normal growth, reproduction, and maintenance of health. Vitamins differ from carbohydrates, fats, and proteins because they do not provide calories or serve as structural elements for our bodies. Vitamins serve as *coenzymes*. By facilitating the action of **enzymes,** vitamins help initiate a wide variety of body responses, including energy production, use of minerals, and growth of healthy tissue.

Types and Sources of Vitamins Discovered just after the turn of the twentieth century, the 13 essential vitamins can be classified as *water-soluble* (capable of being dissolved in water) or *fat-soluble* (capable of being dissolved in fat or lipid tissue). Water-soluble vitamins include the B-complex vitamins and vitamin C. Most of the excess of these water-soluble vitamins is eliminated from the body during urination. The fat-soluble vitamins are A, D, E, and K. These vitamins are stored in the body in the adipose tissue or fat with excessive intake.

Table 5.4 USDA Food Guide at 12 Differe

Daily Amount of Food from Each Group (vegetable subgroup

Food Group	Calorie Level 1,000	1,200	1,400	1,600
	Food group amounts shown in cup (c) or o differs from the other units. Oils are show			
Fruits	1 c (2 srv)	1 c (2 srv)	1.5 c (3 srv)	1.5 c (3 srv)
Vegetables	1 c (2 srv)	1.5 c (3 srv)	1.5 c (3 srv)	2 c (4 srv)
Dark green veg.	1 c/wk	1.5 c/wk	1.5 c/wk	2 c/wk
Orange veg.	.5 c/wk	1 c/wk	1 c/wk	1.5 c/wk
Legumes	.5 c/wk	1 c/wk	1 c/wk	2.5 c/wk
Starchy veg.	1.5 c/wk	2.5 c/wk	2.5 c/wk	2.5 c/wk
Other veg.	4 c/wk	4.5 c/wk	4.5 c/wk	5.5 c/wk
Grains	3 oz-eq	4 oz-eq	5 oz-eq	5 oz-eq
Whole grains	1.5	2	2.5	3
Other grains	1.5	2	2.5	2.5
Lean meat and beans	2 oz-eq	3 oz-eq	4 oz-eq	5 oz-eq
Milk	2 c	2 c	2 c	3 c
Oils	15 g	17 g	17 g	22 g
Discretionary calorie allowance	165	171	171	182

Source: U.S. Department of Health and Human Services and U.S. Departm
.gov/dietaryguidelines).

and fish should be fresh, stored appropriately, and c
adequately to reduce the likelihood of serious food
illnesses. This will be discussed later in this chapter

Breads, Cereals, Rice, and Pasta The nutritiona
efit from the breads, cereals, rice, and pasta grou
in its contribution of B-complex vitamins and e
from complex carbohydrates. Some nutritionists b
that foods from this group promote protein intake,
many of them are prepared as complete-protein fo
for example, macaroni and cheese, cereal and mill
bread and meat sandwiches.

This group is referred to as the "grain group"
USDA, and there is a particular emphasis on consu
at least 3 of the 6 ounces of this group from whole g
Whole grains can reduce the risk of chronic diseas
help with weight maintenance.

Whole grains consist of the entire grain seed,
kernel, and can't be identified by the color of the
The FDA requires that food contain 51 percent or
whole-grain ingredients by weight and be low-fat
der to be called "whole grain." On food labels, "
grain" should be the first ingredient listed. Avo
fined grains, because the grain-refining process typ
removes most of the bran and some of the germ, r
ing in the loss of dietary fiber, minerals, vitamins

Considering C

Antioxidant Supplem

Chocolate may actually
that dark chocolate cont
antioxidants than does
tective effect against he
antioxidant properties. I
antioxidants than was b

Antioxidants are sai
which are highly excite
produced in cells during
ing free radicals is cons
reducing the chances o
Alzheimer's disease, ar
people believe that free
age-related changes se

The foods that are a
chocolate, coffee, gree
popular source of antio

colorless means yo
fluids. Of course, p
fruits, vegetables,
noncaffeinated soft
sugar and calories.
tion by persons of
tion by infants, ca
and aspiration pne

Fiber

Although not cons
an important com
sists of plant mater
through the diges
fruits, and vegetab

Fiber can be
basis of water solu
absorb water from
ter, the insoluble
the time it takes t
tract. In contrast,
intestinal tract an
has cholesterol at
removing (or lowe
cause foods high i
and saturated fats
ing blood sugar lo
associated with d
day this latter con

How much
from 21–38 g of
can adults eat on

Dietary Reference Intakes for Vitamins It is possible
to consume and retain too many fat-soluble vitamins,
particularly A and D. All the fat-soluble vitamins, however, hold the potential for toxicity if taken in amounts
that far exceed Dietary Reference Intakes (see Table
5.2). Most toxicity results from the use of supplements
by adults or through excessive food intake of particular
sources in very small children. When toxicity develops,
the condition is referred to as **hypervitaminosis.**

People often think taking megadoses of vitamins
such as vitamin C can be health-enhancing, but the reverse is true. Taking large doses of vitamin C from a
dietary supplement can put a strain on your kidneys,
causing kidney stones and diarrhea. Too much niacin, vitamin B_6, and folate can also be harmful.[7]

Because water-soluble vitamins dissolve rather
quickly in water, you should be cautious in the preparation of fresh fruits and vegetables. One precaution is to
avoid overcooking fresh vegetables. The longer fresh vegetables are steamed or boiled, the more water-soluble vitamins will be lost. More vitamins are retained with microwave cooking than with stove-top cooking. Even soaking
sliced fresh fruit or vegetables can result in the loss of
vitamin C and B-complex vitamins.

To ensure an adequate vitamin intake, do not rely
on bottled vitamins sold in grocery stores or health food
stores. The best way is really the simplest and least expensive way: eat a variety of foods. Unless there are special circumstances, such as pregnancy, infancy, or an existing health problem, virtually everyone in our society
who eats a reasonably well-rounded diet consumes appropriate levels of all vitamins. The validity of this was
recently substantiated by a study of 42,000 women in
which it was demonstrated that those women with a sustained history of eating a balanced diet were significantly
less likely to die prematurely from a variety of chronic
conditions than were those women who ate less balanced
diets.[14]

Should I Take a Supplement? While conducting research to formulate the new dietary guidelines, the USDA
found that most Americans are consuming too many
calories but are not meeting their nutritional needs. How
can this be? We eat too many nutrient-deficient foods
such as junk food and not enough nutrient-dense foods
(which will be discussed later in this chapter). The USDA
and the American Dietician Association recommend following the food pyramid guidelines, particularly eating
4½ cups of fruits and vegetables a day, rather than taking
supplements to rectify this problem. Most Americans
do not consume this amount of fruit and vegetables on
a daily basis and don't meet their DRIs. We discuss the
food pyramid guidelines in a later section.

Some believe that additional vitamin intake will prevent or delay the onset of chronic health conditions such

---

as cancer and cardiovascular disease. To date there seems
to be no absolute consensus regarding the effectiveness of
most supplements in chronic disease prevention. (See the
box "Vitamin E" on page 138). This said, there is at least
one well-established success story regarding vitamin
supplementation. That success story is the effectiveness
of folic acid supplementation in assuring the appropriate closure of the neural tube during embryonic development, thus preventing the development of spina bifida.[15]
In spite of widespread awareness of the necessity for folic
acid, however, nearly one-third of women of childbearing
age do not take this B vitamin on a daily basis.

The DRI for folic acid for adults is 300–400 µg daily;
however, for pregnant women it is 600 µg a day and for
lactating women it is 500 µg daily. There has been some
suggestion that folic acid can prevent cardiovascular disease, cancer, and Alzheimer's disease (similar to promises made about vitamin E); however, experts say there still
isn't enough evidence to make these claims. Vitamin B_{12}

Key Terms

Dietary Reference Intakes (DRIs) Measures that refer
to three types of reference values: Estimated Average
Requirement, Recommended Dietary Allowance, and
Tolerable Upper Intake Level.

Estimated Average Requirement (EAR) The intake
value that is estimated to meet the requirement in
50 percent of an age- and gender-specific group.

Recommended Dietary Allowance (RDA) The dietary
intake level sufficient to meet the nutrient requirements
of nearly all individuals in an age- and gender-specific
group.

Tolerable Upper Intake Level (UL) The maximum
level of daily nutrient intake that is unlikely to pose
risks of adverse health effects for almost all of the
individuals in the group for whom it is designed.

**Acceptable Macronutrient Distribution Range
(AMDR)** The range of intakes for energy sources
associated with adequate nutrient intake and reduced
risk of chronic disease.

vitamins Organic compounds that facilitate the action
of enzymes.

enzymes Organic substances that control the rate of
physiological reactions but are not altered in the
process.

hypervitaminosis Excessive accumulation of vitamins
within the body; associated with the fat-soluble
vitamins.

vegetables), polyph
(from cruciferous
garlic, chives, and
play an important
slow the developn
At this time, how
which the various
of cancer cells is n
agreed that these
selections, no pr
amounts of variou
made.

Minerals

Nearly 5 percent
materials, the *mi*
structural elemer
thyroid hormone
tion of a number
ance, nerve imp
tion, blood clotti
synthesis. Appro
nized as being e:
mins, minerals a
heat or food proc
Macronutrie
als that are seen
tissues. Example
phorus, sodium,
of *micronutrien*

Table 5.3 Find Your Calorie Count

			Activity Level	
Gender	Age	Sedentary	Moderately active	Active
Child	2–3	1,000	1,000–1,400	1,000–1,4(
Female	4–8	1,200	1,400–1,600	1,400–1,8(
	9–13	1,600	1,600–2,000	1,800–2,2(
	14–18	1,800	2,000	2,4(
	19–30	2,000	2,000–2,200	2,4(
	31–50	1,800	2,000	2,2(
	51+	1,600	1,800	2,000–2,2(
Male	4–8	1,400	1,400–1,600	1,600–2,0(
	9–13	1,800	1,800–2,200	2,000–2,6(
	14–18	2,200	2,400–2,800	2,800–3,2(
	19–30	2,400	2,600–2,800	3,0(
	31–50	2,200	2,400–2,600	2,800–3,0(
	51+	2,000	2,200–2,400	2,400–2,8(

Sedentary means a lifestyle that includes only the light physical ac
ity associated with typical day-to-day life.

Moderately active means a lifestyle that includes physical activity
equivalent to walking about 1.5 to 3 miles per day at 3 to 4 miles p
hour, in addition to the light physical activity associated with typica
day-to-day life.

Active means a lifestyle that includes physical activity equivalent t
walking more than 3 miles per day at 3 to 4 miles per hour, in addit
to the light physical activity associated with typical day-to-day life.

Source: U.S. Department of Health and Human Services and U.S. Departme
Agriculture. Dietary Guidelines for Americans, 2005 (www.healthierus
.gov/dietaryguidelines).

function of this group is to provide vitamin A, vit
C, complex carbohydrates, and fiber. Because Amer
tend to eat only a few vegetables, such as potatoes,
and carrots, the new guidelines give specific recom:
dations about the types of vegetable. One general r
to "eat your colors," meaning you should consume
riety of vegetables over the course of a week. The U
recommends:

- Dark green vegetables (such as broccoli, spinach
  3 cups/week

- Orange vegetables (such as carrots, sweet potato
  2 cups/week

- Legumes (such as soy, kidney, lentil, pinto beans
  3 cups/week

- Starchy vegetables (such as corn, potatoes, green
  peas)—3 cups/week

- Other vegetables (such as cauliflower, asparagus,
  celery)—6½ cups/week

Again, avoid drinking vegetable juices as a wa
meeting these requirements because they can be
in salt and sugar and don't provide the fiber intake
whole vegetables do. **Cruciferous vegetables,** suc
broccoli, cabbage, brussels sprouts, and cauliflower,

*MyPyramid recommends that half of all grain servings come
from whole grains. Because whole grains can't always be
identified by color, it is important to check food labels for
whole-grain content.*

are returned to the food; however, only three B vitamins
(thiamine, niacin, riboflavin) and iron are replaced.

For a 2,000-calorie diet, MyPyramid recommends
6 ounces of grains daily, with at least 3 ounces coming
from whole grains. One ounce is equivalent to:

- 1 slice bread

- 1 cup dry cereal

- ½ cup cooked rice, pasta, cereal

The food industry has risen to the challenge of providing nutritious whole-grain foods with improved taste
and texture. For example, ConAgra has spent millions of
dollars over the past five years to develop "white wheat"
made from a naturally occurring albino variety of flour.
It has 3½ times more dietary fiber, 11 times more vitamin E, 5 times more magnesium, and 4 times more niacin than does refined, unenriched wheat flour. It also
tastes milder and sweeter than most whole grains do. It
combines the best of both worlds—the nutrition of whole
wheat with the taste of white flour.[27]

Oils The USDA defines oils as fats that are liquid at
room temperature, such as vegetable oils used in cooking. Oils come from many different plants and from fish.
Some common oils are canola oil, corn oil, cottonseed
oil, olive oil, safflower oil, soybean oil, and sunflower oil.
Canola and olive oil are preferred over other types of oils.
Some foods, such as nuts, olives, fish, and avocados, are
naturally high in oils. Foods that are mainly oil include
mayonnaise, salad dressings, and soft margarine with no
trans fats. A limit of 24 grams, or 6 teaspoons, of oils is
the daily recommendation. One teaspoon is equal to:

- 1 teaspoon margarine

- 1 tablespoon low-fat mayonnaise

Table 5.5 Sample Menu for a 2,000-Calorie Food Plan

Breakfast

1 cup cold cereal topped with 1 cup fat-free milk and 1 small banana
1 slice whole-wheat toast with 1 teaspoon soft margarine
1 cup orange juice

Lunch

Tuna sandwich (2 slices rye bread, 3 ounces water-packed tuna, 2
  teaspoons mayonnaise, 1 tablespoon diced celery, ¼ cup romaine
  lettuce, and 2 tomato slices)
1 medium pear
1 cup fat-free milk

Dinner

3-ounce boneless, skinless chicken breast
1 baked sweet potato
½ cup peas with onions with 1 teaspoon soft margarine
1 whole-wheat dinner roll (1 ounce) with 1 teaspoon soft margarine
1 cup leafy greens salad with 1 tablespoon sunflower oil and vinegar
  dressing

Snacks

1 cup low-fat fruited yogurt
¼ cup dried apricots

Source: MyPyramid.gov.

- 2 tablespoons light salad dressing

- 1 teaspoon vegetable oil

Discretionary Calories Where do such items as beer,
butter, candy, sodas, cookies, corn chips, and pastries fit
into your diet? Most of these items contribute relatively
little to healthful nutrition; they provide additional calories, generally from sucrose and significant amounts of
salt and fat. Fats, salt, sugar, and alcohol are referred to
as "discretionary calories" and are limited to 100–300
calories a day by the MyPyramid food guide. As described earlier in this chapter, the recommended total
daily fat intake should be 20–35 percent of total calories,
with most fats coming from sources of polyunsaturated
and monounsaturated fatty acids. Less than 10 percent of
total calories should be from saturated fats, and less than
300 mg/day should come from cholesterol. Trans-fatty
acid consumption is to be kept "as low as possible."

The USDA also suggests that we choose and prepare
foods and beverages with little added sugars or caloric
sweeteners. The new food guide recommends no more
than 8 teaspoons of added sugars per day, which is equivalent to ½ ounce of jelly beans or an 8-ounce glass of lem-
onade. Eating too much sugar has been thought to be a major contributor to the increase in obesity in Americans.

Table 5.5 provides a sample 2,000-calorie menu
based on the MyPyramid food guide.

Dietary Guidelines for Americans 2005

The Dietary Guidelines for Americans are science-based and summarize the analysis of the most current information regarding nutrition, health, physical activity, and food safety. The goal of these guidelines is to lower the risk of chronic disease and promote health through diet and physical activity. Taken together, these guidelines encourage Americans to eat fewer calories, make wiser food choices, and be more physically active.

Focus on Nutrient Density Many Americans consume too many calories and too much saturated and trans fat, cholesterol, added sugar, and sodium. At the same time, many people do not meet the recommended intakes for fiber and a number of vitamins and minerals. Therefore, people should choose mostly **nutrient-dense foods,** which provide substantial amounts of vitamins and minerals and comparatively few calories. Junk foods typically are not nutrient-dense, because they are high in sugar and saturated and trans fat, high in calories, and low in vitamins and minerals. Choosing nutrient-dense foods can be especially challenging when eating out; see the box "Healthy Restaurant Eating" for suggestions.

Following the recommendations in the MyPyramid plan can help you choose nutrient-dense foods. In general, Americans are advised to consume more dark green and orange vegetables, legumes, fruits, whole grains, and low-fat milk and milk products. These choices can be substituted for refined grains and foods high in fat

(especially saturated and trans fats), added sugars, and calories. Meet your dietary needs by consuming healthy food choices, not dietary supplements.

Physical Activity Of course, part of managing your weight in a healthy manner includes physical activity. The Dietary Guidelines have emphasized the important role that physical activity plays in our lives by including it in the food pyramid. It is proposed that Americans engage in at least 30 minutes of moderate-intensity physical activity, in addition to the usual activities of daily life, at work or home on most days of the week to reduce the risk of chronic disease. However, to prevent gradual, unhealthy weight gain in adulthood, we are advised to engage in approximately 60 minutes of moderate-to vigorous-intensity activity on most days of the week while not exceeding caloric intake requirements. To lose weight, you need to spend 60–90 minutes each day in physical fitness activities, which include cardiovascular conditioning, stretching exercises for flexibility, and

> ### Key Terms
>
> **nutrient-dense foods** Foods that provide substantial amounts of vitamins and minerals and comparatively few calories.

The Dietary Guidelines for Americans recommend that we increase our intake of fruits, vegetables, whole grains, and fat-free or low-fat dairy products. Fruit can be easily incorporated into the daily diet as part of a meal or as a snack.

resistance exercises or calisthenics for muscle strength and endurance (see Chapter 4).

Weight Management The Dietary Guidelines for Americans define weight management as meaning "to maintain body weight in a healthy range, balance calories from foods and beverages with calories expended, and to prevent gradual weight gain over time, make small decreases in food and beverage calories and increase physical activity." The dietary guidelines were designed with the goal of weight management in mind, and the recommendations for the different food groups were developed to reach this goal. Chapter 6 will go into further detail on how to identify a healthy weight and manage your weight effectively.

Food Groups to Encourage: Fruits, Vegetables, and Milk Americans are advised to consume more fiber-rich whole grains, fruits and vegetables, and milk products. Specifically, it is suggested that we consume 3 to 6 ounce-equivalents of whole-grain products per day, with the rest of the recommended grains coming from enriched or whole-grain products. In general, at least half the grains should come from whole grains. Americans are also encouraged to choose a variety of fruits and vegetables, selecting from all four vegetable subgroups: dark green, orange, legumes, and starchy vegetables. Drinking three cups of fat-free or low-fat milk or the equivalent is also encouraged, especially because milk consumption has been decreasing over the past 30 years.

Foods to Limit: Fats, Sugars, Sodium, and Alcohol

Choose Your Fats Wisely According to the USDA, we should limit our total fat intake to 20–35 percent of calories, with most fat calories coming from polyunsaturated and monounsaturated fatty acids. Less than 10 percent of our calories should come from saturated fatty acids, keeping our consumption of trans-fatty acids as low as possible. Also, we need to limit our cholesterol intake to less than 300 mg/day, getting our protein from low-fat, fat-free, or lean meat, poultry, milk, and bean products.

Sugar Consumption Americans eat more than 140 pounds of sugar per person per year, which is 19 percent more than 30 years ago.[24] This follows the upward trend in soda consumption, as well as the increased consumption of flavored coffees. The Dietary Guidelines for Americans suggest that we choose and prepare foods and beverages with little added sugar or noncaloric sweeteners. Shopping for foods that limit sugar (and fat) can be a challenge, however; see the box "If You See It, You Will Buy It."

Sodium Intake Something new to the USDA guidelines is the limitation on salt intake. They advise consuming less than 2,300 mg, or 1 teaspoon, of sodium each day and to choose and prepare foods with little salt. Most of our salt intake comes from processed or prepared foods. Many people are unaware of the high sodium content in prepared foods, sauces, soups, and canned foods, and so reading the labels for ingredients is extremely important. You might be surprised by some of the foods that contain salt—cookies, minute rice, canned green beans, soft drinks, and cereal. It is also difficult to know how to make healthy choices when eating out if you don't know the sodium content in the menu items. Too much sodium is linked to hypertension, and about 30 percent of Americans have sodium-sensitive high blood pressure, which can lead to heart attack or stroke. It is estimated that about 150,000 deaths each year are caused by consumption of too much salt.

Alcohol Consumption Another difference in the new dietary guidelines is the recommendation concerning alcohol consumption. The USDA states that "those who choose to drink alcoholic beverages should do so sensibly and in moderation." *Moderation* is defined as the consumption of up to 1 drink per day for women and up to 2 drinks per day for men. One drink is defined as either 12 fluid ounces of regular beer, 5 fluid ounces of wine, or 1½ fluid ounces of 80-proof distilled spirits.

If You See It, You Will Buy It: The Strategy of Product Placement

From Coca-Cola cups in front of the judges on *American Idol* to computer-generated first-down lines with advertisements for Ruby Tuesday on CBS during the Auburn vs. Louisiana college football game, product placement is cropping up in more and more unique places. In 2005, $21 million was spent to place products in video games, and $13 billion was spent to place these ads on the Internet. The Internet figure is expected to double to $26 billion by 2011.

Product placement is a type of advertising in which a product is intentionally included in a movie or television program. The product is mentioned by name or used by a character, or might just be seen as a prop in the set. Some familiar examples are Pepsi in *Back to the Future,* Pepsi and Starbucks in *Austin Powers,* and Burger King in *Men in Black.* Research shows that people tend to associate the product with the character or situation where it's displayed, and sales of the product increase dramatically. Product placement is a less expensive form of advertising than traditional commercials, and sometimes it is much more effective.

Some question the ethics of product placement advertising, particularly in movies, television shows, and video games that cater to children. Childhood obesity is on the rise, and it might not help children learn how to eat healthfully when their Play Taxi video game suggests they go to KFC or Pizza Hut. Children ages 8–12 see an average of 21 food ads a day on television but only one public service announcement (PSA) on fitness or nutrition every 2–3 days; this translates into a yearly average of 7,600 food ads and 160 health PSAs. Food products in ads targeting children and teens are primarily candy and snacks (34 percent), cereal (28 percent), and fast food (10 percent).

Product placement is also found in grocery store aisles. Grocery stores purposefully put the most popular items, such as milk and bread, at the back of the store so that you have to go through the entire store to get them—and then perhaps you will pick up some chips, cookies, and other things you weren't planning to get but just happened to see on the way. This strategy relies on impulse buying, and it has been shown that sales of a product can be effectively increased just by changing the product's placement in the store. How often have you gone into the store for one or two items, only to leave with a grocery bag full of things? Here are some strategies to help you avoid impulse buying:

- Make a list before you go to the store, and stick to it.
- Eat before you shop, and don't take hungry kids to the store with you.
- Compare unit prices across brands and sizes; larger packages are not always the best buy.
- Keep an eye out for product placement. The most expensive items and those most subject to impulse buying are likely to be found in flashy packaging at eye level in store aisles, in endcap displays, and near the checkout. Look elsewhere in the store; for example, look higher or lower than eye level to find less-expensive store and generic brands.
- Buy specials and economy-size products only when appropriate. An extra-large package may have a lower per unit cost, but that won't reduce your overall spending if you wind up throwing half the package away because it spoiled before you could finish it.

Sources: Kaiser Family Foundation, "Food for Thought: Television Food Advertising to Children in the United States," March 2007; "Product Placement: You Can't Escape It," *USA Today,* October 11, 2006; Supermarket Psychology 101, Colorado State University Cooperative Extension, www.ext.colostate.edu/PUBS/columnnn/nn060407.html, June 2006.

Because alcoholic beverages tend to contribute calories but little nutrition, they are counterproductive to taking in sufficient nutrients while not going over the daily caloric allotment. However, there are some indications that moderate alcohol consumption, such as having a glass of red wine each day, decreases the risk of coronary heart disease.

Food Safety   Food safety has become a more prominent issue with the recent *E. coli* outbreaks, mad cow disease, and concerns about bird flu in poultry. The dietary guidelines suggest commonsense safety measures, such as making sure your hands and work surfaces are clean before you prepare food. Food should be cooked or chilled at appropriate temperatures (see the section on food safety on page 158). It is further suggested that we *not* wash meat or poultry prior to preparing them, which is the opposite of what has been advised in the past. Avoid unpasteurized juices, milk, and milk products; raw or partially cooked eggs, or foods containing raw eggs; undercooked meat and poultry; and raw sprouts. This will be discussed in more detail in the food safety section later in this chapter.

Recommendations for Special Populations   There are also some special recommendations for specific population groups. For people over 50, consuming vitamin B_{12} in its crystalline form (such as fortified foods or supplements) is recommended. Women of childbearing age need to eat iron-rich plant food or iron-fortified food with an enhancer for iron absorption, such as vitamin-C-rich foods. Taking in adequate amounts of folic acid daily from fortified foods or supplements is important for pregnant women and women who may become pregnant. Older adults, people with dark skin, and those not exposed to enough sunlight need to consume extra vitamin D from vitamin-D-fortified foods and/or supplements.

Good nutrition can make a tremendous difference in increasing your endurance, preventing dehydration, avoiding injury, and enhancing performance. Even small losses of 1–2 percent of your body weight can diminish your physical performance significantly. While water is generally the drink of choice, research shows that sports drinks may offer some performance benefits for high-intensity activity lasting 30 minutes or more. Temperature, intensity, body size, duration of activity, and fitness level all play a role in determining the appropriate fluid intake.

An increase in carbohydrate intake is generally appropriate for the majority of endurance athletes. In comparison to the nonathlete who most likely is well served by a carbohydrate intake of 5 g/kg of body weight, the endurance athlete may require 8–10 g/kg of body weight. This higher carbohydrate intake should be obtained through foods high in complex carbohydrates rather than foods characterized by a high carbohydrate/high fat composition. Carbohydrates should generally supply 60–70 percent of daily caloric intake.

Protein intake for athletes may exceed that of nonathletes by a factor of two (1.2–1.6 g/kg of body weight for athletes versus 0.8 g/kg for nonathletes). This increase in protein intake can, in most cases, be achieved without supplementation. For athletes in the early phase of weight training, when increased muscle mass is the focus, a threefold increase in protein intake can be justified on a relatively short-term basis.

Athletes may also increase their intake of vitamin E and vitamin C above that seen in the general population. The antioxidant/free radical scavenger contribution of these two vitamins is thought by some to contribute to more sustainable health during periods of intense training and competition. Intakes greater than 150 percent of daily values are not, however, recommended.

In addition to vitamins, an increased intake of iron and calcium is often noted among endurance athletes, particularly among women athletes. Increased iron can assist in red blood cell replacement and increase oxygen transportation, thus offsetting to some degree the loss of iron through menstruation and high-impact training (foot pounding) that physically damages red blood cells. In terms of increased calcium, an intake of 1,500 mg per day will help sustain acceptable levels of bone density in women athletes who menstruate, but the supplement alone will not sustain bone health in athletes whose menstrual periods are suppressed by the rigors of training. In this latter group of women athletes, osteoporosislike changes, including stress fractures, are common.

The dietary changes noted here are only a few of the adjustments commonly seen among serious athletes. Additional changes are likely to be even more highly personalized and based on careful laboratory and performance-based testing.

Dietary modifications may also be recommended for athletes and other active individuals. See the box "Nutrition for the Athlete" for specific guidelines.

Additional Eating Plans and Recommendations

Other eating plans are consistent with the Dietary Guidelines for Americans and appropriate for different groups. This section describes the DASH diet, introduces different types of vegetarian diets, and provides nutritional guidelines for older adults. The box "Diverse Food Pyramids" describes food group plans based on different ethnic dietary patterns.

Dietary Approaches to Stop Hypertension (DASH)

The DASH diet is not a weight loss program but an example of how to eat in accordance with the new Dietary Guidelines for Americans. The DASH diet is constructed across a range of calorie levels to meet the needs of various age and gender groups. Originally developed to study the effects of an eating pattern on the prevention and treatment of hypertension, DASH is a balanced eating plan consistent with the new dietary guidelines. You can view examples of the DASH program on the National Institutes of Health website at www.nhlbi.nih.gov/health/public/heart/hbp/dash. Table 5.6 on page 150 also shows how the DASH diet varies by caloric intake requirements.

Vegetarian Diets

For some, vegetarianism is a way of eating, and for others, it is a way of life. In the sections that follow, various forms of vegetarianism will be addressed. The MyPyramid food guide described earlier in this chapter can be used as a guide for all types of vegetarian diets.

A *vegetarian diet* relies on plant sources for most of the nutrients the body needs. Studies show that vegetarians who eat a balanced diet don't seem to have any more iron-deficiency problems than do meat eaters. Although the iron in plant food is not as well absorbed as the iron in animal food is, vegetarians tend to eat more iron-containing foods and more vitamin C foods, which help with the absorption of the iron.[22] In addition, vegetarians tend to get enough calcium from dairy foods, tofu, beans, soybeans, calcium-fortified cereals, and vegetables such as broccoli. There has been some concern about a vitamin B_{12} deficiency, because animal foods are the best source for B_{12} and plant foods don't naturally contain this vitamin. However, soy foods such as tempeh may contain vitamin B_{12}, although it is not as biologically active as the source in animal foods. Many soy products are fortified with vitamin B_{12} as well. Note also that the liver stores so much B_{12} that it would take years to become deficient in this vitamin.[22] Vegetarian diets encompass a continuum from diets that allow some animal sources of nutrients to those that exclude all animal sources. We briefly describe

Learning from Our Diversity

Diverse Food Pyramids

Besides MyPyramid discussed earlier in this chapter, other food pyramids exist. The Mediterranean food pyramid emphasizes fruits, beans, legumes, nuts, vegetables, whole grains, and breads. In fact, the latest version of the USDA pyramid and dietary guidelines are in keeping with what had already been suggested by the Mediterranean food pyramid—for example, using more olive oil, limiting consumption of alcohol, eating more whole grains, fruits, and vegetables, choosing lean meat, and exercising daily.

The Asian food pyramid limits meat consumption even more by recommending consumption of meat on a monthly basis and daily consumption of fish, shellfish, and dairy products. The Asian diet,

like the Mediterranean diet, encourages daily intake of fruit, legumes, vegetables, and whole grains. In addition, the Asian diet includes rice and noodles and suggests eating poultry, eggs, and sweets only once a week.

The Latin American food pyramid also advises consumption of meat, sweets, and eggs only once a week. Like the Asian diet, it encourages eating fish and shellfish on a daily basis, and, unlike the Mediterranean and Asian diets, it advises consumption of poultry on a daily basis. As in the other food pyramids, fruit, vegetables, beans, and whole grains are to be consumed every day, and physical exercise is emphasized by all three food pyramids.

The Mediterranean Diet Pyramid

Source: © Oldways Preservation and Exchange Trust. www.oldwayspt.org

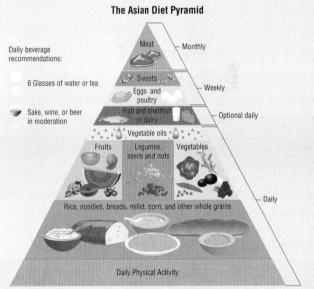

The Asian Diet Pyramid

Source: © Oldways Preservation and Exchange Trust. www.oldwayspt.org

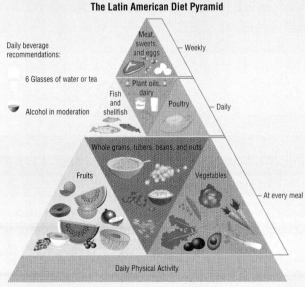

The Latin American Diet Pyramid

Source: © Oldways Preservation and Exchange Trust. www.oldwayspt.org

Table 5.6 DASH Eating Plan

Food Groups	Servings/day		
	1,600 calories/day	2,600 calories/day	3,100 calories/day
Grains*	6	10–11	12–13
Vegetables	3–4	5–6	6
Fruits	4	5–6	6
Fat-free or low-fat milk and milk products	2–3	3	3–4
Lean meats, poultry, and fish	3–6	6	6–9
Nuts, seeds, and legumes	3/week	1	1
Fats and oils	2	3	4
Sweets and added sugars	0	Less than 2	Less than 2

*Whole grains are recommended for most grain servings as a good source of fiber and nutrients.
Source: National Heart, Lung, and Blood Institute. Your Guide to Lowering Your Blood Pressure with DASH, 2006 (www.nhlbi.nih.gov/health/public/heart/hbp/dash/how-make-dash.html).

three vegetarian diets, beginning with the least restrictive in terms of food sources.

Ovolactovegetarian Diet Depending on the particular pattern of consuming eggs (*ovo*) and milk (*lacto*) or using one but not the other, ovolactovegetarianism can be an extremely sound approach to healthful eating during the entire course of the adult years. An **ovolactovegetarian diet** provides the body with the essential amino acids while limiting the high intake of fats seen in more conventional diets. The exclusion of meat as a protein source lowers the total fat intake, while the consumption of milk or eggs allows for an adequate amount of saturated fat to remain in the diet. The consistent use of vegetable products as the primary source of nutrients supports the current dietary recommendations for an increase in overall carbohydrates, an increase in complex carbohydrates, and an increase in fiber. Most vegetarians in the United States fit into this category.

Meatlike products composed of textured vegetable protein are available in supermarkets. Nonmeat bacon strips, hamburger and chicken patties, and link sausage can be used by people who want to restrict their meat intake but still want a meatlike product. Soybeans are a primary source of this textured vegetable protein.

Vegetarians who do consume dairy products face challenges when making food choices if they wish to avoid other animal products in their food. Because most cheese is made with rennet, a coagulating agent that usually comes from stomachs of slaughtered newly born calves, many vegetarians eliminate cheese from their diet or opt for rennetless cheese. Vegetarian cheeses are manufactured using rennet from either fungal or bacterial sources. Similarly, yogurt is often made with gelatin derived from animal ligaments, skins, tendon, and bones (gelatin is also found in marshmallows, candy such as jelly beans, and candy corn, poptarts, and a variety of other foods).

It has become easier to follow a vegetarian diet since stores have begun offering organic vegetarian items that do not contain these animal products. However, it can be difficult to avoid all animal products without being an avid and knowledgeable label reader.

Lactovegetarian and Ovovegetarian Diets People who include dairy products in their diet but no other animal products, such as eggs and meat, are *lactovegetarians*. In contrast, people who exclude dairy products such as milk and cheese, yet consume eggs, are *ovovegetarians*. Both diets carry the advantages of ovolactovegetarianism.

Soy foods are an important source of protein and other nutrients for vegetarians.

Vegan Vegetarian Diet A **vegan vegetarian diet** is one in which not only meat but also other animal products, including milk, cheese, and eggs, are excluded from the diet. When compared with the ovolactovegetarian diet, the vegan diet requires a higher level of nutritional understanding to avoid nutritional inadequacies.

One potential difficulty is that of obtaining all the essential amino acids. Since a single plant source does not contain all the essential amino acids, the vegan must learn to consistently employ a complementary diet. By carefully combining various grains, seeds, and legumes, amino acid deficiency can be prevented.

In addition to the potential amino acid deficiency, the vegan could have some difficulty in maintaining the necessary intake of vitamin B_{12}. Possible ramifications of inadequate B_{12} intake include depression, anemia, back pain, and menstrual irregularity. Vegans often have difficulty maintaining adequate intakes of iron, zinc, and calcium.[1] Calcium intake must be monitored closely by the vegan. In addition, vitamin D deficiencies can occur. Supplements and daily exposure to sunshine will aid in maintaining adequate levels of this vitamin.

A final area of potential difficulty for the vegan is that of an insufficient caloric intake because of the satiation resulting from the nature of the diet. Early satiation caused by a large amount of fiber may lower carbohydrate intake to the point that protein stores (muscle mass) are used for energy.

When practiced knowledgeably, vegan vegetarianism is sound for virtually all people, including pregnant and breastfeeding women, infants and children, older adults, and athletes.

Semivegetarian Diets People become vegetarians for many reasons. Some avoid meat and animal products for ethical or spiritual reasons. Others choose vegetarianism for health or environmental reasons. In recent years, however, some people have found a middle ground between the two eating styles. These so-called **semivegetarians** are increasing their intake of vegetables and cutting back greatly on meat consumption but not necessarily eliminating meat entirely. Semivegetarians add occasional servings of fish and poultry to the ovolactovegetarian diet, and some even eat red meat on occasion. **Pesco-vegetarians** eat fish, dairy products, and eggs along with plant foods.

A semivegetarian diet is much healthier than the typical meat-laden Western diet. The American Cancer Society, the American Heart Association, and the National Academy of Science all recommend dietary changes that are closely related to the typical semivegetarian diet. The health benefits of such a diet are well documented.

The semivegetarian diet may be desirable to some people because the limited consumption of meat products may help ward off some nutrient deficiencies, and

such a diet can be healthier than that of the typical American.

 TALKING POINTS What do you think about vegetarian diets? If you were to follow a vegetarian diet, which one would you be likely to choose?

Nutrition and the Older Adult

Nutritional needs change as adults age. Age-related alterations to the structure and function of the body are primarily responsible for this. Included among the changes that alter nutritional requirements and practices are changes in the teeth, salivary glands, taste buds, oral muscles, gastric acid production, and peristaltic action (movement of food through the gastrointestinal tract). Older adults can find food less tasteful and harder to chew. Chronic constipation resulting from changes in gastrointestinal tract function can also decrease interest in eating.[28]

The progressive lowering of the body's basal metabolism is another factor that eventually influences dietary patterns of older adults. As energy requirements fall, the body gradually senses the need for less food. This gradual recognition of lower energy needs results in a lessened food intake and loss of appetite in many older adults. Because of this decreased need for calories, nutrient density—the nutritional value of a food relative to the number of calories supplied—is an important factor for older adults. The USDA dietary guidelines make some specific suggestions for people over 50. They include consuming more vitamin B_{12}, because older people tend to have difficulty absorbing this vitamin. Older adults are also encouraged to consume extra vitamin D–fortified foods, since this vitamin may be lacking in this group.

Besides the physiological factors that influence dietary patterns among the elderly, several psychosocial factors alter the role of food in the lives of many older

---

Key Terms

ovolactovegetarian diet (oh voe **lack** toe veg a **ter** ee in) A diet that excludes all meat but does allow the consumption of eggs and dairy products.

vegan vegetarian diet (**vee** gun *or* **vay** gun) A vegetarian diet that excludes the consumption of all animal products, including eggs and dairy products.

semivegetarian diet A diet that significantly reduces but does not eliminate meat consumption and allows consumption of dairy products and eggs.

pesco-vegetarian diet A vegetarian diet that includes fish, dairy products, and eggs along with plant foods.

adults. Social isolation, depression, chronic alcohol consumption, loss of income, transportation limitations, and housing restrictions are factors in lifestyle patterns that can alter the ease and enjoyment associated with the preparation and consumption of food.

Special Nutrition Concerns: Challenges and Tools for Consumers

Food Labels

Since 1973, food manufacturers have been required by the FDA to provide nutritional information (labels) on products to which one or more nutrients have been added or for which some nutritional claim has been made. Despite the presence of these labels, there was concern about whether the public could understand the labels as they appeared and whether additional information was required. Accordingly, the FDA, in consultation with individual states and public interest groups, developed new labeling regulations. Revised labels began appearing on food packages in 1993. The currently used label is shown in Figure 5-4. Specific types of information contained on the new label are highlighted. Additionally, newly developed definitions for nutrition-related terms are shown in the box "Speaking Label-ese" on page 154.

Proposals for the labeling of raw foods, including fresh produce, meat, and seafood, are now being studied. Concern for consumer protection stems from recent disclosures regarding inadequate meat inspection, undercooking of hamburgers, and the risk of contaminated seafood. Processed meat, fish, and poultry products, such as hot dogs, fish sticks, and chicken patties, must be labeled. Produce, such as vegetables and fruit, is not required to be labeled. Currently, single-ingredient meat, fish, and poultry products are not required to have a label. However, in conjunction with the National Nutrition Summit meetings held in the spring of 2000, it was announced that food labels for meats, including information on fat, saturated fat, cholesterol, and other nutrients, would be forthcoming.

As of January 1, 2006, foodmakers are required by the FDA to put the amount of trans fat on food labels, sparking some companies such as Frito-Lay and Kraft to start reducing and even eliminating trans fat from its products. The FDA has further recommended that food labels list calories in larger type print, list the percentage of the consumer's daily allotment of calories, and list the total amount of calories in the container, not just the calories per serving. For example, pretzels might be listed as having 100 calories per serving and approximately 15 servings per bag, leaving it up to you to compute how many servings and calories you have consumed. The FDA is also urging restaurants to list calories on their menus. The FDA prohibits any nutrient claim that it has not defined. For example, the FDA defines *low-fat* as containing 3 grams or less of fat per serving. The FDA has not yet defined what can be considered to be low-carb even though many foodmakers and restaurants use this term in their advertising. Consumers need to know what is meant by claims such as *low-calorie, low-fat*, and *low-carb*; having a standard definition makes it much easier to make healthy and informed nutritional choices.

As of January 1, 2006, the FDA began requiring food labels to clearly state if food products contain any proteins derived from any of the eight major food allergens. In addition, the Food Allergen Labeling and Consumer Protection Act of 2004 (FALCPA) requires manufacturers to clearly identify the presence of ingredients that contain protein derived from milk, eggs, fish, crustacean shellfish, tree nuts, peanuts, wheat, or soybeans in the list of ingredients or to say "contains" followed by name of the food allergen after or adjacent to the list of ingredients. This is very important for those who suffer from food allergies, and there is a discussion of this topic later in this chapter.

Fast Foods

Fast foods are convenience foods usually prepared in walk-in or drive-through restaurants. The nutritional values of fast foods can vary considerably (see Table 5.7 on page 155), and **fat density** remains a serious limitation of fast foods. In comparison to the recommended standard (20–35 percent of total calories from fat), 40–70 percent of the calories in fast foods are obtained from fats. The restaurant and fast-food industry has received strong criticism lately for its contribution to creating overweight Americans. In response, KFC, Wendy's, Ruby Tuesday, Chili's, and some other national restaurant chains are going trans-fat-free, although KFC still uses trans fat in its pot pies and biscuits. Table 5.7 shows how many fast foods are high in sodium and saturated and trans fat.

Although many fast-food restaurants have broadened their menus to include whole-wheat breads and rolls, salad bars, fruit, and low-fat milk, a recent study showed that those who said they ate out at fast-food restaurants at least twice a week or more gained 10 pounds more than those who did not. A recent study showed that most people underestimate how many calories they have eaten when they eat fast food, often by as much as 500 calories. Also, sit-down chain restaurants such as

---

> **Key Terms**
>
> **fat density** The percentage of a food's total calories that are derived from fat; above 35 percent reflects high fat density.

Nutrition Facts

Serving Size 1 cup (228g)
Servings Per Container 2

Amount Per Serving

Calories 250   Calories from Fat 110

	% Daily Value*
Total Fat 12g	18%
Saturated Fat 3g	15%
Trans Fat 3g	
Cholesterol 30mg	10%
Sodium 470mg	20%
Potassium 700mg	20%
Total Carbohydrate 31g	10%
Dietary Fiber 0g	0%
Sugars 5g	
Protein 5g	
Vitamin A	4%
Vitamin C	2%
Calcium	20%
Iron	4%

* Percent Daily Values are based on a 2,000 calorie diet. Your Daily Values may be higher or lower depending on your calorie needs.

	Calories:	2,000	2,500
Total Fat	Less than	65g	80g
Sat Fat	Less than	20g	25g
Cholesterol	Less than	300mg	300mg
Sodium	Less than	2,400mg	2,400mg
Total Carbohydrate		300g	375g
Dietary Fiber		25g	30g

Check the serving size and number of servings.

- The Nutrition Facts Label information is based on ONE serving, but many packages contain more. Look at the serving size and how many servings you are actually consuming. If you double the servings you eat, you double the calories and nutrients, including the % DVs.
- When you compare calories and nutrients between brands, check to see if the serving size is the same.

Calories count, so pay attention to the amount.

- Fat-free doesn't mean calorie-free. Lower-fat items may have as many calories as full-fat versions.
- If the label lists that 1 serving equals 3 cookies and 100 calories, and you eat 6 cookies, you've eaten 2 servings, or twice the number of calories and fat.

Know your fats and reduce sodium for your health.

- The % DV for total fat includes all different kinds of fats.
- Trans fat doesn't have a % DV, but consume as little as possible because it increases your risk of heart disease.
- To help lower blood cholesterol, replace saturated and trans fats with monoun-saturated and polyunsaturated fats found in fish, nuts, and liquid vegetable oils.
- Limit sodium to help reduce your risk of high blood pressure.

Reach for healthy, wholesome carbohydrates.

- Whole grain foods can't always be identified by color or name, such as multi-grain or wheat. Look for the "whole" grain listed first in the ingredient list, such as whole wheat, brown rice, or whole oats.
- There isn't a % DV for sugar, but you can compare the sugar content in grams among products.
- Limit foods with added sugars, which add calories but not other nutrients. Make sure that added sugars are not one of the first few items in the ingredients list.

For protein, choose foods that are lower in fat.

- When choosing a food for its protein content, such as meat, poultry, dry beans, milk and milk products, make choices that are lean, low-fat, or fat-free.

Look for foods that are rich in these nutrients.

- Some Americans don't get enough vitamins A and C, potassium, calcium, and iron, so choose the brand with the higher % DV for these nutrients.
- Get the most nutrition for your calories—compare the calories to the nutrients you would be getting to make a healthier food choice.

The % Daily Value is a key to a balanced diet.

The % DV is a general guide to help you link nutrients in a serving of food to their contribution to your total daily diet. It can help you determine if a food is high or low in a nutrient—5% or less is low, 20% or more is high. You can use the % DV to make dietary trade-offs with other foods throughout the day. The * is a reminder that the % DV is based on a 2,000-calorie diet. You may need more or less, but the % DV is still a helpful gauge.

Figure 5-4 Nutrition Facts Label

Source: U.S. Department of Agriculture, Nutrition Facts Label, August 2006.

Applebee's, Outback Steakhouse, Chili's, Cracker Barrel, Denny's, Olive Garden, and Red Lobster offer children's meals that are adult-sized in calories and fat content. For example, the Boomerang Cheeseburger with fries at Outback Steakhouse has 840 calories and 31 grams of saturated-plus-trans fat. The Applebee's grilled cheese sandwich with fries has 900 calories and 14 grams of saturated fat in the grilled cheese alone.

Some fast-food restaurants seem to be turning away from their healthy food offerings and reinstating high-fat and high-calorie meals. For example, Burger King has a Double Whopper with cheese containing 1,060 calories and 69 grams of fat, 30 of these being from trans fat. Add King Fries and Coke for a "Meal Deal," and this totals 2,050 calories and 99 grams of fat, 46 grams from trans fat.

Hardee's has a Monster Thickburger, with 1,400 calories and 107 grams of fat. The Meat Lover's breakfast at Denny's, which comes with three pancakes, two eggs, two strips of bacon, and two sausage links, has 1,250 calories and 68 grams of fat, according to the Denny's website. The Fabulous French Toast Platter—with three slices of French toast, two bacon strips, and two sausage links—contains 1,261 calories and 79 grams of fat. Many of the "meal deals" offered by restaurants, such as Burger King's King Value Meal and Wendy's Classic Triple with Cheese plus Great Biggie Fries and a Biggie Cola, supply more than a day's worth of calories and sodium and two days of saturated and trans fats.

Who are these restaurants appealing to with these menu items? Research shows that men ages 18 to 24 make fast-food choices based on getting the most for the least amount of money, not on nutritional value. And don't be fooled by thinking that if it's salad, it's healthy; that can be far from the truth. Wendy's Garden Sensations Salads, for example, have half the daily fat allowance and one-third of the day's sodium. Burger King's

TenderCrisp salads have 530 calories and 32 grams of fat, and McDonald's salads have 510 calories, 31 grams of fat, and half the day's allotment of sodium.

On the other side of the coin, some healthy fast-food choices are Burger King's Veggie Burger with 380 calories (although it contains 930 mg of sodium), Wendy's Ultimate Chicken Grill (360 calories), McDonald's Chicken McGrill (400 calories), McDonald's Hamburger (260 calories), and McDonald's Fruit and Yogurt Parfait (160 calories).

See the box "Eating on the Run" on page 156 for more suggestions on healthier fast-food choices.

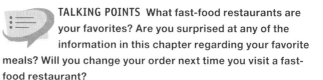

TALKING POINTS What fast-food restaurants are your favorites? Are you surprised at any of the information in this chapter regarding your favorite meals? Will you change your order next time you visit a fast-food restaurant?

Functional Foods

At the forefront of healthful nutrition is the identification and development of foods intended to affect a particular health problem or to improve the functional capability of the body. **Functional foods** contain not only recognized nutrients but also new or enhanced elements that impart medicinelike properties to the food. Alternative labels

> **Key Terms**
>
> **functional foods** Foods capable of contributing to the improvement/prevention of specific health problems.

Table 5.7 Nutritional Facts for Popular Fast-Food Menu Items

	Calories	Total Fat (g)	Saturated Fat (g)	Trans Fat (g)	Sodium (mg)
Burgers					
McDonald's Hamburger	250	9	3.5	0.5	520
McDonald's Cheeseburger	300	12	6	0.5	750
McDonald's Quarter Pounder	410	19	7	1	730
McDonald's Quarter Pounder with Cheese	510	26	12	1.5	1,190
McDonald's Double Quarter Pounder with Cheese	740	42	19	2.5	1,380
McDonald's Big Mac	540	29	10	1.5	1,040
Burger King Hamburger	290	12	4.5	0	560
Burger King Cheeseburger	330	16	7	0.5	780
Burger King Whopper with Cheese	760	47	16	1.5	1,100
Burger King Veggie Burger	420	16	2.5	0	1,100
Burger King Double Stacker	610	39	16	1.5	1,100
Burger King Triple Stacker	800	54	23	2	1,450
Burger King Quad Stacker	1,100	68	30	3	1,800
Wendy's Single with Everything	430	20	7	1	900
Wendy's Double with Everything	700	40	16	2.5	1,500
Chicken					
McDonald's McChicken	360	16	3.5	1	790
McDonald's Premium Grilled Chicken Classic Sandwich	420	10	2	0	1,190
McDonald's Premium Crispy Chicken Club Sandwich	660	28	8	1.5	1,860
McDonald's Chicken McNuggets (10 piece)	420	24	5	2.5	1,120
Burger King TenderGrill Chicken Sandwich	450	10	2	0	1,210
Burger King TenderCrisp Chicken Sandwich	780	43	8	4	1,730
Burger King Chicken Tenders (8 piece)	340	20	5	3	960
Wendy's Ultimate Chicken Grill Sandwich	320	7	1.5	0	950
Wendy's Crispy Chicken Sandwich	360	14	2.5	0	730
Wendy's Chicken Nuggets (10 piece)	460	30	6	0	1,040
Fish					
McDonald's Filet-O-Fish	380	18	4	1	660
Burger King BIG FISH Sandwich	630	30	6	2.5	1,380
Long John Silver's Fish Sandwich	470	23	5	4.5	1,210
Long John Silver's Ultimate Fish Sandwich	530	28	8	5	1,400
Salads (without dressing)					
McDonald's Southwest Salad with Grilled Chicken	320	9	3	0	970
McDonald's Southwest Salad with Crispy Chicken	400	16	4	1.5	1,110
McDonald's Asian Salad with Grilled Chicken	300	10	1	0	890
McDonald's Caesar Salad with Chicken	220	6	3	0	890
Burger King TenderGrill Chicken Garden Salad	240	9	3.5	0	720
Burger King TenderCrisp Chicken Garden Salad	400	21	7	3.5	1,170
Wendy's Mandarin Chicken Salad	360	15	1.5	0	720
Wendy's Chicken Caesar Salad	260	7.5	2.5	0	745
Wendy's Southwest Taco Salad	600	29	15.5	1	1,290
French Fries					
McDonald's Medium French Fries	380	20	4	5	220
Burger King Medium French Fries	360	20	4.5	4.5	380
Wendy's Medium French Fries	420	20	3	1	430
Desserts and Shakes					
McDonald's Chocolate Triple Thick Shake (16 ounces)	580	14	8	1	250
Burger King Chocolate Milk Shake (Medium)	690	20	12	0	480
Wendy's Chocolate Frosty (Medium)	430	11	7	0	299
McDonald's Fruit'n Yogurt Parfait	160	2	1	0	85
McDonald's McFlurry with M & M's Candies	620	20	12	1	190
McDonald's McFlurry with OREO Cookies	560	16	9	2	250

Visit the company websites for the most current menu items and nutritional information.

Sources: McDonald's USA Nutritional Facts for Popular Menu Items, www.mcdonalds.com, April 20, 2007; Burger King Nutritional Information, www.burgerking.com, May 9, 2007; Long John Silver's Nutritional Analysis, www.ljsilvers.com, February 2007; Wendy's U.S. Nutrition Information, www.wendys.com, May 2007. From Nutrition Action Healthletter. Copyright © 2005 by Center for Science in the Public Interest. Reproduced with permission of Center for Science in the Public Interest in the format Textbook via Copyright Clearance Center.

also exist for various subclasses of functional foods, such as *nutraceutics,* or food elements that may be packaged in forms appearing more like medications (for example, pills or capsules), and *probiotics.*[29] **Probiotics,** "for life," are living bacteria (good bugs) that are thought to help prevent disease and boost the immune system. Probiotic bacteria have been associated with the alleviation of allergies, irritable bowel, respiratory infections, and urinary infections, and with cancer prevention. They make the environment in the digestive system inhospitable for harmful bacteria (the bad bugs). More than 400 types of bacteria reside in and on our bodies and outnumber human cells 10 to 1. Yogurt is one example of a food that gives you a dose of these good bugs—lactobacillus bulgaris.

Examples of functional foods include garlic (believed to lower cholesterol), olive oil (thought to prevent heart disease), foods high in fiber (which prevent constipation and lower cholesterol), and foods rich in calcium (which help prevent osteoporosis). In addition, foods that contain high levels of vitamins A, C, and E—primarily fruits and vegetables—and provide the body with natural sources of antioxidants are functional foods.

Other functional foods are those that contain or are enriched with folic acid. These vitamin B family foods aid in the prevention of spina bifida and other neural tube defects (see Chapter 12) and the prevention of heart disease. Foods that are rich in selenium are sometimes categorized as functional foods because of selenium's potential as an agent in cancer prevention. Most recently, the FDA approved a "heart healthy" label for foods that are rich in soy protein.[30] All the functional foods discussed here are approved to carry **health claims** on the basis of current FDA criteria.[31] Phytosterols are another example of a functional food. Phytosterols are found in plants and help lower cholesterol levels. In the past they had been found only in margarine spreads such as Benecol and Take Control, but now they are found in Yoplait Heart Healthy Yogurt, Rice Dream Heartwise Rice Drink, and Lifetime Low-Fat Cheese.[31]

One category of functional foods being researched is vegetables that are genetically engineered to produce a specific biological element that is important to human health. An example is tomatoes that are high in lycopene. Food technologists are interested in expanding the functional food family to include a greater array of health-enhancing food items.

Dietary Supplements

In 2005 it was estimated that Americans spent $20 billion on a wide array of over-the-counter (OTC) products known collectively as *dietary supplements.* These nonprescription products are legally described as:

- Products (other than tobacco) that are intended to supplement the diet, including vitamins, amino acids, minerals, glandular extracts, herbs, and other plant products such as fungi.
- Products that are intended for use by people to supplement the total daily intake of nutrients in the diet.
- Products that are intended to be ingested in tablet, capsule, softgel, gelcap, and liquid form.

- Products that are not in themselves to be used as conventional foods or as the only items of a meal or diet.

Unlike prescription medications, dietary supplements have been available in the marketplace for years almost without restriction. However, dietary supplements now must be deemed safe for human use on the basis of information supplied to the FDA by the manufacturers. In addition, the labels on these products cannot make a direct claim, with the exception of calcium and folic acid supplements, that they can cure or prevent illnesses. However, other materials with such claims may be displayed close to the dietary supplements themselves. Further, the labels on dietary supplements must remind consumers that the FDA has not required these products to undergo the rigorous research required of prescription medications, and so the FDA cannot attest to their effectiveness. Beyond this, consumers are left to themselves to decide whether to purchase and use dietary supplements.

As we mentioned, probiotic products, dietary supplements with live bacteria, are gaining in popularity. The U.S. sales of probiotic supplements have increased 19 percent since 2003, with total sales of $714 million in 2005. Actimel is one of the biggest sellers, claiming to "help to strengthen your body's natural defenses" and enhance your immune system.[32]

Easily accessible to anyone, over 15,000 different dietary supplements can be purchased in grocery stores, drugstores, and discount stores, through mail-order catalogs, and over the Internet. Because of the great demand for these products, major pharmaceutical companies are now entering the dietary supplement field. Whether this trend leads to the development of more effective products, or to a greater effort on the part of the FDA to demand proof of effectiveness, remains to be seen. By definition, supplements are not foods but simply "supplements." Therefore, they remain free from requirements to substantiate their claims of effectiveness (as is now required for functional foods).

 TALKING POINTS A friend asks you about the advantages and disadvantages of taking a dietary supplement. What would you point out to your friend?

Food Allergies

Foods enjoyed by the vast majority of people may be harmful and even deadly to others because of their unique food allergies. For some people, peanuts, the familiar snacks once served on many plane flights, are such a food. Today, U.S. airlines are replacing peanuts with pretzels in order to provide "peanut-free" flights and to protect people known to be allergic to peanuts and peanut-based products. Many schools have already established peanut-free tables in their lunchrooms for the same purpose.

Being intolerant to certain foods is not the same as being allergic to particular foods. **Food intolerance** means that a food upsets your intestines, usually because of an enzyme deficiency. A lactase deficiency, for example, causes lactose intolerance. Lactose intolerance affects 20 percent of Caucasian Americans, 75 percent of African Americans, and 50 percent of Hispanic Americans. Intolerance of gluten (found in wheat, rye, barley, and perhaps oats) affects 1 of every 150 Americans and can cause malnutrition, premature osteoporosis, colon cancer, thyroid disease, diabetes, arthritis, miscarriage, and birth defects.

A **food allergy** mistakenly calls the body's disease-fighting immune system into action, creating unpleasant and sometimes life-threatening symptoms. Peanuts, milk, eggs, shellfish, tree nuts, fish, soy, and wheat account for 90 percent of food allergies. Eight percent of children and 2 percent of adults have food allergies. For some members of this group, food-based allergies may be serious or even life threatening.

Because food allergies generally develop slowly, initial symptoms may not be fully recognized or even associated with the food. It takes three exposures to the allergic food to obtain a significant food allergy reaction. The first time a person eats a food she is allergic to, she may have little or no reaction. The second time she eats this food, she will most likely have a more observable reaction, such as breaking out in hives, itching, runny nose, burning in the mouth, and wheezing. The third exposure can bring on a full-blown reaction, which, for peanut allergies among others, can result in death within minutes. There is no cure for food allergies, and the treatment is for the food-allergic person to avoid these foods and carry an EpiPen (epinephrine) at all times.

Key Terms

probiotics Living bacteria (good bugs) that help prevent disease and strengthen the immune system.

health claims Statements authorized by the FDA as having scientific proof of claims that a food, nutrient, or dietary supplement has an effect on a health-related condition.

food intolerance An adverse reaction to a specific food that does not involve the immune system; usually caused by an enzyme deficiency.

food allergy A reaction in which the immune system attacks an otherwise harmless food or ingredient; allergic reactions can range from mildly unpleasant to life threatening.

For the first time, an experimental drug has proven highly effective against potentially deadly peanut allergies. The once-a-month shots don't cure peanut allergy, which affects about 1.5 million Americans and kills 50 to 100 people each year. Xolair, a drug currently patented for patients with asthma, may hold promise in preventing or reducing the severity of reactions for people who suffer from peanut allergy. Xolair, an anti-IgE therapy, blocks a protein called *immunoglobulin E* from causing an asthmatic reaction. Genentech and Novartis Pharmaceuticals are currently conducting clinical trials for use with people who suffer from peanut allergy in hope that anti-IgE therapy can be used to diminish or eliminate the reaction caused by peanut allergy in the same way it treats asthma. However, Xolair is not a cure or a vaccine. It just adds protection against a fatal reaction in case of accidental ingestion of peanut-containing food. Scientists also are working on treatments that could suppress peanut allergy permanently, but those developments are probably 5 to 10 years in the future.

Food Safety

Technological advances in food manufacturing and processing have done much to assure that the food we eat is fresh and safe. Yet concern is growing that certain recent developments may also produce harmful effects on humans. For example, the preparation, handling and storage of food, irradiation of foods, and genetic engineering of foods all contribute to the safety of our food. Environmental contaminants are another risk; see the box "Fishy Choices" for more information.

Preventing Foodborne Illness

Foodborne illness or food poisoning is the result of eating contaminated food. The symptoms of food poisoning can be easily mistaken for the flu—fatigue, chills, mild fever, dizziness, headaches, upset stomach, diarrhea, and severe cramps. Illness develops within 1 to 6 hours following ingestion of the contaminated food, and recovery is fairly rapid.[33] Bacteria are the culprits in most cases of food poisoning, which can be the result of food not being cooked thoroughly to destroy bacteria or not keeping food cool enough to slow their growth. In addition, nearly half of all cases of food poisoning can be prevented with proper hand washing so as to not contaminate food by viruses, parasites, or toxic chemicals. Food safety is such an important issue that the USDA incorporated it into the new dietary guidelines. Food should be refrigerated below 40 degrees F or kept warm above 140 degrees F. Between 40 degrees F and 140 degrees F, bacteria can double in number in as little as 20 minutes, so it is important to keep food at safe temperatures. (See Figure 5-5 on temperature rules for safe cooking and handling of foods.)

It is estimated that 76 million Americans are the victims of food poisoning each year, and about 5,000 of these people die. *Salmonella* bacteria are the most common cause of foodborne illness and are found mostly in raw or undercooked poultry, meat, eggs, fish, and unpasteurized milk. *Clostridium perfringens,* also called the "buffet germ," grows where there is little to no oxygen and grows fastest in large portions held at low or room temperatures. For this reason, buffet table servings should be replaced often and leftovers should be refrigerated quickly. Refrigerated leftovers may become harmful

180°F	Whole poultry
170°F	Poultry breasts
165°F	Stuffing, ground poultry, reheated leftovers
160°F	Meats (medium), egg dishes, pork, and ground meats
145°F	Beef steaks, veal, lamb (medium rare)
140°F	Hold hot foods
DANGER ZONE	
40°F	Refrigerator temperature
0°F	Freezer temperature

Figure 5-5 Temperature Rules for Cooking and Safe Handling of Food Keep food out of the danger zone between 40 degrees F and 140 degrees F, in which bacteria can multiply rapidly.

Source: U.S. Department of Health and Human Services and U.S. Department of Agriculture. Dietary Guidelines for Americans, 2005 (www.healthierus.gov/dietaryguidelines).

Table 5.8 Cold Storage Limits

Apples	3 weeks
Apricots, peaches, nectarines, pears	3–4 days
Bacon	1 week
Beans, green	3–4 days
Berries, cherries	1–2 days
Butter	1–3 months
Carrots	2 weeks
Cheese, hard	3–4 weeks
Cheese, soft	1 week
Chicken or turkey (fresh)	1–2 days
Chicken or turkey (cooked)	3–4 days
Citrus fruit	1–2 weeks
Deli and vacuum-packed products	3–5 days
Eggs (fresh, in shell)	3–5 weeks
Eggs (hard cooked)	1 week
Fish or seafood (fresh)	1–2 days
Fish (cooked)	3–4 days
Fish (canned, after opening)	3–4 days
Gravy and meat broth	1–2 days
Hot dogs (after opening)	1 week
Lettuce, leaf	3–7 days
Luncheon meat (after opening)	3–5 days
Margarine	4–5 months
Mayonnaise (after opening)	2 months
Milk (after opening)	5 days
Meat (fresh, ground)	1–2 days
Meat (fresh; steak, chops, roasts)	3–5 days
Meat (cooked)	3–4 days
Pizza (cooked)	3–4 days
Soups and stews	3–4 days
Spinach	1–2 days
Yogurt	7–14 days

Sources: Food Safety and Inspection Service, U.S. Department of Agriculture. Basics for Handling Food Safely, September 2006; Food Marketing Institute. A Consumer Guide to Food Quality and Safe Handling.

to eat after 3 days (Table 5.8). The old adage "If in doubt, throw it out" applies to any questionable leftovers. A third type of food poisoning is botulism, which is rare but often fatal. It is caused by home-canned or commercially canned food that hasn't been processed or stored properly. Some warning signs are swollen or dented cans or lids, cracked jars, loose lids, and clear liquids turned milky. Can you tell if meat is spoiled by looking at it? Not necessarily. Some supermarkets package their meat with carbon monoxide, which reacts with the pigment in the meat to make it redder.

The Center for Science in the Public Interest found that fruits and vegetables account for the majority of foodborne illnesses. Salads are by far the biggest culprit. The reason for this seems to be because some of the water used to irrigate and wash produce is contaminated with human and animal feces. *Escherichia coli* has historically been a harmless bacterium that resides in the guts of animals, including humans. A new and pathogenic strain called *E. coli* O157:H7 was identified in 1982 and now causes an estimated 73,000 cases of infection and 60 deaths in the United States each year. *E. coli* can be found in uncooked produce, raw milk, unpasteurized juice, contaminated water, and meat. Dozens of people contracted food poisoning from the green onions in food served at some Taco Bell restaurants in 2006. This same strain of *E. coli* was linked to the spinach that sickened 200 people in 2006. This problem can be difficult to regulate or correct,

because produce comes from all over the world, not just from the United States. Even the ready-to-eat bags of produce that boast they have been "thoroughly" or "triple" washed cannot be guaranteed to be bacteria-free. Washing the produce yourself may not solve the problem, either. Produce washes such as veggie wash don't claim to kill *E. coli* but only to clean off wax, pesticides, and dirt. The best way to avoid getting sick from produce is to cook it so that you kill any remaining bacteria.

What do you do if you suspect food poisoning?

1. Contact a medical professional immediately. Don't wait to see if you feel better.
2. Report the incident to your local health department as soon as possible if the suspected food came from a public place.
3. Preserve the suspected food including any packaging to give to the health department for investigation and possible prevention of further poisoning.

Handle food properly to avoid food poisoning. Frequent handwashing is at the top of the list of food safety tips (see the box "Dos and Don'ts for Food Safety"). Bacteria live and multiply on warm, moist hands, and hands can inadvertently transport germs from one surface to another. It is also important to clean work surfaces with hot, soapy water and keep nonfood items such as the mail, newspapers, and purses off the countertops. Some people advocate the use of antibacterial products, whereas others maintain that if they are overused, these products can lose their effectiveness, and bacteria then become resistant to them. Utensils, dishes, cutting boards, cookware, and towels and sponges need to be washed in hot, soapy water and rinsed well.

Food Irradiation

Because of the increasing concern about contaminated meat and meat products, the first irradiated meat, ground beef, arrived in American supermarkets in early 2000. Irradiated frozen chicken was introduced more recently. Irradiation is a process that causes damage to the DNA of disease-causing bacteria such as salmonella and *E. coli* as well as of insects, parasites, and other organisms so that they can't reproduce. While irradiated meat

has much lower bacteria levels than regular meat does, irradiation doesn't destroy all bacteria in meat. In fact, irradiation actually destroys fewer bacteria than does proper cooking.[34] There is also some concern that irradiation will lull consumers into a false sense of security so that they erroneously believe that they don't have to take the usual precautions in food handling and preparation. For example, undercooking, unclean work surfaces or cooking utensils, and improper storage can still contaminate meat. Some also claim that irradiated meat has a distinct off-taste and a smell like "singed hair."

Safe Farming Techniques

In recent decades, there has been an increased push toward ensuring better treatment of animals raised for slaughter and for dairy production in the United States. As a result of recent reforms, more than half of beef cattle in North America meet their end at slaughterhouses based on innovative designs that consider the fears and inclinations of herd animals. The cages of laying hens are nearly one-third larger than the old ones were, and the practice of starving hens for weeks at a time to stimulate egg production is beginning to be phased out. These reforms are important to ensure more humane treatment of these animals, but they are also proving beneficial to human health and food quality. It has been suggested that there is an increase in the quality of meat when animals are treated humanely, with less bruising, improved tenderness, lower incidence of dark-cutting beef, and lessened occurrence of pale, soft, and dry pork. Furthermore, the taste of eggs is said to be significantly better if they come from humanely treated hens.

One important component in these reforms—some of which have been government mandated and others voluntarily adopted by the agricultural industry—relates to the feed given to beef cattle. The spread of bovine spongiform encephalopathy, more commonly known as mad cow disease, has largely been attributed to the use of animal feed containing the protein-rich by-products of slaughtered cows, including nerve tissue, the tissue most likely to harbor the disease. Such feed—which is believed to be the primary, if not the only, way the disease can be transmitted—was banned in the United States and Canada in August 1997.[35] However, from August 1997 to March 2004, fifty-two companies recalled 410 feed products because of suspected infectious prions, the proteins thought to spread mad cow disease. While the disease had been restricted to European cows, a number of cases of mad cow detected in American cattle in late 2003 encouraged the U.S. government to impose even stricter rules to protect the nation's beef supply from the disease, including banning the butchering of sick or injured cows, banning certain animal parts from the food supply, and increased testing on suspect animals.[35]

Eliminating animal products from feed has also proven beneficial in hens. Many consumers choose to eat only poultry and eggs from free-range, vegetarian-fed chickens, for health and safety reasons. Several companies (such as Eggland's Best) claim that their vegetarian-fed hens produce eggs that have seven times more vitamin E, are lower in cholesterol, have a higher unsaturated/saturated fat ratio, and contain more omega-3 fatty acids than do factory-farmed eggs.[36]

There has also been increasing concern about giving chickens Roxarsone (3-Nitro) because it contains arsenic. It is given to chickens to fatten the birds faster and kill microbes. Human antibiotics are also fed to chickens to increase growth, but the bacteria in the chickens' intestines can develop resistance to the antibiotics. This can result in the antibiotic-resistant bacteria being passed along to people who consume this poultry, causing them to become ill and not respond to drugs typically prescribed to treat this illness.

Organic Foods

The new USDA organic food labels went into effect in October 2002 to standardize regulations for foods grown without synthetic pesticides or other chemicals. Under the new USDA rules, organic means:

- Meat, poultry, and eggs are from animals given no growth hormones or antibiotics. Vitamin and mineral supplements are allowed. Livestock are given organic feed and live in conditions that allow for "exercise, freedom of movement, and reduction of stress."
- Products are not genetically engineered or irradiated to kill germs.
- Crops are grown on land that has not been fertilized with sewage sludge or chemical fertilizers.
- Pests and plant diseases are treated primarily with insect predators, traps, natural repellants, and other nonchemical methods.
- Weeds are controlled by mulching, mowing, hand weeding, or mechanical cultivation, not chemical herbicides.

There are different types of organic foods: "100 percent organic," meaning the food contains all organic ingredients; "organic," which means at least 95 percent of the product is organic; and "made with organic ingredients," which means at least 70 percent of the food is organic as previously defined.[36]

Organic foods have enjoyed a 20 percent annual growth rate over the past several years. One-hundred and twenty new organic snacks were introduced to meet the needs of people trying to find healthier snacks.

Organic products have grown in popularity in recent years and are now available in many major grocery stores.

It is projected that the now $10.4-billion organic food industry will increase to $32 billion by 2009, owing to its increasing popularity. See Chapter 20 for more information on the benefit of organic foods for health and food safety.

Food Additives

Food additives refers to substances added to food to provide color or flavor, replace sugar or fat, or improve nutritional content, texture, or shelf life. Food additives must undergo FDA testing and approval to ensure that the benefits outweigh any risks associated with these additives. For example, emulsifiers help to give peanut butter a more consistent texture and prevent separation while stabilizers and thickeners can give ice cream a smooth, uniform texture. Preservatives such as antioxidants prevent apples from turning brown from exposure to air and fats and oils in baked goods from spoiling. The three most common additives are sugar, salt, and corn syrup.[37]

Genetically Modified Foods

Biotech crops increased 20 percent in 2004, with the United States, Argentina, and Canada being the frontrunners.[38] The success of American agriculture, in terms of food quality and marketability, has been based on the ability to genetically alter food sources to improve yield, reduce production costs, and introduce new food characteristics. Today, however, genetic technology is so sophisticated that changes are being introduced faster than scientists can fully evaluate their effects. For example, the genetic makeup of plant seeds and animals is being modified while scientists are still trying to determine whether human consumption of these products will be safe over extended periods. Concerned individuals and agencies in the United States and abroad are calling for more extensive long-term research into safety issues and stricter labeling requirements for genetically altered foods. The label *GM* (for genetically modified) is appearing on some food items. Some food manufacturers have announced that they will discontinue the use of genetically modified ingredients in their products. The American public appears about equally divided in believing that genetically modified foods are safe (44 percent) or unsafe (20 percent) or that they are uncertain (36 percent) about the safety of such foods.[39]

Taking Charge of Your Health

- Take the Personal Assessment "Are you feeding your feelings?" at the end of this chapter to determine if you are an emotional eater.
- Look on MyPyramid.gov to find your personal food pyramid.

- Assess your physical activity level using MyPyramid.gov.
- Keep track of your food intake for a week, using the pyramid tracker on MyPyramid.gov, and see how well your intake reflects the new dietary guidelines.

- Make one change per week in your eating patterns, such as drinking skim milk or including a new fruit or vegetable.
- Use the tips in the box "Healthy Restaurant Eating" when you eat out.

SUMMARY

- Carbohydrates are composed of sugar units and are the major source of energy for the body. About 45–65 percent of our calories should come from carbohydrates.
- Fats provide a concentrated source of energy for the body and keep us from feeling hungry. No more than 20–35 percent of our calories should come from fats, and most of these fats should be polyunsaturated or monounsaturated.
- Foods containing trans fats should be avoided as much as possible, and less than 10 percent of our calories should come from saturated fats, according to the current dietary guidelines.
- Protein primarily promotes growth and maintenance of body tissue, and is also a source of energy.
- Vitamins serve as catalysts for the body and are found in either water-soluble or fat-soluble forms.
- Minerals are incorporated into various tissues of the body and also participate in regulatory functions within the body.

- Adequate water and fluids are required by the body on a daily basis and are obtained from a variety of food sources, including beverages.
- Fast foods should play a limited role in daily food intake because of their high fat density, as well as their high levels of sugar and sodium.
- Preventive strategies such as hand washing and proper preparation, cooking, and storage of food can help to decrease foodborne illnesses.
- The USDA Dietary Guidelines for Americans focus on the role that trans fat, saturated fat, sugar, sodium, and alcohol play in weight management and health and disease. The current Dietary Guidelines for Americans address the importance of daily physical activity.

REVIEW QUESTIONS

1. What unique contributions do carbohydrates, fats, and protein each make to overall nutrition?
2. What role do vitamins play in the body? What is the most current perception regarding the need for vitamin supplementation?
3. What roles do minerals play in the body? What is a trace element?
4. What is the current recommendation regarding daily fluid intake? Why is water considered an essential nutrient?
5. What are the two principal forms of fiber, and how does each of them contribute to health?
6. What are functional foods, and what contribution do they make to health beyond supplying various nutrients as do all foods?

7. Identify each of the food groups in the current food pyramid. What is the additional group? Explain the nutritional benefit of each food group and the recommended daily adult allotments. What are discretionary calories?
8. What are the specific areas of nutritional concern addressed by the current Dietary Guidelines for Americans?
9. What do the current dietary guidelines suggest in terms of physical activity, and what are the benefits of such physical activity?
10. What is the principal concern regarding excessive fast-food consumption? How can food selection at a fast-food restaurant be made nutritionally healthier?

ANSWERS TO THE "WHAT DO YOU KNOW?" QUIZ

1. True   2. True   3. False   4. False   5. True   6. False   7. False

Should Food Safety Be Regulated by State or Federal Government?

The National Uniformity Food Act was passed by the U.S. House of Representatives on March 2006. This bill put food safety laws entirely under the jurisdiction of the FDA and is intended to provide consistency and alleviate confusion regarding food labeling. Currently all 50 states have their own food safety standards and label requirements. The idea of changing to national standards sounds good, right?

There has been strong opposition to this idea from the Consumers Union, which contends that nationalization would make the standards lower and weaken current practices. The Consumers Union claims that the FDA will base its standards on the lowest common denominator of all the states, eliminating 200 state laws that are more stringent than the FDA laws. Proponents of the bill, such as the National Uniformity for Food Coalition, claim that states will still have the ability to set higher standards by petitioning the FDA for permission and that the bill would let consumers know that the minimum standards are consistent across all states.

Currently the bill has lost momentum due to this hot debate. Lawmakers are going back to the drawing board to see what the need was for this change in the first place. It was thought that labels varied so much from state to state that they contradicted each other, but this has not been substantiated. There is also concern about how this change would impact food inspections, which are currently being carried out by state inspectors. Some say that the inspections would become more lax, making food less safe rather than more safe.

Source: "Alert: Putting Food Safety in the Hands of the Federal Government May Expose Us to Health Hazards," *Vegetarian Times*, November/December, 2006.

ENDNOTES

1. Wardlaw GM. *Perspectives in Nutrition* (5th ed.). New York: Mc-Graw-Hill, 2002.
2. Sweeteners: Not all sweeteners are equal. *Nutrition Action,* May 2004.
3. *USDA Agricultural Outlook.* Washington, DC: U.S. Department of Agriculture, April 2000.
4. U.S. Department of Health and Human Services. *Report of the Expert Panel on Population Strategies for Blood Cholesterol Reduction.* NIH Pub No 9-3049. Washington, DC: Author, 1990.
5. Lichtenstein AH. Dietary trans fatty acid. *J Cardiopulm Rehabil;* 20(3):143–146, 2000.
6. Willer WC, Ascherio A. Trans fatty acids: Are the effects only marginal? *Am J Public Health;* 84:722, 1994.
7. Duyff R. *American Dietetic Association Complete Food and Nutrition Guide* (2nd ed.). Hoboken, NJ: Wiley, 2002.
8. Katan MB. Trans fatty acids and plasma lipoproteins. *Nutr Rev;* 58(6):188–191, 2000.
9. National Insutitutes of Health. *Practical Guide to the Identification, Evaluation and Treatment of Overweight and Obesity in Adults,* 2001.
10. Cheskin LJ, et al. Gastrointestinal symptoms following consumption of Olestra or regular triglyceride potato chips score. *JAMA;* 279(2): 150–152, 1998.
11. Wardlaw GM. *Contemporary Nutrition: Issues and Insights.* New York: McGraw-Hill, 1999.
12. Soyonara: Tough times for the miracle bean. *Nutrition Action,* October 2006.
13. National Academy of Sciences, *Dietary Reference Intakes,* 2004.
14. Kant AK. A prospective study of diet quality and mortality in women. *JAMA;* 283(16): 2109–2115, 2000.
15. Czeizel AE, Dudaz I. Prevention of the first occurrence of neural-tube defects by periconceptional vitamin supplementation. *N Eng J Med;* 327(26): 1832–1835, 1992.
16. Antioxidants: Still hazy after all these years. *Nutrition Action,* November 2005.
17. Good cup, bad cup: How to survive in latte land. *Nutrition Action,* September 2006.
18. Garigan TP, Ristedt DE. Death from hyponatremia as a result of acute water intoxication in an Army basic trainee. *Mil Med;* 164(3):234–238, 1999.
19. Arieff AI, Kronlund BA. Fatal child abuse by forced water intoxication. *Pediatrics;* 103(6 Pt 1): 1292–1295, 1999.
20. Chandalia M, et al. Beneficial effects of high dietary fiber intake in patients with type 2 diabetes mellitus. *N Engl J Med;* 342(19): 1392–1398, 2000.
21. Schatzkin A, et al. Lack of effect of a low-fat, high-fiber diet on the recurrence of colorectal adenomas. Polyp prevention Trial Study Group. *N Engl J Med;* 342(16): 1149–1115, 2000.
22. Sears W, Sears M. *The Family Nutrition Book.* New York: Little, Brown and Co, 1999.
23. FDA allows whole oat foods to make health claim on reducing the risk of heart disease. *FDA Talk Paper,* January 1998.
24. The changing American diet. *Nutrition Action,* April 2006.
25. www.health.gov/dietaryguidelines/dga, 2005.
26. American Cancer Society. *Cancer Facts and Figures—2000.* The Association, 2000.
27. Flour power: A slice of multigrain can taste like bread. *USA Today,* August 9, 2004.

28. Williams S, Schlenker E. *Essentials of Nutrients and Diet Therapy* (8th ed.). St. Louis, MO: Mosby, 2003.

29. Fransworth ER. What we are trying to do? *Medicinal Food News;* 1(1):1–6, 1999. www.medicinalfoodnews.com/vol01/issue1.html.

30. U.S. Food and Drug Administration Center for Food Safety and Applied Nutrition. *FDA Approves New Health Claim for Soy Protein and Coronary Heart Disease* [FDA talk paper]. October 1999, www.fda.gov/fdac/bbs/topics/ANSWERS/ANS00980.html.

31. Kurtzweil P. Staking a claim to good health. *FDA Consumer,* November–December 1998. www.fda/gov/fdac/features/1998,689-labl.html.

32. A bug for what's bugging you. *USA Today,* July 9, 2003, D-1.

33. Oppel RA, Jr. Infected cow old enough to have eaten now-banned feed. *New York Times,* December 30, 2003.

34 The truth about irradiated meat. *Consumer Reports,* 34–37, August 2003.

35. Grady D. U.S. Imposes stricker safety rules for preventing mad cow disease. *New York Times,* December 31, 2003.

36. USDA gives bite to organic label. *USA Today,* October 16, 2002. Corporate website, www.eggland.com.

37. Insel P, Turner E, Ross D. *Nutrition.* Sudbury, MA: Jones and Barlett, 2002.

38. Biotech crops gained ground across globe. *USA Today,* January 13, 2005.

39. Americans are iffy on genetically modified foods. *USA Today,* September 18, 2003.

Personal Assessment

Rate Your Plate

Take a closer look at yourself, your current food decisions, and your lifestyle. Think about your typical eating pattern and food decisions.

Do You . . .

	Usually	Sometimes	Never
Consider nutrition when you make food choices?	❏	❏	❏
Try to eat regular meals (including breakfast), rather than skip or skimp on some?	❏	❏	❏
Choose nutritious snacks?	❏	❏	❏
Try to eat a variety of foods?	❏	❏	❏
Include new-to-you foods in meals and snacks?	❏	❏	❏
Try to balance your energy (calorie) intake with your physical activity?	❏	❏	❏

Now for the Details

Do You . . .

Eat at least 6 ounces of grain products daily?	❏	❏	❏
Eat at least 2½ cups of vegetables daily?	❏	❏	❏
Eat at least 2 cups of fruits daily?	❏	❏	❏
Consume at least 3 cups of milk, yogurt, or cheese daily?	❏	❏	❏
Go easy on higher fat foods?	❏	❏	❏
Go easy on sweets?	❏	❏	❏
Drink 8 or more cups of fluids daily?	❏	❏	❏
Limit alcoholic beverages (no more than 1 daily for a woman or 2 for a man)?	❏	❏	❏

Score Yourself

Usually = 2 points
Sometimes = 1 point
Never = 0 points

If you scored . . .

24 or more points—Healthful eating seems to be your fitness habit already. Still, look for ways to stick to a healthful eating plan—and to make a "good thing" even better.

16 to 23 points—You're on track. A few easy changes could help you make your overall eating plan healthier.

9 to 15 points—Sometimes you eat smart—but not often enough to be your "fitness best."

0 to 8 points—For your good health, you're wise to rethink your overall eating style. Take it gradually—step by step!

TO CARRY THIS FURTHER . . .

Whatever your score, make moves for healthful eating. Gradually turn your "nevers" into "sometimes" and your "sometimes" in "usually." Try some of the suggestions from the discussion of MyPyramid and the Dietary Guidelines for Americans.

Source: Adapted from *The American Dietetic Association's Monthly Nutrition Companion: 31 Days to a Healthier Lifestyle*, Chronimed Publishing, 1997.

Personal Assessment

Are you feeding your feelings?

Sometimes people use food as a way of coping with their emotions and problems. To identify how you might be using food as a coping strategy and what feelings you tend to associate with eating, complete the following inventory.

0 = Never

1 = Rarely

2 = Occasionally

3 = Often

4 = Always

1. _____ Do you eat when you are angry?
2. _____ When you feel annoyed, do you turn to food?
3. _____ If someone lets you down, do you eat to comfort yourself?
4. _____ When you are having a bad day, do you notice that you eat more?
5. _____ Do you eat to cheer yourself up?
6. _____ Do you use food as a way of avoiding tasks you don't want to do?
7. _____ Do you view food as your friend when you are feeling lonely?
8. _____ Is food a way for you to comfort yourself when your life seems empty?
9. _____ When you are feeling upset, do you turn to food to calm yourself down?
10. _____ Do you eat more when you are anxious, worried, or stressed?
11. _____ Does eating help you to cope with feeling overwhelmed?
12. _____ Do you eat more when you are going through big changes or transitions in your life?
13. _____ Do you reward yourself with food?
14. _____ When you think you have done something wrong, do you punish yourself by eating?
15. _____ When you are feeling badly about yourself, do you eat more?
16. _____ When you feel discouraged about your efforts to improve yourself, do you eat more, thinking "what's the use of trying"?

_____ **TOTAL SCORE**

Interpretation

If your total score is . . .

0 to 16 You don't eat to cope with your emotions. Your eating may not be related to your emotional state. However, you may avoid eating when you are upset or having trouble coping with your feelings. You may run away from food rather than running to food to cope.

17 to 47 Although you fall in the average range, you may use food to deal with specific situations or feelings such as anger, loneliness, or boredom. See the breakdown of scores below to identify how you may be using food to cope with particular feelings.

48 to 64 You run to food to cope with your emotions, and you may want to consider developing other ways of appropriately expressing your feelings.

Next, look more closely at your specific responses . . .

If you answered "3" or "4" to most of questions #1–#4, this can be indicative of eating when you are angry.

If you answered "3" or "4" to most of questions #5–#8, this can be indicative of eating when you are lonely or bored.

If you answered "3" or "4" to most of questions #9–#12, this can be an indication that you are a stress eater.

If you answered "3" or "4" to most of questions #13–#16, this can be an indication that you are using food to cope with feelings of low self-esteem and self-worth.

TO CARRY THIS FURTHER . . .

- Use the assessment scores to help you learn to recognize the triggers for your emotional eating.
- Make a list of things to do when you get the urge to eat and you're not hungry. Try going for a walk or calling a friend to distract yourself.
- Do something fun if you are tempted to eat to avoid work or a dreaded task.
- Reward yourself with things other than food.

Source: Adapted from *Nutrition for a Healthy Life*. Courtesy of March Leeds.

Maintaining a Healthy Weight

What Do You Know about Weight Management?

◉ The number of Americans who are overweight or obese has been increasing over the past few years. True or False?

◉ Body mass index (BMI) is a good way to assess body composition to determine if you are under- or overweight or in the normal weight range. True or False?

◉ Socioeconomic status is not a contributing factor to developing obesity. True or False?

◉ Most diets are effective for long-lasting weight management if you follow them correctly. True or False?

◉ A goal of losing 5 pounds per week is a reasonable goal. True or False?

◉ Diet pills and supplements are effective methods to manage your weight. True or False?

◉ Bulimia nervosa is more common than anorexia nervosa. True or False?

Check your answers at the end of the chapter.

Online Learning Center Resources
www.mhhe.com/payne10e

Visit the Online Learning Center for tools to improve your grade and get the most out of your course—chapter objectives, practice quizzes, key terms flashcards, chapter summaries for your digital audio player, Web activities, self-assessments, and many other study aids.

Body Weight and Wellness

Weight management has become an obsession in American culture as well as a significant health problem. In the United States, obesity has risen at an epidemic rate during the past 20 years (Figure 6-1). One of the national health objectives for the year 2010 is to reduce the prevalence of obesity among adults to less than 15 percent.[1] Research indicates that the situation is worsening rather than improving. According to the National Center for Chronic Disease Prevention and Health Promotion, an estimated 66 percent of adult Americans are either overweight or obese.[2] Currently 30 percent, or 60 million, adult Americans are obese with more women (35 percent) than men (31 percent) meeting the criteria for obesity. Up 74 percent since 1991, the number of overweight children and adolescents has tripled in the past 20 years.[3] These people face an increased risk of developing serious health problems, independent of other risk factors not directly related to weight. People who are overweight are 40 percent more likely to die prematurely than those of average weight. Obesity may account for as many as 400,000 deaths annually.[4]

zone begins when a woman's BMI is about 18 or below. Women tend to store fat in their pelvic region, around their hips and thighs ("pears"). Not only does this fat help to protect vital reproductive organs, it also acts as a source of stored energy for pregnancy and breastfeeding. As women enter menopause, they produce less estrogen. This leads to a change in body shape and fat distribution. During a woman's fertile years, the female hormones estrogen and progesterone are responsible for maintaining the female shape of a narrow waist and rounded hips. During and after menopause, the female waist thickens and fat is deposited around the stomach area similar to the male's pattern of fat distribution ("apples"). In addition, as in men, the metabolic rate slows and fewer calories are required. So if a woman continues to eat the same amount of food as she has throughout her fertile years, without increasing her exercise, weight and fat gain are likely to occur.[17]

Electrical impedance, the Bod Pod, skinfold measurement, and hydrostatic weighing are some of the most common methods for assessing body fat composition.

Electrical Impedance **Electrical impedance** is a relatively new method to determine body composition. This assessment procedure measures the electrical impedance or resistance to a weak electrical flow directed through the body. Because adipose tissue resists the passage of the electrical current more than muscle tissue does, electrical impedance can be used to calculate the percentage of body fat. However, in addition to high cost and limited availability, psychological variables, such as fear or discomfort associated with the electrical current flow, can reduce the practicality of electrical impedance.

Bod Pod (Body Composition System) The newest method of determining body composition involves the use of the Bod Pod, an egg-shaped chamber that uses computerized pressure sensors to determine the amount of air displaced by the person's body (larger people displace more air than smaller people). The person is allowed to breathe normally during the test, and the amount of air in the lungs can either be measured directly in the Bod Pod or is estimated. A complete test, with printed results, can be achieved in less than 4.5 minutes.[18] Body density can itself be used to determine the percentage of the subject's body that is composed of fat. Upon knowing the percent body fat, the percent of lean body mass can be calculated, again using a mathematical formula.[19] The Bod Pod is highly accurate and much more comfortable for subjects than is hydrostatic weighing.

Skinfold Measurements A **skinfold measurement** provides another way to measure body fat percentage. Skinfold measurements rely on constant-pressure **calipers** to measure the thickness of the layer of fat beneath the skin's surface. Skinfold measurements of subcutaneous fat are taken at several key places on the body. Measurements of skinfold thickness can then be used to calculate the percentage of body fat, and then a relatively simple conversion can be made to determine desired body weight. There are some drawbacks to this type of measure: First, a second person may be required to perform the test, because it is sometimes difficult to get an accurate measurement on yourself. Second, skinfolds are notoriously hard to locate precisely, and being just a few millimeters off can make a significant difference. Research recommends that 50–100 tests are needed before an examiner can be classified as "competent" with body fat calipers. Body fat calipers used correctly are accurate to within 4 percent at best.[5]

Hydrostatic Weighing **Hydrostatic weighing** (underwater weighing) is a precise method for determining the relative amounts of fat and lean body mass that make up body weight. A person's percentage of body fat is determined by comparing the underwater body weight with the body weight out of the water and dry. The necessity for expensive equipment and trained technicians makes the use of this method impractical for the average person. Traditionally, hydrostatic weighing has been considered the most accurate or sensitive means of determining body composition, with a 97 percent accuracy rate. The Bod Pod appears to be just as accurate and certainly more comfortable to use than underwater weighing.

Additional techniques used to determine body composition include computerized axial tomography (CT) scans, magnetic resonance imaging (MRI), infrared light transmission, and neutron activation. These techniques have limited application because of cost and availability.

The Bod Pod measures air displacement, which can be used to calculate percentage of body fat.

in humans, it still remains unclear as to how this research can be utilized in the treatment of obesity.

Physiological and Hormonal Factors

Building on the new information about the genetic and neuropsychological basis of obesity, researchers have identified centers for the control of eating within the hypothalamus of the central nervous system (CNS). These centers—the feeding center for hunger and the satiety center for fullness—tell the body when it should begin consuming food and when food consumption should stop. It takes 20 minutes on average for these signals to go from the stomach to the brain to relay the message "stop eating." These centers are thought to continuously monitor a variety of factors regarding food intake.[29]

Causes of Obesity

Genetic, physiological, metabolic, environmental, psychological, and other factors may all play a part. In the past decade, the overall prevalence of obesity has increased so that currently one-third of all Americans are obese. Moreover, in the last 20 years, the number of overweight children in the United States has tripled to one in five children.[20] Genetics, dietary practice, and activity level seem to all play a role in this dramatic increase.

Four additional factors seem to play a significant role in the prevalence of obesity: sex, age, socioeconomic status, and race. Biology accounts for only 33 percent of the variation in body weight, so the environment can also exert an enormous influence. According to the Centers for Disease Control and Prevention, prevalence rates for obesity in women is 35 percent and 31 percent among men and is found mainly in the 20–55 age group. Among women, obesity is strongly associated with socioeconomic status, being twice as common among those with lower socioeconomic status as it is among those with higher status.[21] Although prevalence among black and white men does not differ significantly, obesity is far more common among black than among white women, affecting 66 percent of black women compared with 58 percent of white women.

While the precise cause of obesity remains unclear, we do know that obesity is a complex condition caused by a variety of factors. Until we are sure what causes obesity, it will remain difficult to develop effective ways of managing weight.

Calorie Balance: Energy Intake versus Energy Output

What accounts for the high percentage of Americans defined as overweight or obese? Experts point to two salient factors: greater daily caloric consumption and a relatively low level of consistent physical activity. Women eat 335 more calories, and men eat 168 more calories, per day than they did 30 years ago. In addition, nearly two-thirds of Americans are not physically active on a regular basis and 25 percent are completely sedentary.[22] (See Chapter 4.)

The increase in weight occurs, of course, when the body is supplied with more energy than it can use and the excess energy is stored in the form of **adipose tissue,** or fat. This is called a **positive caloric balance.** Consuming about 3,500 calories a week more than is needed results in a weight gain of 1 pound of fat per week.[23] Weight remains constant when caloric input and caloric output are equal. This is called **caloric balance.** To maintain a specific weight, people must balance their energy intake with the energy expenditure. To lose weight, an individual must achieve a **negative caloric balance,** which involves expending more calories than are taken in. A negative

caloric balance can be created by reducing caloric intake, increasing physical activity, or both. The key to losing weight and keeping it off is engaging in regular aerobic exercise and eating a balanced diet that is consistent with the current dietary guidelines as described in Chapter 5. In other words, eat healthfully and exercise regularly.

What are our energy needs? How many calories should we consume (or expend) to achieve a healthy weight? There is no single answer for everyone. The new USDA dietary guidelines are based on consuming 2,000 calories a day.[24] (See Chapter 5.) Age and gender both affect the amount of calories people need. In addition, people may need fewer or more calories than the USDA recommendation depending on these three factors: (1) basal metabolism, (2) activity requirements, and (3) the thermic effect of food. Of these factors, basal metabolism is the most important determinant of the total calories required by an individual.

Basal Metabolic Rate **Basal Metabolic Rate (BMR)** is a measure of resting energy expenditure that is taken upon awakening, 10–12 hours after eating, or 12–18 hours after significant physical activity. A closely related construct, resting metabolic rate (RMR), is often used

Key Terms

electrical impedance A method used to measure the percentage of body fat using a harmless electrical current.

skinfold measurement A measurement to determine the thickness of the fat layer that lies immediately beneath the skin; used to calculate body composition.

caliper A device used to measure the thickness of a skinfold from which percentage of body fat can be calculated.

hydrostatic weighing Weighing the body while it is submerged in water.

adipose tissue Tissue made up of fibrous strands around which specialized cells designed to store liquified fat are stored.

positive caloric balance Caloric intake greater than caloric expenditure resulting in weight gain.

caloric balance Caloric intake and caloric expenditure are equal and body weight remains constant.

negative caloric balance Caloric intake is less than caloric expenditure, resulting in weight loss.

basal metabolic rate (BMR) The amount of energy, expressed in calories, that the body requires to maintain basic functions.

interchangeably with BMR. In comparison with t BMR, the RMR is measured at rest, without the string controls on physical activity required as with measuri BMR. RMR measures the calories needed for functic ing such as blood circulation, respiration, brain activi muscle function, body temperature, and heartbeat.[25]

Basal metabolism changes as people age. For bc males and females, the BMR is relatively high at bir and continues to increase until the age of 2. Except 1 a slight rise at puberty, the BMR gradually declin throughout the remainder of life. A variety of oth variables also affect BMR, including body compositic (muscular bodies are associated with higher BMR physical condition (fit people have higher BMRs), s (males have 5 percent higher BMRs), hormone secr tions (people with excessively active thyroid and adr nal glands have higher BMRs), sleep (BMRs are abo 10 percent lower during sleep), pregnancy (a 20 perce increase in BMR is typical, especially in the last trime ter), body temperature (a 1 degree rise in body temper ture increases BMR about 7 percent), and environment temperature (deviations above and below 78 degrees result in increased BMRs).[26]

The most important variables related to BMR are ag body composition, activity level, and caloric intake. Fc example, if people fail to recognize that BMR declin with aging, they might fail to adjust food intake accorc ingly, and weight gain will occur. Also, for those who al thinner, the presence of lean tissue favors a higher bas: metabolic rate with greater resistance to weight gai Finally, an increase in physical activity fosters a faste BMR, which contributes to weight loss. In contrast, i those people with above-average levels of body fat, BM rates are lower, thus providing the body with excess calc ries that will be stored as fat.

Activity Requirements Each person's caloric *activit requirements* vary directly according to the amount c daily physical work completed. When weight manage ment experts are asked to identify the single most im portant reason that obesity is so high in today's society they are most certain to point to inactivity. People of al ages tend to be less active and burn fewer calories thai did their ancestors only a few generations ago (see th box "The Growing Problem of Obesity"). Both adults anc children spend less time devoted to exercise as a result o longer work hours at sedentary jobs, a decline in physica education programs in school, and increased participa tion in sedentary recreational activities, such as brows ing the Internet, playing video games, and watching tele vision. In addition, many of the laborsaving devices anc increased automation in the home and workplace have contributed to increased inactivity. Physical activity use: between 20 and 40 percent of caloric intake. According to some studies, nearly two-thirds of Americans are not physically active on a regular basis, and 25 percent are

and as many as 10 percent of women may have some degree of thyroid hormone deficiency. In such individuals, the underactive thyroid makes burning up food difficult, and so weight gain is common. As we acquire greater understanding of the hormones and neurotransmitters that influence hunger and satiety, drugs designed to influence their actions will be developed. Some of these drugs already exist and will be described later in this chapter.

The effects of hormonal changes on eating can be seen each month just before a woman's menstrual cycle; many women say that they crave salty and sugary foods during this time. Pregnancy brings about another host of hormonal and metabolic changes. During a normal pregnancy, a woman requires an extra 300 calories a day to support the developing fetus and supportive tissues, and to fuel her elevated maternal metabolic rate. In addition, pregnant women will develop approximately 9 extra pounds of adipose tissue that will be used as an energy source during lactation. The average woman is expected to gain 25–35 pounds during pregnancy.[5] Many women express concern about their ability to lose this weight following the birth of the child, and some women do gain much more than the recommended amount of weight. However, the majority of women lose their pregnancy weight within 6 months to a year after having a baby. Nevertheless, obesity is one of the most frequent causes for complications in pregnancy. Women who are obese during pregnancy have a much higher risk of hypertension and gestational diabetes. Obesity has also been associated with infertility, poor pregnancy outcomes, and miscarriage.[30]

Typically, breast-feeding can help women to burn more calories and return to their prepregnancy weight, although extra fat may linger, since nature intended this to be a store of energy for breast-feeding. Breast-feeding requires an additional 500 calories a day.[31] Mothers who breast-feed tend to lose more weight when their babies are 3 to 6 months old than do formula-feeding mothers who consume fewer calories. Infants who are breast-fed also have a lower chance of developing obesity and asthma in childhood and adolescence.[32, 33]

Many researchers believe that the number of fat cells a person has is initially determined during the first two years of life. Babies who are overfed will develop a greater number of fat cells than will babies who receive a balanced diet of appropriate, infant-sized portions. Overfed babies, especially those with a family history of obesity, tend to develop **hypercellular obesity.** When these children reach adulthood, they will have more fat cells. An increase in fat cells during infancy and childhood can increase the chances of developing obesity. This increase can result in five times as many fat cells in obese people as in people of normal weight. Dieting reduces only the size of fat cells, not the number of fat cells. People who have hypercellular obesity have an abnormally high number of fat cells and are biologically limited in their ability to lose weight.[34]

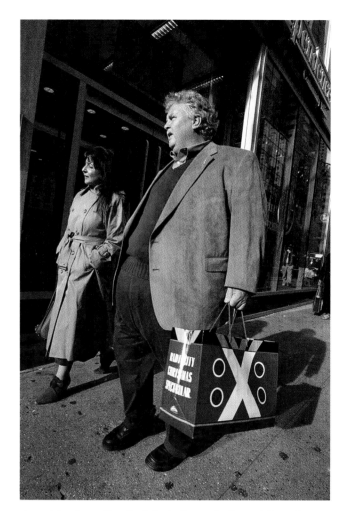

A variety of genetic, physiological, metabolic, social, environmental, and lifestyle factors contribute to the development of obesity.

Hypercellular obesity in adulthood can also result from excessive weight gain in late childhood and adolescence. If an individual's weight is 75 percent above the desirable weight, this can stimulate an increase in the number of fat cells, resulting in eventual obesity.

Hypertrophic obesity is the result of a pattern of overeating for a long period of time. Over a period of years, the existing fat cells increase in size to accommodate excess fat intake. Note that, after puberty, as your body stores more fat, the number of fat cells remains the same but each fat cell can get bigger. Hypertrophic obesity is generally associated with excessive fat around the waist and is thought to contribute to conditions such as type 2 diabetes, high levels of fat in the blood, high blood pressure, and heart disease. Hypertrophic obesity generally appears during middle age when physical activity tends to decline, whereas caloric intake remains the same.[34]

Metabolic Factors

Traditional theory has suggested that the energy expenditure and energy storage centers of the body possess a genetically programmed awareness of the body's most physiologically desirable weight, called **set point.** [35] However, the term *set point* is somewhat misleading in that it does not refer to a certain number or point but a weight range that the body is genetically programmed to maintain. When the body falls below its natural set point, one's metabolism reacts by slowing down the body's functioning in order to conserve energy. In other words, the body senses that it is not receiving enough calories to maintain healthy functioning and so it sends calories to essential areas of the body and uses the energy as efficiently as possible. Alternatively, when someone consumes more calories than are needed, the body begins to increase the rate of metabolism in an effort not to gain weight above the set point. The process of storing or burning more energy to maintain the body's "best" weight is called **adaptive thermogenesis.** This process also explains the reason that 90 percent of people who go on any diet gain all the weight back plus more within a year of going off the diet. When dieting, people reduce their caloric intake, which in turn lowers their metabolism. When they discontinue the diet, they typically eat more calories and foods with higher fat content on a lowered metabolism. This is a good formula for weight gain. In addition, dieters tend to lose muscle and regain their weight as fat.

It has also been found that weight as early as infancy is predictive of obesity in adulthood. Babies who gain weight rapidly tend to develop obesity in childhood as well. In fact, a study found that by age 2 babies who gained weight more quickly from birth than what is typical were overweight regardless of what and how much they were fed. Babies born smaller than the norm are more likely to be obese, as are children who are overweight by age 2. Some believe that there may be a metabolic switch activated in the fetus during pregnancy that causes babies to be born small and store extra calories efficiently as a way to survive. [36]

There is a great deal of debate on how an individual's set point can be altered. The number of fat cells in the body, the blood level of insulin, and regions of the brain such as the hypothalamus all seem to play a role in determining the set point. Certain drugs such as amphetamines and other diet pills and herbal supplements can act on the brain to temporarily lower the set point. However, once these drugs are discontinued, the set point returns to the previous level or perhaps an even higher level and weight increases as a result. Healthier and more permanent methods of changing one's set point are through regular exercise and healthy eating patterns. In fact, a recent study of 8,000 successful dieters found that the majority of them used "my own diet and exercise regimen" and did not follow any formal weight reduction program. [37]

The body's requirement for energy to maintain basic physiological processes decreases progressively with age. This change reflects the loss of muscle tissue as both men and women age. This loss of muscle mass eventually alters the ratio of lean body tissue to fat. As the proportion of fat increases, the energy needs of the body are more strongly influenced by the lower metabolic needs of the fat cells. [38] This excess energy is then stored in the fat cells of the body. A gradual decrease in caloric intake and a conscious effort to expend more calories can effectively prevent this gradual increase in weight leading to obesity.

Family, Social, and Cultural Factors

Ethnic and cultural differences also relate to the incidence of obesity and what is considered to be a healthy weight. The statistics are startling: 66 percent of African American women are overweight, and 33 percent are obese. For Mexican Americans, 75 percent of women and 76 percent of men are overweight or obese. Fifty-eight percent of Caucasian women and 70 percent of Caucasian men are overweight or obese. [39] Until recently Asian Americans had a lower rate of obesity than the general population; however, new figures now show that 8 percent of Chinese children 10 to 12 years of age are obese and 15 percent are overweight, which is closer to the overall 19 percent of 6- to 11-year-old American children who are overweight.

Obesity is second only to tobacco as the leading cause of premature deaths and disproportionately affects women of color and women of lower socioeconomic classes. On the positive side, African American women report less pressure to be thin than do their white counterparts and tend to be less self-conscious about their weight. [40] Acculturation also has a significant effect on the rates of obesity—the more an ethnic group has adapted to and absorbed Western culture, the higher the rate of obesity within that group. [41]

Key Terms

hypercellular obesity A form of obesity that results from having an abnormally high number of fat cells.

hypertrophic obesity A form of obesity in which there is a normal number of fat cells, but the individual fat cells are enlarged.

set point A genetically programmed range of body weight, beyond which a person finds it difficult to gain or lose additional weight.

adaptive thermogenesis The physiological response of the body to adjust its metabolic rate to the presence of food.

Table 6.2 Top Ten States for Weight

Percentage of Obese Adult Americans

1. Mississippi	29.5
2. Alabama	28.7
3. West Virginia	28.6
4. Louisiana	27.4
5. Kentucky	26.7
6. Tennessee	26.6
7. Arkansas	26.4
8. Indiana	26.2
8. South Carolina	26.2
10. Texas	25.8

Source: Trust for America's Health, *F is for Fat, 2006,* www.healthyamericans .org/reports/obesity2006.

Socioeconomic status is also an important influence on obesity. Upper socioeconomic women tend to be thinner than lower socioeconomic women; however among men there is not such a pattern.[42] Limited access to health care, lower education levels, lower income levels, and increased stress are some of the reasons cited for this disparity. In addition, children's weight gain has been associated with the cost of fruits and vegetables where they live—the higher the cost, the higher the weight of children who live in that area. Interestingly, higher obesity levels are also related to marriage, parenthood, and geographical location; married men, parents, and people living in rural areas tend to have a higher incidence of obesity.[43] Table 6.2 lists the states with the highest percentages of obese Americans, citing hunger and lack of accessibility to healthy, safe food as the major reasons for this.

The information, values, traditions, and messages you receive from your family also have a significant impact on your dietary habits. If an infant's cries for food are immediately responded to, that child will likely learn what the sensation of hunger is and what the appropriate response is. If crying unrelated to hunger is responded to by the offer of a cookie or candy, the child will learn to soothe himself or herself with food. Studies show that children become confused about what hunger is and how to satisfy it if their hunger needs are neglected or overindulged in infancy.[44]

Some of the first power struggles between parents and their children revolve around issues of food. A child who has little power in her life can exert some power and control through refusing to eat certain foods and demanding other foods and determining when she wants to eat. Parents who use food as a reward for good behavior ("If you get an 'A' on your test, I will treat you to ice cream"); as punishment ("You weren't behaving so you can't have dessert"); or as a guilt trip ("Don't waste food. Clean your plate. Children are starving in the world") may inadvertently be creating negative dietary practices

that will continue throughout the child's life. Interestingly, research has shown that children are extraordinarily adept at meeting their nutritional needs when left to their own devices. One study allowed children to eat whatever they wanted for a week. Did they always pick high-fat, high-sugar foods? No. Actually, when we look at each day's intake, they didn't eat a balanced diet. However, when one takes the full week into consideration, they met their nutritional needs perfectly.

What your parents say to you not only has a tremendous influence on your eating behavior; what they do, their own eating practices, can have even a greater impact. Children are exposed to different foods and model what their parents eat. If a parent makes comments such as "I shouldn't eat that because I will get fat" or doesn't eat fruits or vegetables, or sits down with a bag of chips in front of the television every night, the child will probably do the same. In the same vein, when parents exercise regularly, eat a balanced diet, and make positive comments about their weight, children tend to mimic this behavior.

 TALKING POINTS What were the messages you received in childhood regarding food? What positive and negative eating habits have you learned from your family?

Environmental Factors

Certainly environmental factors such as the smell or sight of freshly made cookies, or an advertisement for a candy bar, can affect your eating habits. Even the clock signaling it is "time to eat" can encourage us to eat even when we aren't hungry. While this may seem adaptive and helpful in regulating our food intake, Dr. Kelly D. Brownell, a professor of psychology at Yale and an expert on eating disorders, has gone so far as to label American society a "toxic environment" when it comes to food. Researchers contend that the local environment has a powerful effect on eating (see the box "The Freshman 15 Has Lost Weight"). Factors such as portion size, price, advertising, the availability of food, and the number of food choices presented all can influence the amount the average person consumes. For example, moviegoers will eat 50 percent more popcorn if given an extra-large tub of popcorn instead of a container one size smaller, even if the popcorn is stale. If a tabletop in the office is stocked with cookies and candy, coworkers tend to nibble their way through the workday, even if they are not hungry. One study showed that when the candy was in plain sight on workers' desks, they ate an average of nine pieces each. Storing the candy in a desk drawer reduced consumption to six pieces, as compared to putting the candy a couple of yards from the desk, cutting the number to three pieces per person.[45]

Another study found that half of children stop on their way to and from school each day to spend about $2 a day on junk food, increasing their caloric intake by 610 calories each day. Hamburgers, pizza, French fries, cookies, candy, and pastries are the top-selling foods for school-age children. In response to these and other findings, many public schools have begun offering only healthy foods in their cafeterias, replacing soft drinks, candy, and chips with juice, milk, fruit, and granola bars.

Packaging and price can also influence the amount people consume, a concept of which advertisers, restaurants, and grocery stores are well aware. Dropping the price of the low-fat snacks by even a nickel resulted in dramatically increased sales. In contrast, stickers signaling low-fat content or cartoons promoting the low-fat alternatives had little influence over which snacks were more popular. This is true not only of food but also of beverages: people tend to drink *more* from short, wide glasses than from thin, tall ones, thinking they are drinking less.[45]

Having more choices also appears to make people eat more. In one study, people ate more when offered sandwiches with four different fillings than they did when they were given sandwiches with their single favorite filling. In another study, participants who were served a four-course meal with meat, fruit, bread, and a pudding ate 60 percent more food than did those served an equivalent meal of only their favorite course. Even the cup holders in automobiles have grown larger to make room for giant drinks. Note that these findings apply to people of all body sizes not just people who are overweight or obese, as is often the misconception. However, one difference seems to relate to the age of the individuals studied. One study found that 3-year-olds who were served three different portion sizes of macaroni and cheese for lunch on three different days ate the same amount each time. Five-year-olds, however, ate more when more was put in front of them.[46]

This phenomenon is referred to as unit bias or the tendency to think that a single unit of food is the right amount to eat or drink, no matter what size it is. So we often don't make a conscious decision about how much to eat, as the choice is made for us by the portion size that is offered to us. We mindlessly eat food without questioning the amount.[45] We also tend to eat or drink whatever is offered to us, one large cookie or a small one, and still think of it as the same amount of calories because it is one cookie.

 TALKING POINTS Do you think there should be more regulation of the food industry? If so, what recommendations would you make? What food would you include for regulation and how should this be determined?

 The Freshman 15 Has Lost Weight

Most people have heard about the "Freshman 15," which refers to the 15 pounds freshmen can expect to gain in their first year of college. However, research has shown that this is a myth, as the average college freshman gains 8 pounds not 15. This is better news, but still, college students are probably not excited about the prospect of gaining 8 pounds in their first year of college. These same students are being referred to as the cohort group "Generation XL."

Most freshmen gain 5–10 pounds their first year in college, usually in the first semester. Sophomores tend to gain 2 to 3 more pounds. Men gain more than women, on average. Researchers speculate that having easy access to large amount of high-sugar, high-fat foods, late-night snacking, an increase in alcohol consumption, and less physical activity may contribute to college students' weight gain. Some students have become so concerned about gaining the "freshmen 15" that they go the other extreme, becoming underweight, some to the point of developing an eating disorder.

So what can you do to maintain a healthy weight at college? Don't skip breakfast, choose healthy snacks such as fruit, watch your portion sizes, and limit your alcohol consumption. Exercise regularly in addition to walking or riding your bike to class. And if you order pizza at midnight, limit yourself to one slice!

Sources: "Freshmen 15 Down to Just 8," *USA Today*, October 23, 2006; "Studies: College Kids Packing on Pounds," www.comcast.net, October 23, 2006.

Psychological Factors

Psychological factors related to overeating concern the reasons people eat other than physiological hunger. Individuals with eating disorders often report that they don't know when they are hungry and often eat when they are not hungry and don't eat when they have a biological reason for doing so. Why do people eat if not in response to hunger? Frequently people eat in response to their emotions—for example, to comfort themselves or when bored, tired, stressed, or depressed. Some people say they use food as a way of coping with hurt, sadness, and anger, "swallowing" their feelings and putting food on top of them. Others eat out of habit and associate food with certain activities, such as eating popcorn at a movie, eating chips in front of the television, and having dessert after dinner. Certainly many people think of chocolate when they want to cheer themselves up. Food is also part of celebrations, holidays, and family bonding, as well as a mainstay of socialization. It is difficult to think about social activities we engage in that don't involve food in some way.

Some people develop relationships with food that substitute for real human relationships or to fill other

Faith-Based Weight Loss Programs

Faith-based weight loss programs have increased in popularity over the years. These programs are different from other weight loss programs in that they have a spiritual or biblical component to them. There seems to be a market sector for these types of groups, as a 1998 Purdue University study found that religious Americans were more likely to be overweight than those who were nonreligious, with Baptists being the heaviest religious group.[*] Most of the faith-based weight loss programs encourage a relationship with God rather than with food or have some other spiritual component, such as prayer, losing weight in 40 days as in the "Body by God" program, or eating a raw vegan diet similar to the diet followed by Adam and Eve. Other programs view some foods as sinful and involve following a strict regimen.

Some modern diets promote spiritual components, and some food has been referred to as sinful. *The Weigh Down Diet* by Gwen Shamblin approaches weight loss from a religious perspective, advising people to feed the human soul with a relationship with God rather than with food. Holding meetings in local churches, Shamblin teaches you "God's rules for eating." She advocates allowing your stomach to become empty before eating and to give your appetite to God to control. In fact, she suggests waiting to eat until your stomach is growling and to focus on making the desire for eating go away. This is counter to what many nutritionists, physicians, and psychologists suggest in terms of healthy eating. She states that exercise is not important for weight management, writing in her book that "The only exercises we insist on are getting down on your knees to pray and getting the muscle of your will to surrender some of the extra food you have been eating."[†] Again, this advice is not consistent with the USDA's guidelines of engaging in daily physical exercise for 30–90 minutes.

There are a number of other religious or spiritually based approaches to weight loss. For example, the *Hallelujah Diet* by Rev. George Malkmus suggests that we eat a vegan diet. He states, "The Lord gave us everything we need in the Garden of Eden; fruits, vegetables, nuts, and seeds." He calls this the "Hallelujah diet" to

"celebrate its true creater." Dr. Don Colbert wrote a book based on a similar philosophy called *What Would Jesus Eat?* which encourages the consumption of non-animal-derived living foods rather than dead or processed foods. Another Christian weight-management book is *The Maker's Diet* by Jordan S. Rubin. He warns against a vegan diet and suggests eating meat and dairy products instead. He further recommends eating foods in their most organic and least-processed states and consuming food in the form the body was designed by God to eat them. For example, he doesn't think milk should be pasteurized nor should the fat be removed to make skim or low-fat milk.[‡] Stephen Arterburn, author of the "Lose It for Life Diet," suggests that people should lose weight so that "people can look at us and see Jesus." His diet combines the South Beach Diet with the self-help aspect of the book *The Purpose-Driven Life.*[*]

While Shamblin is a registered dietitian and has a master's degree in food and nutrition, most of the diet ministries are led by people without these types of degrees and credentials. There has been some concern raised about food safety issues with unprocessed dairy products, meat, and other foods as well as how these diets contradict the new dietary guidelines released by the USDA, particularly those concerning exercising daily and eating a balanced diet. Some critics say that God is being used as a gimmick to get in on the $50 billion diet industry, while others view giving dietary advice as part of God's ministry. Although faith-based diets have been in existence since the 1957 "Pray Your Weight Away Diet," there has been no research to substantiate the effectiveness of any of these programs.[§]

[*]"HWJD: How Would Jesus Diet?" *New York Times,* May 13, 2005.
[†]Shamblin, G. *The Weigh Down Diet.* New York: Bantam Doubleday Dell, 1997.
[‡]"What Would Jesus Eat? Diets Grapple with God's Gastronomic Will," *Muncie Star Press,* June 2004.
[§]"Can You Pray Your Pounds Away?" *Vegetarian Times,* March 2006.

psychological or spiritual needs (see the box "Faith-Based Weight Loss Programs"). Comments such as "Food is my best friend" and "A great meal is better than sex" are indicative to the degree to which many people rely on food to fill their needs. As we'll learn in our discussion of eating disorders later in the chapter, psychological issues with food can become serious, even life-threatening problems.

Weight-Management Strategies

Weight loss occurs when the calories consumed are fewer than required by the body for physiological maintenance and activity. This may sound overly simplified, and certainly the $50 billion-a-year weight loss industry would like us to think it is much more complicated than this.

Weight loss followed by weight gain may be less healthy and certainly more frustrating than maintaining body weight, even at weight above the desirable levels. When a diet or weight loss strategy fails, the person, not the diet, is blamed. This causes people to jump to another weight loss method and then another, and a vicious cycle has begun. However, a commitment to a lifestyle change of eating in healthy ways and engaging in regular exercise seems to be the most effective strategy for weight loss and weight maintenance.

Lifestyle Approaches for Lifetime Healthy Weight Management

In order to maintain a healthy weight, you will need to eat a balanced diet supported by portion control, participate

Lifestyle approaches to weight management address two key components of energy balance—energy in as food and energy out as physical activity. Strategies for creating a negative energy balance include reducing your intake of large portions of high-calorie foods (such as fast food) and increasing your level of physical activity.

in regular physical activity, get consistent, sufficient sleep, and develop healthy ways of coping and problem solving.

Balanced Diet Supported by Portion Control A diet that reduces caloric intake is the most common approach to what seems to be a national obsession with weight loss. The choice of foods included in the diet and the amount of food that can be consumed are the two factors that distinguish the wide range of diets currently available. However, dieting alone usually does not result in long-term weight loss. Effective and long-lasting weight management requires a lifestyle change, not just going on a diet for a specific time period only to return to your old patterns of eating. This is the problem many people face when they go on strict diets and overly restrict their calories. Because the diet is so restrictive and demanding, they are unable to continue to follow it for very long and return to their previous eating patterns. In addition, people tend to overeat the foods they denied themselves while dieting, because they feel deprived and the forbidden food seems even more alluring. This can also lead to binge eating. Thus diets tend not to work in the long run.

A healthy and successful approach to weight loss and subsequent management of that loss is to establish a nutritionally sound balanced diet (see Chapter 5) that controls portions. The food pyramid outlines the breakdown of daily caloric intake for each food group. You can get a personalized dietary guideline by inputting your gender, age, and activity level at MyPyramid.gov. One study showed that people cut 256 calories a day just by trimming their portion sizes by 25 percent.

Maintaining a balanced diet and watching your portion sizes is especially important on the weekends. Many people throw their good eating habits out the window on the weekends, as evidenced by a recent study that found that Americans eat an average of 115 extra calories per day from Friday to Sunday as compared to the rest of the week. Most of these calories came from alcohol and increased fat consumption. These extra calories can result in a gain of 5 pounds over the course of a year.

 TALKING POINTS Have you ever tried to lose weight? What methods were effective for you? What is the longest time you have stuck to a particular weight management strategy?

Physical Activity Many experts now believe that the most important component of weight management is regular physical activity. Physical activity contributes to weight loss and the maintenance of weight loss because activity burns calories (Table 6.3). Remember, the need for calories decreases with age and with decreased activity.

An additional benefit derived from physical activity is that proportionately more fat is lost than is lost through dieting alone. Studies suggest that the weight loss achieved through physical activity is 95 percent fat and 5 percent lean tissue, such as muscle, in comparison with a loss of 75 percent fat and 25 percent lean tissue when dieting alone is used. Exercise also offers the benefits of increased heart and lung endurance, muscular strength, and flexibility.

How much exercise is enough? The current USDA dietary guidelines (see Chapter 5) advise American adults to engage in at least 60 minutes of moderately intense aerobic exercise almost every day for weight maintenance and 90 minutes of this type of exercise for weight loss. Weight training has become a more important factor in weight management. (See Chapter 4 for further recommendations on physical fitness.)

Table 6.3 Calories Expended during Physical Activity

To determine the number of calories you have spent in an hour of activity, simply multiply the *calories per hour per pound* column by your weight (in pounds). For example, after an hour of archery, a 120-pound person will have expended 209 calories; a 160-pound person, 278 calories; and a 220-pound person, 383 calories.

Activity	Calories/Hour/Pound	Activity	Calories/Hour/Pound
Archery	1.74	Marching (rapid)	3.84
Baseball	1.86	Painting (outside)	2.10
Basketball	3.78	Playing music (sitting)	1.08
Boxing (sparring)	3.78	Racquetball	3.90
Canoeing (leisure)	1.20	Running (cross-country)	4.44
Cleaning	1.62	Running	
Climbing hills (no load)	3.30	11 min 30 sec per mile	3.66
Cooking	1.20	9 min per mile	5.28
Cycling		8 min per mile	5.64
5.5 mph	1.74	7 min per mile	6.24
9.4 mph	2.70	6 min per mile	6.84
Racing	4.62	5 min 30 sec per mile	7.86
Dance (modern)	2.28	Scrubbing floors	3.00
Eating (sitting)	0.60	Sailing	1.20
Field hockey	3.66	Skiing	
Fishing	1.68	Cross-country	4.43
Football	3.60	Snow, downhill	3.84
Gardening		Water	3.12
Digging	3.42	Skating (moderate)	2.28
Mowing	3.06	Soccer	3.54
Raking	1.44	Squash	5.76
Golf	2.34	Swimming	
Gymnastics	1.80	Backstroke	4.62
Handball	3.78	Breaststroke	4.44
Hiking	2.52	Free, fast	4.26
Horseback riding		Free, slow	3.48
Galloping	3.72	Butterfly	4.68
Trotting	3.00	Table tennis	1.86
Walking	1.14	Tennis	3.00
Ice hockey	5.70	Volleyball	1.32
Jogging	4.15	Walking (normal pace)	2.16
Judo	5.34	Weight training	1.90
Knitting (sewing)	0.60	Wrestling	5.10
Lacrosse	5.70	Writing (sitting)	0.78

Source: From Bannister and Brown, "The Relative Energy Requirements of Physical Activity." In H. B. Falls, editor. *Exercise Physiology*, Academic Press, 1988, Table 6.5. Used with permission by Elsevier.

As a result, exercise boot-camp workouts are becoming more popular in gyms. These military-style exercise programs involve drills with running, jumping jacks, push-ups, squats, sit-ups, and weight lifting shouted from a trainer who looks and acts more like a drill sergeant.

As with most things, too much or too little exercise is not beneficial and can be unhealthy. As will be discussed in a later section, some people with eating disorders tend to overexercise, resulting in diminishing returns.

Sleep   Research has recently discovered that not getting enough sleep doesn't just make you grumpy and sluggish—it can make you gain weight as well! People who sleep 2 to 4 hours a night have been found to be 73 percent more likely to be obese than those who sleep 7 to 9 hours. Sleeping 5 hours a night results in a 50 percent chance of being obese compared to those consistently sleeping 7 to 9 hours. Twenty-three percent of people who sleep 6 hours tend to be obese. In other words, the higher the BMI, the less sleep the person got.[47]

Why does less sleep equal more weight? We used to think that sleeping too much made us gain weight and staying up meant we were more active and so burned calories, but this has been disproved. People tend to watch television, read, or be online late at night, and so they are not active. In addition, people tend to eat high-fat, high-sugar foods while they are engaging in these activities. Some people say that they eat sugary foods in order to give themselves more energy to stay up late to study or to get work done.

Learning to Eat Mindfully

Have you had the experience of eating out of a bag of chips or munching on a sandwich and finding that you have eaten the entire thing without even realizing it? Do you tend to eat "on the run" or very quickly without tasting your food? Do you eat while doing other things, such as watching TV, reading, or in front of the computer? These are all examples of eating mindlessly—not paying attention and not enjoying the food you are eating.

There is a growing trend of eating mindfully. This means giving your undivided attention to the experience of eating, focusing on the present, and having a nonjudgmental perspective about what you are eating. Eating mindfully is the opposite of dieting, because you eat when you are hungry, pay attention to feeling full, and don't view any foods as "good" or "bad." In the wake of the fast-food craze that consumes us, mindful eating and its cousin, the Slow Food movement, emphasize taking your time when eating and consuming

unprocessed, healthy foods. It also incorporates guided imagery, deep breathing, and meditation to become more aware of your feelings of hunger and fullness and your emotions related to eating and food. This approach helps some people stop using food to cope and develop other ways of coping with stress rather than eating away their problems. Mindful eating can be an effective tool for weight management, because it helps you learn to eat when you are hungry and stop when you are full, and not feel deprived. It is a lifestyle, not a diet, and can be permanently incorporated into your daily life. Mindful eating also emphasizes body acceptance and how to build a healthy mind/body connection.

Source: Albers, S. *Eating Mindfully,* Oakland, CA. New Harbinger Publications Inc. 2003. Used with permission by Susan Albers.

Two hormones, ghrelin and leptin, have been found to regulate both sleep and hunger. A sleep study at the University of Chicago found that leptin levels were 18 percent lower and ghrelin levels 28 percent higher after subjects slept 4 hours. Sleep-deprived subjects reported feeling the most hungry and craved carbohydrates, the energy food. Ghrelin has been referred to as the accelerator for eating. When ghrelin levels are up, people feel hungrier. Leptin is the brake for eating; higher levels are associated with feeling full and decreased appetite.

These sleep studies seem to indicate that a hormonal relationship exists between sleep and hunger. The ghrelin level in people who routinely slept 5 hours a night was 15 percent higher, compared to 15 percent lower leptin levels in people who slept 8 hours a night. The first group had higher BMIs than did individuals sleeping 8 hours at night. Studies have also found that children are not getting the 10 to 11 hours of sleep a night they require, which may also help explain the increase in childhood obesity.[48]

So, one way for us to manage our weight is to manage our sleep better. This means managing our time better—prioritizing our commitments and activities and not overloading our schedules, so that we can get the rest we need.

Lifestyle Support and Problem Solving   Not only do you need to be committed to a lifestyle of regular physical activity and healthy food choices, but you also need to build a support group that will encourage you in these endeavors. Inform family, friends, classmates, and co-workers about your intent to rely on them for support and encouragement. Perhaps you will inspire others to make similar lifestyle changes.

It may be helpful for you to reevaluate your perception of food and eating. Do you use food as a way of coping with stress, boredom, or other feelings? Consider, instead, coping with stressors with nonfood options such as talking with friends or family, exercising, or journaling. You may want to take the Personal Assessment at the end of this chapter to see if you are eating mindlessly (see also the box "Learning to Eat Mindfully"). Additionally, if you tend to use food as a way to reward yourself for hard work or completing something, you might want to choose other types of rewards, such as engaging in a hobby or another activity you enjoy. Take care that you don't adopt other unhealthy methods of coping (see the box "Smoking and Weight").

The lifestyle choices suggested here will significantly help reduce your chances of developing a weight problem or a weight-related health problem in your lifetime. Again, genetics will exert its effects to some degree on weight and body composition, but you can counteract these effects by employing the methods discussed here.

Specific Dietary Approaches

There are many different strategies for losing weight, and they vary in effectiveness, harmfulness, cost, and ease of use. The next section will cover the most popular weight loss methods: temporary caloric restriction, low-calorie foods and controlled serving sizes, controlled fasting, formal or commercial weight reduction programs, weight loss drugs, herbal supplements, and surgical interventions.

Temporary Calorie Restriction   People use a variety of fad diets in an attempt to achieve rapid weight loss. Currently there are over 150 popular diets, often promoted by celebrities or people who claim to be nutrition experts.

Table 6.4 Rating the Diets

	Overall Score	Nutritional Analysis	Short-Term Weight Loss	Long-Term Weight Loss
Volumetrics	Good	Excellent	Good	Good
Weight Watchers	Good	Excellent	Fair	Fair
Jenny Craig	Good	Excellent	Good	Good
Slim Fast	Good	Excellent	Good	Good
eDiets	Good	Excellent	Below Avg	Below Avg
Zone Diet	Good	Excellent	Fair	Below Avg
Ornish Diet	Fair	Fair	Fair	Fair
Atkins Diet	Below Avg	Poor	Good	Fair

Source: "New Diet Winners," *Consumer Reports*, June 2007.

With few exceptions, these approaches are both ineffective and potentially dangerous. In addition, some require far greater expense than would be associated with weight loss or management techniques using portion control and regular physical activity. (See Table 6.4.)

The main problem with dieting is that it is a temporary, quick fix. Most diets will result in temporary weight loss if followed correctly, and they usually make the promise of losing weight rapidly. Of course, much of the weight lost initially is water weight and not fat. Research shows that 90 percent of all people who diet gain back their weight, plus more, within a year. Oprah Winfrey is a good example of what happens to most dieters. She lost 67 pounds in four months consuming only Optifast. She kept this weight off for only one day. The first day she went off her diet and went back to her old eating patterns, she began gaining weight. She weighed 211 pounds pre-diet and she weighed 226 pounds post-diet. Look at Figure 6-2 to see why people struggle with losing weight.

Diets don't teach us how to eat; they teach us how not to eat! The restriction of calories is the basis of all diets. Some suggest limiting the consumption of fat, others sugar, or the caloric intake is dangerously low for all food groups. Many diet plans, such as the South Beach diet and the Atkins diet, advocate the restriction of carbohydrates, which can cause ketosis. Ketosis can cause the blood to become too acidic, and dehydration can occur. The body requires a minimum of 50–100 grams of carbohydrate per day to avoid ketosis.[26] Low-carbohydrate diets are characterized by initial rapid weight loss, which is appealing to most people, but this loss is primarily due to water and not fat loss. Complications associated with low-carbohydrate, high-protein diets include dehydration, hypertension, heart disease, cancer, electrolyte loss, calcium depletion, weakness due to inadequate dietary carbohydrates, nausea due to ketosis, vitamin and mineral deficiencies, and possible kidney problems. Gout (painful inflammation of the joints) and kidney failure are potential side effects. The risk of coronary heart disease may be higher in those who stay on the diet a long time, owing to the increased consumption of foods high in saturated fat and cholesterol.

Most diets are temporary in nature because they are medically unhealthy and potentially harmful. They are also too restrictive, and people end up craving the very foods they are being told to avoid. Dieters begin feeling deprived and resentful, and respond by retaliating against the diet and bingeing on the "forbidden" foods.

Low-Calorie Foods and Controlled Serving Sizes Recently, a variety of familiar foods have been developed in a reduced-calorie form. By lowering the carbohydrate content with the use of nonnutritive sweeteners, reducing the portion size, reducing the fat content of the original formulations, or removing fat entirely (see the discussion of Olestra in Chapter 5), manufacturers have produced "lite" versions of many food products. For example, many frozen entrees, such as Healthy Choice Oriental Beef with Vegetables (290 calories), Weight Watchers Lasagna Florentine (210 calories), and Healthy Choice Fettucine with Turkey and Vegetables (350 calories), are low in calories. Because fat helps us to feel satiated or not hungry, these low-fat, low-calorie meals tend not to satisfy our hunger for very long, and we may find ourselves wanting to snack or binge by late afternoon.

 TALKING POINTS Your best friend is trying to follow a low-fat, low-calorie diet in order to lose weight but is finding herself constantly hungry. What can you tell her about the diet plan she's chosen? What changes might she make to increase her chances of success?

Figure 6-2 Why Weight Loss Is Often Pie-in-the-Sky *USA Today* surveyed 126 of the nation's top registered dietitians about trends in obesity and weight loss. Selected findings are shown here.

Source: From *USA Today*, December 29, 2004. Reprinted with permission.

What's the major reason people want to lose weight?

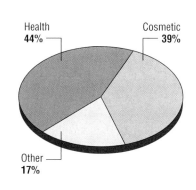

Health **44%**
Cosmetic **39%**
Other **17%**

What's the main reason people resist changing their eating habits?

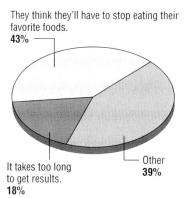

They think they'll have to stop eating their favorite foods. **43%**
It takes too long to get results. **18%**
Other **39%**

What's the biggest mistake people make when trying to lose weight?

Going on a fad diet **27%**
Other **25%**
Not exercising **13%**
Not limiting portions **20%**
Setting inappropriate goals, such as wanting to lose quickly **15%**

What's the main reason people don't exercise or increase physical activity to manage weight?

They hate exercise. **44%**
Lack of time **37%**
They think weight loss is mostly about diet, not activity. **5%**
Other **14%**

Controlled Fasting In cases of extreme obesity, some patients are placed on a complete fast in a hospital setting. The patient consumes only water, electrolytes, and vitamins. Weight loss is substantial because the body is forced to begin **catabolizing** its fat and muscle tissue. Complete fasting is such an extreme approach to weight loss that it must be done in an institutional setting so that the patient can be closely monitored. Inadequate protein and sodium and potassium loss are particular health concerns.

Today some people regularly practice short periods of modified fasting. Solid foods are removed from the diet for a number of days. Fruit juices, water, supplements, and vitamins are used to minimize the risks associated with total fasting. However, unsupervised short-term fasting can be dangerous and is not recommended.

In addition to the controlled fasting just discussed, a somewhat different version of this practice is appearing with the long-term use of readily available, low-calorie, nutrient-dense food supplementation products such as Ensure, Boost, SlimFast, and Sustical. Regardless of whether they are marketed as nutrient-dense supplements for older adults or as adjuncts to weight loss diets,

these drinks should not be viewed, or used, as meal replacements. Because these products contain no more than 400 calories (and the lite versions contain as few as 200 calories), their routine use as meal replacements could move even a young, healthy adult dangerously close to caloric inadequacy in a short time. Perhaps if used in place of a high-calorie snack or as a very occasional substitute for breakfast, these supplements may not present the dangers that their routine use does.

Formal or Commercial Weight Reduction Programs In virtually every area of the country, at least one version of the popular weight reduction programs, such as TOPS (Take Off Pounds Sensibly), Jenny Craig, and Nutri-System Weight Loss Centers, can be found. Pioneered by Weight Watchers, these programs generally feature a

> **Key Terms**
>
> **catabolizing** The metabolic process of breaking down tissue for the purpose of converting it to energy.

format consisting of (1) a well-balanced diet emphasizing portion control and low-fat, low-saturated fat, and high-complex carbohydrate foods, (2) specific weight loss goals to be attained over a set period of time, (3) encouragement from supportive leaders and fellow group members, (4) emphasis on regular physical activity, and (5) a maintenance program (follow-up program). The box "Choosing a Diet Plan" presents some guidelines for choosing a weight loss program.

Although in theory these programs offer an opportunity to lose weight for people who cannot or will not participate in a physical activity program, their effectiveness is very limited. The minimal success of these programs and the difficulty that working adults have in attending meetings has resulted in falling enrollment and the development of home-based programs, such as those developed by hospital-based wellness programs, many YMCAs and YWCAs, and even Weight Watchers. Further, these programs can be costly when compared with self-directed approaches, especially when the program markets its own food products. The pros and cons of a variety of weight loss programs are presented in Table 6.4.

The Weight Loss Industry In response to our nation's near obsession with thinness, a thriving weight loss industry exists to assist us in our attempts to lose weight.

Americans are spending in excess of $50 billion each year in an attempt to achieve and maintain weight loss.

The weight loss industry has capitalized and profited on the meaning that thinness has in the American culture, including a bias against large people. These programs are promising not just weight loss but happiness and success in life as well. Thinness is associated not only with beauty but also with one's ability to have successful relationships, careers, and self-worth. A study was conducted asking 32,000 women what they would choose: a successful career, a satisfying romantic relationship, or a loss of 10–15 pounds. The majority of these women chose to lose weight, believing that they would also have a successful career and relationship if they lost 10–15 pounds.[9]

Another study showed children pictures of a minority child, a disabled child, and an overweight child and asked them to choose who they would like to be their friend. Overwhelmingly, the overweight child was their last choice. The American Association of University Women conducted a study to examine the changing attitudes children and adolescents have of themselves in terms of their body image. While 60 percent of elementary school girls said, "I am always happy with the way I am," only 29 percent of high school girls said the same thing. For boys, 67 percent of elementary school boys liked how they looked, and 46 percent of high school boys continued to feel this way. It is these attitudes that play into the measures to which individuals will go and the price they will pay to achieve the cultural ideal.

The financial success of the weight loss industry in this country has in part been because of its effective television advertising. Skillfully produced commercials featuring successful program members suggest likely success for the viewer willing to sign on. Before 1994, these commercials were regular fare on daytime television. Today, however, commercials for diet programs such as Jenny Craig, NutriSystem, Weight Watchers, and others are considerably more restrained in their messages about success. Under directives issued by the Federal Trade Commission (FTC), today's advertisements cannot misrepresent program performance. They must disclose that most weight loss is temporary, and they now inform the viewer that their loss will most likely not approximate that of the successful subjects featured in their commercials.

Most recently some nationally franchised weight loss programs have added a "medical" component to their format that involves prescribing medications. Consumers should find out if medical supervision will be a regular component of the program or a brief, one-time physician visit involving little more than basic screening.

Weight Loss Drugs

Another approach to weight loss involves over-the-counter weight loss drugs, herbal supplements, and prescription drugs. These are designed to either suppress hunger, increase metabolism, or block fat absorption in order to manage weight.

Over-the-Counter (OTC) Weight Loss Drugs and Herbal Supplements

Most OTC and herbal supplements are designed to suppress hunger and increase metabolism. None of them are recommended for long-term use, as they can cause serious health problems and can be addictive. It is difficult to stop taking these pills because weight loss only occurs while taking them and weight gain usually occurs once the drug or supplement is discontinued. Most of these contained ephedra or ephedrine until it was banned by the FDA in 2003[49] following the death of 23-year-old Baltimore Orioles pitcher Steve Bechler, whose death was linked to an ephedra supplement. Ephedra has been associated with at least 155 deaths and dozens of heart attacks and strokes, and it can cause high blood pressure, seizures, heart irregularities, insomnia, anxiety, and tremors.

Herbal weight loss supplements come as pills, bars, teas, and powders to mix in liquids. Some people see herbal supplements such as stackers, mini thins, hoodia, and fat burners as safe because they are "natural," and yet they can be more dangerous and deadly than prescription medications because they are not inspected for purity and accuracy of the contents or the potency of the ingredients. The Dietary Supplement Health and Education Act (DSHEA) of 1994 relegated herbal supplements to the category "dietary supplements," limiting the FDA's power to regulate these products to ensure that they meet certain standards or are safe and effective. In fact, it is difficult to stop the sale of dietary supplements that appear dangerous because there must be enough proof to substantiate the health risks.

However, there is some evidence linking these diet pills to heart attacks, strokes, hepatitis, headaches, tremors, anxiety, extreme irritability, and insomnia in consumers of all ages. After the FDA banned ephedra, other supplements with questionable safety took its place. For example, supplements with bitter orange contain the compound syndephrine, which is chemically similar to ephedrine and affects blood pressure and heart rate in ways similar to ephedra.[50] Aristolochia fangchi, another herb used in weight loss pills, has been associated with kidney damage, renal failure, and kidney cancer.

Some diet supplements, such as cascara and aloe, act as strong stimulant laxatives, others, often derived from caffeine, act as diuretics. Juniper seeds, dandelion, equistine, horsetail, and shave grass are examples of these and have been linked to renal damage, brain damage, and convulsions. Other diet pills, such as glucomannan and guar gum, create a feeling of fullness because of their dietary fiber content and have been associated with gastrointestinal and esophageal obstructions.

There is also a danger in the potential interactions between prescription medications and herbal agents.

Most people are unaware of these and physicians may overlook them because 70 percent of patients do not disclose their use of herbal supplements to their physicians. Chromium, pyruvate, 5-hydroxytryptophan (5-HTP), chitosan, and carnitine are some common herbal supplements used for weight loss; however, there are hundreds of herbal supplements, and so it is impossible to list them all. It is important to look at the labels and read the ingredients in diet pills to see what you are really ingesting and to know how these herbs may affect your body. In addition, these dietary supplements have not been shown to be effective in helping to lose weight!

One particular over-the-counter weight loss medication containing **phenylpropanolamine (PPA)** merits mentioning, as drug companies making these products were asked to stop manufacturing it in 2000 because of PPA's association with an increased risk for stroke. The FDA issued a public health advisory telling consumers not to use any products containing PPA for this reason. PPA was also found in OTC cough and cold medications.

Prescription Weight Loss Drugs

Some prescription medications have also been shown to produce serious side effects. Two such medications, *phentermine* and *fenfluramine*, have been prescribed for patients who wanted to lose weight. Both drugs affect levels of serotonin, the neurotransmitter associated with satiety. This combination, referred to as *phenfen*, gradually raised concern among health experts because of the side effects it produced in people with angina, glaucoma, and high blood pressure. In addition, reports began to surface that some patients had developed a rare but lethal condition called *pulmonary hypertension*.

During the mid-1990s, a new serotonin-specific weight loss drug, *dexfenfluramine* (Redux), was approved for use in the United States. Some patients began to take dexfenfluramine with fenfluramine in an attempt to find a new combination that would be even more effective than phenfen or Redux used alone, and death resulted in some cases.

In September 1997, the FDA requested voluntary withdrawal of fenfluramine and dexfenfluramine from the market because of reports of heart valve damage in those using these drug combinations.[51] Manufacturers responded by ceasing all distribution of the drugs. In October 1999, a $4.8 billion class-action settlement was

---

Key Terms

phenylpropanolamine (PPA) (**fen** ill **pro** puh **nol** uh meen) The active chemical compound found in some over-the-counter diet products and associated with increased risk of stroke.

proposed, through which patients whose use of the drugs resulted in heart valve damage would receive monetary compensation and continuing medical care. Phentermine remains on the market and is used in combination with various antidepressants, such as Prozac, Zoloft, and Paxil. For those people whose use of the diet drug combinations led to heart valve damage, a study reported at the end of 1999 indicated that once medication use ceased, damage did not progress, and some indication of improvement was noted.[52]

At the same time of the initial concern over the use of phentermine and fenfluramine, the FDA approved yet another obesity drug, *sibutramine* (brand name Meridia), even though an advisory committee within the FDA recommended against approving it. Meridia acts on serotonin in the body similarly to how phenfen and Redux functioned and, like its predecessors, has been linked to heart attacks, high blood pressure, strokes, and death; however, it still remains on the market in the United States. Italy recently pulled Meridia from the market following reports of death linked to this drug.

Fat-Blocking Drugs   *Orlistat* (brand name Xenical) has also been used for weight loss. Unlike phentermine and sibutramine, which influence the neurotransmitter serotonin, orlistat reduces fat absorption in the small intestine by about 30 percent. The drug is intended for use among people who are 20 percent or more over their ideal weight. In persons who tolerate the drug's side effects, a 10 percent reduction of weight without significant dietary restriction is possible.

For the first time, the FDA has approved a prescription diet pill, Xenical (orlistat), as an OTC medication called Alli.[53] Costing about $50 for a two-month supply, Alli contains half the dosage of Xenical. Alli is not without its risks, as it has the same problematic side effects as Xenical, including sudden diarrhea, commonly referred to as "alli-oops" because of the lack of warning and soiled pants Alli users have reported experiencing. Some have intense stomach pain when taking this pill, and it has also been linked with precancerous lesions in the colon.[53]

Some concerns related to the use of orlistat include anal leakage, severe abdominal cramping, excessive flatulence, and inhibition of the absorption of vitamins and minerals in the body. Olestra has been used in fat-free chips such as "Wow!" potato chips and there have been complaints of stomach discomfort among people who ate them. In addition, people erroneously believe that they can eat as much as they want since it is fat-free, but it is not calorie-free and so they may end up gaining weight as a result.

Surgical Interventions

It used to be that surgical measures were undertaken only if the person's weight was severely endangering his or her

An over-the-counter version of the prescription drug orlistat (Xenical) was approved by the FDA in 2007.

health and other less invasive methods had been unsuccessful. Now surgeries such as liposuction, tummy tucks, gastric bypass surgery, and gastric band surgeries are becoming increasingly popular and commonplace, especially among teenagers. Gastric bypass surgery, vertical banded gastroplasty, and laparoscopic adjustable gastric banding all involve major surgery. They can also be very expensive, costing upward of $25,000, and some insurance companies will not pay for this, claiming it is cosmetic surgery even though there are significant medical risks associated with obesity. Even so, the number of obesity surgeries being performed has increased 600 percent over the past five years.[54] Although obesity surgeries are not approved for patients under age 18, in 2004 there were 350 of them performed on children as test cases. With the increase in obesity among children, along with improved surgical techniques, there has been a push for the FDA to approve these surgeries for children.

All three operations limit the amount of food a person can eat at one time, because overeating results in vomiting or severe diarrhea. Because the stomach is made smaller, individuals who have undergone these procedures must limit their food intake to half a cup to a cup of food at each "meal." However, it is possible to regain weight by eating small portions of high-calorie foods on a consistent basis. Individuals lose weight because this type of surgery limits the amount of food that can be digested, therefore decreasing the amount of calories that they can eat at one time.

Gastric Bypass Surgery   Gastric bypass is the most common type of weight loss surgery, and it has gained interest since celebrities such as singer Carnie Wilson, *American Idol* judge Randy Jackson, and weatherman Al Roker have gone public about their experiences with this surgery. It is a major operation and involves dividing the stomach into two compartments to create a pouch, the size of a thumb, for food to enter. The small intestine

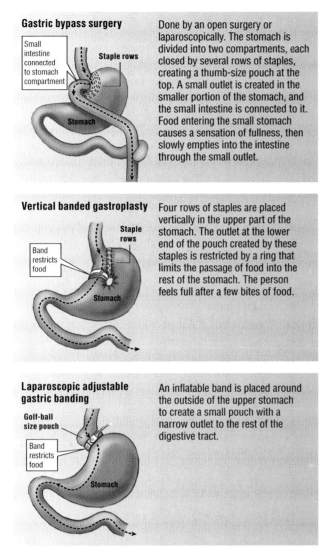

Gastric bypass surgery

Small intestine connected to stomach compartment

Staple rows

Stomach

Done by an open surgery or laparoscopically. The stomach is divided into two compartments, each closed by several rows of staples, creating a thumb-size pouch at the top. A small outlet is created in the smaller portion of the stomach, and the small intestine is connected to it. Food entering the small stomach causes a sensation of fullness, then slowly empties into the intestine through the small outlet.

Vertical banded gastroplasty

Staple rows

Band restricts food

Stomach

Four rows of staples are placed vertically in the upper part of the stomach. The outlet at the lower end of the pouch created by these staples is restricted by a ring that limits the passage of food into the rest of the stomach. The person feels full after a few bites of food.

Laparoscopic adjustable gastric banding

Golf-ball size pouch

Band restricts food

Stomach

An inflatable band is placed around the outside of the upper stomach to create a small pouch with a narrow outlet to the rest of the digestive tract.

Figure 6-3 Three Types of Obesity Surgery
Source: From *USA Today,* May 5, 2004. Reprinted with permission.

is cut below the stomach and connected to a smaller portion of the stomach, bypassing the larger stomach and a section of the intestine, which are no longer used (see Figure 6-3). According to the American Society for Bariatric Surgery, an average of 171,000 people each year now undergo gastric bypass surgeries (also referred to as *bariatric surgeries*), compared to just 16,800 people in 1993. The average cost per surgery is $26,000 to $35,000, and the average death rate is 1 in 200. Candidates for this surgery typically have a BMI above 40 or are 100 pounds or more (men) or at least 80 pounds (women) overweight. People with a BMI between 35 and 40 who suffer from type 2 diabetes or life-threatening cardiopulmonary problems may also be candidates for surgery.

Gastric bypass surgery tends to result in greater weight loss (93.3 pounds on average) than does gastroplasty (67 pounds on average) after one year. Over two years, gastric bypass surgery patients have been shown to lose two-thirds of excess weight. These surgeries are not without their risks: hernias, ulcers, liver damage, infection, internal leaks, and even death. These surgeries are not a cure-all for weight management; individuals who have these operations must continue to exercise regularly, take nutritional supplements, eat small portions very slowly, and decrease intake of high-sugar foods in order to maintain their weight loss.

Gastric Band Surgery There are two types of gastric band surgery: vertical banded gastroplasty and laparoscopic adjustable gastric banding. Vertical banded gastroplasty uses both a band and staples to create a small stomach pouch, limiting the passage of food into the rest of the stomach. This results in a feeling of fullness after only a few mouthfuls of food. This used to be the most common weight loss surgery, but it has decreased in popularity with the rise of gastric bypass surgery. Weight loss is not as rapid as with gastric bypass surgery. However, some insurance companies will pay for gastric band surgery because it costs half as much as gastric bypass. Laparoscopic adjustable gastric banding, a less invasive procedure, involves an inflatable band being placed around the upper end of the stomach, again creating a small pouch. A narrow passage is also made into the rest of the stomach. The band is inflated with a salt solution through a tube that connects the band to an access port positioned under the skin. In this way, the band can be tightened or loosened over time to change the size of the passageway into the stomach.

This procedure is reversible. It too can involve complications following surgery, such as band slippage, erosion and deflation, obstruction of the stomach, dilation of the esophagus, infection, nausea, stomach wall deterioration, ulcers, vomiting, heartburn, and difficulty swallowing.

Cosmetic Surgeries and Procedures Cosmetic surgeries have increased 38 percent since 2000, with over 10 million Americans undergoing these surgeries. Forty-four percent more men and forty-two percent more women had cosmetic surgery in 2005 as compared to 2000. Some call it "addictive," because once they have one procedure, they notice other parts of their bodies that they want to change. In her book *Beauty Junkies: Inside Our $15 Billion Obsession With Cosmetic Surgery*, Alex Kuczynski talks about her pursuit of perfection through plastic surgery. Some believe that changing their bodies will improve their body image and their overall satisfaction with their lives. With the convenience and ease of being able to do some of the more minor procedures over the lunch hour, some people now view cosmetic surgery as being similar to getting a haircut. The most common cosmetic surgeries are liposuction, breast augmentation, eyelid surgery, abdominoplasty (tummy tuck), and breast reduction (Table 6.5).

Table 6.5 Most Common Cosmetic Procedures Performed in 2006

Surgical Procedures

Liposuction	400,000
Breast augmentation	380,000
Eyelid surgery	210,000
Abdominoplasty ("tummy tuck")	170,000
Breast reduction	150,000

Nonsurgical Procedures

Botulinum toxin injections*	3,180,000
Hyaluronic acid injections*	1,590,000
Laser hair removal	1,480,000
Microdermabrasion*	990,000
Laser skin resurfacing*	580,000

*Injections of botulinum toxin or hyaluronic acids are designed to reduce facial lines; microdermabrasion and laser skin resurfacing remove layers of skin to reduce wrinkles, age spots, acne scars, and other skin conditions.

Source: Data from the American Society for Aesthetic Plastic Surgery, "Top Surgical and Non-surgical Cosmetic Procedures Among All Americans in 2006," www.surgery.org/public/consumer/trends/cosmetic_surgery_trends.

Liposuction and Abdominoplasty Liposuction is the most frequent cosmetic operation in the United States in which fat tissue is removed. Liposuction involves removing unwanted fat from specific areas, such as the abdomen, hips, buttocks, thighs, knees, upper arms, chin, cheeks, and neck. A small tube is inserted through the skin, and adipose tissue is vacuumed out. This is more of a sculpting or contouring operation than a weight loss surgery, because little weight is lost. Potential risks and outcomes include infection; the formation of fat clots or blood clots, which may travel to the lungs and cause death; excessive fluid loss, which can lead to shock or fluid accumulation that must be drained; friction burns or other damage to the skin or nerves; numbness; skin discoloration; irregular body contours; and sagging skin. Approximately 400,000 people undergo liposuction each year. The cost of liposuction ranges from $3,000 to $8,500, depending upon the part of the body receiving the surgery and the size of the patient.

People considering these procedures should carefully investigate all aspects, including the training and experience of the surgeon, to determine whether they are appropriate for them.

There exists a growing concern regarding the safety of liposuction based on a comparison of surgery-related deaths during liposuction and the death rates for all surgery, including trauma-based cases. In the case of all types of surgery, the mortality rate is reported to be between 1 death for every 100,000 cases and 1 death for every 300,000 surgical cases, whereas for liposuction the rate may be 20 to 60 times higher.[55] In spite of these figures, the Society of Plastic and Reconstructive

Surgeons believes the procedure is still acceptably safe, explaining that an office-based procedure often carries a higher mortality rate than do procedures conducted in hospitals.

Abdominoplasty, known more commonly as a tummy tuck, is a major surgical procedure to remove excess skin and fat from the middle and lower abdomen and to tighten the muscles of the abdominal wall. It leaves a permanent scar, which can extend from hip to hip. Infection and blood clots are some of the potential risks. A balanced diet and regular exercise are required to maintain the results from this surgery.

 TALKING POINT Do you think that having cosmetic surgery would bring you more happiness and improve the quality of your life?

Body Wrapping Although not a surgical procedure or weight loss technique, *body wrapping* is another form of body contouring. In this procedure, various areas of the body are tightly wrapped with 6-inch strips of material soaked in a solution of amino acids that are claimed to draw toxins out of the underlying tissue, shrink fatty deposits, diminish **cellulite,** lighten stretch marks, and eliminate inches of fat. Once the wrapping is removed, the newly contoured body area may remain this way for 4 to 10 weeks. Although the secret to the success of a particular spa's body wrapping approach is supposed to lie in its uniquely formulated soaking solution, the contouring effect probably results from dehydration of the underlying tissue and redistribution of extracellular fluids through pressure from the wrapping.

Regarding cellulite, note that no product or noninvasive procedure currently in the marketplace has been shown to be effective in removing or reducing this tissue. Thus, the dimpled appearance of the buttocks, back of the arm, and upper leg seems destined to remain, despite cosmetic companies' advertisements of lotions and creams that claim to eliminate cellulite.

Approaches for Weight Gain

For some, the lack of adequate body weight, called **underweight,** can be a serious concern. These people would likely fall into a BMI category of less than 18.5 and be 10–20 percent below normal on a standard height/weight table. One population that tends to struggle more with being too thin is the elderly. The CDC found that extreme thinness is associated with death in people over the age of 70. Also significant, unintentional weight loss has been associated with later development of Alzheimer's disease. A weight loss of 5 percent or more in a month is considered significant.

Nutritionists believe that the healthiest way to gain weight is to increase the intake of "calorie-dense" food (see the box "Weight Management Tips"). These foods are characterized by high fat density resulting from high levels of vegetable fats (polyunsaturated fats). Particularly good foods in this regard are dried fruits, bananas, nuts, granola, and cheeses made from low-fat milk. The current recommendation is to eat three calorie-dense meals of moderate size per day, interspersed with two or three substantial snacks. Using MyPyramid in Chapter 5, one should increase intake for each group.[56]

A second component of weight gain for those who are underweight is an exercise program that uses weight training activities intended to increase muscle mass. For all the reasons detailed in Chapter 4, the use of anabolic drugs in the absence of highly competent medical supervision has no role in healthful weight gain. In addition, carefully monitored aerobic activity should be undertaken in sessions adequate to maintain heart-lung health, while at the same time one should restrict unnecessary activity that expends calories.

For those who cannot gain weight in spite of having tried the preceding approaches, a medical evaluation could supply an explanation for being underweight. If no medical explanation can be found, the person must begin to accept the reality of his or her unique body type. Five percent of the population are naturally underweight. When individuals fall below 80 percent of their desirable weight on standard height/weight tables and have BMIs below 16, it is highly probable that they are not only underweight but, more important, undernourished. This condition suggests clinically significant dietary deficiencies in both the quantity and the quality of the food being consumed. Whether the undernourishment is associated with anorexia nervosa, other medical conditions characterized by weight loss (such as inflammatory bowel disease), or poverty or famine, affected people are in danger of death from starvation.

Key Terms

cellulite Tissue composed of fat cells intertwined around strands of fibrous connective tissue.

underweight A condition in which the body is below the desirable weight.

Eating Disorders

Given the pressure most people feel to maintain the cultural ideal of beauty, and being bombarded with images of very thin actresses models, and such as Portia de Rossi, Kate Bosworth, Mary-Kate Olsen, and Nicole Richie, it is no wonder that some people develop serious medical and psychological disorders associated with body image, weight, and food. It is also not surprising that many of the very models we are trying to emulate also have eating disorders, as they succumb to the pressure to be ever thinner. Anorexia nervosa, bulimia nervosa, binge eating, and disordered eating are frequently found in college populations. We have included these topics in the chapter on weight management because most eating disorders begin with dieting. However, most eating disorders also involve inappropriate food choices, as well as psychological issues. Those issues are discussed in Chapters 2 and 5.

A recent survey showed that dieting has become the norm for females starting at an early age. Fifty percent of 9-year-olds and 80 percent of 10-year-olds have reported dieting.[22] While eating disorders involve a preoccupation with food and weight, much deeper psychological issues underly these conditions.

In the United States, conservative estimates indicate that after puberty 5 to 10 million females and 1 million males struggle with eating disorders such as anorexia, bulimia, or binge eating disorder. It is estimated that approximately 8 percent of college women will develop an eating disorder, and the population most at risk for developing bulimia is college freshmen women. Ninety to ninety-five percent of people with eating disorders are women, although the prevalence of eating disorders in men is on the rise. Athletes such as dancers, gymnasts, swimmers, runners, and wrestlers are at risk for developing eating disorders because of the focus on weight and appearance for successful performance. In fact, any group in which success is influenced by weight or attractiveness is at risk for the development of an eating disorder, such as those involved in the performance arts, theatre, television, and modeling.

Anorexia Nervosa

Anorexia nervosa is an eating disorder in which a person denies his or her own feelings of hunger and avoids food, with marked weight loss occurring. Anorexics tend to run from food in the relentless pursuit of thinness, although they never perceive themselves as thin enough. To meet the diagnostic criteria for anorexia nervosa, the individual has an intense fear of gaining weight, even though he or she weighs less than 85 percent of the expected weight for his/her age, gender, and height, and, in females, menstruation ceases for at least three consecutive months.[57] In addition, people with anorexia perceive

Preoccupation with weight and shape, inappropriate dieting, and perfectionism are factors associated with the development of eating disorders.

themselves as overweight and much larger than they really are. Anorexics lose their ability to recognize when they are hungry and have difficulty eating even if they want to do so. Depression, irritability, withdrawal, perfectionism, and low self-esteem are some of the psychological problems associated with anorexia. In addition, anorexics tend to feel cold most of the time because they have very little body fat (2–10 percent) and also suffer from lightheadedness, dizziness, insomnia, hair loss, muscle cramps, stress fractures, fatigue, decreased memory and concentration, and gastrointestinal problems. More serious complications include heart and kidney failure, hypothermia, osteoporosis, infertility, and, in 25 percent of cases, death. See the box "Recognizing Anorexia Nervosa and Bulimia Nervosa" for more information.

As with other eating disorders, anorexia nervosa also involves a sense of feeling out of control in one's life and attempting to find control through food and weight loss. It is not a coincidence that anorexia nervosa typically begins around puberty: most individuals with anorexia have a fear of growing up and all that goes with being an adult, such as financial responsibility, sexual relationships, leaving one's family, and becoming more autonomous and independent.

Anorexia often begins with dieting but may also begin as a result of an illness such as the stomach flu, a relationship that breaks up, or after dental surgery, when it might be expected that one would temporarily eat less. However, anorexics will tell you that the disorder begins to take on a life of its own after what started as wanting

★ Recognizing Anorexia Nervosa and Bulimia Nervosa

The American Psychological Association uses the following diagnostic criteria to identify anorexia nervosa and bulimia nervosa.

Anorexia	Bulimia
• Body weight is 15 percent or more below desirable weight	• Binge eating two or more times a week for at least three months
• Fear of weight gain	• A lack of control over bingeing
• Distorted body image	• Engaging in inappropriate compensatory behavior purging two or more times a week for at least three months to prevent weight gain
• In women, the absence of three or more menstrual periods young girls may not start menstruating at the appropriate age); men, sex hormones decrease	• Overly concerned about body image

Characteristic symptoms include the following. Note that it is unlikely that all the symptoms will be evident in any one individual.

Anorexia	Bulimia
• Looks thin and keeps getting thinner	• Bathroom use immediately after eating
• Skips meals, cuts food into small pieces, moves food around plate to appear to have eaten	• Eating in secret
• Loss of menstrual periods and possible infertility	• Excessive time (and money) spent food shopping
• Wears baggy clothes in an attempt to disguise weight loss and to keep warm	• Shopping for food at several stores instead of one store
• Significant hair loss; lanugo (fine downy body hair)	• Menstrual irregularities and possible fertility problems
• Extreme sensitivity to cold	• Excessive constipation
• Dizziness, lightheadedness, headaches	• Swollen and/or infected salivary glands, sore throat
• Withdrawn, irritable, depressed	• Bursting blood vessels in the eyes
• Insomnia, fatigue, loss of energy	• Dental erosion in teeth and gums
• Decreased sex drive	• Dehydration and kidney dysfunction
• Dehydration, kidney dysfunction	• Significant hair loss; dry, brittle hair and nails
• Decreased concentration	• Increased acne and skin problems
• Heart irregularities, heart failure	• Heart irregularities, heart failure

to lose a few pounds turns into losing 15 percent or more of body weight and still not feeling satisfied with one's appearance. Friends and family might initially encourage the person on his or her weight loss and say complimentary things about his or her appearance but soon become concerned when the person's weight continues to dramatically decrease.

Anorexia has become more common as changing cultural ideals for beauty have changed. Our standards have gone from Marilyn Monroe who was a voluptuous 5 feet 5 inches and 140-pounds to Kate Moss who has been reported to be 5 feet 7 inches and 105 pounds.[9] Now the "lollipop look" is considered the "in look" in Hollywood, with actresses and models having stick-thin bodies, making their heads seem huge. More attention has been drawn to this disorder since Mary-Kate Olsen went public with her battle with anorexia in the summer of 2004. She is not alone; other stars have admitted to having anorexia—for example, Tracey Gold (*Growing Pains* sitcom), Spice Girl Victoria Beckham, singer Whitney Houston, and actresses Christina Ricci and Portia de Rossi. Because many of these stars are seen as the

> **Key Terms**
>
> **anorexia nervosa** An eating disorder in which the individual weighs less than 85 percent of the expected weight for his or her age, gender, and height; has an intense fear of gaining weight; and, in females, ceases to menstruate for at least 3 consecutive months. People with anorexia perceive themselves as overweight, even though they are underweight.

standard for the American body ideal, they may be inadvertently increasing the number of women with eating disorders.

Recently researchers have found a significant difference in the brain chemistry of anorexics, compared to those who don't have this disorder. Anorexics have a higher level of serotonin activity in their brains, which is believed to be linked to feelings of anxiety and obsessional thinking. It is further believed that starvation may act to decrease the amount of serotonin in the brain, creating a sense of calm for anorexics. Further research is being done to investigate this biochemical link to anorexia, which will have implications for treatment and recovery.

Denial of problems plays a major role in eating disorders in that the individual refuses to acknowledge that there is anything wrong, even though she is becoming thinner and wasting away, and family and friends are expressing great concern. Anorexia nervosa is considered a serious medical and psychological disorder; however, some anorexics argue that "Anorexia is a lifestyle not a disorder." Heated debates and discussions often occur on pro-anorexia websites. With names like "Thinspiration," "Stick Figures," and "Anorexic and Proud," these pro-anorexia forums have become very popular and deadly in the past few years. These websites show computer-enhanced pictures of models and actresses such as Calista Flockhart and Lara Flynn Boyle making them appear thinner and more skeletal than they really are.[58] Messages on these websites include tips on how to starve, how to purge, and ways of hiding one's disorder, as well as encouragement to lose more weight. There has been a push among health providers, educators, and health organizations to eliminate these types of websites, and they have been somewhat successful. However, these sites still do exist, although somewhat disguised and underground.[59]

Three groups that have traditionally been overlooked in the incidence of anorexia are women of color, female athletes (see the Female Athlete Triad in Chapter 4), and men. The research shows a significant increase in the incidence of anorexia among these three groups. More focus has been given to anorexia among women of color, and it has been proposed that this group might be more vulnerable to developing eating disorders than Caucasian women are because of ethnocultural identity issues. It has been suggested that the more pressure women of color feel to fit into the dominant culture's standards of beauty and thinness, the more likely they are to develop eating disorders.

Often female athletes are not diagnosed with eating disorders because the symptoms of anorexia—absence of menses, low body fat and weight, and osteoporosis—are referred to as the female athlete triad and are not uncommon among athletes, and so they don't necessarily signify the presence of an eating disorder.

The incidence of anorexia nervosa (as well as bulimia nervosa, which we'll cover later) has traditionally been much lower in men than in women. Today, however, the incidence of both conditions is increasing in men as they begin to feel some of the same pressures that women feel to conform to the weight and body composition standards imposed by others. The "lean look" of young male models serves as a standard for more and more young men, whereas the requirements to "make weight" for various sports drives others. Runners, jockeys, swimmers, and gymnasts frequently must lose weight quickly to meet particular standards for competition or the expectations of coaches and trainers. Researchers report that men are less inclined than women are to admit that they may have an eating disorder, thinking it is a "woman's illness." Thus they are less likely to seek treatment. In addition, physicians tend not to suspect men of having eating disorders, and so they go untreated.

Fortunately, psychological treatment in combination with medical and dietary interventions can return the person with anorexia nervosa to a more life-sustaining pattern of eating. The person with anorexia needs to receive the care of professionals experienced in the treatment of this disorder. It is not uncommon for this treatment to take three to five years. If others, including friends, coworkers, roommates, and parents, observe this condition, they should consult a health care provider for assistance.

 TALKING POINTS What would you do if you suspected that a friend of yours had an eating disorder? Would you share your concern with him or her? If so, what would you say?

Bulimia Nervosa

Whereas anorexics are underweight, people with **bulimia nervosa** often are of a normal weight. These individuals use food and weight as a way of coping with stress, boredom, conflict in relationships, and low self-esteem. It is not uncommon in our society to comfort ourselves with food, to have social activities based on food, and to eat as a way of procrastinating a dreaded activity. However, people with bulimia take this to the extreme, engaging in recurrent bingeing, consuming unusually large amounts of food, and feeling out of control with their eating.[57]

While anorexics run away from food, bulimics run to food to cope with their emotions, problems, and stress. Because they feel so guilty, ashamed, and anxious about the food they have consumed, people with bulimia **purge** by self-induced vomiting, taking an excessive number of laxatives and diuretics, or excessively exercising or fasting. There is a strong preoccupation with weight, calories, and food among sufferers of bulimia. Most people with bulimia constantly count calories, weigh themselves throughout the day, and frequently make negative statements concerning different parts of their bodies, primarily focusing on the thighs, stomach, and waist. As with

Resources for Anorexia and Bulimia Treatment

Local Resources

- College or university counseling and health centers
- Comprehensive mental health centers
- Crisis intervention centers
- Mental health associations

Organizations and Self-Help Groups

National Association of Anorexia Nervosa and Associated Disorders (ANAD)
Hotline: 847-831-3438
www.anad.org

American Psychological Association (APA) HelpCenter
www.helping.apa.org

Academy for Eating Disorders (AED)
847-498-4274
www.aedweb.org/index.cfm

Anorexia Nervosa and Related Eating Disorders, Inc. (ANRED)
541-344-1144
www.anred.com

National Eating Disorder Association
206-382-3587
www.NationalEatingDisorders.org

Bulimia Anorexia Nervosa Association (BANA)
519-969-2112
www.bana.ca

Laureate Eating Disorders Program
800-322-5173
www.eatingdisorders.laureate.com

---

anorexia, bulimia is associated with depression, isolation, anxiety, perfectionism, and low self-esteem. Dental erosion, hair loss, esophageal lesions, blood in the vomit and stools, loss of voluntary gag reflex, kidney damage, heart failure, gastrointestinal problems, ketosis, edema, infertility, parotid gland swelling, depression, and insomnia are just some of the medical problems associated with bulimia nervosa.

The publicity surrounding Terri Schiavo's death highlights the lethality of this disorder—she entered a persistent vegetative state following a heart attack possibly caused by bulimia. She had developed a potassium deficiency that was reportedly caused by bulimia nervosa. Many public figures have acknowledged struggling with this disorder, including Jane Fonda, Paula Abdul, Katharine McPhee (*American Idol*), Felicity Huffman (*Desperate Housewives*), Joan Rivers, and the late Princess Diana. All these individuals have talked about the pressures to be thin in order to be successful in their careers and how they succumbed to this pressure by developing an eating disorder.

Bulimia often begins around 17 to 18 years of age when young adults are separating from their families and are forging lives of their own; some conflict arises around issues of independence, autonomy, and relationships with family. There is a higher incidence of bulimia than anorexia, although some bulimics may have had anorexia in the past. There is also a higher rate of bulimia among female college students as compared to their peers who are not attending college. Treatment for bulimia nervosa involves nutritional counseling, psychological counseling, and consultation with a physician. Often people with bulimia recover from this disorder within a year of beginning treatment. See the box "Resources for Anorexia and Bulimia Treatment" for sources of help for eating disorders.

Binge Eating Disorder

Binge eating disorder is the newest term for what was previously referred to as compulsive overeating. It is also the most common of all of the eating disorders, affecting 3.5 percent of women and 2 percent of men. It is also strongly linked to obesity. Binge eaters use food to cope in the same way that bulimics do and also feel out of control and unable to stop eating during binges. People with this disorder report eating rapidly and in secret or may snack all day. They tend to eat until they feel uncomfortably full, sometimes hoarding food and eating when they aren't physically hungry.[57] Like people with bulimia, they feel guilty and ashamed of their eating habits and have a great deal of self-loathing and body hatred. People who have binge eating disorder do not engage in purging behavior, which differentiates them from people with bulimia nervosa. Typically, binge eaters have a long history

Key Terms

bulimia nervosa An eating disorder in which individuals engage in episodes of bingeing, consuming unusually large amounts of food and feeling out of control, and then engaging in some compensatory purging behavior to eliminate the food.

purging Using vomiting, laxatives, diuretics, enemas, or other medications, or means such as excessive exercise or fasting, to eliminate food.

binge eating disorder An eating disorder formerly referred to as compulsive overeating disorder; binge eaters use food to cope in the same way that bulimics do and also feel out of control, but do not engage in compensatory purging behavior.

of diet failures, feel anxious, are socially withdrawn from others, and are overweight. Heart problems, high blood pressure, joint problems, abnormal blood sugar levels, fatigue, depression, and anxiety are associated with binge eating. The treatment of this eating disorder involves interventions similar to those described for treating bulimia nervosa.

Chewing and Spitting Out Food Syndrome

Chewing and spitting out food without swallowing it has also been used as a method for weight loss or weight management. This is a common eating disorder and falls within the "Eating Disorder Not Otherwise Specified" diagnosis. It differs from bulimia nervosa, and researchers contend that chewing and spitting out food without swallowing may indicate a more severe eating disorder.[60]

Night Eating Syndrome

Night eating syndrome has not yet been formally defined as an eating disorder. The signs and symptoms of this syndrome include eating more than half of one's daily food intake after dinner and before breakfast; feeling tense, anxious, and guilty while eating; difficulty falling or staying asleep at night; and having little to no appetite in the morning. Unlike binge eating, night eating involves eating throughout the evening hours rather than in short episodes. There is a strong preference for carbohydrates among night eaters. Some researchers speculate that night eating may be an unconscious attempt to self-medicate mood problems, because eating carbohydrates can trigger the brain to produce so-called "feel good" neurochemicals. About 60 percent of women and 40 percent of men suffer from night eating syndrome. It is also related to obesity. Research is underway in examining the underlying causes of this syndrome and developing subsequent treatment interventions. It seems likely that a combination of biological, genetic, and psychological factors contribute to this problem.

Body Dysmorphic Disorder

Body dysmorphic disorder (BDD) is a secret preoccupation with an imagined or slight flaw in one's appearance. Sometimes, people become almost completely fixated on concerns regarding body image, leading to repeatedly weighing themselves and checking mirrors throughout the day, compulsively dieting, exercising, and undergoing cosmetic surgery.[61] Perceptions of an imperfect body may lead to psychological dysfunction, such as not wanting to leave the house because of imagined defects. People with this disorder are 45 times more likely to commit suicide than the general population, demonstrating how their self-loathing can take a devastating toll on them.

Bigorexia

Bigorexia has been characterized as a "reverse anorexia nervosa" in which people want to be more muscular but see themselves as puny and scrawny.[5] Some say a better term for this would be "muscle dysmorphia" because they can never be muscular enough to satisfy their self-esteem. It has also been referred to as the "Adonis complex," but women also suffer from this disorder, though not as frequently as men. Many people take anabolic steroids (see Chapter 4) or diet supplements to get bigger and more buff. People with this preoccupation obsessively lift weights for hours each day, sometimes sacrificing important social relationships, jobs, or physical health. They can also become preoccupied with decreasing fat as they increase muscle and may develop eating disorders. Similar to people with anorexia, they tend to wear bigger clothes to hide their bodies, tend not to be seen in public, and avoid social situations because they see themselves in a distorted, negative way.

Treating Eating Disorders

The treatment for eating disorders is multimodal and multidimensional involving nutritionists, psychologists, physicians, family, and friends. There are different treatment modalities, such as individual, group, and family counseling. Sometimes treatment requires inpatient hospitalization to medically stabilize the individual. In extreme cases, a feeding tube may be inserted to treat starvation, especially if the person refuses to eat. Behavioral modification and cognitive therapy are utilized in counseling people with eating problems. Medications such as antidepressants are often used to decrease obsessive-compulsive behavior, reduce anxiety, alleviate depression, and improve mood. Some medications can stimulate or reduce appetite as well. There is some debate over the efficacy of using an addictions model, similar to the 12-step Alcoholics Anonymous philosophy, with eating disorders. Overeaters Anonymous utilizes this model in helping people with eating problems, and many hospital programs employ this model in their treatment programs. While there seems to be some overlap of eating disorders with substance abuse problems, such as denial of problems, feeling out of control of one's behavior, and

---

Key Terms

body dysmorphic disorder (BDD) A secret preoccupation with an imagined or slight flaw in one's appearance.

bigorexia An obsession with getting bigger and more muscular, and thinking that your body is never muscular enough.

using food or drugs or alcohol to cope with problems, this is where the similarities end—obviously one needs food to live, which is not the case with drugs and alcohol.

A Final Thought about Health and Weight Management

Recognizing the attention placed on physical attractiveness and its relationship to thinness, ask yourself if you are healthy enough to accept your unique body even if it does not match the cultural ideal. As you recall from Chapter 1, it is important to develop every dimension of health, not simply the physical dimension. We hope that focusing on all dimensions of health, including the psychological aspects outlined in Chapter 2, will balance the pressure most of us feel to strive for a body image that is unrealistic and obtainable by only a few.

Taking Charge of Your Health

- Investigate the resources available on your campus that you could use to determine your healthy weight and body composition profile.

- Evaluate your eating behaviors to find out if you are using food to cope with stress. If you are, develop a plan to use nonfood options, such as exercise or interaction with friends or family members, to deal with stress.

- Formulate a realistic set of goals for changing your weight and body composition in a time frame that allows you to do so in a healthful way.

- Establish a daily schedule that lets you make any necessary dietary and physical activity adjustments.

- Keep a daily journal of your weight-management efforts.

- Monitor your progress toward meeting your weight-management goals.

- Design a reward system for reaching each goal.

- Learn to accept your body including the imperfections.

- Focus on other aspects of yourself that you like that are not related to appearance.

SUMMARY

- Weight management has become an obsession in American culture as well as a significant health problem; an estimated 66 percent of U.S. adults are either overweight or obese.

- Doctors usually define "overweight" as a condition in which a person's weight is 1 to 19 percent higher than "normal," as defined by a standard height/weight chart. Obesity is usually defined as a condition in which a person's weight is 20 percent or more above normal weight. "Morbid obesity" refers to being 50 to 100 percent over normal weight, more than 100 pounds over normal weight, or sufficiently overweight to interfere with health or normal functioning.

- Some of the methods for assessing one's weight are: body mass index, current height/weight tables, waist to hip ratios, electrical impedance, the Bod Pod, skinfold measurements, hydrostatic weighing, and home scales.

- Basal metabolic rate (BMR) is a measure of resting energy expenditure that is taken upon awakening, 10–12 hours after eating, or 12–18 hours after significant physical activity.

- Four factors seem to play a significant role in the prevalence of obesity: sex, age, socioeconomic status, and race.

- Weight loss occurs when the calories consumed are fewer than the energy the body needs for physiological maintenance and activity.

- The primary types of weight-management technique include dietary alterations, surgical interventions, medications, weight loss programs, and physical activity.

- A commitment to a lifestyle change of eating in healthy ways and engaging in regular aerobic exercise seem to be the most effective strategy for weight loss and weight maintenance.

- Anorexia nervosa is a psychological condition in which the individual weighs less than 85 percent of his or her expected weight for his or her age, gender, and height.

- People with bulimia nervosa use food and weight as a way of coping with stress, boredom, conflict in relationships, and low self-esteem. They engage in recurrent bingeing and purging to eliminate the food from their bodies.

- Binge eaters use food to cope in the same way that bulimics do and also feel out of control and unable to stop eating during binges, but they do not engage in purging behaviors.

REVIEW QUESTIONS

1. What percentage of U.S. adults are either overweight or obese?
2. How has the average caloric intake and physical activity level for Americans changed over the past two decades?
3. Define *overweight, obesity,* and *morbid obesity.*
4. List at least four of the methods used for assessing weight.
5. Define Basal Metabolic Rate (BMR).
6. What are four factors that seem to play a significant role in the prevalence of obesity?
7. Give four examples of how environmental factors can influence the amount the average person consumes.
8. Give examples of four different types of weight-management techniques.
9. What is the most effective strategy for weight loss and weight maintenance?
10. Describe the symptoms of anorexia nervosa, bulimia nervosa, and binge eating disorder.

ANSWERS TO THE "WHAT DO YOU KNOW?" QUIZ

1. True   2. True   3. False   4. False   5. False   6. False   7. True

As We Go to Press

A Vaccine for Obesity?

Currently, there is an experimental study being conducted with overweight and obese people that involves injecting a natural hormone into their gut for weight loss. The hormone, oxyntomodulin, was given 30 minutes prior to each meal, three times a day, and the experimental group lost an average of five pounds a month. This hormone is purported to promote a feeling of fullness, and so people feel full but are eating less than they typically would.

Something else that may be coming in the near future to the weight loss industry is an anti-obesity vaccine that targets the hormone ghrelin. Ghrelin regulates the body's energy balance and has an effect on appetite, weight gain, and energy expediture. The vaccine blocks the binding of ghrelin, keeping more ghrelin circulating in the blood and less in the brain and CNS. This is purported to increase energy expenditures and decrease the amount of fat that is stored. Currently, research is being conducted in mice using this anti-obesity vaccine with promising results. Perhaps, in the near future, people will have an opportunity to be vaccinated against obesity. Would you line up for this type of shot?

Sources: "Anti-Obesity Vaccine Comes Closer to Reality," *USA Today,* August 1, 2006; "Hormone Injection May Trigger Weight Loss," WebMD Medical News, August 26, 2005.

ENDNOTES

1. National Research Council. *Healthy People 2010.* www.healthypeople.com.
2. National Center for Chronic Disease Prevention and Health Promotion. *Defining Overweight and Obesity.* October 2006.
3. National Center for Health Statistics, Centers for Disease Control and Prevention. *Obesity Still a Major Problem, New Data Show.* October 6, 2004.
4. *USDA Revamps Food Pyramid to Unveil New Symbol.* www.usda.gov .April 18, 2005.
5. Brownell KD, Fairburn CG. *Eating Disorders and Obesity: A Comprehensive Handbook.* New York: Guilford Press, 1995.
6. Pope M, Phillips K, Olivardia T. *The Adonis Complex.* New York: Simon & Schuster, 2000.
7. National Institutes of Health. Clinical guidelines on the identification, evaluation, and treatment of overweight and obesity in adults. As reported in *First Federal Obesity Clinical Guidelines* (NIH News Advisory). June 17, 1998.
8. American Heart Association. *Heart and Stroke Facts.* 2003.
9. Poulton T. *No Fat Chicks.* Secaucus, NJ: Carol Publishing Group, 1997.
10. Anderson A. *Males with Eating Disorders.* Philadelphia: Brunner/Mazel, 1990.
11. Anderson A, Cohn L, Holbrook T. *Making Weight: Men's Conflicts with Food, Weight, Shape, and Appearance.* Carlsbad, CA: Gurze Books, 2000.
12. Cash T, Henry P. Women's body images: The results of a national survey in the U.S.A. *Sex Roles Res* 33 (1): 19–29. 1995.
13. Gaesser G. *Big Fat Lies.* Carlsbad, CA: Gurze Books, 2002.
14. U.S. Department of Agriculture/U.S. Department of Health and Human Services. Nutrition and your health: Dietary guidelines for Americans. *Home and Garden Bulletin* 232. 2000.
15. Waist management: Gauging your risks. *Consumer Reports,* p. 48. August 2003.
16. Thelen MH, Powell AL, Lawrence C, Kuhnent ME. Eating and body image concerns among children. *Journal of Consulting and Clinical Psychology* 21: 41, 46. 1992
17. Lindzey G, Thompson R, Spring B. *Psychology* (3rd ed.). New York: Worth, 1988.
18. International Health Racquet and Sportsclub Association. BOD POD body composition system to descend on San Francisco's IHRSA convention. As reported in the 29th Anniversary Exhibition in San Francisco's Moscone Convention Center, March 22–24, 2001.
19. Dempster P, Aitkens S. A new air displacement method for the determination of human body composition. *Med Sci Sports Exer* 27 (2): 1692–97. 1995.
20. U.S. Department of Health and Human Services. *The Surgeon General's Call to Action to Prevent and Decrease Overweight and Obesity.* Rockville, MD: USDHHS, Public Health Service, Office of the Surgeon General. 2001. www.surgeongeneral.gov/topics/obesity/calltoaction/CalltoAction.pdf.

21. Sobal J. Obesity and socioeconomic status: A framework for examining relationships between physical and social variables. *Med Anthro* 13: 231–247. 1991.

22. Harvard Women's Health Watch: Panel issues new guidelines for healthy eating. *Harvard Medical School* 10 (3). November 2002.

23. Kirby J. *Dieting for Dummies.* New York: Wiley, 1998.

24. *Dietary Guidelines for Americans,* www.health.gov/dietaryguidelines. 2005.

25. Insel P, Turner RE, Ross D. *Nutrition* (4th ed.). Sudbury, MA: Jones & Bartlett, 2002.

26. Wardlaw GM. *Perspectives in Nutrition* (4th ed.). New York: McGraw-Hill, 1999.

27. Halaas J et al. Weight-reducing effects on the plasma protein encoded by the obese gene. *Science* 269 (5223): 543–546. 1995.

28. Folsom AR et al. Serum leptin and weight gain over eight years in African American and Caucasian young adults. *Obesity Research* 7 (1): 1–8. 1999.

29. Sakurai T et al. Orexins and orexin receptors: A family of hypothalamic neuropeptides and G protein-coupled receptors that regulate feeding behavior. *Cell* 92 (4): 573–585. 1998.

30. Pettigrew R, Hamilton FD. Obesity and female reproductive function. *Brit Med Bull* 53:2, 341–358. 1997.

31. La Leche League International. *The Womanly Art of Breast-Feeding.* 1997.

32. Dell S, To T. Breastfeeding and asthma in young children. *Arch Ped Adol Med* 155:1261–65. 2001.

33. Hediger ML, et al. Association between infant breast-feeding and overweight in young children. *JAMA* 285 (19): 2453–60. 2001.

34. Gillman MW, et al. Risk of overweight among adolescents who were breastfed as infants. *JAMA* 285 (19): 2461–67. 2001.

35. Set point: What your body is trying to tell you. *National Eating Disorders Information Centre Bulletin* 7 (2). June 1992.

36. Stettler N, Zemel BS, Kumaniyika S, Stallings VA. Infant weight gain and childhood overweight status in a multicenter, cohort study. *Pediatrics* 109 (2): 194–99. February 2002.

37. The truth about dieting. *Consumer Reports.* June 26–31, 2002.

38. Saladin KS. *Anatomy and Physiology: The Unity of Form and Function.* Dubuque, IA: William C. Brown/McGraw-Hill, 1998.

39. Statistics related to overweight and obesity. National Institutes of Health, August 2005.

40. Sorbara M, Geliebter A. Body image disturbance in obese outpatients before and after weight loss in relation to race, gender and age of onset of diabetes. *Int J Eating Disorders* (May 2002): 416–23.

41. Sobal J, Stunkard AJ. Socioeconomic status and obesity: A review of the literature. *Psych Bull* 105: 260–75. 1989.

42. Stunkard AJ, Wadden TA. *Obesity: Theory and Therapy.* New York: Raven Press, 1993.

43. Sobal J, Rauschenbach B, Frongillo E. Marital status, fatness and obesity. *Social Science and Medicine* 35: 915–23. 1992.

44. Weight Watchers. *Stop Stuffing Yourself: Seven Steps to Conquering Overeating.* New York: Wiley, 1988.

45. Study: People taking eating clues from portion size. *The Star Press,* July 31, 2006.

46. Obesity in America: The gorge yourself movement. *New York Times,* August 19, 2003.

47. Sleep loss may equal weight gain. *USA Today,* December 7, 2004.

48. One more reason to get enough sleep. *Harvard Women's Health Watch,* May 2005.

49. Ephedra ban puts herb industry on notice. *New York Times,* December 31, 2003.

50. Ephedra-free doesn't mean risk-free. WebMD Health, September 9, 2005.

51. Center for Drug Evaluation and Research, FDA. FDA announces withdrawal of fenfluramine and dexfenfluramine. News Release no. 97–32. September 15, 1997.

52. Hensrud DD et al. Echocardiographic improvement over time after cessation of use of fenfluramine and phentermine. *May Clin Pro 74* (12): 1191–97. 1999.

53. Taking the diet pill . . . Alli. *People,* July 9, 2007.

54. Obesity surgery increases 600 percent. ABC News. May 31, 2006.

55. Grazer FM, de Jong RH. Fatal outcomes from liposuction: Census survey of cosmetic surgeons. *Plastic Reconstructive Surgery* 105 (1): 436–46. 2000.

56. American Dietetic Association. Gaining weight: A healthy plan for adding pounds. *Hot Topics,* www.eatright.org/nfs10html. 1998.

57. *Diagnostic and Statistical Manual of Mental Disorders IV-TR* Washington, DC: American Psychiatric Association. 2000.

58. Gotthelf M. The new anorexia outrage. *Self Magazine,* August 2001, 82–84.

59. Lilenfeld L. Academy members debate over pro-anorexia websites. *Academy of Eating Disorders Newsletter,* June 2001.

60. Update: Chewing and spitting out food. *Eating Disorders Review,* July/August 2002.

61. A dangerous duo: Body dysmorphic disorder with anorexia nervosa. *Eating Disorders Review,* November/December 2002, 4–5.

Personal Assessment

Do you eat mindlessly or mindfully?

Below is a collection of statements about your everyday experiences. Using the 1–6 scale, indicate how frequently or infrequently you currently have each experience. Answer according to what really reflects your experience rather than what you think your experience should be. Treat each item separately from every other item.

1	2	3	4	5	6
Almost always	Very frequently	Somewhat frequently	Somewhat infrequently	Very infrequently	Almost never

1. I could be experiencing some emotion and not be conscious of it until sometime later. 1 2 3 4 5 6
2. I break or spill things because of carelessness, not paying attention, or thinking of something else. 1 2 3 4 5 6
3. I find it difficult to stay focused on what's happening in the present. 1 2 3 4 5 6
4. I tend to walk quickly to get where I'm going without paying attention to what I experience along the way. 1 2 3 4 5 6
5. I tend not to notice feelings of physical tension or discomfort until they really grab my attention. 1 2 3 4 5 6
6. I forget a person's name almost as soon as I've been told it for the first time. 1 2 3 4 5 6
7. It seems I am "running on automatic," without much awareness of what I'm doing. 1 2 3 4 5 6
8. I rush through activities without being really attentive to them. 1 2 3 4 5 6
9. I get so focused on the goal I want to achieve that I lose touch with what I'm doing right now to get there. 1 2 3 4 5 6
10. I do jobs or tasks automatically, without being aware of what I'm doing. 1 2 3 4 5 6
11. I find myself listening to someone with one ear, doing something else at the same time. 1 2 3 4 5 6
12. I drive places on "automatic pilot" and then wonder why I went there. 1 2 3 4 5 6
13. I find myself preoccupied with the future or the past. 1 2 3 4 5 6
14. I find myself doing things without paying attention. 1 2 3 4 5 6
15. I snack without being aware that I'm eating. 1 2 3 4 5 6

Interpretation

To get score your, add up the numbers you circled for the 15 items and divide the total by 15. (This gives you the mean.) The higher your mean score, the higher your level of mindfulness.

TO CARRY THIS FURTHER . . .

If you scored low on this assessment, try some of the suggestions in the box "Learning to Eat Mindfully" to become a more mindful eater.

Source: From K. W. Brown and R. M. Ryan. "The Benefits of Being Present: The Role of Mindfulness in Psychological Well-Being," *Journal of Personality and Social Psychology*, 84, 822–848. Copyright © 2003 by the American Psychological Association. Adapted with permission.

Personal Assessment

Body love or body hate?

When you catch a glimpse of yourself in a mirror, do you smile at what you see or grimace? The following quiz will help you to assess your body self-esteem associated with your appearance. Please answer using the following rating scale:

1 = Rarely or never

2 = Sometimes

3 = Almost always or always

Add up your scores to determine your total score, and look at the interpretation of your scores.

_____ 1. I worry about my weight and weighing "too much."

_____ 2. I prefer to eat by myself and not with other people.

_____ 3. My mood is determined by the scale and how I feel about my appearance.

_____ 4. I make negative comments about my appearance to myself and others.

_____ 5. I think I look less attractive on days that I haven't exercised.

_____ 6. I have a difficult time accepting compliments about my appearance from others.

_____ 7. I compare myself to other women and find myself lacking.

_____ 8. I ask other people how I look.

_____ 9. I avoid social situations, activities, and events involving food.

_____10. I feel more anxious about my body in the summertime because of the need to wear bathing suits and clothing suitable for warmer temperatures.

_____ **TOTAL POINTS**

Interpretation

If you scored between 10 and 15, you have positive body self-esteem and are accepting of yourself and your appearance.

If you scored between 16 and 23, you scored in the average range.

If your score was between 24 and 30, you have poor or low body self-esteem.

TO CARRY THIS FURTHER . . .

If you scored in the average range: While you are in good company, feeling about your body the way most people do, you may want to reframe your body image and develop more of an appreciation for your body and appearance.

If you have poor body self-image: Your self-esteem in general is probably driven by how you see yourself, and you may be putting too much emphasis on your appearance and are too self-critical. You may feel as though you never are thin enough or look good enough and can always find a flaw when looking in the mirror. To improve your body self-esteem, focus on other aspects of yourself, focus on the positive aspects of your body, and be more accepting of yourself and less perfectionistic.

Preventing Drug Abuse and Dependence

Health educators have no doubt that the use, misuse, and abuse of many drugs can impair health. These substances not only alter the functioning of the body and mind but also affect the other dimensions of health. In Part Three, we take a look at addictive substances and their effects on the user.

1. **Physical Dimension**
   The effects of substance use, especially the long-term use of tobacco and alcohol, are well understood. These substances cause illness and death. Alcohol abuse can destroy the structure and function of many body systems. Tobacco use damages the cardiovascular system and the tissues of the respiratory tract and can cause cancer in many sites throughout the body. Chronic abuse of psychoactive drugs impairs many central nervous system functions. Even the experimental use of these drugs carries the danger of toxic overdose.

2. **Emotional Dimension**
   Because psychoactive drugs alter nervous system functioning, many users experience depression and mood swings. Some people use drugs to avoid emotional expression or to numb their feelings. When psychological dependence combines with physical dependence, the addict may begin to lose touch with reality.

3. **Social Dimension**
   Psychoactive drug use often takes place in social settings. For some people, drinking or using other drugs is perceived as a necessary first step toward enjoying the company of others. However, most people have little tolerance for inappropriate substance use, such as use of illegal drugs, excessive alcohol intake, and smoking in public places where tobacco use is banned.

4. **Intellectual Dimension**
   Intellectual impairment is one consequence of chemical abuse. People cannot perform well intellectually when they are feeling high or low or when their senses are dulled. Some people prefer to disregard information about the dangers of substance abuse, a choice that could prove extremely harmful to their health.

5. **Spiritual Dimension**
   Although drug use has long played a role in the religious practices of people throughout the world, the nonceremonial use of drugs conflicts with the principles of service to others. Substance abuse can hinder spiritual growth by turning a person's focus inward, making it impossible to develop the other-directedness that is essential to a rich spiritual life.

6. **Occupational Dimension**
   Use of both legal and illegal drugs clearly stands in the way of occupational health. Most workplaces are smoke-free, forcing smokers to stand outside or walk to the smoker's lounge to have a cigarette. These continual interruptions lower a worker's productivity. Illegal drug use can keep a job candidate from being hired and can result in being fired. And use of illegal drugs or alcohol on the job can be dangerous and will certainly lower a worker's level of performance.

part three

Making Decisions about Drug Use

What Do You Know about Drug Use?

◉ Intravenous drug injection is the most efficient and fastest way to administer a drug. True or False?

◉ Socioeconomic status is not predictive of drug use. True or False?

◉ Drug use is highest for 18- to 25-year-olds, compared to any other age group. True or False?

◉ The use of all drugs has been increasing over the years. True or False?

◉ Marijuana can be legally used for medical reasons in some states. True or False?

◉ Energy drinks such as Red Bull can have dangerous effects on the heart. True or False?

◉ Self-help groups are the most popular type of drug treatment. True or False?

Check your answers at the end of the chapter.

What does the word **drug** mean? Each of us may have different ideas about what a drug is. Although a number of definitions are available, we consider a drug to be "any substance, natural or artificial, other than food, that by its chemical or physical nature alters structure or function in the living organism."[1] Included in this broad definition is a variety of psychoactive drugs, medicines, and substances that many people do not usually consider to be drugs.

Psychoactive drugs alter the user's feelings, behavior, perceptions, or moods when using stimulants, depressants, hallucinogens, opiates, or inhalants. Prescribed medications function to heal unhealthy tissue as well as ease pain, prevent illness, and diagnose health conditions. Although some psychoactive drugs are used for medical reasons, as in the case of tranquilizers and some narcotics, the most commonly prescribed medicines are antibiotics, hormone replacement drugs, sulfa drugs, diuretics, oral contraceptives, and cardiovascular drugs. Legal substances not usually considered to be drugs (which certainly are drugs) include caffeine, tobacco, alcohol, aspirin, and other over-the-counter (OTC) drugs. These common substances are used so frequently in our society that they are rarely perceived as true drugs.

Does "Just Say No" Really Make a Difference?

"Just Say No." "This is your brain [picture of an egg]. This is your brain on drugs [picture of fried eggs]. Any questions?" Public service announcements (PSAs) have been used to prevent drug abuse since World War II. A PSA is "any announcement (including network) for which no charge is made and which promotes programs, activities, or services of federal, state, or local governments (e.g., recruiting, sale of bonds, etc.) or the programs, activities, or services of nonprofit organizations (e.g., United Way, Red Cross blood donations, etc.) and other announcements regarded as serving community interests, excluding time signals, routine weather announcements, and promotional announcements."[†] But how effective are they?

Research suggests that some PSAs have a positive effect, some have no effect, and some actually do the opposite of what they intend in that they result in encouraging people to use drugs. For example, there was a PSA featuring a woman "who looked like Winona Ryder" in a tight tank top in an expensive-looking kitchen—she smashed an egg with a skillet and then smashed up the kitchen with the skillet. This was intended to demonstrate how destructive heroin can be.[*] The target audience thought she looked sexy when she was mad and did not receive the intended message. It is important to know your target audience in terms of their attitudes, beliefs about the consequences of some behavior, perceived norms, and self-efficacy.[†] Unfortunately this type of research is rarely done.

One study did find that viewers paid more attention to PSAs related to methamphetamine and heroin than to PSAs about marijuana or drugs in general. The PSAs that specifically pointed out negative consequences of drug use were more effective than ones with messages such as "Just Say No [because we say so]." PSAs that used humor had negative consequences (increased the likelihood of drug use). Those that were more realistic and were related to perceptions of harm, danger, or violating social norms were most effective in preventing drug use. The "Friends Don't Let Friends Drive Drunk" series of PSAs presented more realistic depictions of how allowing friends to drink and drive violates social norms and has negative consequences.

Also, the more print and air time effective PSAs receive, the more likely they are to have an impact in changing behavior. Studies have shown that when media time and space were devoted to PSAs, smoking, drinking, and drug use declined—and when less PSA advertising was donated, these rates increased.[†] Unfortunately, with demands for greater profit margins, less print and air time have been given to PSAs in recent years. What PSAs do you remember? Did they influence your behavior? Why or why not?

[*]Rich, F. "Just Say $1 Billion," *New York Times*, July 15, 1998.
[†]"Avoiding the Boomerang: Testing the Relative Effectivenss of Antidrug Public Service Announcements Before a National Campaign," *American Journal of Public Health* 92(2), February 2002.

The use of psychoactive drugs can be tremendously disruptive in many people's lives, from causing tragic deaths or the loss of employment opportunities (most Fortune 500 companies use preemployment drug testing) to causing personal relationships to deteriorate and babies to be born with profound birth defects. Perhaps realizing this, college students have generally moved away from using the most dangerous illegal drugs.

However, it is safe to say that drug use remains a significant problem and area of concern for both college students and the general population (see the box "Does 'Just Say No' Really Make a Difference?"). Alcohol is the most important problem drug for most college students, but other drugs pose risks for certain students (Table 7.1). Additionally, many nontraditional-age students see the destructive effects of drug use on their neighborhoods and worry about their children being exploited by drug dealers.

For organizational reasons, this chapter primarily deals with psychoactive drugs. Alcohol is covered in Chapter 8. The effects of tobacco are delineated in Chapter 9. Prescription and OTC drugs and medicines are discussed at length in Chapter 18. Anabolic steroids, drugs used primarily for increasing muscle growth, are discussed in Chapter 4.

Addictive Behavior

This chapter explores the health consequences of drug use, misuse, and abuse. Before we talk about specific drugs, however, we need to put drug use in the broader context of addictive behavior. The use and abuse of drugs is just one of the many forms of addictive behavior. Addictive behavior includes addictions to shopping, gambling, sex, television, video games, Internet use, or work, as well as addictions to alcohol or other drugs.

TALKING POINTS How would you approach a friend and tell him he has a gambling addiction that needs to be controlled?

Key Terms

drug Any substance, natural or artificial, other than food, that by its chemical or physical nature alters structure or function in the living organism.

psychoactive drug Any substance capable of altering feelings, moods, or perceptions.

Drug use by peers, identification with youth subculture, weak academic performance, and truancy are all associated with higher rates of drug use and abuse.

indicates that a higher rate of drug abuse occurs among 18- to 25-year-olds.[5] Nevertheless, the drug abuse that does occur among those in the younger age group is of concern because patterns that are established at an early age can carry over into later life. In fact, 13 percent of those who first tried marijuana at age 14 abused or were dependent on illicit drugs after age 18, as compared to 2 percent of those who first tried marijuana after age 18.[6] In fact, during this period, experimentation with a **gateway drug** (alcohol, nicotine, or marijuana) often begins, which may lead to heavier drug use later.[1]

Modeling and Advertising **Modeling** of drug use within the peer group and family has already been presented. However, celebrities, musicians, and athletes also serve as models of behavior.

When models are employed by the media to sell products, advertising becomes an important factor in fostering drug use. The marketing of tobacco and alcohol products is perhaps the best example. "Beautiful people" are depicted enjoying a social drug, such as alcohol, coffee, tea, or tobacco, in opulent surroundings that most viewers can only dream of being in. Celebrities participate in events sponsored by alcohol or tobacco companies.

The Self-Medication Movement People's ability to engage in medical self-management makes drug use easier and more socially acceptable than in the past. In a society conditioned by the effectiveness and availability of OTC and prescription medications, the use of other drugs, both legal and illegal, to make ourselves feel better seems more acceptable than ever before. This attitude can fosters drug misuse and, for some, drug abuse. See the box "Improving Your Mood without Drugs" for non-drug strategies for reducing stress and negative feelings.

Drug Classifications

Drugs can be categorized according to the nature of their physiological effects. Most psychoactive drugs fall into one of six general categories: stimulants, depressants,

---

Changing for the Better

Improving Your Mood without Drugs

It's tempting to reach for a pill when I feel stressed, but I don't want to get into that habit. What can I do to improve my mood without using drugs?

Talk with a trusted friend. Confide your feelings to a close, trusted friend or family member. By opening up to another person, you'll gain insights into how you can get beyond your negative feelings without resorting to drug use.

Get moving. Go for a walk, ride your bike, or swim a few laps. Physical activity is a natural way to enhance your mood. Nearly every college provides recreation programs such as aerobics, swimming, dancing, or weight lifting.

Give yourself a break. If you're tired, take a quick power nap. If you're overworked, set aside some personal time—just for yourself. Read, watch TV, surf the Net, or call a friend. Decide what you like to do, and then do it. You'll return to your responsibilities with renewed enthusiasm.

Reexamine your spiritual health. Many people find comfort by making connections to their spiritual life. Through activities

such as meditation, spiritual reflection, and renewal of faith, people often gain reassurance and a sense of calmness.

Restructure your daily activities. If you have one hectic day after another but feel as though you're not accomplishing anything, try reorganizing your daily activities. Experiment with new patterns. Plan to get sufficient sleep, eat regular meals, and set aside specific times for work, family activities, and pleasure. Find out what works best for you.

Seek professional guidance. If you've tried these strategies but your mood still isn't improving, consider seeking professional help. This important first step is up to you. Visit your college health center or counseling center, and talk with people who are trained to help you learn how to become a happier person.

Do volunteer work. One way to feel good is to help others. Teach reading to adults, become a Big Brother or Big Sister, work in a soup kitchen, or drive a van for the elderly in your community.

Table 7.2 Psychoactive Drug Categories

Drugs and Examples of Commercial (Street) Names	Intoxication Effects	Potential Health Consequences
Stimulants		
Amphetamine Dexedrine *(black beauties, speed, uppers, bennies)* **Cocaine** *(Blow, C, coke, crack, flake, rock, snow, toot)* **Methamphetamine** *(Chalk, crank, crystal, glass, ice, meth, fire, zip)* **MDMA** *(Ecstasy, X, Eve, clarity, lover's speed, Adam)* **Methylphenidate** Ritalin *(JIF, MPH, Skippy, vitamin R, R-ball)* **Nicotine** Cigarettes, cigars, spit tobacco, bidis	Increased heart rate, blood pressure, breathing rate, metabolism; feelings of energy, exhilaration; increased mental alertness; reduced appetite *Additional specific effects:* *For cocaine*—increased temperature *For methamphetamine*—aggression, violence, psychotic behavior *For MDMA*—mild hallucinogenic effects, increased empathy and tactile sensitivity	Tolerance, dependence; rapid or irregular heart beat; weight loss; irritability, nervousness, impulsiveness, insomnia; panic, paranoia; heart failure *For cocaine*—chest pain, respiratory failure, seizures, strokes; withdrawal symptoms *For methamphetamine*—cardiac and neurological damage, impaired memory/learning, violent behavior, stroke, teeth and organ damage *For MDMA*—impaired memory and learning, hyperthermia, cardiac and liver toxicity, kidney failure *For nicotine*—see Chapter 9
Depressants		
Alcohol Beer, wine, liquor *(booze, hooch, sauce)* **Barbiturates** Amytal, Seconal *(barbs, reds, red birds, yellows)* **Flunitrazepam** Rohypnol *(forget-me pill, roofies, rope, R2)* **GHB** *(G, Georgia home boy, liquid X, grievous bodily harm, easy lay)* **Methaqualone** Quaalude, Sopor *(ludes, quay)* **Tranquilizers** Ativan, Valium, Xanax *(downers, tranks, candy)*	Slowed heart rate, breathing rate, blood pressure; reduced anxiety; lowered inhibitions; impaired judgment; mood changes (feelings of well-being or euphoria or irritability and abusiveness); slurred speech; reduced concentration, reflexes, coordination; sedation, drowsiness, loss of consciousness	Tolerance, dependence; respiratory depression and arrest; injuries due to reduced coordination and judgment; coma, death; some depressants have life-threatening withdrawal symptoms *For flunitrazepam*—visual disturbances, memory loss for the time under the drug's effects *For GHB*—headache, loss of consciousness and reflexes, seizures
Hallucinogens		
LSD *(Acid, blotter, boomers, microdot, yellow sunshines)* **Mescaline** *(Buttons, mesc, peyote)* **Psilocybin** *(Shrooms, magic mushroom, purple passion)*	Altered states of feeling and perception; nausea; increased body temperature, heart rate, blood pressure; loss of appetite; sleeplessness; weakness, numbness; tremors; nervousness, paranoia	Persisting perception disorder (flashbacks), memory loss, depression *(continued)*

hallucinogens, cannabis, narcotics, and inhalants (Table 7.2). According to the 2005 National Survey on Drug Use and Health (NSDUH), American Indians had the highest rate of substance abuse and dependence (21 percent) while Asians had the lowest rate (4.5 percent). Eleven percent of Pacific Islanders, 9.3 percent of Hispanics, and 8.5 percent of African Americans reported substance abuse or dependence in 2005; these were similar to 2004 rates. Marijuana was the most commonly used illegal drug, followed by nonmedical use of prescription drugs (Figure 7-2).

Stimulants

In general, **stimulants** excite or increase the activity of the CNS. Also called "uppers," stimulants alert the CNS by increasing heart rate, blood pressure, and the rate of brain function. Users feel uplifted and less fatigued.

Examples of stimulant drugs include caffeine, amphetamines, and cocaine. Most stimulants produce psychological dependence and tolerance relatively quickly, but

> **Key Terms**
>
> **gateway drug** An easily obtainable legal or illegal drug that represents a user's first experience with a mind-altering drug; this drug can serve as the "gateway" to the use of other drugs.
>
> **modeling** The influence others have on us by example of their own behavior.
>
> **stimulants** Psychoactive drugs that stimulate the function of the central nervous system.

Table 7.2 Psychoactive Drug Categories (continued)

Drugs and Examples of Commercial *(Street)* Names	Intoxication Effects	Potential Health Consequences
Cannabis		
Hashish *(Hash, hemp, boom, chronic gangster)* ***Marijuana*** *(Pot, dope, weed, reefer, Mary Jane, grass, ganja)*	Euphoria, slowed thinking and reaction time, confusion, impaired balance and coordination See Table 7.3	Cough, frequent respiratory infections; impaired memory and learning; increased heart rate, anxiety; panic attacks; tolerance and dependence
Narcotics (Opiates)*		
Heroin *(Dope, H, junk, smack, brown sugar)* ***Morphine*** *(M, monkey, Miss Emma)* ***Opium*** Laudanum, paregoric *(big O, gum, hop)* ***Oxycodone*** Oxycontin *(Oxy, OC, killer)*	Pain relief, euphoria, reduced pulse and blood pressure, pinpoint pupils, drowsiness, confusion, staggering gait, sedation, nausea, constipation	Tolerance, dependence; respiratory depression and arrest; unconsciousness, coma, death; unpleasant but not life-threatening withdrawal *For injection use*—risk of skin infections and transmission of HIV, hepatitis
Inhalants		
Solvents, gases, petroleum products Paint thinner, gasoline, glues, propane, aerosol propellant, nitrites *(laughing gas, poppers, snappers, whippets)*	Stimulation; loss of inhibition; headache; nausea, vomiting; slurred speech; loss of motor coordination; wheezing; hallucinations, delusions; possible aggressiveness	Muscle weakness; depression, memory impairment; damage to the cardiovascular and nervous systems; unconsciousness; sudden death
Dissociative Anesthetics		
Ketamine Ketalar SV *(cat Valium, K, Special K, vitamin K)* ***PCP*** Phencyclidine *(angel dust, hog, love boat, peace pill)*	Increased heart rate and blood pressure, impaired motor function, rapid and involuntary eye movements, memory loss, numbness, nausea, vomiting *For PCP*—possible acute anxiety, aggression, violence	Delirium; depression; decreased respiration, blood pressure, heart rate

*Additional narcotics with similar effects include codeine, fentanyl, meperidine (Demerol), methadone, and hydrocodone (Vicodin).
Sources: National Institute on Drug Abuse, Commonly Abused Drugs, www.drugabuse.gov/DrugPages/DrugsofAbuse.html, March 2007; U.S. Drug Enforcement Agency, Drug Briefs and Backgrounds, www.usdoj.gov/dea/concern/concern.htm, March 2007.

they are unlikely to produce significant physical dependence when judged by life-threatening withdrawal symptoms. The important exception is cocaine, which seems to be capable of producing psychological dependence and withdrawal so powerful that continued use of the drug is inevitable for some users.

Caffeine The methylxanthines are a family of chemicals that includes three compounds: caffeine, theophylline, and theobromine. Of these, caffeine is the most heavily consumed.

Caffeine is a tasteless drug found in coffee, tea, chocolate, many soft drinks, energy drinks, and several groups of over-the-counter drugs (see the box "Energy Drinks"). It is a relatively harmless CNS stimulant when consumed in moderate amounts. Fifty percent of Americans drink coffee daily, drinking 330 millions cups per day, earning the United States the name "Caffeine Nation."[7]

The chronic effects of long-term caffeine use are less clear. Chronic users show evidence of tolerance and withdrawal, indicating that they are physically dependent. Researchers have attempted to link caffeine to coronary heart disease, pancreatic cancer, and fibrocystic breast disease. So far, the results have been inconclusive.

For the average healthy adult, moderate consumption of caffeine is unlikely to pose any serious health threat. However, excessive consumption (equivalent to eight or more cups of coffee daily) could lead to anxiety, diarrhea, restlessness, delayed onset of sleep or frequent awakening, headache, and heart palpitations. Pregnant women are advised to avoid caffeine consumption.

Amphetamines Amphetamines produce increased activity and mood elevation in almost all users. The amphetamines include several closely related compounds: amphetamine, dextroamphetamine, and methamphetamine. These compounds do not have any natural sources and are completely manufactured in the laboratory. Medical use of amphetamines is limited primarily to the treatment of obesity, **narcolepsy,** and attention deficit hyperactivity disorder (ADHD).

Amphetamines can be ingested, injected, or snorted (inhaled). At low-to-moderate doses, amphetamines elevate mood and increase alertness and feelings of energy

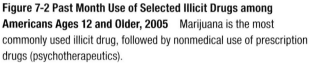

Figure 7-2 Past Month Use of Selected Illicit Drugs among Americans Ages 12 and Older, 2005 Marijuana is the most commonly used illicit drug, followed by nonmedical use of prescription drugs (psychotherapeutics).

Source: Substance Abuse and Mental Health Services Administration. (2006). *Results from the 2005 National Survey on Drug Use and Health: National Findings* (Office of Applied Studies, NSDUH Series H-30, DHHS Publication No. SMA 06-4194). Rockville, MD.

by stimulating receptor sites for two naturally occurring neurotransmitters. They also slow the activity of the stomach and intestine and decrease hunger. In the 1960s and 1970s, amphetamines were commonly prescribed for dieters, but when it was discovered that the appetite suppression effect of amphetamines lasted only a few weeks, most physicians stopped prescribing them. At high doses, amphetamines can increase heart rate and blood pressure to dangerous levels. As amphetamines are eliminated from the body, the user becomes tired.

When chronically abused, amphetamines produce rapid tolerance and strong psychological dependence. Other effects of chronic use include impotence and episodes of psychosis. When use is discontinued, periods of depression may develop.

Methamphetamine Today the abuse of amphetamines is a more pressing concern than it has been in the recent past because of the sharp increase in the abuse of methamphetamine. Known by a variety of names and forms, including "crank," "ice," "crystal," "meth," "speed," "crystal meth," "chalk," "fire," "glass," and "zip," methamphetamine has a high potential for abuse and is produced in illegal home laboratories with over-the-counter ingredients (see the box "Meth Lab Warning Signs").[8]

Methamphetamines can be smoked, ingested orally, snorted, or injected. **Crystal methamphetamine,** glass or ice, is among the most dangerous forms of methamphetamine. Ice is a very pure form of methamphetamine that looks like rock candy.[9] When smoked or injected,

the effects of ice are felt in about seven seconds as a wave of intense physical and psychological exhilaration. This effect lasts for several hours (much longer than the effects of crack), until the user becomes physically exhausted. The user experiences a rush of pleasure that is the result of the drug telling the brain to release large amounts of dopamine.[10] When ingested orally or snorted, methamphetamine induces euphoria, which may result in quick addiction for the user.

Abuse can lead to memory loss, violence, anxiety, paranoia, euphoria, hyperthermia, convulsions, increased wakefulness and physical activity, and cardiac and neurological damage. Chronic use can result in Parkinsonlike symptoms, rotten teeth ("meth mouth"),

---

Key Terms

narcolepsy A sleep-related disorder in which a person has a recurrent, overwhelming, and uncontrollable desire to sleep, often at inappropriate times.

crystal methamphetamine A dangerous form of methamphetamine that quickly produces intense physical and psychological exhilaration when smoked.

stroke, anorexia, increased heart rate and blood pressure, death,[11] nutritional difficulties, weight loss, reduced resistance to infection, and damage to the liver, lungs, and kidneys. Psychological dependence is quickly established. Withdrawal causes acute depression and fatigue but not significant physical discomfort.

Recent data from the National Survey on Drug Use and Health (NSDUH) shows that use of methamphetamine declined between 2002 and 2005 among persons 12 years old or older. Those living in the western United States were more likely to have used methamphetamine in the past year than those living in any other part of the country. The study also found that the number of people who used methamphetamine for the first time decreased between 2004 and 2005.

Ritalin

There is an increasing concern about misuse and abuse of methylphenidate (Ritalin) as 8 million prescriptions were written for children and adolescents.

Ritalin is typically prescribed to help focus attention in those who are hyperactive or cannot concentrate. Critics argue that the drug is being prescribed to treat a variety of problems. Studies suggest that access to health care may influence a diagnosis of ADHD, when the better course of treatment would be to identify and treat the root cause of the problems.[12] Supporters respond that Ritalin enables them to succeed in school and work (see the box "Ritalin and Adderall Abuse on College Campuses").

Cocaine

Cocaine, perhaps the strongest of the stimulant drugs, has received much media attention. Cocaine is the primary psychoactive substance found in the leaves of the South American coca plant.[13] The effects of cocaine last only briefly—from 5 to 30 minutes. Regardless of the form in which it is consumed, cocaine produces an immediate, near-orgasmic "rush," or feeling of exhilaration. This euphoria is quickly followed by a period of marked depression. Used only occasionally as a topical anesthetic, cocaine is usually inhaled (snorted), injected, or smoked (typically as crack). There is overwhelming scientific evidence that users quickly develop a strong psychological dependence on cocaine. Considerable evidence suggests that physical dependence also rapidly develops. Cocaine users risk a weakened immune system making them "more susceptible to infections, including HIV."[14] However, physical dependence on cocaine does not lead to death on withdrawal.

Crack Cocaine Crack is made by combining cocaine hydrochloride with common baking soda. When this pastelike mixture is allowed to dry, a small rocklike crystalline material remains. This crack is heated in the bowl of a small pipe, and the vapors are inhaled into the lungs.[13] Some crack users spend hundreds of dollars a day to maintain their habit.

The effect of crack is almost instantaneous. Within 10 seconds after inhalation, cocaine reaches the CNS and influences the action of several neurotransmitters at specific sites in the brain. As with the use of other forms of cocaine, convulsions, seizures, respiratory distress, and cardiac failure have been reported with this sudden, extensive stimulation of the nervous system.

Within about 6 minutes, the stimulating effect of crack has been completely expended, and users frequently become depressed. Dependence develops within a few weeks, because users consume more crack in response to the short duration of stimulation and rapid onset of depression.

Intravenous administration has been the preferred route for cocaine users who are also regular users of heroin and other injectable drugs. Intravenous injection results in an almost immediate high, which lasts about 10 minutes. A "smoother ride" is said to be obtained from a "speedball," the injectable mixture of heroin and cocaine (or methamphetamine).[4] However, such a mixture can be volatile and even fatal.

Freebasing As inhaling crack did, freebasing developed as a technique for maximizing the psychoactive effects of cocaine. Freebasing first requires that the common form of powdered cocaine (cocaine hydrochloride) be chemically altered (alkalized). This altered form is then dissolved in a solvent such as ether or benzene. This liquid solution is heated to evaporate the solvent. The heating process leaves the freebase cocaine in a powder form that can then be smoked, often through a water pipe. Because of the large surface area of the lungs, smoking cocaine facilitates fast absorption into the bloodstream.

One danger of freebasing cocaine is the risk related to the solvents used. Ether is a highly volatile solvent capable of exploding and causing serious burns. Benzene is a known carcinogen associated with the development of leukemia. Clearly, neither solvent can be used without increasing the level of risk typically associated with cocaine use.

Depressants

Depressants (or sedatives) sedate the user, slowing down CNS function. Drugs included in this category are alcohol (see Chapter 8), barbiturates, and tranquilizers. Depressants produce tolerance in abusers, as well as strong psychological and physical dependence.

Barbiturates Barbiturates are the so-called sleeping compounds that function by enhancing the effect of inhibitory neurotransmitters. They depress the CNS to the point where the user drops off to sleep or, as is the case with surgical anesthetics, the patient becomes anesthetized. Medically, barbiturates are used in widely varied dosages as anesthetics and for treatment of anxiety, insomnia, and epilepsy.[1] Regular use of a barbiturate quickly produces tolerance—eventually such a high dose is required that the user still feels the effects of the drug throughout the next morning. Some abusers then begin to alternate barbiturates with stimulants, producing a vicious circle of dependence. Other misusers combine alcohol and barbiturates or tranquilizers, inadvertently producing toxic or even lethal results. Abrupt withdrawal from barbiturate use frequently produces a withdrawal syndrome that can involve seizures, delusions, hallucinations, and even death.

Methaqualone (Quaalude, Sopor, "ludes") was developed as a sedative that would not have the dependence properties of other barbiturates.[1] Quaaludes were occasionally prescribed for anxious patients. Today,

compounds resembling Quaaludes are manufactured in home laboratories and sold illegally so that they can be combined with small amounts of alcohol for an inexpensive, drunklike effect.

Tranquilizers Tranquilizers are depressants that are intended to reduce anxiety and to relax people who are having problems managing stress. Because of their sedating effects, they have also been prescribed to treat insomnia. Lorazepam (Atavan), alprazolam (Xanax), diazepam (Valium), and chlordiazepoxide (Librium) are some of the most commonly prescribed. Unfortunately, some people become addicted to these and other prescription drugs.[15] All tranquilizers can produce physical and psychological dependence and tolerance.

"Date Rape" Drugs "Date rape" drugs or **club drugs** are commonly used on college campuses. These drugs are usually slipped into the drink of an unsuspecting person and can result in a coma or even death.

Common "date rape" drugs include GHB (gamma-hydroxybutyrate), also known as G, Liquid Esctasy, Easy Lay, Georgia Home Boy, and Rohypnol ("roophies"). When these drugs are consumed they cause a drunklike or sleepy state that can last for hours. During this time is when unsuspecting individuals are taken advantage

> ### Key Terms
>
> **depressants** A category of drugs that sedate the user by slowing CNS function; they produce tolerance and strong psychological and physical addiction in users.
>
> **club drug** One of a variety of psychoactive drugs typically used at raves, bars, and dance clubs.

of, against their will and without their knowledge. (For additional information, see the box "Club Drugs.")

As a rule, it is wise not to accept drinks from people you do not know or leave your drink unattended. This recommendation extends to all parties where drinkers do not know what has been added to the punch or other drinks.[16]

Hallucinogens

As the name suggests, hallucinogenic drugs produce hallucinations—perceived distortions of reality. Also known as *psychedelic drugs* or *phantasticants,* **hallucinogens** reached their height of popularity during the 1960s. At that time, young people were encouraged to use hallucinogenic drugs to "expand the mind," "reach an altered state," or "discover reality" (see the box "Drugs and Spirituality"). Not all the reality distortions, or "trips," were pleasant. Many users reported "bummers," or trips during which they perceived negative, frightening distortions.

Hallucinogenic drugs include laboratory-produced lysergic acid diethylamide (LSD), mescaline (from the peyote cactus plant), and psilocybin (from a particular genus of mushroom). Consumption of hallucinogens seems to produce not physical dependence but mild levels of psychological dependence. The development of tolerance is questionable. **Synesthesia,** a sensation in which users report hearing a color, smelling music, or touching a taste, is sometimes produced with hallucinogen use.

The long-term effects of hallucinogenic drug use are not fully understood. Questions about genetic abnormalities in offspring, fertility, sex drive and performance, and the development of personality disorders have not been fully answered. One phenomenon that has been identified and documented is the development of flashbacks—the unpredictable return to a psychedelic trip that occurred months or even years earlier. Flashbacks are thought to result from the accumulation of a drug within body cells.

LSD The most well-known and powerful hallucinogen is lysergic acid diethylamide (LSD). LSD was first isolated in 1938 by Albert Hoffmann, who was studying a group of chemicals that were extracted from a fungus that infects rye and other cereal grains. Five years later, he accidentally discovered its hallucinogenic effects.

Dr. Timothy Leary helped to spread the popularity of LSD in the 1960s by promoting the use of LSD in mind expansion and experimentation. LSD helped define the counterculture movement of the 1960s. During the 1970s and the 1980s, this drug lost considerable popularity. LSD use peaked in 1996, with an annual prevalence of 8.8 percent.[18] There was sharp decline in the use of LSD between the years 2002 and 2003, which was attributed to the increase in Ecstasy use. However, the rates haven't changed since that time.[18] Part of the appeal of LSD is its low cost and easy availability.

LSD is manufactured in home laboratories and frequently distributed in absorbent blotter paper or gelatin squares. It is odorless, colorless, and tasteless.[18] Users place the paper on their tongue or chew the paper to ingest the drug. LSD is similar in structure to the neurotransmitter serotonin and produces psychedelic effects by interfering with the normal activity of this neurotransmitter. Although the typical doses ("hits") today are about half as powerful as those in the 1960s, users still tend to rapidly develop a high tolerance of LSD. The effects of LSD depend upon the dose. Physical dependence does not occur. The effects can include altered perception of shapes, images, time, sound, and body form. Synesthesia is common to LSD users. LSD is metabolized in the liver and excreted. Its effects last an average of six to nine hours.

Users may describe LSD experiences as positive and "mind-expanding," or negative and "mind-constricting," depending on the user's mood and the social setting in which the drug is taken. Positive sensations include feelings of creativity, deep understanding of oneself and the universe, and feelings of grandeur. Although LSD users report feelings of increased insight and creativity, a real increase in these skills has not been demonstrated. At the same time, some reports of bad trips on LSD are thought to have been caused by other substances, such as PCP, that were sold to the user as LSD. Deaths resulting from bizarre behavior after taking LSD have been reported. Dangerous side effects include panic attacks, flashbacks, and occasional prolonged psychosis.

Ecstasy and Designer Drugs   In recent years, chemists who produce many of the illicit drugs in home laboratories have designed versions of drugs listed on FDA Schedule 1. Under the Controlled Substances Act, substances regulated by the Food and Drug Administration are placed in one of five schedules. Schedule 1 contains the most dangerous drugs that have no medical use.[19] Designer drugs are similar to the controlled drugs on the FDA Schedule 1 but are sufficiently different so that they escape governmental control. The designer drugs are either newly synthesized products that are similar to already outlawed drugs but against which no law yet exists, or they are reconstituted or renamed illegal substances. Designer drugs are said to produce effects similar to their controlled drug counterparts.

People who use designer drugs do so at great risk because the manufacturing of these drugs is unregulated. The neurophysiological effect of these homemade drugs can be quite dangerous. So far, a synthetic heroin product (MPPP) and several amphetamine derivatives with hallucinogenic properties have been designed for the unwary drug consumer.

DOM (STP), MDA (the "love drug"), and MDMA ("Ecstasy" or "XTC") are examples of amphetamine-derivative, hallucinogenic designer drugs. These drugs

Key Terms

hallucinogens Psychoactive drugs capable of producing hallucinations (distortions of reality).

synesthesia A sensation of combining of the senses, such as perceiving color by hearing it or perceiving taste by touching it.

FDA Schedule 1 A list of drugs that have a high potential for abuse but no medical use.

MDMA (Esctasy) is a designer drug that has both stimulant and hallucinogenic effects. Heavy or long-term use has a number of negative effects, including memory impairment, possibly caused by depletion of the neurotransmitter serotonin.

produce mild LSD-like hallucinogenic experiences, positive feelings, and enhanced alertness. They also have a number of potentially dangerous effects. These dangers include increased heart rate and blood pressure, muscle tension, involuntary teeth clenching, nausea, blurred vision, faintness, and chills or sweating. MDMA use can also cause hyperthermia from a sharp increase in body temperature, which can result in kidney, liver, and cardiovascular system failure.[20] Experts are particularly concerned that MDMA can produce strong psychological dependence and can deplete serotonin, an important excitatory neurotransmitter associated with a state of alertness and mood. Heavy or long-term users can experience depression, anxiety, paranoia, hallucinations, panic attacks, and hostility. Memory loss is commonly experienced in heavy MDMA users, who are therefore sometimes called "E-tards."[21] Permanent brain damage is possible. As with LSD, there was a decline in MDMA use from 2002 to 2003, but its use rate has remained the same since then: On average, people first tried this drug at age 20.[22]

Phencyclidine Phencyclidine (PCP, "angel dust") is a complicated drug because it not only produces hallucinogenic effects but also acts as an analgesic, a depressant, a stimulant, and an anesthetic. This makes the typical PCP experience impossible to predict or describe. The physical effects of PCP begin a few minutes after consumption and continue for four to six hours. PCP was studied for years during the 1950s and 1960s and was found to be an unsuitable animal and human anesthetic.[23]

Manufactured in tablet or powder form, PCP can be injected, inhaled, taken orally, or smoked. Some users report mild euphoria, although most report bizarre perceptions, paranoid feelings, and aggressive behavior.

It can increase blood pressure and body temperature and decrease coordination. People also report feeling an increased state of drowsiness, a decreased sensitivity to pain, and a sense of disconnection from reality. PCP overdose may cause convulsions, cardiovascular collapse, and damage to the brain's respiratory center.

In a number of cases, the aggressive behavior caused by PCP has led users to commit brutal crimes against both friends and innocent strangers. PCP accumulates in cells and may stimulate bizarre behavior months after initial use.

PCP is an extremely unpredictable and dangerous drug. Although PCP has been blamed in many reports of bizarre, even homicidal, behavior, it continues to be abused. Because PCP is easily and cheaply manufactured in home laboratories, authorities have difficulty limiting its availability.

Cannabis

Cannabis (marijuana) is the most widely used illicit drug among college students (see the box "Who Uses Marijuana?"). Marijuana has been labeled a mild hallucinogen for a number of years. However, most experts now consider it to be a drug category in itself. Marijuana produces mild effects like those of stimulants and depressants. Marijuana has been implicated as contributing to a large number of traffic fatalities.

Products and Potency Marijuana is actually a wild plant (*Cannabis sativa*) whose fibers were once used in the manufacture of hemp rope. When the leafy material and small stems are dried and crushed, users can smoke the mixture in rolled cigarettes ("joints"), cigars ("blunts"), or pipes. The resins collected from scraping the flowering tops of the plant yield a marijuana product called hashish, or hash, commonly smoked in a pipe.[24]

The potency of marijuana's hallucinogenic effect is determined by the percentage of the active ingredient, tetrahydrocannabinol (THC), present in the product. The concentration of THC averages about 3.5 percent for regular grade marijuana, 7–9 percent for higher quality marijuana (sinsemilla), 8–14 percent for hashish, and as high as 50 percent for hash oil.[1] Today's marijuana has THC levels that are higher than in past decades.

Short-Term Effects THC is a fat-soluble substance and thus is absorbed and retained in fat tissues within the body. Before being excreted, THC can remain in the body for up to a month. With the sophistication of today's drug tests, trace metabolites of THC can be detected for up to 30 days after consumption.[3] It is possible that the THC that comes from passive inhalation of high doses (for example, during an indoor rock concert) can also be detected for a short time after exposure.

Once marijuana is consumed, its effects vary from person to person (see Table 7.3). Being "high" or "stoned" means different things to different people. Many people report heightened sensitivity to music, cravings for particular foods, and a relaxed mood. There is widespread consensus that marijuana's behavioral effects include four probabilities: (1) Users must learn to recognize what a marijuana high is like, (2) marijuana impairs short-term memory, (3) users overestimate the passage of time, and (4) users lose the ability to maintain attention to a task.[3]

Long-Term Effects The long-term effects of marijuana use are still being studied. Chronic abuse may lead to an amotivational syndrome in some people. Heavy marijuana users have trouble paying attention and retaining new information for at least a day after last using the drug, according to a recent study.

The irritating effects of marijuana smoke on lung tissue are more pronounced than those of cigarette smoke, and some of the more than 400 chemicals in marijuana are now linked to lung cancer development. In fact, one of the most potent carcinogens, benzopyrene, is found in higher levels in marijuana smoke than in tobacco smoke. Marijuana smokers tend to inhale deeply and hold the smoke in the lungs for long periods. It is likely that at some point the lungs of chronic marijuana smokers will be damaged.

Long-term marijuana use is also associated with damage to the immune system and to the male and female reproductive systems and with an increase in birth defects in babies born to mothers who smoke marijuana. Chronic marijuana use lowers testosterone levels in men, but the effect of this change is not known. The effect of long-term marijuana use on a variety of types of sexual behavior is also not fully understood.

Medical Uses Marijuana has been used to relieve the nausea caused by chemotherapy, to improve appetite in AIDS patients, and to ease the pressure that builds up in the eyes of glaucoma patients. However, a variety of other drugs, many of which are nearly as effective, are also used for these purposes. The U.S. Supreme Court recently struck a blow to the proponents of the medical use of marijuana. In 2005 the U.S. Supreme court outlawed the use of medical marijuana. However, 13 states have state laws that allow terminally ill patients to legally use marijuana for medical purposes.

Narcotics

The **narcotics,** or opiates, are among the strongest dependence-producing drugs. Overdose can be lethal and can occur the first time taking the drug. People using narcotics experience a rush of pleasure followed by a dreamy, drowsy state in which they feel little pain. Breathing slows, sometimes to the point of respiratory failure. Users also report that their skin flushes, their pupils become

> **Key Terms**
>
> **narcotics** Opiates; psychoactive drugs derived from the Oriental poppy plant. Narcotics relieve pain and induce sleep.

Table 7-3 Effects of Marijuana

Short-Term Effects	Long-Term Effects
• Increased heart rate and blood pressure • Feeling of elation • Drowsiness and sedation • Increased appetite • Red eyes • Food cravings • Slow reaction time • Feelings of depression, excitement, paranoia, panic, and euphoria • Problems with attention span, memory, learning, problem-solving, and coordination • Sleeplessness*	• Lung damage • Increased risk of bronchitis • Emphysema • Lung cancer • Heart attack[†] • Loss of motivation and short-term memory • Increased panic or anxiety • May become tolerant to marijuana • Damage to lungs, immune system, and reproductive organs • Can remain in the body for up to a month • Can cause birth defects • Five times more damaging to the lungs than tobacco products*

*National Institute on Drug Abuse. National Institutes of Health, *NIDA Research Report-Marijuana Abuse,* www.nida.nih.gov/ResearchReports/Marijuana/default.html, February 15, 2005.
[†]"Stronger Marijuana Is Major Health Risk," *The Independent,* February 1, 2001.

pinpointed, and they feel nauseous and may vomit. Depending upon how quickly the drug is metabolized in the liver, the effects of most narcotics are experienced for 4 to 6 hours. The effects from taking methadone can last 12 to 24 hours.[21] Medically, narcotics are used to relieve pain and induce sleep. On the basis of origin, narcotics can be subgrouped into the natural, quasisynthetic, and synthetic narcotics.

Natural Narcotics Naturally occurring substances derived from the Oriental poppy plant include opium (the primary psychoactive substance extracted from the Oriental poppy), morphine (the primary active ingredient in opium), and thebaine (a compound not used as a drug). Morphine and related compounds have medical use as analgesics in the treatment of mild to severe pain.

Quasisynthetic Narcotics Quasisynthetic narcotics are compounds created by chemically altering morphine. These laboratory-produced drugs are intended to be used as analgesics, but their benefits are largely outweighed by a high dependence rate and a great risk of toxicity. The best known of the quasisynthetic narcotics is heroin. Although heroin is a fast-acting and very effective analgesic, it is extremely addictive. Heroin can be inhaled ("snorted"), smoked, injected into a vein, or "skin-popped" (injected beneath the skin surface). Heroin produces dreamlike euphoria and, like all narcotics, strong physical and psychological dependence and tolerance.

Most new heroin users are smoking or snorting heroin, rather than injecting the drug. One-quarter of the new users of heroin are under age 18, and nearly half are ages 18 to 25.[25]

Heroin users who inject the drug face an additional risk. As with the use of all other injectable illegal drugs, the practice of sharing needles increases the likelihood of transmission of various communicable diseases, including hepatitis C and HIV (see Chapter 13). Abrupt withdrawal from heroin use is rarely fatal, but the discomfort during **cold turkey** withdrawal is reported to be excruciating.

Synthetic Narcotics Meperidine (Demerol) and propoxyphene (Darvon), common postsurgical painkillers, and methadone, the drug prescribed during the rehabilitation of heroin addicts, are synthetic narcotics. These opiatelike drugs are manufactured in medical laboratories. They are not natural narcotics or quasisynthetic narcotics because they do not originate from the Oriental poppy plant. Like true narcotics, however, these drugs can rapidly induce physical dependence. One important criticism of methadone rehabilitation programs is that they merely shift the addiction from heroin to methadone. See the box "From OxyContin to Fentanyl and Dextromethorphan" for more on abuse of synthetic narcotics and other prescription and OTC medications.

Inhalants

Inhalants constitute a class of drugs that includes a variety of volatile (quickly evaporating) compounds that generally produce unpredictable, drunklike effects in users and feelings of euphoria.[26] Users of inhalants may also have some delusions and hallucinations. Some users may become quite aggressive. Drugs in this category include anesthetic gases (chloroform, nitrous oxide,

Emergency room visits to treat overdoses on fentanyl have increased 14 times in the last few years. The fentanyl patch is a prescription painkiller intended for cancer patients and those with chronic pain; the patch dispenses the medication slowly through the skin. Abusers are putting it under their tongues, chewing it, or injecting it, releasing three days' worth of medication at one time, often resulting in death. There have also been more deaths related to mixing heroin and fentanyl. Fentanyl is a synthetic narcotic and has seen an increase in abuse since the government has been cracking down on oxycodone (OxyContin), a similar prescription painkiller. Fentanyl has also been referred to as "Apache," "China girl," "China white," "dance fever," "friend," "goodfella," "jackpot," "murder 8," "TNT," and "Tango and Cash." Federal drug agents believe fentanyl is being made in labs in Mexico and smuggled into the

United States. Both oxycodone and fentanyl have the side effects, tolerance, addiction, and withdrawal symptoms associated with narcotics.

Dextromethorphan (DXM), a drug found in over-the-counter cough medications, has also been increasingly abused. It is absorbed quickly into the body, metabolizing in 15 to 60 minutes after ingestion. Slang terms for DXM often correlate to the brands of cough medicine used, such as "tussin," "robo," "Red Baron," "dex," "Red Devils," "RDs," "White Angels," and "skittles." Recreational users report that, at high doses, DXM has effects similar to those of narcotics and hallucinogens. Recreational use of DXM is frequently referred to as "dexing," "floating," "getting a float," "tussing," "robofrying," or "doing the robot." It can cause psychosis and irreversible damage in the body, and can also be lethal at high doses.

"Syrup," "Sizzurp," "Sir," "Purple Drank," "Purple Tonic," "Lean," "Southern Lean," "Drank," "Robo," and "Cherry Syrup" are some of the common names for a codeine-laced cough syrup mixed with a soft drink or sports drinks. "Purple" drink refers to the color of the cough syrup. In 2004, 8.3 percent of secondary school students reported having taken 25 times the prescribed amount in order to get high.

The FDA continues to monitor the abuse of these drugs and other prescription and OTC medications. There is increasing concern over the nonmedical use of prescription and OTC drugs, which may bring further FDA regulations and control.

Sources: "Deaths Rise from Addiction, Misuse of Painkiller Patch," *Contra Costa Times*, June 16, 2006; "FDA Strengthens Warnings for OxyContin," U.S. Food and Drug Administration, www.fda.gov/bbs/topcs/ANSWERS/2001/ANS01091.html, July 25, 2001.

---

and ether), vasodilators (amyl nitrite and butyl nitrite), petroleum products and commercial solvents (gasoline, kerosene, plastic cement, glue, typewriter correction fluid, paint, and paint thinner), and certain aerosols (found in some propelled spray products, fertilizers, and insecticides).

Most of the danger in using inhalants lies in the damaging, sometimes fatal effects on the respiratory and cardiovascular systems.[26] Furthermore, users may unknowingly place themselves in dangerous situations because of the drunklike hallucinogenic effects. Aggressive behavior might also make users a threat to themselves and others.

For more information about inhalants, contact the National Inhalant Prevention Coalition at www.inhalants.org.

Combination Drug Effects

Drugs taken in various combinations and dosages can alter and perhaps intensify effects.

A **synergistic effect** is a dangerous consequence of taking different drugs in the same general category at the same time. The combination exaggerates each individual

drug's effects. For example, the combined use of alcohol and tranquilizers produces a synergistic effect greater than the total effect of each of the two drugs taken separately. In this instance, a much-amplified, perhaps fatal sedation will occur. In a simplistic sense, "one plus one equals four or five."

When taken at or near the same time, drug combinations produce a variety of effects. Drug combinations have additive, potentiating, or **antagonistic effects.** When two or more drugs are taken and the result is

> ## Key Terms
>
> **cold turkey** Immediate, total discontinuation of use of a drug; associated with withdrawal discomfort.
>
> **inhalants** Psychoactive drugs that enter the body through inhalation.
>
> **synergistic effect** A heightened, exaggerated effect produced by the concurrent use of two or more drugs.
>
> **antagonistic effect** The effect produced when one drug reduces or offsets the effects of a second drug.

merely a combined total effect of each drug, the result is an **additive effective.** The sum of the effects is not exaggerated. In a sense, "one plus one plus one equals three."

When one drug intensifies the action of a second drug, the first drug is said to have a **potentiated effect** on the second drug. One popular drug-taking practice during the 1970s was the consumption of Quaaludes and beer. Quaaludes potentiated the inhibition-releasing, sedative effects of alcohol. This particular drug combination produced an inexpensive but potentially fatal drunklike euphoria in the user. More recently, the combined use of various "club drugs" results in unpredictable potentiated drug effects.

An antagonistic effect, on the other hand, is a drug's action in reducing another drug's effects. Knowledge of this principle has been useful in the medical treatment of certain drug overdoses, as in the use of tranquilizers to relieve the effects of LSD or other hallucinogenic drugs.

Because of these possible synergistic drug effects, patients should always inform their doctors and dentists of any illegal drugs they have taken.

Society's Response to Drug Use

During the last 25 years, society has responded to illegal drug use with growing concern. Most adults see drug abuse as a clear danger to society. This position has been supported by the development of community, school, state, and national organizations interested in the reduction of illegal drug use. These organizations have included such diverse groups as Parents Against Drugs, Parents for a Drug-Free Youth, Drug Abuse Resistance Education (DARE), Mothers Against Drunk Driving (MADD), Narcotics Anonymous, and the federal Drug Enforcement Administration. Certain groups have concentrated their efforts on education, others on enforcement, and still others on the development of laws and public policy.

The personal and social issues related to drug abuse are very complex. Innovative solutions continue to be devised. Some believe that only through early childhood education will people learn alternatives to drug use. Starting drug education in the preschool years may have a more positive effect than waiting until the upper elementary or junior high school years. The focus on reducing young people's exposure to gateway drugs (especially tobacco, alcohol, and marijuana) may help slow down the move to other addictive drugs. Some people advocate much harsher penalties for drug use and drug trafficking.

Others support legalizing all drugs and making governmental agencies responsible for drug regulation and control, as is the case with alcohol. Advocates of this position believe that drug-related crime and violence would

virtually cease once the demand for illegal products is reduced.

Unless significant changes in society's response to drug use take place soon, families and communities will continue to be plagued by drug-related tragedies. Law enforcement officials will be pressed to the limits of their resources in their attempts to reduce drug flow. Our judicial system will be heavily burdened by thousands of court cases. Health care facilities could face overwhelming numbers of patients.

Currently, approximately $19.2 billion is spent to fight the drug war in the United States—$13 billion on law enforcement (supply reduction) and $6.2 billion on education, prevention, and treatment (demand reduction).[27] In comparison with other federally funded programs, the "war on drugs" is less expensive than farm support, food stamps, Medicare, and national defense. However, it remains to be seen whether any amount of money spent on enforcement, without adequate support for education, treatment, and poverty reduction, can reduce the illegal drug demand and supply.

Prevention: The Best Solution

We combat the drug problem in the United States on two fronts: the demand side and the supply side. The U.S. government attempts to reduce the supply of illegal (illicit) drugs through drug interdiction efforts at our borders, through joint efforts with countries such as Mexico and Colombia, and through law-enforcement measures within our own borders.

However, the best way to avoid the immense costs of drug abuse is simply to reduce the demand. We do this by helping people develop the tools needed to avoid the use of illegal drugs. Experts are currently mounting prevention efforts on three levels: primary, secondary, and tertiary. Take a look at each of these three levels. Which level is most familiar to you?

Primary Prevention **Primary prevention** means reaching people who have not yet used drugs and reducing their desire to try drugs. Primary prevention programs can target individuals, families, peer groups, neighborhoods, schools, workplaces, colleges, and the community. Examples of primary prevention include the DARE program, teaching assertiveness and refusal skills to children and teens, having drug-free schools, using student leaders from schools as role models and as presenters of peer programs, debunking the myths associated with drug use (such as that smoking is sexy), and community programs for drug education. The key to primary prevention is to keep potential users from starting to use drugs.

Secondary Prevention **Secondary prevention** targets those who are beginning to experiment with drugs and uses detection, screening, intervention, and treatment of early drug abuse to help avoid further drug use and identify people at risk for developing addictions. These programs do not prevent initial drug use but instead involve detection and early treatment of drug problems before they become severe. Popular methods include crisis telephone hotlines, peer counseling, individual and family counseling, school and worksite drug screening programs, and student and employee assistance programs.[28]

Tertiary Prevention **Tertiary prevention** (third-level prevention) targets drug-dependent people, such as cocaine abusers, heroin addicts, or alcoholics. These individuals require specialized, intensive help that includes rehabilitation and maintenance. Such intensive treatments may require temporary hospitalization. Additional treatment methods include intensive outpatient care, support groups, and after-care programs. Relapse prevention is designed to help people recovering from drug abuse maintain their drug-free lifestyles.[28]

Drug Testing

Drug testing is one of society's responses to drug use and is becoming an increasingly popular prevention tool. In 1986 the federal government instituted drug-testing policies for federal employees in safety-sensitive jobs. In 1988 the Drug Free Workplace Act extended the drug-free federal policy to include all federal grantees (including universities) and most federal contractors. Although this act did not mandate drug testing, it encouraged tougher approaches to prevent and deal with drug problems at the work site.

Private companies have developed drug-testing procedures similar to those used with federal agencies. Most Fortune 500 companies use drug testing to screen applicants or monitor employee drug use.

Drug tests commonly search for amphetamines, barbiturates, benzodiazepines (the chemical bases for prescription tranquilizers such as Valium and Librium), cannabinoids (THC, hashish, and marijuana), methaqualone, opiates (heroin, codeine, and morphine), and PCP. With the exception of marijuana, most traces of these drugs are eliminated by the body within a few days after use. Marijuana can remain detectable for up to 30 days after use.

How accurate are the results of drug testing? At typical cutoff standards, drug tests are likely to identify 90 percent of recent drug users. This means that about 10 percent of recent users will pass undetected. (These 10 percent are considered *false negatives.*) Nonusers whose drug tests indicate drug use (*false positives*) are quite rare. (Follow-up tests on these false positives would nearly always show negative results.) Human errors are probably more responsible than technical errors for inaccuracies in drug tests.

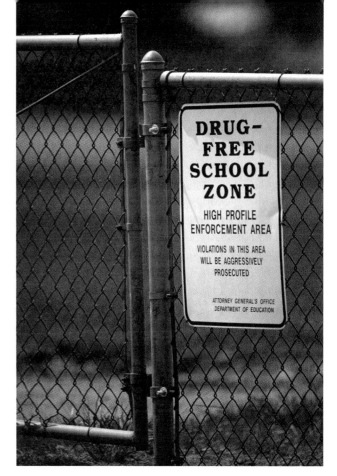

A drug-free school program is an example of a primary prevention measure designed to prevent potential drug users from ever trying drugs.

Recently, scientists have been refining procedures that use hair samples to detect the presence of drugs. These procedures seem to hold much promise, although certain technical obstacles remain. Watch for refinements in hair-sample drug testing in the near future.

Key Terms

additive effect The combined (but not exaggerated) effect produced by the concurrent use of two or more drugs.

potentiated effect A phenomenon whereby the use of one drug intensifies the effect of a second drug.

primary prevention Measures intended to deter first-time drug use.

secondary prevention Measures aimed at early detection, intervention, and treatment of drug abuse before severe physical, psychological, emotional, or social consequences can occur.

tertiary prevention Treatment and rehabilitation of drug-dependent people to limit physical, psychological, emotional, and social deterioration or prevent death.

Alcohol and Its Immediate Effects on the Body

As described in Chapter 7, alcohol is a depressant that slows the function of the central nervous system. Like for other depressants, consuming too much alcohol can lead to intoxication, sedation, and even death. Its effects on the user depend on the type of beverage, the circumstances under which it is consumed, and factors related to the individual user.[1]

The Nature of Alcoholic Beverages

Alcohol (also known as *ethyl alcohol* or *ethanol*) is the principal product of **fermentation.** In this process, yeast cells act on the sugar content of fruits and grains to produce alcohol and carbon dioxide.[2]

The alcohol concentration in beverages such as whiskey, gin, rum, and vodka is determined through a process called **distillation.** These distilled beverages are expressed by the term *proof*, a number that is twice the percentage of alcohol by volume in a beverage. Thus 70 percent of the fluid in a bottle of 140-proof gin is pure alcohol. Most proofs in distilled beverages range from 80 to 160. The pure grain alcohol that is often added to fruit punches and similar beverages has a proof of almost 200. Beer, wine, and hard liquor contain different concentrations of ethanol, which means they affect an individual in different ways. The alcohol content in beer is about 4 percent, for wine it is 10–14 percent, and for port and sherry it is 20 percent because they have alcohol added to them.

Lite and Ice Beers

"Lite" beer and low-calorie wines have been introduced in response to concerns about the number of calories in alcoholic beverages. These beverages are not low-alcohol beverages but merely low-calorie beverages. Only beverages marked "low alcohol" contain a lower concentration of alcohol than do the usual beverages of that type.

Ice beers actually contain a higher percentage of alcohol than do other types of beer. The term *ice* refers to the way in which this beer is processed. After brewing and fermentation, it is deep-chilled at 24 to 28 degrees F, which causes ice crystals to form in the mixture. When these ice crystals are removed, the remaining liquid contains a higher percentage of alcohol. Most regular and light beers contain less than 5 percent alcohol, whereas ice beer generally contains 5–6 percent alcohol. Do you think beer drinkers are choosing this beer for its reportedly rich flavor or simply because it contains more alcohol?

Nutritional Content: Empty Calories

The nutritional value of alcohol is extremely limited. Alcoholic beverages produced today through modern processing methods contain nothing but empty calories—about 100 calories per fluid ounce of 100-proof distilled spirits and about 150 calories per each 12-ounce bottle or can of beer. Therefore, alcohol consumption can significantly contribute to your weight and little else. Pure alcohol contains only simple carbohydrates; it has no vitamins and minerals, and no fats or protein.

Researchers have suggested that drinking red wine (no more than two glasses for men and one glass for women, daily) can increases levels of HDL cholesterol (the good cholesterol), reduce LDL (the bad cholesterol), and reduce blood clotting. This is because of the antioxidants in the flavonoids. Resveratrol, another antioxidant found in the skin of red grapes, is thought to help fight cancer, Alzheimer's disease, and Parkinson's disease.[3]

Physiological Effects of Alcohol Consumption

First and foremost, alcohol is classified as a drug—a very strong CNS depressant. The primary depressant effect of alcohol occurs in the brain and spinal cord. Many people think of alcohol as a stimulant because of the way most users feel after consuming a serving or two of their favorite drink. Any temporary sensations of jubilation, boldness, or relief are attributable to alcohol's ability as a depressant drug to release personal inhibitions and provide temporary relief from tension.

How Is Alcohol Absorbed in the Body?

Eighty percent of alcohol is absorbed by the small intestine, and the stomach absorbs the other 20 percent. Then the alcohol enters the bloodstream, where it is carried throughout the body to all the organs. More than 90 percent of the alcohol is **metabolized** in the liver. Less than 2 percent of alcohol is excreted unchanged through the skin, breath, and urine.

Factors That Influence the Absorption of Alcohol

The rate of **absorption** of alcohol is influenced by several factors, most of which can be controlled by the individual.

Type of Beverage and Circumstances of Consumption

- *Alcohol concentration.* The stronger the concentration of alcohol in the beverage, the more alcohol is absorbed. Also, carbonated liquids such as sodas or champagne speed up absorption, whereas water will dilute the concentration and slow the rate of absorption.[4]

- *Number of drinks consumed.* As more drinks are consumed, more alcohol is absorbed.

- *Speed of consumption.* If consumed rapidly, even relatively few drinks will result in a large

Alcohol is a strong central nervous system depressant. In social situations, it may appear to act as a stimulant because it depresses the inhibitory centers of the brain.

concentration gradient that leads to high blood alcohol concentration.

- *Presence of food.* Food can compete with alcohol for absorption into the bloodstream, thus slowing the absorption of alcohol. When you slow your alcohol absorption, your body can remove alcohol already in the bloodstream.

Individual Body Chemistry   Each person has an individual pattern of physiological functioning that may affect the ability to process alcohol. For example, in some conditions, such as that marked by "dumping syndrome," the stomach empties more rapidly than is normal, and alcohol seems to be absorbed more quickly. The emptying time may be either slowed or quickened by anger, fear, stress, nausea, and the condition of the stomach tissues.

Race/Ethnicity   Research suggests that alcohol tolerance levels may range from weak to strong based on an individual's race/ethnic origin. These ethnic differences may have a genetic link. Genetics may also help protect some Asians from developing alcoholism. About half of all Far East Asians produce low levels of an important enzyme that helps metabolize alcohol. These people cannot tolerate even small amounts of alcohol. In addition, genetic factors influencing the absorption rates of alcohol in the intestinal tract have been hypothesized to predispose some Native Americans to alcoholism. More research is needed about the role of genetic factors in all forms of chemical dependence.

Gender   Women absorb about 30 percent more alcohol into the bloodstream than men do, despite an identical number of drinks and equal body weight. The reason for this is that women produce much less alcohol dehydrogenase than men do.[4] This enzyme is responsible for

breaking down alcohol in the stomach—less alcohol dehydrogenase means more alcohol absorption.

Other reasons also help explain why women tend to absorb alcohol more quickly than do men of the same body weight: (1) Women have proportionately more body fat than men do. Since alcohol is not stored easily in fat, it enters the bloodstream relatively quickly. (2) Women's bodies have proportionately less water than do men's bodies of equal weight, thus consumed alcohol does not become as diluted as it does in men. (3) Alcohol absorption is influenced by a woman's menstrual cycle. Alcohol is more quickly absorbed during the premenstrual phase of a woman's cycle. Also, there is evidence that women using birth control pills absorb alcohol more quickly than usual.[5]

With the exception of a person's body chemistry, race/ethnicity, and gender, all factors that influence absorption can be moderated by the alcohol user.

Blood Alcohol Concentration   The amount of alcohol that can be metabolized is the same no matter how much alcohol is in the blood. This rate is about 0.25 to 0.30 ounce per hour. As previously mentioned, the activity of the enzyme alcohol dehydrogenase is the major factor in determining the rate of alcohol metabolism.[4] So doing things like drinking coffee or exercising have no effect on alcohol metabolism. A person's **blood alcohol concentration (BAC)** rises when alcohol is consumed faster than it can be removed (oxidized) by the liver.[6] A fairly predictable sequence of events takes place when a person drinks alcohol at a rate faster than one drink every hour. When the BAC reaches 0.05

Key Terms

fermentation A chemical process whereby plant products are converted into alcohol by the action of yeast cells on carbohydrate materials.

distillation The process of heating an alcohol solution and collecting its vapors into a more concentrated solution.

metabolism The chemical process by which substances are broken down or synthesized in a living organism to provide energy for life.

absorption The passage of nutrients or alcohol through the walls of the stomach or the intestinal tract into the bloodstream.

blood alcohol concentration (BAC) The percentage of alcohol in a measured quantity of blood; BAC can be determined directly, through the analysis of a blood sample, or indirectly, through the analysis of exhaled air.

Table 8.1 Blood Alcohol Concentration Effects*

Approx. No. Drinks per Hour	BAC (%)	Typical Effects
1	0.02	Relaxed, body feels warmer
2–3	0.05	Decreased inhibition, impaired judgment, less alert
4	0.08	Legally drunk, poor muscle coordination, impaired perception, difficulty detecting danger, slower response
5	0.10	Slurred speech, slowed thinking, poor coordination
7	0.15	Vomiting, loss of balance, less muscle control
9	0.20	Double vision, nausea, memory loss
14	0.30	Tremors, blackouts, lowered body temperature
18	0.40	Difficulty breathing, coma, possible death
22	0.50 and above	Death

Note: 1 drink = 1.5 ounces of liquor (80 proof), 5 ounces of wine, or 12 ounces of beer.

*Estimates are for a 160-pound man.

Source: From J. B. Wyngardener and L. H. Smith, *Cecil Textbook of Medicine*, 18th Ed. Copyright 1988 by Elsevier. Used with permission.

percent, initial measurable changes in mood and behavior take place. Inhibitions and everyday tensions appear to be released, while judgment and critical thinking are somewhat impaired. This BAC would be achieved by a 160-pound person drinking about two drinks in an hour (see Table 8.1).

At a level of 0.10 percent (one part alcohol to 1,000 parts blood), the drinker typically loses significant motor coordination. Voluntary motor function becomes quite clumsy. At this BAC, most states consider a drinker legally intoxicated and thus incapable of safely operating a vehicle. Although physiological changes associated with this BAC do occur, certain users do not feel drunk or appear impaired.

As a person continues to elevate the BAC from 0.20–0.50 percent, the health risk of **acute alcohol intoxication** increases rapidly. A BAC of 0.20 percent is characterized by the loud, boisterous, obnoxious drunk person who staggers. A 0.30 percent BAC produces further depression and stuporous behavior, during which time the drinker becomes so confused that he or she may not be capable of understanding anything. The 0.40 percent or 0.50 percent BAC produces unconsciousness. At this BAC a person can die, because brain centers that control body temperature, heartbeat, and respiration may virtually shut down.

An important factor influencing the BAC is the individual's blood volume. The larger the person, the greater the amount of blood into which alcohol can be distrib-

uted. Conversely, the smaller person has less blood into which alcohol can be distributed, and as a result, a higher BAC will develop. To find out what a BAC level would be for your age and gender and the type and number of alcoholic drinks, go to this website: www.healthstatus.com/calculate/bac.

Alcohol Oxidation: Sobering Up Alcohol is removed from the bloodstream principally through the process of **oxidation.** Oxidation occurs at a constant rate (about one-fourth to one-third ounce of pure alcohol per hour) that cannot be appreciably altered. Because each typical drink of beer, wine, or distilled spirits contains about one-half ounce of pure alcohol, it takes about 2 hours for the body to fully oxidize one typical alcoholic drink.[4]

After a night of drinking alcohol, the next morning people may experience uncomfortable symptoms such as headache, nausea, fatigue, diarrhea, loss of appetite, or an overall feeling of being sick. These symptoms are commonly known as a *hangover* and are the result of the body reacting to too much alcohol in its system. These symptoms may be intensified by dehydration, poor nutrition, an empty stomach, lack of sleep, poor health, or increased physical activity while drinking.

Although people have attempted to sober up by drinking hot coffee, taking cold showers, or exercising, the oxidation rate of alcohol is unaffected. Thus far the FDA has not approved any commercial product that can help people achieve sobriety. Since alcohol causes dehydration, rehydration and the passage of time remain the only effective way to sober up.

Alcohol Poisoning

Not everyone who goes to sleep, passes out, or even becomes unconscious after drinking has a high BAC. People who are already sleepy, have not eaten well, are sick, or are bored may drink a little alcohol and quickly fall asleep. However, people who drink heavily in a short time may be setting themselves up for an extremely unpleasant, toxic, potentially life-threatening experience because of their high BAC.

What are the danger signs of alcohol poisoning (also referred to as acute alcohol intoxication)? The first sign is **shock,** signaling that the body is not getting enough blood flow. The drinker will already have become unconscious. He or she cannot be aroused from a deep stupor. A person's BAC level can continue to rise even when she or he has stopped drinking, is sleeping, or is unconscious. The person will probably have a weak, rapid pulse (over 100 beats per minute). The skin will be cool and damp, and breathing will be increased to once every three or four seconds. These breaths may be shallow or deep but will certainly occur in an irregular pattern. The skin will be pale or bluish. (In a person with dark skin, these color changes will be more evident in the fingernail beds or in the mucous membranes inside the mouth or under the eyelids.) Whenever any of these signs are present, seek emergency medical help immediately. (See the box "Are You Ready for an Alcohol-Related Emergency?" for a summary of these signs.)

Involuntary regurgitation (vomiting) can be another potentially life-threatening emergency for a person who has drunk too much alcohol. When a drinker has consumed more alcohol than the liver can oxidize, the pyloric valve at the base of the stomach tends to close. Additional alcohol remains in the stomach. This alcohol irritates the lining of the stomach so much that involuntary muscle contractions force the stomach contents to flow back through the esophagus. By removing alcohol from the stomach, vomiting may be a life-saving mechanism for conscious drinkers.

An unconscious drinker who vomits, however, may be lying in such a position that the airway becomes obstructed with the vomitus from the stomach. This person is at great risk of dying from **asphyxiation.** As a first-aid measure, unconscious drinkers should always be rolled onto their sides to minimize the chance of airway obstruction. If you are with a person who is vomiting, make certain that his or her head is positioned lower than the rest of the body. This position minimizes the chance that vomitus will obstruct the air passages.

Also keep a close watch on anyone who passes out from drinking. Unfortunately, partygoers sometimes make the mistake of carrying these people to bed and then forgetting about them. You should do your best to monitor the physical condition of anyone who becomes unconscious from drinking because of the risk of death. If you really care about these people, you will observe them at regular intervals until they appear to be clearly out of danger. Although this may mean an evening of interrupted sleep for you, you might save someone's life.

Alcohol's Interaction with Other Drugs

Consuming alcohol when you have taken other drugs can change how these drugs normally act in your system. Some of these interactions, like those that occur when sedatives are taken with alcohol, can be potentially dangerous. Because sedatives and alcohol are both depressants, taken together they can induce coma, unconsciousness, and death. Anti-anxiety medications, the benzodiazepines, and antihistamines are also sedating and cause increased drowsiness. Alcohol taken with some antibiotics can cause nausea, vomiting, and seizures. Acetaminophen, such as Tylenol, can interact in a dangerous manner with alcohol, causing liver damage. Ibuprofen and aspirin can be taken with alcohol but may cause stomach upset. Antidepressants combined with alcohol can impair both mental and physical skills. The action of some antidepressants is increased with alcohol; others have decreased action when taken with alcohol. Antipsychotic medications, such as Thorazine, taken with alcohol can cause drowsiness, impaired coordination, and potentially fatal respiratory suppression. It is advisable to avoid consuming alcohol if taking any other type of drugs or medications.

Patterns of Alcohol Use

Although alcohol is a widely used drug, many people choose not to drink. Among drinkers, there is a great deal of variation in the amount and circumstances of their alcohol consumption. It is important to distinguish between light, responsible drinking and patterns of alcohol use that are potentially harmful in the short or long term.

Key Terms

acute alcohol intoxication A potentially fatal elevation of BAC, often resulting from heavy, rapid consumption of alcohol.

oxidation The process that removes alcohol from the bloodstream.

shock Profound collapse of many vital body functions; evident during acute alcohol intoxication and other serious health emergencies.

asphyxiation Death resulting from lack of oxygen to the brain.

have suffered from physical, sexual, or mental abuse, and may not want to deal with or think about their personal situation.

Following are some of the behaviors that a dysfunctional family typically experiences.[23] The family:

- Lives in fear and fears others different from them.
- Depends on family members to the exclusion of the outside world. An exception can be made for outsiders who are very similar to the family members.
- Believes that, to be successful, you must have money, make money, or marry into money.
- Believes that the authority figures in the family are always right.
- Teaches every member of the family to adapt to the emotional sickness present and feels threatened when a member attempts to recover.
- Teaches conditional love.
- Teaches that to have a worthwhile identity you must gain the approval of the outside world, and especially of the family itself.
- Feels threatened and abandoned at the death or departure of a member of the group.
- Tries to maintain the group through guilt and pity, which it calls "love."
- Expects all members to like the same things and people.
- Thrives on chaos and conflict and sees this as excitement.

As a result of these constant dysfunctional behaviors, the person living with an alcoholic can develop many of the following problems:

- Become isolated and afraid of people and authority figures.
- Become an approval-seeker and lose his or her identity in the process.
- Become frightened by angry people and any criticism.
- Become an alcoholic, marry one, or find another compulsive personality such as a workaholic to continue the sickness.
- Develop a victim mentality and be attracted by weakness in potential friends or loved ones.
- Have an extreme sense of responsibility and focus on others to the detriment of himself or herself.
- Feel guilty when being assertive or saying no.
- Become addicted to excitement.
- Confuse pity with love.
- Lose the ability to feel or express feelings.
- Be terrified of abandonment and be willing to tolerate abuse to hold on to a relationship.

- Develop all the symptoms of an alcoholic without actually drinking.

The good news is that many resources, such as recovery and support groups, are now available for both the alcoholic and those who live with the alcoholic. Those who have lived with an alcoholic will face their own issues as they work through their own recovery. They may find that they learned compulsions from the alcoholic, or they may transfer the compulsions to other behaviors, such as excessive eating, gambling, house cleaning, or taking up lost causes or people. Those who know, or are still living with, an active alcoholic also can consider intervention to urge the alcoholic to seek help.

Enabling   Problem drinkers and alcoholics frequently use the psychological defense mechanism of denial to maintain their drinking behavior. By convincing themselves that their lives are not affected by their drinking, problem drinkers and alcoholics are able to maintain their drinking patterns. A person's denial is an unconscious process that is apparent only to rational observers.

Formerly, alcoholics were required to admit that their denial was no longer effective before they could be admitted to a treatment program. This is not the case today. Currently, family members, friends, and coworkers of alcohol-dependent people are encouraged to intervene (with the help and supervision of a professional) and force an alcohol-dependent person into treatment.

During treatment, chemically dependent people must break through the security of denial and admit that alcohol controls their lives. This process is demanding and often time consuming, but there is no alternative path to recovery.

For family and friends of chemically dependent people, denial is part of a process known as *enabling*. In this process, people close to the problem drinker or alcoholic inadvertently support drinking behavior by denying that a problem really exists. Enablers unconsciously make excuses for the drinker, try to keep the drinker's work and family life intact, and in effect make the continued abuse of alcohol possible. For example, college students enable problem drinkers when they clean up a drinker's messy room, lie to professors about a student's class absences, and provide class notes or other assistance to a drinker who cannot perform academically. Even the use of designated drivers has been criticized as enabling behavior.

Alcohol counselors contend that enablers can significantly delay the onset of effective therapy. Do you know of a situation in which you or others have enabled a person with alcohol problems?

Codependence   A new term was coined in the 1980s to describe the relationship between drug-dependent people and those around them—*codependence*. This term implies a kind of dual addiction. The alcoholic and the person close to the alcoholic are both addicted, one to

Common Traits of Adult Children of Alcoholics

Adult children of alcoholics may:

- Have difficulty identifying normal behavior
- Have difficulty following a project from beginning to end
- Lie when it would be just as easy to tell the truth
- Judge themselves without mercy
- Have difficulty having fun
- Take themselves very seriously
- Have difficulty with intimate relationships

- Overreact to changes over which they have no control
- Constantly seek approval and affirmation
- Feel that they are different from other people
- Be super-responsible or super-irresponsible
- Be extremely loyal, even in the face of evidence that the loyalty is undeserved
- Tend to lock themselves into a course of action without considering the consequences

Experts agree that adult children of alcoholics who believe they have come to terms with their feelings can sometimes face lingering problems. Support groups to contact include Al-Anon (www.al-anon.alateen.org), Adult Children of Alcoholics (www.adultchildren.org), and Children of Alcoholics Foundation (www.coaf.org).

Source: JG Woititz, *Adult Children of Alcoholics,* Health Communications, Inc., 1990. Used with permission.

---

alcohol and the other to the alcoholic. People who are codependent often find themselves denying the addiction and enabling the alcohol-dependent person.

Unfortunately, this kind of behavior damages both the alcoholic and the codependent. The alcoholic's intervention and treatment may be delayed for a considerable time. Codependent people often pay a heavy price as well. They often become drug or alcohol dependent themselves, or they may suffer a variety of psychological consequences related to guilt, loss of self-esteem, depression, and anxiety. Codependents may be at increased risk for physical and sexual abuse.

Fortunately, researchers continue to explore this dimension of alcoholism. Many students have found some of the sources listed at the end of this chapter to be especially helpful. (To determine whether you could benefit from a support program such as Al-Anon or Alateen, answer the questions in the Personal Assessment "Does Someone's Drinking Trouble You?" at the end of this chapter.)

Adult Children of Alcoholic Parents In recent years a new dimension of alcoholism has been identified—the unusually high prevalence of alcoholism among adult children of alcoholics (ACOAs). It is estimated that these people are about four times more likely to develop alcoholism than are persons whose parents are not alcoholics. Even the ACOAs who do not become alcoholics may have a difficult time adjusting to everyday living. The box "Common Traits of Adult Children of Alcoholics" describes 13 traits that, to some degree, most ACOAs exhibit.

In response to this concern, support groups have been formed to prevent the adult sons and daughters of alcoholics from developing the condition that afflicted their parents. If a stronger link for an inherited genetic predisposition to alcoholism is found, these groups may play an even greater role in the prevention of alcoholism.

Women and Alcohol For decades, women have consumed less alcohol and had fewer alcohol-related problems than men. Evidence is mounting that a greater percentage of women are choosing to drink and that some subgroups of women, especially young women, are drinking more heavily. A greater number of admissions of women to treatment centers may also reflect that alcohol consumption among women is on the rise. Special approaches for women to use for staying sober are discussed in the box "Women and Alcohol."

Studies show that there are now almost as many female as male alcoholics. However, differences appear to exist between men and women when it comes to alcohol abuse.[20] Some of the more pronounced differences are: (1) More women than men can point to a specific triggering event, such as a divorce, death of a spouse, a career change, or children leaving home, that started them drinking heavily. (2) Alcoholism among women often starts later and progresses more quickly than alcoholism among men. (3) Women tend to be prescribed more mood-altering drugs than men are; thus, women face a greater risk of drug interaction or cross-tolerance. (4) Nonalcoholic men tend to divorce their alcoholic spouses nine times more often than nonalcoholic women divorce their alcoholic spouses; thus, alcoholic women are not as likely to have a family support system to aid them in their recovery attempts. (5) Female alcoholics do not tend to receive as much social support as men in their treatment and recovery. (6) Although men outnumber women entering treatment programs by almost four to one, women alcoholics tend to come into treatment earlier than men. (7) Women alcoholics are more likely than male alcoholics to have medical complications. This may result from the differences in the metabolism of alcohol between men and women. Women are particularly susceptible to diseases of the liver. (8) Unmarried or divorced single-parent women often have economic problems that

Learning from Our Diversity

Women and Alcohol

Do women drink for the same reasons men do? The research says no—there are some important differences in alcohol use for men and women. Women with low self-esteem are twice as likely to drink alcohol, whereas no such relationship exists for men. This was true for teenage girls as well as for college women. Women who were sexually or physically abused in childhood are much more likely than men to have alcohol-related problems. Peer pressure, a family history of alcohol abuse, and maternal drinking during pregnancy are more predictive of a likelihood to have alcohol problems for women than for men. Genetics plays a role to some degree in the variation between the genders; however, this does not account for all of these differences.

There are critical periods in women's lives where they are more likely to develop alcohol-related problems. For instance, more female college freshmen than female high school seniors reported binge drinking. Compared to men, women have more late-onset alcoholism (developing alcoholism after age 59). Life transitions, stressful life events, experiencing a crisis or a loss, loneliness, and boredom are triggers for women to develop problems with alcohol.

Because women have different triggers for their alcohol-related problems, they require different treatment approaches for alcohol treatment. We are now beginning to see specialized groups and treatment facilities that focus on women's issues related to alcohol abuse and dependence. One such group, Women for Sobriety (WFS), is a mutual aid organization for women with alcohol problems that was founded in 1975 by Dr. Jean Kirkpatrick. The WFS program focuses on improving self-esteem; members achieve sobriety by taking responsibility for their actions and by learning not to dwell on negative thoughts. Another alternative, Rational Recovery, is open to both men and women. RR, which is based on the theories of psychologist Albert Ellis's Rational Emotive Therapy, also uses a cognitive, nonspiritual approach that fosters cohesiveness and provides the emotional support sought by people who seek to gain and maintain sobriety.

Particularly for "marginalized" alcoholic women such as lesbians, members of racial and ethnic minorities, and those of non-Christian religious backgrounds, alcoholism treatment professionals increasingly are being encouraged to present the full range of support-group options, including but not emphasizing the approach of Alcoholics Anonymous.

Sources: Galanter M, et al. Rational recovery: Alternative to AA for addiction? *American Journal of Drug and Alcohol Abuse,* 1993, vol. 19, p. 499; Hall J, Lesbians' participation in Alcoholics Anonymous: Experience of social, personal, and political tensions, *Contemporary Drug Problems,* Spring 1996, vol. 23, no. 1, p. 113; Kaskutas L. A road less traveled: Choosing the "Women for Sobriety" program, *Journal of Drug Issues,* Winter 1996, vol. 26, no. 1, p. 77, Women for Sobriety, Inc. www.womenforsobriety.org/, March 10, 2005; California J, *Women Under the Influence,* Baltimore: Johns Hopkins University Press, 2006.

make entry into treatment programs especially difficult. In light of the generally recognized educational, occupational, and social gains made by women during the last two decades, it will be interesting to see whether these male-female differences continue.

Responsible Use of Alcohol

The responsible use of alcohol involves keeping your own drinking safe and moderate as well as being a responsible host. On a social and community level, we all need to be concerned about the messages sent about alcohol in both advertisements and public service announcements. A number of organizations work to prevent the potentially dangerous effects of alcohol use, including some that focus specifically on drinking among college students.

Becoming a Responsible Drinker

As you learned in Chapter 7, "Making Decisions about Drug Use," being able to decline drugs and alcohol when others around are using these substances is a challenge that you can learn to meet. For example, participating in a long bicycle ride or run can leave you with an excellent sense of well-being produced by endorphins, natural painkillers produced by the brain. Such a "high" is enhanced by the knowledge that you have earned the good feeling through your efforts. Consider some additional techniques for avoiding alcohol:

- Avoid parties where you can expect heavy drinking.
- Avoid people who are drinking heavily or becoming erratic or threatening.
- Request a nonalcoholic beer, soft drink, or glass of water instead of alcohol (see the box "Cool, Calm, and Collected").
- Participate in activities that can provide a nonchemical high. See the Personal Assessment at the end of Chapter 7 on page 234 for a variety of suggestions.
- Cultivate friends who find their highs through natural, positive activities in which you share an interest.

Hosting a Party Responsibly

Fortunately, an increasing awareness of the value of responsible party hosting seems to be spreading among college communities. The impetus for this awareness has come from various sources, including respect for an individual's right to choose not to drink alcohol, the growing recognition that many automobile crashes are alcohol related, and the legal threats posed by **host negligence.** Responsibly hosting parties at which alcohol is served is becoming a trend, especially among college-educated young adults. For guidelines for hosting a social event at which alcoholic beverages are served, see the box "Partying 101."

In addition to these suggestions, the use of a **designated driver** is an important component of responsible alcohol use. By planning to abstain from alcohol or to carefully limit their own alcohol consumption, designated drivers are able to safely transport friends who have been drinking. Designated drivers have indisputably saved many lives. However, there may be a downside. Some health professionals are concerned that the use of designated drivers allows the nondrivers to drink more heavily than they might otherwise. In effect, designated drivers "enable" drinkers to be less responsible for their own behavior. This freedom from responsibility might eventually lead to further problems for the drinkers.

 TALKING POINTS Have you noticed an increased use of designated drivers in your community? Would you be willing to be a designated driver?

Organizations That Support Responsible Drinking

The serious consequences of the irresponsible use of alcohol have led to the formation of a number of concerned-citizen groups. Although each organization has a unique approach, all attempt to deal objectively with two indisputable facts: alcohol use is part of our society, and irresponsible alcohol use can be deadly.

> **Key Terms**
>
> **host negligence** A legal term that reflects the failure of a host to provide reasonable care and safety for people visiting the host's residence or business.
>
> **designated driver** A person who abstains from or carefully limits alcohol consumption to be able to safely transport other people who have been drinking.

Mothers Against Drunk Driving is one of many organizations working against the irresponsible use of alcohol.

Mothers Against Drunk Driving Mothers Against Drunk Driving (MADD) is a national network of over 600 local chapters in the United States and Canada. This organization attempts to educate people about alcohol's effects on driving and to influence legislation and enforcement of laws related to drunk drivers. For more information about MADD, visit its website at www.madd.org.[17]

Students Against Destructive Decisions Many students have known the acronym *SADD* to stand for the youth group Students Against Driving Drunk or Students Against Destructive Decisions. Recently, the group has restructured itself to expand beyond drunk driving to include other high-risk activities that are detrimental to youth, such as underage drinking, drug use, drugged driving, and failure to use seat belts. Founded in 1981, this organization now has millions of members in thousands of chapters throughout the country. Remaining central to the drunk driving aspect of SADD is the "Contract for Life," a pact that encourages students and parents to provide safe transportation for each other if either is unable to drive safely after consuming alcohol. This contract also stipulates that no discussions about the incident are to be started until both can talk in a calm and caring manner. For more information about SADD, visit its website at www.saddonline.com.[24]

BACCHUS and GAMMA Peer Education Network BACCHUS (Boost Alcohol Consciousness Concerning the Health of University Students) began in 1975 as an alcohol-awareness organization at the University of Florida. Run by student volunteers, this organization promoted responsible drinking among college students who chose to drink. It was not an anti-alcohol group, but a "harm reduction" group. Over the years, hundreds of chapters were formed on campuses across the country.

When supporters of BACCHUS realized that many students interested in alcohol awareness were from fraternities and sororities, they developed GAMMA (Greeks Advocating Mature Management of Alcohol) to join BACCHUS to form a peer education network. Campuses are now able to choose BACCHUS, GAMMA, or any other acronym or name for their groups.

With the broadening of the original BACCHUS organization has come an expansion of the health issues this group addresses. Originally, the focus was on alcohol abuse and prevention. Now the BACCHUS and GAMMA Peer Education Network confronts a variety of student health and safety issues. For additional information about this organization, check out its website at www.bacchusgamma.org.[25]

Other Approaches Other responsible approaches to alcohol use are surfacing nearly every day. Even among college fraternity organizations, attitudes toward the indiscriminate use of alcohol are changing. Most fraternity rush functions are now conducted without the use of alcohol, and growing numbers of fraternities are alcohol-free.

Another encouraging sign on college campuses is the increasing number of alcohol use task forces. Although each of these groups has its own focus and title, many are meeting to discuss alcohol-related concerns on their particular campus. These task forces often try to formulate detailed, comprehensive policies for alcohol use across the entire campus community.

Alcohol Advertising

Every few years, careful observers can see subtle changes in the ways the alcoholic beverage industry markets its products. Recently, the marketing push appears to be directed toward minorities (through advertisements for malt liquor and fortified wines), women (through wine and wine cooler ads), and youth (through trendy, young adult-oriented commercials). See the box "Do Alcohol Ads Target Young People—and Does It Matter?" for more on the issue of targeted marketing campaigns.

On the college campus, aggressive alcohol campaigns have used rock stars, beach party scenes, athletic

Do Alcohol Ads Target Young People—and Does It Matter?

Recent studies have shown that television and radio advertisements have a disproportionate amount of alcohol ads aimed at youth (defined as 12- to 20-year-olds) compared to any other age group. Youths drink alcohol more than they smoke or use other drugs, so there is a growing concern that these ads are contributing to an increase in underage drinking. Researchers at the Center on Alcohol Marketing and Youth (CAMY) evaluated the placement of radio and television advertisements for the most-advertised U.S. alcohol brands. They found that alcohol advertising is common on programs that have disproportionately large youth audiences. In addition, this advertising accounts for a substantial proportion of all alcohol radio advertising heard by underage youth. This contradicts the alcohol industry's voluntary standard to not advertise alcohol on radio or television programs that have an audience that is 30 percent or more youth. This study also found that almost half of the 67,404 alcohol ads were placed in youth-oriented programming. In 2005, 8 percent of alcohol ads on television were aired on programming with underage audiences, down from 11 percent in 2001. Most of these were on cable channels.

Does it really make a difference if youth are exposed to ads selling alcohol? Yes. Studies show that, compared to people who started drinking later in their lives, people who start drinking before age 15 are 4 times more likely to become alcohol dependent, 7 times more likely to be involved in an alcohol-related motor vehicle crash, and at least 10 times more likely to experience alcohol-related violence at some point in their lives. Numerous studies have shown that the more alcohol advertising young people are exposed to, the more likely they are to drink or drink more.

The National Research Council and the Institute of Medicine (NRC/IOM) recommend that the alcohol industry voluntarily restrict its advertising to programs for which the audience is 25 percent or less youth, with the goal of decreasing this to programs with 15 percent or less youth instead of its current 30 percent threshold. The Federal Trade Commission (FTC) reviewed the alcohol industry's efforts at self-regulation of its marketing practices in 1999 and 2003, and will examine their efforts again in 2007. If the alcohol industry does not start complying with its own standards, the FTC may begin efforts to force them to do so.

Sources: "CAMY: Alcohol Ads on the Radio Continue to Reach Youth," Georgetown University, September 2006; The Center for Alcohol Marketing for Youth, Georgetown University Executive Summary, "Still Growing After All These Years: Youth Exposure to Alcohol Advertising on Television, 2001–2005," December 2006.

event sponsorships, and colorful newspaper supplements to encourage the purchase of alcohol. Critics claim that most of the collegiate advertising is directed at minors and that the prevention messages are not strong enough to offset the potential health damage to this population. As a college student, how do you feel about alcohol advertising on your campus? If you are a nontraditional-age student, do you find the advertising campaigns amusing or potentially dangerous?

Some beer and liquor companies have begun using websites on the Internet to promote their products. Critics contend that the colorful graphics, hip language, games, chat rooms, and "virtual bars" are designed to recruit underage drinkers.

Alcohol Advertising in Ethnic Communities A literature review by the Trauma Foundation at San Francisco General Hospital[26] reports some interesting facts concerning alcohol availability and alcohol advertising in ethnic communities. In the United States, low-income Latino and African American communities have a disproportionate number of alcohol outlets compared to white communities. This concentration of alcohol outlets seems to be related to an increase in traffic injuries and assaults. Additionally, as the number of alcohol outlets increases, the likelihood of increased crime and violence rises. Crime and violence drive out existing business establishments and discourage new businesses from locating in the area. Economic development can become thwarted.

The Trauma Foundation also reports that alcohol is more heavily advertised in low-income African American and Latino communities than in other neighborhoods. The advertisements are found on billboards as well as the displays inside and around the alcohol outlets. Advertising frequently exploits important cultural symbols, and promotions are targeted toward specific ethnic groups. For example, malt liquor is marketed especially to African Americans. Thus, rap singers are frequently featured in promotions and advertisements for malt liquor.

Alcohol Prevention Messages

The first successful national campaign against drunk driving, "Designated Driver," began in 1998. Besides targeting specific audiences and using well-timed and strategically placed public service announcements, its developers convinced TV producers and writers to work references to the designated driver into the dialogue of their shows. Gradually, the message got through to young people.

In contrast, the "Campaign for Alcohol Free Kids" relied heavily on dramatic graphics, such as grisly photos

Acupuncture as Treatment for Alcoholism

For over 30 years, practitioners have used acupuncture to treat patients coping with alcohol and other substance abuse. The discovery of the connection between drug addiction and acupuncture began in the early 1970s, when a neurosurgeon in South China was preparing a patient for surgery by using acupuncture as a preoperative procedure. The patient, who was experiencing opium withdrawal symptoms, reported to the physician that the acupuncture made his symptoms go away.

Acupuncturists began using their tiny needles for detoxification from tobacco, alcohol, and other drug addictions. Acupuncture today is seen as an adjunct to other therapeutic programs. Thus, it is used in combination with 12-step programs and individual counseling.

Acupuncture can produce many physical and mental changes in a patient. Among these changes are relief of the physical symptoms of withdrawal, including body aches, cravings, headache, nausea, sweating, and muscle cramps. Acupuncture also provides relief from depression, anxiety, and insomnia. These body changes permit the patient to be relaxed, comfortable, and more receptive to counseling and treatment protocols. Acupuncture can be used safely on an outpatient basis and is a "drug-free" form of treatment.

Most commonly, five acupuncture needles are placed in each of the patient's outer ears. The needles are positioned at specific points that correspond to the lungs, liver, kidneys, and nervous system, and one needle is placed at a point that produces relaxation. While the patient quietly rests and meditates for about 45 minutes, the needles produce the release of endorphins, known neurotransmitters that produce feelings of pleasure. This pleasure reduces cravings, eases withdrawal symptoms, and promotes relaxation. The desire for alcohol and/or other drugs decreases.

The benefits from acupuncture can be noticed immediately for some persons. For others, it may take multiple sessions before they begin to see improvement. A typical treatment regimen recommends daily treatment sessions for 2 weeks, then three treatments each week for several weeks, followed by weekly treatments. Additional treatments are recommended if the client experiences a relapse or major emotional setback.

Over 100 drug treatment centers in the United States are presently offering acupuncture as an optional, valuable form of complementary medicine. Some insurance companies are even covering the costs of acupuncture treatment in their policies. With the rapid growth of alternative and complementary medicine being used in the United States, it is likely that more drug clinics will start using acupuncture as an adjunct to traditional alcohol and drug treatments.

Sources: Otto K. Acupuncture and substance abuse: A synopsis, with indications for further research. *The American Journal on Addictions/American Academy of Psychiatrists in Alcoholism and Addictions* 1, 43–51, 2003; Acupuncture treatment for substance abuse. www.acupuncture.com, June 19, 2003; Woititz JG, *Adult Children of Alcoholics,* Health Communications, Inc., 1990.

of car crash scenes on prom night.[27] Although the overall visual impact was powerful, the campaign lacked a practical element. Worse, the ads seemed to be preaching.

The Ad Council's "Friends Don't Let Friends Drive Drunk" is based on the idea that we all have responsibility for one another. If someone is your friend, you want to take care of that person, so don't let your friend do something dangerous.

The "You Drink & Drive, You Lose" campaign, a part of the National Public Education Campaign, targets two high-risk groups, 21- to 34-year-olds and repeat offenders. The message is simple: make the right choice—don't drink and drive. The "Don't Lose It!" TV spot focuses on the fact that it's inconvenient to be stopped, but the time spent at the checkpoint is for your own safety. It seems to be saying: "Sure, you're in a hurry, but this is important, so be patient." The graphics range from a serious-looking police officer talking to a motorist to hands locked in handcuffs.

What the successful campaigns have in common is a message that is simple, believable, and acceptable. Rather than scolding or preaching, the ads emphasize the fact that you have a choice and ask you to make the right one.

Treatment for Alcohol Problems

Similar to the treatment approaches for drug use described in Chapter 7, treatments for problem drinking, alcohol abuse, and alcohol dependence can involve outpatient individual counseling, group counseling, intensive outpatient treatment, or even nontraditional approaches (see the box "Acupuncture as Treatment for Alcoholism"). In-patient hospitalization may be required for those with alcohol dependence, particularly in addressing the physical withdrawal symptoms. Counseling focuses on understanding the triggers and high-risk situations and developing healthier ways of coping with stress and life's problems. However, alcohol recovery can often require lifestyle changes as well, including finding new friends, social activities, and habits, drinking soda or water if at a bar, playing golf or watching sports without drinking, and rewarding yourself with something other than a drink when relaxing at the end of a long week.

Often people who have been in treatment are considered in recovery rather than cured. This comes from a belief that once an alcoholic, always an alcoholic, as the individual can never drink alcohol without risking relapse. There is another philosophy about treatment,

The Spiritual Component in Alcoholics Anonymous

Alcoholics Anonymous (AA) is a self-help support group for people with problems with alcohol. It was started by Bill Wilson and Dr. Robert Smith in 1935, who were recovering alcoholics themselves. Together they also wrote the "Big Book," a 400-page book outlining the 12 steps to recovery. These steps include acknowledging you have no control over your alcohol use, asking for help, admitting your imperfections, confessing to the damage you have caused other people as a result of your alcohol use, making amends where harm has been done, and working with others who want to recover. Fellowship and "spiritual awakening" are important components of this program.

Following are the 12 steps that AA believes an individual must go through to gain sobriety:

1. We admitted we were powerless over alcohol—that our lives had become unmanageable.
2. Came to believe that a Power greater than ourselves could restore us to sanity.
3. Made a decision to turn our will and our lives over to the care of God as we understood Him.
4. Made a searching and fearless moral inventory of ourselves.
5. Admitted to God, to ourselves and to another human being the exact nature of our wrongs.
6. Were entirely ready to have God remove all these defects of character.
7. Humbly asked Him to remove our shortcomings.
8. Made a list of all persons we had harmed, and became willing to make amends to them all.
9. Made direct amends to such people wherever possible, except when to do so would injure them or others.
10. Continued to take personal inventory and when we were wrong promptly admitted it.
11. Sought through prayer and meditation to improve our conscious contact with God as we understood Him, praying only for knowledge of His will for us and the power to carry that out.
12. Having had a spiritual awakening as the result of these steps, we tried to carry this message to alcoholics, and to practice these principles in all our affairs.

As you can see, 6 of the 12 steps refer to *God*, and there are religious references and overtones throughout the steps. While AA does have roots in evangelical Christianity, the modern-day AA groups claim that it is a nonreligious organization and is not affiliated with any specific religion. AA certainly has a spiritual component, but people can choose their own definitions of their greater power, including their own personal power or the power of the AA group.

Abstaining from alcohol, finding support with a group of people who share similar struggles, taking an honest introspective look into one's flaws, and finding ways to make peace within oneself and with others are part of the AA process of spiritual awakening. AA has helped millions of people recover from alcoholism, and AA groups are found all over the world.

Source: The Twelve Steps are reprinted with permission of Alcoholics Anonymous World Services, Inc. Permission to reprint the Twelve Steps does not mean that A.A.W.S. has reviewed or approved the contents of this publication or that A.A.W.S. necessarily agrees with the views expressed herein. A.A. is a program of recovery from alcoholism only—use of the Twelve Steps in connection with programs and activities which are patterned after A.A., but which address other problems, or in any other non-A.A. context, does not imply otherwise.

called the Marlatt method, that suggests that people with alcoholism or alcohol-related problems can decrease their drinking to a moderate level and don't have to abstain from alcohol to recover. There is debate about which method is more effective.

Helping the Alcoholic: Rehabilitation and Recovery

When an alcoholic realizes that alcoholism is not a form of moral weakness but rather a clearly defined illness, the chances for recovery are remarkably good. It is estimated that as many as two-thirds of alcoholics can recover. Recovery is especially improved when the addicted person has a good emotional support system, including concerned family members, friends, and employer. When this support system is not well established, the alcoholic's chances for recovery are considerably lower.

Alcoholics Anonymous (AA) is a voluntary support group of recovering alcoholics who meet regularly to help one another get and stay sober. There are over 100,000 groups in 150 countries worldwide.[28] AA encourages alcoholics to admit their lack of power over alcohol and to turn their lives over to a higher power (although the organization is nonsectarian; see the box "The Spiritual Component in Alcoholics Anonymous"). Members of AA are encouraged not to be judgmental about the behavior of other members. They support anyone with a problem caused by alcohol.

Al-Anon and Alateen are parallel organizations that give support to people who live with alcoholics. Al-Anon is geared toward spouses and other relatives, whereas Alateen focuses on children of alcoholics. Both organizations help members realize that they are not alone and that successful adjustments can be made to nearly every situation. AA, Al-Anon, and Alateen chapter organizations are usually listed in the telephone book or in the classified sections of local newspapers. You can locate Al-Anon and Alateen on the Web at www.al-anon.alateen.org.[29]

For people who feel uncomfortable with the concept that their lives are controlled by a higher power, secular recovery programs are becoming popular. These programs maintain that sobriety comes from within the alcoholic. Secular programs strongly emphasize self-reliance, self-determination, and rational thinking about one's drinking. Secular Organizations for Sobriety (SOS) and Rational Recovery are examples of secular recovery programs.

Medical Treatment for Alcoholism

Could there be a medical cure for alcoholism? For nearly 50 years, the only prescription drug physicians could use to help drinkers stop drinking was antabuse. Antabuse would cause drinkers to become extremely nauseated whenever they used alcohol.

In 1995 the Food and Drug Administration approved a drug called naltrexone that works by reducing the craving for alcohol and the pleasurable sensations felt when drinking. Combining naltrexone with conventional behavior modification has been shown to reduce alcohol relapse significantly.

Taking Charge of Your Health

- Determine whether you are affected by someone's drinking by doing the Personal Assessment "Does someone's drinking trouble you?" at the end of this chapter.

- Review the box "Are You Ready for an Alcohol-Related Emergency?"

- Assess your level of social responsibility by reviewing the box "Partying 101."

- If you think that you are a problem drinker or an alcoholic, join a support group to get help.

- Enter into a "Contract for Life" with your parents or closest friends, a pact that says that you will provide safe transportation for one another if any of you are unable to drive safely after consuming alcohol.

- Make a commitment to responsible alcohol use by joining a campus group that works toward this goal.

SUMMARY

- As BAC rises, predictable depressant effects take place, and the risk of acute alcohol intoxication increases; people with this condition are in danger and must receive first aid immediately.
- Federal legislation has pushed all states to lower the legal BAC standard to 0.08 percent.
- Alcohol is removed from the bloodstream through the process of oxidation.
- Chronic alcohol use causes a variety of serious health problems for the drinker and can cause fetal alcohol syndrome in infants when a woman drinks during pregnancy.
- Alcohol-related social problems include accidents (motor vehicle crashes, falls, drownings, and fires and burns), crime and violence, and suicide.

- Problem drinking is an alcohol use pattern in which a drinker's behavior creates personal difficulties or problems for others.
- Alcoholism or alcohol dependence is a primary, chronic disease characterized by addiction to alcohol; it has a variety of possible causes and manifestations.
- Enabling is a behavior pattern in which people close to the problem drinker or alcoholic make the continued use of alcohol possible by keeping the drinker's work and family life intact.
- Alcoholics Anonymous and other support groups can help an alcoholic recover from the disease.
- The drugs antabuse and naltrexone are sometimes prescribed to discourage alcohol use.

REVIEW QUESTIONS

1. What is the definition of an alcoholic drink?
2. What is binge drinking?
3. What is meant by the term *proof*?
4. What is the nutritional value of alcohol? How do "light" and low-alcohol beverages compare?
5. Identify and explain the various factors that influence the absorption of alcohol. Why is it important to be aware of these factors?
6. What is BAC? Describe the general sequence of physiological events that takes place when a person drinks alcohol at a rate faster than the liver can oxidize it.

7. What are the signs and symptoms of acute alcohol intoxication? What are the first-aid steps you should take to help a person with this problem?
8. Describe the characteristics of fetal alcohol syndrome and fetal alcohol effects.
9. Explain the differences between problem drinking, alcohol abuse, and alcoholism.
10. List some ways you can keep alcohol consumption under control.

ANSWERS TO THE "WHAT DO YOU KNOW?" QUIZ

1. True   2. False   3. False   4. True   5. False   6. True   7. False

As We Go to Press

College Binge Drinking on the Rise

Despite the increased efforts on college campuses to educate students about the risks of drug and alcohol abuse, college students have higher rates of drug and alcohol abuse than are found in the general population. A recent study found that 23 percent of college students meet the criteria for alcohol or drug abuse or dependence compared to 8.5 percent of the general population. Half of all college students abuse drugs or binge-drink at least once a month. Eighty-three percent of all recent arrests involving college students also involved alcohol, as compared to 23 percent of arrests in 2001. Caucasian students have higher rates than those found in the minority student population.

Why have drug abuse and alcohol abuse increased over the past few years? Some say there are not enough college administrators to give enough attention or resources to this issue. But the majority of college administrators reported in this study that they thought the responsibility for preventing alcohol and drug abuse lies with students. What do you think?

Sources: College drug use, binge drinking rise, *USA Today*, March 15, 2007; National Center on Addiction and Substance Abuse at Columbia University, *Wasting the Best and the Brightest: Substance Abuse at America's Colleges and Universities*, March 2007, www.casacolumbia.org.

ENDNOTES

1. U.S. Department of Health and Human Services. *Alcohol and Health: Tenth Special Report to the U.S. Congress*, NIH Publication No. 00-1583. Washington, DC: U.S. Government Printing Office, 2000.
2. Zest for Life. *Alcohol and Ethanol Information Page*, www.anyvitamins.com/alcohol-ethanol-info.htm, March 9, 2005.
3. Gaziano JM, et al. Light-to-moderate alcohol consumption and mortality in the Physicians' Health Study enrollment cohort. *Journal of the American College of Cardiology*, 35(1), 2000, 96–105.
4. Ksir C, Hart C, Oakley R. *Drugs, Society and Human Behavior*. 12th ed. New York: McGraw-Hill, 2008.
5. Be Responsible About Drinking. *Women and Alcohol*, www.brad21.org/alcohol_and_women.html, March 9, 2005.
6. Pinger RR, et al. *Drugs: Issues for Today* (3rd ed.). New York: McGraw-Hill, 1998.
7. U.S. Bureau of the Census. *Statistical Abstract of the United States, 1999* (199th ed.). Washington, DC: U.S. Government Printing Office, 1999.
8. Substance Abuse and Mental Health Services Administration. (2006). *Results from the 2005 National Survey on Drug Use and Health: National Findings* (Office of Applied Studies, NSDUH Series H-30, DHHS Publication No. SMA 06-4194). Rockville, MD.
9. American College Health Association Spring 2006 Survey, *Journal of American College Health* 55 (January–February 2007).
10. Brown SA, Tapert SF, Granholm E, et al. Neurocognitive functioning of adolescents: Effects of protracted alcohol use, *Alcoholism, Clinical and Experimental Research*, 24(2), 2000, 164–171.
11. ADA: Division of Drug and Alcohol Abuse. *As a Matter of Fact . . . Fetal Alcohol Syndrome*, www.well.com/user/woa/fsfas.htm, March 9, 2005.
12. Morse RM, et al. The definition of alcoholism, *JAMA* 1992; 268(8): 1012–1014.
13. Burns M. *Delirium Tremens*, emedicine.com, Inc., November 8, 2004.
14. *Diagnostic and Statistical Manual of Mental Disorders*, 4th ed. Washington DC: American Psychiatric Association, 2000.
15. National Institute on Alcohol Abuse and Alcoholism. *Tenth Special Report to the U.S. Congress on Alcohol and Health*, Chapter 6. NIH Publication No. 00-1583. Rockville, MD: U.S. Department of Health and Human Services, 2000.
16. Traffic Safety Facts 2003: *Alcohol*. U.S. Department of Transportation National Highway Traffic Safety Administration.
17. Mothers Against Drunk Driving. *About Us*, www.madd.org, March 9, 2005.
18. The Trauma Foundation. *Alcohol and Unintentional Injury: A Brief Review of the Literature*, www.tf.org/tf/alcohol/ariv/reviews/injurev5.html, June 16, 2003.
19. USLA Lifeguards for Life. *Training Guide for USLA Safety Tips: General Information on Drowning*, www.usla.org/ PublicInfo/Safety_guide.shtml, June 16, 2003.
20. Kinney J. *Loosening the Grip: A Handbook of Alcohol Information* (7th ed.). New York: McGraw-Hill, 2003.
21. Vaughn C. *Children of Alcoholics: At Risk for Family Violence*. U.S. Department of Health and Human Services and SAMHSA's National Clearinghouse for Alcohol and Drug Information, February 10, 2003.
22. *Facts about Suicide*. Centers for Disease Control and Prevention, National Center for Health Statistics, 1998.
23. Adult Children Educational Foundation Computer Bulletin Board. *Sick Families*, www.recovery.org/acoa/families.html, December 24, 1997.
24. SADD History. *Students Against Drunk Driving*, www.saddonline.com, March 1, 2005.
25. Organization History and Mission. The BACCHUS and GAMMA Peer Education Network, www.bacchusgamma. org/, March 1, 2005.
26. Trauma Foundation at San Francisco General Hospital. *The Effects of Alcohol on Different Ethnic Communities: Fact Sheet*, www.tf.org/tf/alcohol/ariv/facts/ethfct25.html, June 20, 2003.
27. Campaign for Alcohol Free Kids: Who We Are, www.alcoholfreekids.com Ad Council, March 8, 2005.
28. Alcoholics Anonymous. *AA At a Glance*, www.alcoholics-anonymous.org, March 1, 2005.
29. Al-Anon/Alateen Web Site Information, www.al-anon.alateen.org/, March 1, 2005.

Personal Assessment

How do you use alcoholic beverages?

Answer the following questions about your own alcohol use. Record your number of yes and no responses at the end of the questionnaire.

Do you:	Yes	No
1. Drink more often than you did a year ago?	_____	_____
2. Drink more heavily than you did a year ago?	_____	_____
3. Plan to drink, sometimes days in advance?	_____	_____
4. Gulp or "chug" your drinks, perhaps in a contest?	_____	_____
5. Set personal limits on the amount you plan to drink but then consistently disregard these limits?	_____	_____
6. Drink at a rate greater than one drink per hour?	_____	_____
7. Encourage or even pressure others to drink with you?	_____	_____
8. Frequently want a nonalcoholic beverage but then end up drinking an alcoholic drink?	_____	_____
9. Drive your car while under the influence of alcohol or ride with another person who has been drinking?	_____	_____
10. Use alcoholic beverages while taking prescription or OTC medications?	_____	_____
11. Forget what happened while you were drinking?	_____	_____
12. Have a tendency to disregard information about the effects of drinking?	_____	_____
13. Feel embarrassed because of your alcohol use?	_____	_____
TOTAL	_____	_____

Interpretation

If you answered yes to any of these questions, you may be using alcohol irresponsibly. Two or more yes responses indicate an unacceptable pattern of alcohol use and may reflect problem drinking behavior.

TO CARRY THIS FURTHER . . .

Ask your friends or roommates to take this assessment. Are they willing to take this assessment and then talk about their results with you? Be prepared to discuss any follow-up questions they might have about their (or your) alcohol consumption patterns. Your willingness to talk about drinking behavior might help someone realize that this topic can and should be discussed openly. Finally, be aware of how people in your area can get professional help with drinking or other drug concerns.

Use the space below to write down important phone numbers where you can find alcohol-related assistance for you or your friends and relatives.

_____

_____

_____

_____

_____

_____

_____

_____

_____

Personal Assessment

Does someone's drinking trouble you?

The following questions are designed to help you decide whether you are affected by someone's drinking and could benefit from a program such as Al-Anon. Record your number of yes and no responses on the total lines at the end of the questionnaire.

	Yes	No
1. Do you worry about how much someone else drinks?	_____	_____
2. Do you have money problems because of someone else's drinking?	_____	_____
3. Do you tell lies to cover up for someone else's drinking?	_____	_____
4. Do you feel that if the drinker loved you, he or she would stop drinking to please you?	_____	_____
5. Do you blame the drinker's behavior on his or her friends?	_____	_____
6. Are plans frequently upset or meals delayed because of the drinker?	_____	_____
7. Do you make threats, such as "If you don't stop drinking, I'll leave you"?	_____	_____
8. Do you secretly try to smell the drinker's breath?	_____	_____
9. Are you afraid to upset someone for fear it will set off a drinking bout?	_____	_____
10. Have you been hurt or embarrassed by a drinker's behavior?	_____	_____
11. Are holidays and gatherings spoiled because of someone's drinking?	_____	_____
12. Have you considered calling the police for help in fear of abuse?	_____	_____
13. Do you search for hidden alcohol?	_____	_____
14. Do you often ride in a car with a driver who has been drinking?	_____	_____
15. Have you refused social invitations out of fear or anxiety that the drinker will cause a scene?	_____	_____
16. Do you sometimes feel like a failure when you think of the lengths to which you have gone to control the drinker?	_____	_____
17. Do you think that if the drinker stopped drinking, your other problems would be solved?	_____	_____
18. Do you ever threaten to hurt yourself to scare the drinker?	_____	_____
19. Do you feel angry, confused, or depressed most of the time?	_____	_____
20. Do you feel there is no one who understands your problems?	_____	_____
TOTAL	_____	_____

Interpretation

If you answered yes to three or more of these questions, Al-Anon or Alateen may be able to help. You can contact Al-Anon or Alateen by looking in your local telephone directory or by writing to Al-Anon Family Group Headquarters, Inc., 1600 Corporate Landing Parkway, Virginia Beach, VA 23454–5617, or you may call (888) 4AL-ANON.

TO CARRY THIS FURTHER . . .

Sometimes the decision to seek help from a support group is a difficult one. If you answered yes to any of the questions above, spend a few moments reflecting on your responses. How long have you been experiencing problems because of someone else's drinking? How would sharing your feelings with others—people who have dealt with very similar problems—help you cope with your own situation? Knowing you're not alone can often be a great relief; it's up to you to take the first step.

Source: From *Are You Troubled by Someone's Drinking?* 1980, by Al-Anon Family Group Headquarters, Inc. Reprinted by permission of Al-Anon Family Group Headquarters, Inc.

Rejecting Tobacco Use

What Do You Know about Tobacco Use?

◉ Until recently there was an inverse relationship between the level of education completed and the level of cigarette smoking. True or False?

◉ Internal documents of the tobacco industry demonstrate that the tobacco industry neither knew of the health risks associated with its products nor intentionally marketed its products to young adolescents. True or False?

◉ Nicotine dependency is easily (and quickly) established in the majority of people who begin cigarette use. True or False?

◉ Carbon dioxide, produced during the combustion of tobacco, is the gaseous element in tobacco smoke that reduces the oxygen-carrying capacity of the blood. True or False?

◉ When homicide and suicide are removed from death-related statistics, the life expectancy of smokers is virtually the same as that of their nonsmoking peers. True or False?

◉ When assessed at the end of one year, well over half of the people who successfully completed a 10- to 12-week smoking cessation program will still be tobacco-free. True or False?

◉ In public places, today's smokers are more likely to be asking, "Where can I smoke?" rather than "Where can't I smoke?" True or False?

Check your answers at the end of the chapter.

Tobacco Use in American Society

If you were to visit certain businesses, entertainment spots, or sporting events in your community, you might leave convinced that virtually every adult is a tobacco user. Certainly, for some segments of society, tobacco use is the rule rather than the exception. You may be quite surprised, however, to find out that the great majority of adults do not use tobacco products.

Table 9.1 displays current cigarette smoking by males and females for each state.[1] Note that Kentucky, a major tobacco-producing state, has the highest percentage of smokers (28.7 percent), whereas

Table 9.1 Current Cigarette Smoking by Sex and State: 2005

[In percent. Current cigarette smoking is defined as persons who reported having smoked 100 or more cigarettes during their lifetime and who currently smoke every day or some days. Based on the Behavioral Risk Factor Surveillance System, a telephone survey of health behaviors of the civilian, noninstitutionalized U.S. population, 18 years old and over; for details, see source]

State/Area	Males	Females	Total	State/Area	Males	Females	Total	State/Area	Males	Females	Total
Alabama	29.5	20.5	24.8	Louisiana	24.6	20.6	22.6	Oklahoma	26.5	23.8	25.1
Alaska	27.9	22.0	25.0	Maine	22.4	19.5	20.9	Oregon	20.6	16.5	18.5
Arizona	22.0	18.8	20.4	Maryland	19.7	18.4	19.0	Pennsylvania	25.0	22.5	23.7
Arkansas	25.2	21.9	23.5	Massachusetts	18.1	18.0	18.1	Puerto Rico	18.1	8.7	13.1
California	19.2	11.3	15.2	Michigan	24.1	20.2	22.1	Rhode Island	19.4	20.1	19.8
Colorado	21.6	18.1	19.9	Minnesota	21.0	19.1	20.0	South Carolina	25.3	20.1	22.6
Connecticut	16.9	16.2	16.5	Mississippi	25.9	21.7	23.7	South Dakota	20.4	19.2	19.8
Delaware	22.5	19.0	20.7	Missouri	24.9	22.1	23.4	Tennessee	29.3	24.5	26.8
District of Columbia	22.9	17.6	20.1	Montana	19.3	19.1	19.2	Texas	23.3	16.8	20.0
Florida	24.8	18.7	21.6	Nebraska	23.4	19.2	21.3	Utah	13.7	9.3	11.5
Georgia	25.0	19.4	22.2	Nevada	25.2	20.9	23.1	U.S. Virgin Islands	10.7	6.1	8.3
Hawaii	19.3	15.0	17.1	New Hampshire	20.4	20.5	20.5	Vermont	21.6	17.0	19.3
Idaho	19.7	16.2	17.9	New Jersey	19.6	16.8	18.1	Virginia	21.5	19.7	20.6
Illinois	21.2	18.7	19.9	New Mexico	24.4	18.8	21.5	Washington	19.1	16.1	17.6
Indiana	29.7	25.1	27.3	New York	23.0	18.2	20.5	West Virginia	27.4	26.0	26.6
Iowa	21.8	19.1	20.4	North Carolina	25.6	19.9	22.7	Wisconsin	22.1	19.5	20.8
Kansas	18.9	16.8	17.8	North Dakota	21.5	18.6	20.0	Wyoming	20.5	22.1	21.3
Kentucky	30.6	26.9	28.7	Ohio	21.9	22.8	22.3				

Source: Centers for Disease Control and Prevention, State-specific prevalence of current cigarette smoking among adults and secondhand smoke rules and policies in homes and workplaces—United States, 2005, *Morbidity and Mortality Weekly Report,* Vol. 55, No. 42, October 27, 2006.

Utah, a state in which nearly three-fourths of the residents are Mormons and thus refrain from tobacco and alcohol use, reports the smallest percentage of tobacco uses (11.5 percent). How does your home state compare?

Only 8.1 percent of the population of the U.S. Virgin Islands are smokers.[1] Whether this reflects the influences of cultural practices, cigarette prices and availability, or preferences for other forms of tobacco is not known. Also, when 14 states were asked what percentage of their households were "totally smoke-free," reports ranged from 63.6 percent in Kentucky to 82.9 percent in Arizona; "totally smoke-free workplaces" ranged from a low of 54.8 percent in Kentucky to a high of 85.5 percent in West Virginia.[2]

Following the Surgeon General's 1964 report (the first official statement of concern by the federal government regarding the dangers of smoking), the prevalence of smoking began a decline that lasted until 1991, when a leveling off was noted that lasted for the next three years. Since 1994 the percentage of the population who smoke has declined slowly but progressively.

Cigarette Smoking among College Students

Until very recently, the rate of cigarette smoking among college graduates was lower than that reported for the population as a whole, and it was significantly lower than the rate for persons with very little formal education. In fact, the prevalence of smoking among college students decreased progressively from 21 percent in 1964 to 14 percent in 1995. However, an upward trend in cigarette use by college students has been noted, with a recent study indicating that 30.6 percent of full-time enrolled students had smoked within the preceding month, while 42.7 percent of part-time enrolled students had smoked.[3] In contrast, a downward trend in smoking by 12th-graders has been reported, with 13.4 percent smoking daily during the past month in 2005.[4] Because the majority of today's college students graduated from high school during a period of decreased smoking by 12th-graders, we could have expected a progressive decline in college student smoking. Such has not been the case, however, suggesting that factors encountered after matriculation are fostering smoking among college students.

When a college community is viewed as a whole regarding which segments of the student body are most likely to smoke, there appears to be a direct relationship between the level of alcohol consumption and cigarette smoking. Additional direct relationships appear between smoking and other drug use and in housing where smoking is permitted. Similar, although perhaps less influential, relationships are seen among tobacco use and coping style, depression, and perceptions of life satisfaction.[5]

The historically predictable relationship between higher levels of completed education and the lessened likelihood of smoking remains clearly evident even today.

Demographic Trends in Smoking

A number of different factors appear to influence smoking rates among Americans (Table 9.2). Among the most important are the following:

- *Gender.* Men have higher rates of smoking than women, a pattern that is consistent for people of different ages and ethnicities.[6]

- *Race/ethnicity.* American Indians and Alaska Natives have the highest smoking rate, while people of Asian descent have the lowest rate.[6]

- *Level of education.* Higher levels of education have historically been associated with lower rates of smoking, a trend that continues today. People with undergraduate or graduate degrees are far less likely to smoke than those with lower levels of education.[6] However, today's college students may be reversing this trend.

- *Age.* The rate of smoking goes down as age goes up; among those age 65 and over, the rate drops below 10 percent. Over the course of time, it is likely that both quitting and premature death reduce the percentage of smokers in the population.[6]

- *Geographical residence.* The Midwest has the highest percentage of smokers, while the West has the lowest percentage.[7]

- *County population density.* People who live outside metropolitan areas are most likely to be smokers, and small metropolitan areas have a higher percentage of smokers than large metropolitan areas.[7]

- *Employment status.* Full-time employees have somewhat higher rates of smoking than people who work part-time, but people who are unemployed have the highest rate of smoking when considering employment status.[8] This pattern may reflect not only the lower level of education found in the unemployed but also the immediate gratification that smoking brings to people who may have few opportunities to seriously pursue long-range goals and who are not encumbered by workplace smoking restrictions.

- *Recent homelessness or incarceration.* People who have spent more than 24 hours on the street or who have lived in a shelter or prison have a high smoking rate (56.2 percent).[9]

- *Place of birth.* In comparison to native-born Americans, people living in the United States who are foreign-born are among the least likely to be current smokers (14.1 percent).[10] For information on smoking rates outside the United States, see the box "Smoking around the World."

Table 9.2 Patterns of Cigarette Smoking

	Percentage of Smokers		
	Men	**Women**	**Total**
All adults*	23.9	18.1	20.9
Race/ethnicity*			
White	24.0	20.0	21.9
Black	26.7	17.3	21.5
Hispanic	21.1	11.1	16.2
American Indian/ Alaskan Native	37.5	26.8	32.0
Asian	20.6	6.1	13.3
Education*			
9–11 years	36.8	29.0	32.6
GED diploma	47.5	38.8	43.2
High school graduate	28.8	20.7	24.6
Associate degree	26.1	17.1	20.9
Some college	26.2	19.5	22.5
Undergraduate degree	11.9	9.6	10.7
Graduate degree	6.9	7.4	7.1
Age (years)*			
18–24	28.0	20.7	24.4
25–44	26.8	21.4	24.1
45–64	25.2	18.8	21.9
65+	8.9	8.3	8.6
Geographical division†			
Midwest			29.9
South			27.3
Northeast			26.0
West			22.5
County type†			
Large metropolitan			24.9
Small metropolitan			27.5
Nonmetropolitan			30.2
Employment status†			
Full-time			28.3
Part-time			25.2
Unemployed			43.8

*Percentage of people who report smoking at least 100 cigarettes during their lifetimes and current smoking every day or some days.

†Percentage of people who report past-month smoking.

Sources: Centers for Disease Control and Prevention, Tobacco use among adults—United States, 2005. *MMWR,* Vol. 55, No. 42, October 27, 2006; Substance Abuse and Mental Health Services Administration. (2006). *Results from the 2005 National Survey on Drug Use and Health: National Findings* (Office of Applied Studies, NSDUH Series H-30, DHHS Publication No. SMA 06-4194). Rockville, MD.

Marketing of Tobacco Products

Shredded plant material, wrapped in paper or leaf, ignited with a flame, and then placed on or near the delicate tissues of the mouth . . . what other human behavior does this resemble? If you answered *None!* to this question, then you appreciate that smoking is unique, and, therefore, that it must be learned. How it is learned is currently a less than fully understood process that most likely requires a variety of stimuli ranging from modeling to actual experimentation. The role of advertising as a source of models has long been suspected and intensely debated. Today, as in the past, controversy surrounds the intent of the tobacco industry's advertising. Are the

Learning from Our Diversity

Smoking around the World

People in less-developed areas of the world are becoming increasingly exposed to the cultural influences of the postindustrial world, including behavioral patterns and access to products. Among the most insidious of these behavioral patterns is cigarette smoking, which is supported by access to imported cigarettes or the technology to manufacture indigenous brands. As the postindustrial countries of the world turn way from cigarette smoking and move toward improved health, the people in less-developed areas of the world are progressing toward levels of smoking exceeding the highest levels ever seen in the United States or Western Europe.

According to the American Cancer Society, the following levels of adult smoking for males and females were reported for 2005. In the United States the rates of cigarette smoking hover slightly above 20 percent—so we can easily imagine the level of smoking-related illnesses being experienced in and projected for the future in less-developed areas of the world.

The data indicate that heavy smoking is more common in males, although levels of smoking for women are distressingly high, particularly in the first countries listed. China has a large effect on the demand for imported and indigenous tobacco—30 percent of all of the world's cigarettes are smoked in China. Needless to say, American tobacco companies consider China one of the "bright spots" in the future economic well-being of their industry.

Countries Reporting Heavy Levels of Smoking for Males and Females

Males (%)		Females (%)	
Yemen	77	Cook Island	71
Djibouti	75	Nauru	59
China	67	Guinea	47
Cambodia	67	Chile	37
Kazakhstan	65	Republic of Serbia	34
Republic of Korea	65	Republic of Montenegro	34
Armenia	62	Kirbati	32
Russian Federation	60	FYR Macedonia	32
Albania	60	Lebanon	31
Samoa	60	Tuvalu	31
Guinea	59	Bosnia and Herzegovina	30

Source: Mackay J, Eriksen M, Shafey O., *The Tobacco Atlas* (2nd ed.), 2006, American Cancer Society.

---

familiar logos seen in a variety of media intended to challenge the brand loyalty of those who have already decided to smoke, as the industry claims? Or are the ads intended to entice new smokers, older children and young adolescents, in sufficient numbers to replace the 3,000 smokers who die each day from the consequences of tobacco use? This latter objective is now known, by admission of the tobacco industry, to have been pursued for decades.

Master Tobacco Settlement Agreement A significant roadblock to the tobacco industry's success in addicting another generation of cigarette smokers began in the early 1990s when previously secret documents of the five largest cigarette manufacturers were leaked to the public. The fortuitous availability of these documents gave rise to a massive suit by all of the attorneys general of the 50 states. Using information regarding the tobacco industry's decades-old knowledge of the health risks of their products, the states brought suit against the industry to recoup Medicaid money paid by the states in treating illness due to smoking. This huge class-action suit was promulgated in 1998, leading to a Master Tobacco Settlement Agreement in 1999.

Although the settlement is multifaceted and is far too complex to detail in this text, two significant components of the settlement are the monetary award to the states of $246 billion, to be paid to the states over 25

years, and the implementation of restrictions on the tobacco industry regarding multiple aspects of their marketing of cigarettes and other tobacco products. The following is a highly abbreviated list of restrictions placed on the tobacco industry's marketing:[11]

- Prohibits brand-name sponsorship of concerts, events with significant youth attendance, and team sports (basketball, football, auto racing, and so on)

- Limits tobacco companies from sponsoring more than one public event per year (music, cultural, artistic events—the tobacco product's brand name cannot appear)

- Bans the use of tobacco product names for stadiums and arenas

- Bans the use of cartoon characters in tobacco advertisements and promotions

- Bans the paid placement of tobacco products in movies, videos, and theater productions; smoking can still be featured in movies (see the box "Smoking in Film")

- Prohibits the distribution and sale of nontobacco products (such as caps and T-shirts) with brand-name logos

- Bans future tobacco products from using previous product names (such as Wings and Old-Golds) or

Theories of Nicotine Addiction

The establishment and maintenance of physical dependence or addiction is less than fully understood. Most experts, however, believe that for a specific individual, addiction has a multifaceted etiology, or cause, with increasing attention being directed toward a genetic basis for addiction. Accordingly, several theories have been proposed to explain the development of dependence. We present a brief account of some of these theories. Readers are reminded that many of these theories are technically sophisticated and only a most basic description can be provided in a personal health textbook. The more emotional aspects of dependence formation are discussed later in the chapter.

Genetic Influences Although the specific genetic pathways that influence both the initiation and maintenance of smoking (or other forms of tobacco use) are less than fully understood, a role for genetic influence is evident. Applying new statistical techniques to earlier studies of smoking patterns in families and between identical twins, it is now believed that initiation and maintenance of initial smoking is 60 percent driven by genetic influences.[15]

Recent research studies have identified specific chromosomes that contribute to the genetic susceptibility of developing nicotine dependence. These include chromosomes 1, 3, 4, 7, 8, 9, 11, 16, 17, and 20,[16] with chromosomes 5 and 10 contributing to dependence in African Americans.[17, 18] Most likely additional genetic markers will soon be included in this lengthening list.

Of course, the smoking of the first few cigarettes is a choice made by beginning smokers. In a yet-to-be-determined percentage of beginning smokers, the *initiation* of smoking, or the desire to continue with this new behavior, is underlined by a genetic predisposition to neurohormonally "appreciate" the stimulating effects of nicotine. Once smoking has been so easily and successfully initiated, the continuation of smoking is then *maintained* by the same, or closely related, genetic predisposition for neurohormonal excitation of the central nervous system. The "hook" for a lifetime of smoking is, thus, set in large part by a genetic susceptibility.[19] The remaining influence needed for initiation and maintenance of initial smoking is 20 percent environmental and 20 percent the unique needs of individuals.[20]

Once the relatively brief period of initial exposure (initiation) and early maintenance is passed, the role of genetic influences may be even more powerful—providing 70 percent of the maintenance stimulus required over decades of smoking. Environmental and personality factors subside accordingly.[20]

Bolus Theory In the **bolus theory** of nicotine addiction, one of the oldest and most general theories of

addiction, each inhalation of smoke releases into the blood a concentrated quantity of nicotine (a ball or bolus) that reaches the brain and results in a period of neurohormonal excitement. The smoker perceives this period of stimulation as pleasurable but, unfortunately, short-lived. Accordingly, the smoker attempts to reestablish this pleasurable feeling by again inhaling and sending another bolus of nicotine on its way to the brain. The 70,000 or more inhalations during the first year of smoking serve to condition the novice smoker, resulting in a lifelong pattern of cigarette dependence. The level needed for arousal is different for each individual smoker, depending on the length of addiction, the level of tolerance, genetic predisposition, and environmental and personal stimuli.

Recognition of two types of smokers emerges from an understanding of the bolus theory of smoking. *Peak smokers* are those smokers who become dependent on the arousal of pleasure centers in the brain (see page 267) that are stimulated by the rapid increase of nicotine levels following inhalation and distribution of nicotine within the CNS. In contrast, *trough maintenance smokers* maintain an even consistently higher level of nicotine titration in order to avoid the negative consequences of withdrawal. In other words, some smokers enjoy the consequences (arousal) caused by arrival of the bolus, whereas others so dislike the feelings caused by dissapation of the bolus that they inhale to avoid these unpleasant feelings.

Adrenocorticotropic Hormone (ACTH) Theory Yet another theory of dependence suggests that nicotine stimulates the release of adrenocorticotropic hormone (ACTH) from the anterior pituitary, or "master gland" of the endocrine system (see Chapter 3), causing the release of **beta endorphins** (naturally occurring opiate-like chemicals) that produce mild feelings of euphoria. Perhaps this stresslike response mechanism involving ACTH accounts for the increased energy expenditure seen in smokers and thus their tendency to maintain a lower body weight.

When these physiological responses are viewed collectively, nicotine may be seen as biochemically influencing brain activity by enhancing the extent and strength of various forms of "communication" between different brain areas and even glands of the endocrine system. If this is the case, it is apparent why, once addicted, the functioning of the smoker's control systems is much altered in comparison with that of nonsmokers.

Self-Medication Theory Another explanation of the addiction to smoking, called *self-medication,* suggests that nicotine, through the effects of mood-enhancing dopamine, may allow smokers to "treat" feelings of tiredness, lack of motivation, or even depression. In other words, a smoke lifts the spirits, if only briefly. Eventually, however, smokers become dependent on tobacco as a "medication" to make themselves feel better. Recent research, however, challenges the role of self-medication (purposeful stimulating of dopamine release) as a causative factor in establishing and maintaining smoking behavior. Some now suggest that, instead, the removal of the depressed level of arousal (being in a period of withdrawal) is the primary player in the establishment of nicotine dependence.

Regardless of the mechanism involved, as tolerance to nicotine develops, smoking behavior is adjusted to either maintain arousal or prevent the occurrence of withdrawal symptoms. At some point, however, the desire for constant arousal is probably superseded by the smoker's desire not to experience withdrawal.

The importance of nicotine as the primary factor in establishing dependence on tobacco is supported by research that demonstrates that smokers will not select a nontobacco cigarette if a tobacco cigarette is available. Even tobacco cigarettes with a very low level of nicotine seem to be unacceptable to most smokers, as do cigarettes with very low nicotine but with high tar content. Interestingly, users of low-nicotine cigarettes tend to inhale more frequently and deeply to obtain as much nicotine as possible.

Even more impressive (and alarming) than the power of nicotine to cause dependency is the small amount of time needed for it to do so. Instruments designed to assess the time required for the onset of dependence on nicotine—such as DANDY[21] (Development and Assessment of Nicotine Dependency in Youths) and HONC[22] (Hooked On Nicotine Checklist; see the Personal Assessment at the end of this chapter)—have established that beginning smokers (recall that most smokers begin during adolescence) become dependent on cigarettes within 3 weeks to 3 months of smoking on as little as two cigarettes per day. Males are more likely to be a bit more resistant to dependency, taking a month or two, whereas females can become dependent in a matter of a very few days of initial experimentation. Additionally, it is now known that for children who try smoking on a very limited basis and then stop, a "sleeper effect" may be put into place that increases their vulnerability to becoming a smoker within the next three years, in comparison to peers who did not experiment with smoking.[23]

 TALKING POINTS A smoker says that she does not consider smoking to be a form of drug use. She becomes angry at the suggestion that cigarettes are part of a drug-delivery system. How would you respond to her position?

Nicotine Dependency and Traumatic Brain Injury Recent findings related to the consequence of strokes occurring in a very specific area of the brain called the insula provide an interesting aside to the discussion of the brain and nervous system's role in nicotine dependence. Located in the brain at ear level, the insula is a small area that plays a critical role in the communication of information to the prefrontal cortex, where behavioral decisions are formulated. In a smoker whose insula has been damaged by the disruption of blood flow (stroke), nicotine dependence often disappears instantly and the individual can immediately stop smoking. In other words, damage to this specific area of the brain appears to disrupt the flow of information from other nicotine-sensitive areas of the brain, disrupting the reward system that would otherwise result in the act of smoking. Perhaps in the future there will be a smoking-cessation technology centered on insula function.

Acute Effects of Nicotine on Nervous System Function

In comparison with the more chronic effects of nicotine on the central nervous system (CNS) that may eventually result in physical dependence or addiction, nicotine also produces changes of short duration. In the CNS, nicotine activates receptors within the nucleus accumbens (a reward center) and the locus caeruleus (a cortical activating center) of the brain. Through the use of EEG (electroencephalography) and MRI (magnetic resonance imaging) technology, the location and extent of brain activity can be assessed. Upon reaching the brain areas mentioned, nicotine induces increased brain activity in a consistent and predictable manner. This is part of a general arousal pattern signaled by the release of the neurotransmitters **norepinephrine,** dopamine, acetylcholine, and serotonin. Heavy use of tobacco products, resulting in high levels of nicotine in the bloodstream, eventually produces a blocking effect as more and more receptor sites for these neurotransmitters are filled. The result is a generalized depression of the CNS.

The level of plasma nicotine associated with normal levels of heavy smoking (one to two packs per day) would not likely produce the depressive effect just described. However, in chain smokers (four to eight packs per day),

---

Key Terms

bolus theory A theory of nicotine addiction based on the body's response to the bolus (ball) of nicotine delivered to the brain with each inhalation of cigarette smoke.

beta endorphins Mood-enhancing, pain-reducing, opiatelike chemicals produced within the smoker's body in response to the presence of nicotine.

norepinephrine (nor epp in **eff** rin) An adrenaline-like neurotransmitter produced within the nervous system.

tobacco users. Carbon monoxide interferes with oxygen transport within the circulatory system.

As described earlier in the chapter, carbon monoxide is a component of the gaseous phase of tobacco smoke and readily joins with the hemoglobin of the red blood cells. Carbon monoxide has an affinity for hemoglobin 206 times that of oxygen. Once the hemoglobin of a red cell has accepted carbon monoxide molecules, the hemoglobin is transformed into carboxyhemoglobin. Thereafter, the carboxyhemoglobin permanently weakens the red blood cell's ability to transport oxygen. So long as smoking continues, these red blood cells remain relatively useless during the remainder of their 120-day lives. Levels of carboxyhemoglobin in heavy smokers are associated with significant increases in the incidence of myocardial infarction.

When a person has impaired oxygen-transporting abilities, physical exertion becomes increasingly demanding on both the heart and the lungs. The cardiovascular system will attempt to respond to the body's demand for oxygen, but these responses are themselves impaired as a result of the influence of nicotine on the cardiovascular system. If tobacco does create the good life, as advertisers claim, it also unfortunately lessens the ability to participate actively in that life.

Smoking and Oral Contraceptive Use   Women who smoke and use oral contraceptives, particularly after age 35, are placing themselves at a much greater risk of experiencing a fatal cardiovascular accident (heart attack, stroke, or embolism) than are oral contraceptive users who do not smoke. This risk of cardiovascular complications increases further for oral contraceptive users 40 years of age or older. Women who both smoke and use oral contraceptives are four times more likely to die from myocardial infarction (heart attack) than are women who only smoke. Because of this adverse relationship, *it is strongly recommended that women who smoke not use oral contraceptives.*

Cancer

Over the past 60 years, research from the most reputable institutions in this country and abroad has consistently concluded that tobacco use is a significant factor in the development of virtually all forms of cancer and the most significant factor in cancers involving the respiratory system.

In describing cancer development, the currently used reference is 20 pack-years, or an amount of smoking equal to smoking one pack of cigarettes a day for 20 years. Thus the two-pack-a-day smoker can anticipate cancer-related tissue changes in as few as 10 years, while the half-pack-a-day smoker may have 40 years to wait. Regardless, the opportunity is there for all smokers to confirm these data by developing cancer as predicted. It

is hoped that most people will think twice before disregarding this evidence.

Data supplied by the American Cancer Society (ACS) indicate that during 2006 an estimated 1,399,790 Americans developed cancer.* These cases were nearly equally divided between the sexes and resulted in approximately 564,830 deaths. In the opinion of the ACS, 30 percent of all cancer cases are heavily influenced by tobacco use. Lung cancer alone accounted for about 172,570 of the new cancer cases and 162,460 deaths in 2006. Fully 87 percent of men with lung cancer were cigarette smokers.[27] A genetic "missing link" between smoking and lung cancer was established, when mutations to an important tumor suppressor gene were identified. If it was necessary to have a final "proof" that smoking causes lung cancer, that proof appears to be in hand.

Cancer of the entire respiratory system, including lung cancer and cancers of the mouth and larynx accounted for about 217,360 new cases of cancer and 174,480 deaths.[27] Despite these high figures, not all smokers develop cancer.

Respiratory Tract Cancer   Recall that tobacco smoke produces both a gaseous and a particulate phase. As noted, the particulate phase contains the tar fragment of tobacco smoke. This rich chemical environment contains more than 4,000 known chemical compounds, hundreds of which are known to be carcinogens.

In the normally functioning respiratory system, particulate matter suspended in the inhaled air settles on the tissues lining the airways and is trapped in mucus produced by specialized *goblet cells*. This mucus, with its trapped impurities, is continuously swept upward by the beating action of hairlike cilia of the ciliated columnar epithelial cells lining the air passages (Figure 9-2). On reaching the throat, this mucus is swallowed and eventually removed through the digestive system.

When tobacco smoke is drawn into the respiratory system, however, its rapidly dropping temperature allows the particulate matter to accumulate. This brown, sticky tar contains compounds known to harm the ciliated cells, goblet cells, and the basal cells of the respiratory lining. As the damage from smoking increases, the cilia become less effective in sweeping mucus upward to the throat. When cilia can no longer clean the airway, tar accumulates on the surfaces and brings carcinogenic compounds into direct contact with the tissues of the airway.

At the same time that the sweeping action of the lining cells is being slowed, substances in the tar are stimulating the goblet cells to increase the amount of mucus they normally produce. The "smoker's cough" is the body's attempt to remove this excess mucus.

With prolonged exposure to the carcinogenic materials in tar, predictable changes will begin to occur within

* Excluding cases of nonmelanoma skin cancer.

Figure 9-2 Development of Lung Cancer   Tissue changes associated with lung cancer (bronchogenic carcinoma).

the respiratory system's basal cell layer (Figure 9-2). The basal cells begin to display changes characteristic of all cancer cells. In addition, an abnormal accumulation of cells occurs. When a person stops smoking, preinvasive lesions do not repair themselves as quickly as once thought.

By the time lung cancer is usually diagnosed, its development is so advanced that the chance for recovery is very poor. Still today, only 15 percent of all lung cancer victims survive for five years or more after diagnosis.[27] Most die in a very uncomfortable, painful way.

Two primary forms of lung cancer are seen in smokers: squamous cell carcinoma and adenocarcinoma. The former is declining in prevalence as the level of smoking in this country declines, but the latter form of lung cancer is increasing. Some experts attribute this increase, in the face of declining smoking, to a change in the chemical nature of cigarette smoke due to subtle changes in the formulation of cigarette tobacco and the ventilation of filters.[29]

Cancerous activity in other areas of the respiratory system, including the larynx, and within the oral cavity (mouth) follows a similar course. In the case of oral cavity cancer, carcinogens found within the smoke and within the saliva are involved in the cancerous changes. Tobacco users, such as pipe smokers, cigar smokers, and users of smokeless tobacco, have a higher (4 to 10 times) rate of cancer of the mouth, tongue, and voice box.

Other Tobacco-Enhanced Cancers   In addition to drawing smoke into the lungs, tobacco users swallow saliva that contains an array of chemical compounds from tobacco. This saliva is retained in the stomach and then passes into the small intestine, where carcinogenic and toxic compounds in the saliva are absorbed into the blood. Contact between this material and the walls of the digestive organs leads to an enhanced risk of cancer in these areas of the gastrointestinal system. Additionally, the breakdown of carcinogens and toxic substances in the liver greatly increases the development of cancer in this critically important organ. Filtering of the blood by the kidneys eventually concentrates toxic materials in the urinary bladder, leading to increases in kidney and bladder cancer. Smoking may also accelerate the rate of pancreatic cancer development.

As reported earlier in the chapter, documents released in 1997 from within the tobacco industry clearly

Key Terms

embolism A potentially fatal condition in which a circulating blood clot lodges in a smaller vessel.

mucus Clear, sticky material produced by specialized cells within the mucous membranes of the body; mucus traps much of the suspended particulate matter within tobacco smoke.

cilia (sill ee uh) Small, hairlike structures that extend from cells that line the air passages.

A healthy lung (right) versus the lung of a smoker (left). Smoking causes shortness of breath and "smoker's cough" and can lead to chronic obstructive lung disease.

show that the major tobacco companies were aware of tobacco's role in the development of cancer and had made a concerted effort to deprive the American public access to such knowledge.

Chronic Obstructive Lung Disease

Chronic obstructive lung disease (COLD), also known as chronic obstructive pulmonary disease (COPD), is a disorder in which the amount of air that flows in and out of the lungs becomes progressively limited. COLD is a disease state that is made up of two separate but related diseases: **chronic bronchitis** and **pulmonary emphysema.**

With chronic bronchitis, excess mucus is produced in response to the effects of smoking on airway tissue, and the walls of the bronchi become inflamed and infected. This produces a characteristic narrowing of the air passages. Breathing becomes difficult, and activity can be severely restricted. With cessation of smoking, chronic bronchitis is reversible.

Emphysema causes irreversible damage to the tiny air sacs of the lungs, the **alveoli.** Chest pressure builds when air becomes trapped by narrowed air passages (chronic bronchitis) and the thin-walled sacs rupture. Emphysema patients lose the ability to ventilate fully.

Key Terms

chronic bronchitis Persistent inflammation and infection of the smaller airways within the lungs.

pulmonary emphysema An irreversible disease process in which the alveoli are destroyed.

alveoli (al **vee** oh lie) Thin, saclike terminal ends of the airways; the sites at which gases are exchanged between the blood and inhaled air.

They feel as though they are suffocating. You may have seen people with this condition in malls and other locations as they walk slowly by, carrying or pulling their portable oxygen tanks.

More than 10 million Americans suffer from COLD. It is responsible for a greater limitation of physical activity than any other disease, including heart disease. COLD patients tend to die a very unpleasant, prolonged death, often from a general collapse of normal cardiorespiratory function that results in congestive heart failure (see Chapter 10).

Smoking and Body Weight

Although not perceived as a health problem by people who continue smoking in order to control weight, smoking does appear to minimize weight gain. In studies using identical twins, twins who smoked were six to eight pounds lighter than their nonsmoking siblings. Current understanding about why smoking results in lower body weight is less than complete. One factor may be an increase in Basal Metabolic Rate (BMR) (see Chapter 6) brought about by the influence of nicotine on sympathetic nervous system function. However, in spite of the modest level of weight management provided by regular cigarette smoking, the overall increase in morbidity and premature death experienced by smokers is in no way "worth" the benefit of weighing a few pounds less.

Additional Health Concerns

In addition to the serious health problems stemming from tobacco use already described, other health-related changes are routinely seen. These include a generally poor state of nutrition, a decline in insulin sensitivity, a decline in short-term memory, the gradual loss of the sense of smell, and premature wrinkling of the skin. Tobacco users are also more likely to experience strokes (a potentially fatal condition), lose bone mass leading to osteoporosis, experience more back pain and muscle injury, and find that fractures heal more slowly. Further, smokers who have surgery spend more time in the recovery room. Additionally, smokers have a fourfold greater risk of developing serious gum (periodontal) disease, now thought to be a risk factor for cardiovascular disease. Also, smokers may need supplementation for two important water-soluble vitamins, vitamin C and vitamin B.

Combining Tobacco and Alcohol Use

Although there are exceptions to every generalization, it is very common to see tobacco and alcohol being used by the same people, often at the same time. Younger people who use both tobacco and alcohol are also more likely to use additional drugs. Accordingly, both tobacco and alcohol are considered *gateway drugs* because they are often introductory drugs that "open the door" for a more broadly based polydrug use pattern (see Chapter 7).

Beyond the potential for polydrug use initiated by the use of tobacco and alcohol is the simple reality that the use of both tobacco products and alcoholic beverages is associated with a wide array of illnesses and with premature death. As you have seen in this chapter and in Chapter 8 regarding alcohol use, the negative health impact of using both is significant. When use is combined, of course, the risks of living less healthfully and dying prematurely are accentuated.

Risks from Specific Tobacco Products

Most tobacco used today in the United States is in the form of standard machine-produced cigarettes. However, there are other forms of tobacco and variations on the standard cigarette in use by Americans. Tobacco products such as bidis, cigars, mentholated cigarettes, and smokeless tobacco have their own special health risks and regulatory challenges. New products developed by the tobacco industry have been marketed as being safer in some way than standard cigarettes, but there is no such thing as a safe cigarette.

Nonmanufactured Forms of Cigarettes

Although the vast majority of American cigarette smokers use familiar brand-name manufactured cigarettes produced in this country, segments of the smoking population use, to some degree, nonmanufactured cigarettes. Nonmanufactured cigarettes (or the supplies for making them) generally are sold in places that might not enforce the legal age restrictions on purchasing manufactured cigarettes. Of course, in terms of dependence

Mentholated cigarettes have been heavily marketed to African American smokers.

and harmfulness, these kinds of cigarettes are no better, if not worse, than manufactured cigarettes. Nonmanufactured cigarettes include roll-your-own cigarettes, bidis, and kreteks.[30]

Roll-Your-Own Cigarettes Hand-filled cigarettes are made by the smoker from fine-cut, loose tobacco, using cigarette paper. This form of cigarette may be "hand-rolled" or a small hand held rolling machine may be used. The tobacco and papers necessary to roll your own cigarettes are widely available; the roll-your-own machine might require more effort to find. Regardless, this type of cigarette is more affordable that the leading brands of manufactured cigarettes. From a health standpoint, roll-your-own cigarettes carry all of the risks of manufactured cigarettes.

Bidis Most often imported from the Indian subcontinent, bidis are small, handmade cigarettes consisting of a small amount of tobacco wrapped in a dried temburni or tendu leaf tied with a small length of colorful string. These cigarettes are particularly dangerous to health because the tobacco used is high in tar and nicotine and these cigarettes' inefficient combustion delivers a high level of carbon monoxide.

Kreteks A popular cigarette from Indonesia, kreteks are hand-wrapped cigarettes made from clove-flavored tobacco or other highly flavored tobacco. A particular health danger of kreteks is that they contain an additive, eugenol, that produces an anesthetic effect in the throat, resulting in a tendency to inhale more deeply, thus delivering more tar and nicotine.

Mentholated Cigarettes

Of the 599 approved additives for use in the manufacturing of cigarettes, one of the most familiar, and most popular, is menthol—which imparts a unique taste and

If one were to judge on the basis of the number of newly opened cigar stores and clubs catering to cigar smokers, as well as the highly visible magazine *Cigar Aficionado,* one could conclude that cigar smoking was the hottest trend in tobacco use. To a degree this contention is true when one considers that in 1991 only 2.2 percent of the adult population smoked cigars on a regular basis, whereas by 1998 the size of the cigar-smoking population had risen to 5.2 percent. However, the most recent data available (2002) suggest only a slight increase, to 5.4 percent. We can hope that this very small increase suggests a possible leveling off of the cigar craze of the 1990s.

In any case, cigar smokers who continue to smoke and those of you who might be interested in this form of tobacco use should consider the following information from the American Lung Association:

- *Secondhand (sidestream) cigar smoke is more poisonous than secondhand cigarette smoke is.* The smoke from one cigar equals that of three cigarettes. Carbon monoxide emissions from one cigar are 30 times higher than those for one cigarette.

- *Cigar smoking can cause cancer of the larynx (voice box), mouth, esophagus, and lungs.* Cancer death rates for cigar smokers are 34 percent higher than those for nonsmokers.

- *Ninety-nine percent of cigar smokers have atypical cells found in the larynx.* These cells are the first step toward malignancy (cancer).

- *Cigar smokers are three to five times more likely to die of lung cancer than are nonsmokers.*

- *Cigar smokers have five times the risk of emphysema compared to nonsmokers.*

- *Nicotine does not have to be inhaled to damage the heart and blood vessels.* It is absorbed into the bloodstream through the mucous membranes of the mouth. Nicotine increases the heart rate and constricts the blood vessels, which reduces blood flow to the heart.

"cooling" sensation in the throat. Menthol-flavored cigarettes have been on the market for decades and have proven highly attractive to African American male smokers.

Health researchers have speculated that there is a relationship between the long-term smoking of mentholated cigarettes among African American males and the high level of lung cancer in this population. A meta-analysis of five large epidemiological studies of African American smokers concluded that the menthol in cigarette tobacco was not a factor in the higher rate of lung cancer in this population. Additionally, menthol did not increase puff number or puff volume, or result in elevated heart rates, higher levels of carbon monoxide in the blood, higher tar intake, or high levels of nicotine-breakdown by-products.[31]

Pipe and Cigar Smoking

Many people believe that pipe or cigar smoking is a safe alternative to cigarette smoking. Unfortunately, this is not the case. All forms of tobacco present users with a series of health threats (see the box "Thanks, but No Cigar").

When compared with cigarette smokers, pipe and cigar smokers have cancer of the mouth, throat, larynx (voice box), and esophagus at the same frequency. Cigarette smokers are more likely than are pipe and cigar smokers to have lung cancer, cancer of the larynx, chronic obstructive lung disease (COLD) also called chronic obstructive pulmonary disease (COPD), and heart disease. The cancer risk of death to pipe and cigar smokers is 4 times greater from lung cancer and 10 times greater from laryngeal cancer than it is for nonsmokers.

In comparison to cigarette smokers, pipe and cigar smokers are considerably fewer in number. Interestingly, cigar smoking enjoyed a resurgence through much of the 1990s. During 1998–1999 there was a substantial decline in sales of premium cigars, but beginning in 1999 an upward trend in cigar imports began. By 2005 (the most recent year for which figures are available), 319.4 million cigars were imported into the United States. This decrease is thought to reflect a growing displeasure with domestically manufactured cigars. Because many people smoke cigars only on occasions, it is difficult to determine the number of regular cigar smokers.

Perhaps because of the increase in cigar smoking noted previously, the National Cancer Institute commissioned the first extensive study of regular cigar smoking. That report confirmed and expanded on the health risks identified in earlier smaller studies.[32]

In response to the recognition of these risks, the FTC now requires that cigar manufacturers disclose the tobacco content and additives in their products. Most recently the FTC announced its intention of requiring five rotating health warnings to appear on cigars, including two that have been currently agreed on by the FTC and major cigar manufacturers: *Cigars Are Not a Safe Alternative to Cigarettes* and *Cigar Smoking Can Cause Cancer of the Mouth and Throat, Even If You Don't Inhale.*

Smokeless Tobacco Use

As the term implies, smokeless tobacco, such as Skoal and Copenhagen, is not burned; rather, it is placed into the mouth. Once in place, the physiologically active nicotine and other soluble compounds are absorbed through the mucous membranes and into the blood. Within a few minutes, chewing tobacco and snuff generate blood levels of nicotine in amounts equivalent to those seen in cigarette smokers.

Chewing tobacco is taken from its foil pouch, formed into a small ball (called a "wad," "chaw," or "chew"), and placed into the mouth. Once in place, the bolus of tobacco is sucked and occasionally chewed, but not swallowed.

Snuff, a more finely shredded smokeless tobacco product, is marketed in small round cans. Snuff is formed into a small mass (or "quid") for dipping or used in prepackaged pouches. The quid or pouch is placed between the jaw and the cheek; the user sucks the quid or pouch, then spits out the brown liquid. Snuff, as once used, was actually a powdered form of tobacco that was inhaled through the nose.

Although smokeless tobacco would seem to free the tobacco user from many of the risks associated with smoking, chewing and dipping are not without their own substantial risks. The presence of *leukoplakia* (white

spots) and *erythroplakia* (red spots) on the tissues of the mouth indicate precancerous changes. In addition, an increase in **periodontal disease** (with the pulling away of the gums from the teeth, resulting in later tooth loss), the abrasive damage to the enamel of the teeth, and the high concentration of sugar in processed tobacco all contribute to dental problems among users of smokeless tobacco. In those who develop oral cancer, the risk is dramatically heightened if the cancer metastasizes from the site of origin in the mouth to the brain. Clearly, users should be aware of any signs of damage being done by their use of smokeless tobacco (see the box "Early Detection of Oral Cancer"). The validity of this warning was made clear in 1998 when about half of smokeless-tobacco-using Major League Baseball players were found to have tobacco-related lesions when oral examinations were performed by team dentists on the first day of spring training.

In addition to the damage done to the tissues of the mouth, the need to process the inadvertently swallowed saliva that contains dissolved carcinogens places both the digestive and urinary systems at risk of cancer.

In the opinion of health experts, the use of smokeless tobacco and its potential for life-threatening disease is very real and should not be disregarded.[33] Consequently, television advertisements have been banned, and the following warnings have been placed in rotation on all smokeless tobacco products:

Use of smokeless tobacco leads to gum disease, tooth loss, and oral cancer.

Key Terms

periodontal disease Destruction of soft tissue and bone that surround the teeth.

WARNING: THIS PRODUCT MAY CAUSE
MOUTH CANCER
WARNING: THIS PRODUCT MAY CAUSE GUM
DISEASE AND TOOTH LOSS
WARNING: THIS PRODUCT IS NOT A SAFE
ALTERNATIVE TO CIGARETTE
SMOKING

Clearly, smokeless tobacco is a dangerous product, and little doubt exists that continued use of tobacco in this form is a serious problem to health in all its dimensions.

New Product Development

The development of new products by the tobacco industry also attests, in an interesting way, to the inherent dangers of tobacco use long known by the industry (and forcibly admitted to the public in the 1999 tobacco settlement). The new products include Eclipse (by R. J. Reynolds), a cigarette that heats rather than burns most of its tobacco. According to its manufacturer, Eclipse is the first cigarette that produces smoke so low in carcinogens that it is the "next best choice" to quitting. This latter contention certainly states in a null manner something about cigarettes marketed before the development of Eclipse. Unfortunately for customers who switched to Eclipse in search of a safe cigarette, the claims made by the company about the cigarette's low carcinogenic composition proved inaccurate (or purposefully false). Most likely the end of the "safe cigarette" is in sight.

Another recently introduced cigarette, Accord, features a "smoking system" intended to reduce the production of sidestream smoke. This system uses a battery-powered device into which a special small cigarette is inserted. The smoker inhales through the device, and the cigarette is electrically ignited only when actively inhaled.

Three relatively new products are Advance cigarettes with "Trionic" filters supposedly capable of extracting more toxins than any filter to date; Omni, a brand advertised to significantly reduce selected carcinogens, nitrosamines, and catechols, the "major causes of lung cancer" according to their advertisements; and Quest, a brand intended to lead smokers to "nicotine free smoking." It should be noted that none of these new brands can deliver anything approaching a safe cigarette, nor are they intended to assist smokers in becoming nonsmokers.

Another addition to the new products recently introduced by the tobacco industry are self-extinguishing (reduced-ignition-propensity, or RIP) cigarettes that are necessary for continuing sales in the state of New York. The technology for this form of fire-risk-reducing cigarette, that largely extinguishes a burning cigarette if not inhaled upon within 60 seconds, has been available for several years, although not introduced by the tobacco industry until required to do so by New York.

A more alarming new product introduced by the tobacco industry is that of flavored cigarettes, such as Camel Exotic Blend. The manufacturer of this brand, R. J. Reynolds, contends that they are on the market to offer established smokers a greater choice of products, but their appeal appears instead to be aiming at young, beginning smokers. In October 2006, R. J. Reynolds agreed to a domestic ban on the sale of its popular flavored cigarettes, including Twista Lime and Mocha Taboo. This decision flowed from strong pressure from the attorneys general in many states following the release of data suggesting that nearly one-fifth of young smokers prefer flavored cigarettes over nonflavored brands. Other companies have remained silent on the Reynolds decision.

Although not related to a new product development per se, concerns have newly arisen over the unexpectedly high nicotine levels in the modern filtered cigarettes that are favored by virtually all smokers. New testing technologies have shown that smokers take in almost twice as much nicotine as previously believed. Part of the reason for this high level of nicotine intake is that the row of ventilation holes in the filter are obstructed by the lips of fingers of the smokers, thus blocking the escape of smoke. Additionally, smokers of filter-tipped low-tar and low-nicotine cigarettes seem strongly inclined to increase their "puff-volume" by inhaling more deeply and more often.[34] In combination, these factors help deliver the nicotine loads that keep smokers dependent and the tobacco industry in business.

Nontobacco Sources of Nicotine

Regardless of whether they are intended as aids to smoking cessation or only supplemental forms of nicotine for use when smoking is not permitted, numerous new forms of nicotine delivery systems have appeared in the marketplace in recent years. An area of growing concern is, of course, that these nontobacco delivery sources of nicotine could provide introductory exposure to nicotine, at a tragically early age, for the next generation of nicotine-dependent youth. Included among these nontobacco sources of nicotine are multiple flavors of nicotine suckers, nicotine-flavored gum, nicotine straws, nicotine-enhanced water (Nico Water), inhalers, sprays, drops, lozenges, and transdermal patches. To date, only Nico Water has been formally addressed by the Food and Drug Administration (and their request for control was rejected by the courts), others came into the marketplace as prescription-only or approved OTC products.

Nicotine Bridge Products   In light of the rapidly expanding restrictions on smoking, how do smokers survive long hours in smoke-free environments? The answer, a nicotine bridge product: a gel, cream, or candy-like piece that contains nicotine for absorption through a body surface to maintain an adequate level of titration until cigarettes can be smoked. These over-the-counter products, bearing names such as Ariva and Stonewall, are more convenient, affordable, tasty, or pleasant smelling than the nicotine step-down products used for smoking cessation. Of course, there is concern that these products enable smokers to continue their nicotine dependence in place of seeking cessation, and that they may be nicotine-introductory products if they become too readily available to children.

Smoking and Reproduction

In all its dimensions, the reproductive process is impaired by the use of tobacco, particularly cigarette smoking and environmental tobacco smoke in close proximity to pregnant women.[35, 36] Problems can be found in association with infertility, problem pregnancy, breast-feeding, and the health of the newborn. So broadly based are reproductive problems and smoking that the term *fetal tobacco syndrome* or *fetal smoking syndrome* is regularly used in clinical medicine. Some physicians even define a fetus being carried by a smoker as a "smoker" and, upon birth, as a "former smoker."

Infertility

Recent research indicates that cigarette smoking by both men and women can reduce levels of fertility. Among men, smoking adversely affects blood flow to erectile tissue, reduces sperm motility, and alters sperm shape, and it causes an overall decrease in the number of viable sperm. Among women, the effects of smoking are seen in terms of abnormal ovum formation, including a lessened ability on the part of the egg to prevent polyspermia, or the fertilization by multiple sperm. Smoking also negatively influences estrogen levels, resulting in underdevelopment of the uterine wall and ineffective implantation of the fertilized ovum. Lower levels of estrogen may also influence the rate of transit of the fertilized egg through the fallopian tube, making it arrive in the uterus too early for successful implantation or, in some cases, restricting movement to the point that an ectopic, or tubal, pregnancy may develop. Also, the early onset of menopause is associated with smoking.

Although causative pathways remain somewhat unclear, the influences of smoking are noted in two aspects of male infertility, sperm degradation and erectile dysfunction. In the former cases, several chemicals in tobacco smoke are able to cross the blood-testis barrier and structurally alter the DNA of the genetic material within the sperm. The presence of abnormal sperm in the male compromises the chances of fertilization. In erectile dysfunction, smoking, most likely through the effects of nicotine on blood-flow dynamics, decreases blood flow into the erectile tissues of the penile shaft, resulting in the inability to obtain or sustain an erection.[37, 38]

Problem Pregnancy

The harmful effects of tobacco smoke on the course of pregnancy are principally the result of the carbon monoxide and nicotine to which the mother and her fetus are exposed. Carbon monoxide from the incomplete oxidation of tobacco is carried in the maternal blood to the placenta, where it diffuses across the placental barrier and enters the fetal circulation. Once in the fetal blood, the carbon monoxide bonds with the fetal hemoglobin to form fetal carboxyhemoglobin. As a result of this exposure to carbon monoxide, the fetus is progressively deprived of normal oxygen transport and eventually becomes compromised by chronic hypoxia.

Nicotine also exerts its influence on the developing fetus. Thermographs of the placenta and fetus show signs of marked vasoconstriction within a few seconds after inhalation by the mother. This constriction further reduces the oxygen supply, resulting in hypoxia. In addition, nicotine stimulates the mother's stress response, placing the mother and fetus under the potentially harmful influence of elevated epinephrine and corticoid levels (see Chapter 3). Any fetus exposed to all of these agents is more likely to be miscarried, stillborn, or born prematurely. Even when carried to term, children born to mothers who smoked during pregnancy have lower birth weights and may show other signs of a stressful intrauterine life.

Breast-Feeding

Women who breast-feed their infants and continue to smoke continue to expose their children to the harmful effects of tobacco smoke. It is well recognized that nicotine appears in breast milk and thus is capable of exerting its vasoconstricting and stress-response influences on nursing infants. Mothers who stop smoking during pregnancy should be encouraged to continue to refrain from smoking while they are breast-feeding.

Neonatal Health Problems

Babies born to women who smoked during pregnancy are, on average, shorter and have a lower birth weight than do children born to nonsmoking mothers. During

---

Key Terms

ectopic (tubal) pregnancy Pregnancy resulting from the implantation of the fertilized ovum within the inner wall of the fallopian tube.

hypoxia Oxygenation deprivation at the cellular level.

the earliest months of life, babies born to mothers who smoke experience an elevated rate of death caused by sudden infant death syndrome (SIDS). Statistics also show that infants are more likely to develop chronic respiratory problems, more frequent colic, be hospitalized, and have poorer overall health during their early years of life. Problems such as those just mentioned may also be seen in children of nonsmoking mothers, when they were exposed prenatally to environmental tobacco smoke. In addition, environmental tobacco smoke exposure extending beyond the home and into the workplace may increase the probability of problem pregnancies and neonatal health problems. Recently, the interest in the effects of tobacco smoke on pregnancy has been extended to include behavioral differences in children born to women who smoked during pregnancy.

Parenting, in the sense of assuming responsibility for the well-being of children, does not begin at birth, but during the prenatal period. In the case of smoking, this is especially true. Pregnant women who continue smoking are disregarding the well-being of the children they are carrying. Other family members, friends, and coworkers who subject pregnant women to cigarette, pipe, or cigar smoke are, in a sense, exhibiting their own disregard for the health of the next generation.

Involuntary (Passive) Smoking

The smoke generated by the burning of tobacco can be classified as either **mainstream smoke** (the smoke inhaled and then exhaled by the smoker) or **sidestream smoke** (the smoke that comes from the burning end of the cigarette, pipe, or cigar that simply disperses into the air without being inhaled by the smoker). When either form of tobacco smoke is diluted and stays within a common source of air, it can eventually be referred to as **environmental tobacco smoke.** All three forms of tobacco smoke lead to involuntary or passive smoking and can present health problems for both nonsmokers and smokers.

Surprisingly, mainstream smoke makes up only 15 percent of our exposure to the harmful substances associated with involuntary smoking. Sidestream smoke

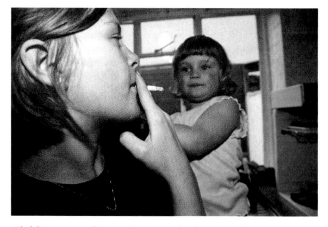

Children exposed to environmental tobacco smoke are at increased risk for wheezing, ear infections, bronchitis, and pneumonia.

is responsible for 85 percent of the harmful substances associated with secondhand smoke exposure. Because it is not filtered by the tobacco, the filter, or the smoker's body, sidestream smoke contains more free nicotine and produces higher yields of carbon dioxide and carbon monoxide. Much to the detriment of nonsmokers, sidestream smoke has a much higher quantity of highly carcinogenic compounds, called *N-nitrosamines,* than mainstream smoke has.

Current scientific opinion suggests that smokers and nonsmokers are exposed to very much the same smoke when tobacco is used within a common airspace. The important difference is the quantity of smoke inhaled by smokers and nonsmokers. It is likely that for each pack of cigarettes smoked by a smoker, nonsmokers who must share a common air supply with the smokers involuntarily smoke the equivalent of three to five cigarettes per day. Even today, because of the small size of the particles produced by burning tobacco, environmental tobacco smoke cannot be completely removed from a workplace, restaurant, or shopping mall by the most effective ventilation system.

Health Risks of Passive Smoking

Recently reported research indicates that involuntary smoke exposure may be responsible for 35,000 to 40,000 premature deaths per year from heart disease among nonsmokers in the United States.[39] Other estimates range upward to 53,000 premature deaths when lung cancer and COPD are included. In addition, large numbers of people exposed to involuntary smoke develop eye irritation, nasal symptoms, headaches, and a cough. Furthermore, most nonsmokers dislike the odor of tobacco smoke.

Involuntary smoking poses some threats to nonsmokers within residential settings.[40] Spouses and children of smokers are at greatest risk for involuntary smoking. Scientific studies suggest that nonsmokers married to smokers are more likely to experience heart attacks than nonsmoking spouses of nonsmokers. This said, a recent meta-analysis of earlier meta-analyses concludes that involuntary smoking carries an increased risk for cardiovascular disease, though the risk for a nonsmoking spouse is less than was once reported.[41] Additionally, a study from China involving over 70,000 nonsmoking women married to smoking spouses found a moderate increase in mortality from both cardiovascular disease and lung cancer in nonsmoking spouses.[42]

In spite of what may or may not be the effects of passive smoking on the nonsmoking partners of smokers, the effects of environmental tobacco smoke on the health of children seems well established. The children of parents who smoke are twice as likely as children of nonsmoking parents to experience bronchitis or pneumonia during the first year of life. In addition, throughout childhood these children will experience more wheezing, coughing, and sputum production than will children whose parents do not smoke. Otitis media (middle ear infection), one of the most frequently seen conditions in pediatric medicine, is also significantly more common in children under age 3 who reside with one or more adults who smoke.

Regarding the relationship between exposure to environmental tobacco and SIDS (sudden infant death syndrome), a recent comprehensive reassessment (meta-analysis) raised important issues about the methodology of nearly 60 earlier studies on this issue. Researchers in New Zealand suggest that currently it is difficult to determine an accurate picture of the relationship. In particular, research needs to better separate the influences of maternal smoking during pregnancy, maternal smoking after pregnancy (in the months immediately following delivery), and other sources of environmental tobacco during the prenatal and postnatal periods.[43]

Regulation of Passive Smoking

In light of the fact that the scientific community has documented to a very substantial degree the inherent dangers of passive or environmental tobacco smoke to the health of nonsmokers and smokers alike, restrictions on public smoking have been large scale and continue to be imposed. Restrictions range from bans on smoking in all public places to bans on smoking in specific places, such as government buildings, retail establishments, public transportation, indoor sports arenas, health care facilities, educational institutions, restaurants, and workplaces. By the end of June 2006, there were statewide bans on smoking (in various configurations) in 17 states, while 461 cities, towns, and counties had smoking bans of various types.[44] Americans traveling outside of the states will increasingly encounter bans on smoking. By the end of 2006, nationwide smoking bans (in

various configurations) were found in Argentina, Armenia, Australia, Belgium, Bhutan, Canada, Cuba, France, India, Ireland, Hong Kong, Italy, Japan, Kenya, Lithuania, Malta, Malay, New Zealand, Norway, Singapore, South Africa, Spain, Sweden, Switzerland, Tanzania, Thailand, Turkey, Uruguay, and Vietnam. The United Kingdom joined this list in the summer of 2007.[45] Smoking is now widely banned in all EU nations.

Many colleges and universities are instituting bans on smoking near the entrances to classroom buildings and residence halls. At Ball State University, cigarettes must be extinguished within 30 feet of an entrance. This restriction on smoking reflects the fact that environmental tobacco smoke accumulates under overhangs and in alcoves.

Most recently, some states are formulating ordinances to ban smoking in selected outdoor venues, such as sidewalk cafes, sports stadiums, and public beaches.

The Cost of Smoking

It is abundantly clear that the 20 percent of the U.S. population that smoke inflict a substantial cost on their nonsmoking neighbors in a multiplicity of ways:[46]

- Smoking causes the premature death of an estimated 440,000 persons annually.

- Smoking costs the American economy an estimated $150 billion annually in health-related expenditures ($75.5 billion in excess health care costs, and $81.9 billion in death-driven losses in productivity).

- Cigarettes alone cost the typical smoker nearly $4,000 annually.

- Life expectancies for adult male and female smokers are reduced nearly 15 years (when passive smoking-related premature deaths are factored out) compared to nonsmokers.

- Nearly 1,000 neonates and infants die unnecessarily during the first year of life due to the effects of other people's smoking.

- Nearly $800 is added to the cost of prenatal care due to smoking during pregnancy.

In more personal ways, smokers also accrue costs that are less easily documented. Smokers lose some independence (nicotine-based needs will structure many aspects of day-to-day living) and may be socially rejected by the nonsmoking majority, including the significant number of young adults who do not want smokers as their life partners (see the box "The Hidden Price Tag of Smoking"). Smokers may experience subtle forms of discrimination when they search for employment (smokers miss more days of work, waste an hour per day on smoking breaks, and eventually raise their employer's health insurance expenditures). Smokers often receive lower

The Hidden Price Tag of Smoking

"I started to hug him but felt myself drawing back. It was almost like a reflex action." Those are the words of a young woman after greeting her brother when he returned home from his first semester at college. The young man had recently become a smoker, and his sister was reacting to the strong smell of smoke on his clothes and hair.

Dramatic as it may sound, smoking does set up barriers between people. First, there's the health issue. Some nonsmokers are adamant about not wanting people they care about to smoke. They also want to protect their children from this danger. And they certainly don't want to breathe in smoke themselves. So, at a family gathering, a smoker may want to have a cigarette after dinner, in the living room with everyone else. But the nonsmokers say no—go outside if you want to smoke. In the process, a birthday dinner or a special holiday is marred by this disagreement.

Whether the person is a family member or a friend, it's difficult to feel close to someone who's doing something you disapprove of—such as smoking. But, from the smoker's point of view, it's hard to feel good about someone who acts superior and doesn't accept you as you are. What do children think about all this? Does a "good" aunt or uncle smoke? If smoking is bad, as a little girl constantly hears at school and at home, why does her favorite uncle smoke?

On the job, smoking has gone the way of the three-martini lunch. It's just not politically correct. In fact, many companies have a no-smoking policy, or smoking is allowed in designated areas only. Ever drive by a big factory or office building and see a group of people standing outside, perhaps huddled under umbrellas? They're not organizing a strike—they're having a smoke. Once again, the smoker

feels isolated. Just as in the family group, the smoker feels the judgment of others—only now it's her boss or secretary who's frowning.

In addition to the more modest work-site restrictions just described, today the hammer has fallen even harder on the heads of smokers—companies are beginning to reject job applications from smokers. (It's hard to hide the telltale signs of smoking and relatively easy to learn from references whether an applicant is a smoker.) Additionally, companies have begun terminating employees who smoke, even when they don't smoke at work. Some companies will pay for smoking-cessation assistance, so long as the employees remain active participants in the program and eventually quit smoking. Countersuits brought by rejected applicants and terminated employees will certainly begin filtering through the court system, but until final rulings are made, smokers should be prepared for increasing discrimination.

The price of smoking is hard to measure. The damage to the smoker's health is beyond dispute. But the spiritual and psychological costs are also real. How does it feel to always be the outsider? The unaccepted? Why does the smoker have to take the chance of missing an exciting play in the stadium to go smoke a cigarette? Or feel the resentment of others at work because he leaves to take a smoking break every hour? Many who have stopped smoking—often after several attempts—say that they thought about more than their health in deciding to quit. They thought about many situations—involving family, outdoor activities, and work—before they threw away the pack and said: "That was my last cigarette."

trade-ins on their vehicles (double detailing is expensive to the dealer) and have a harder time selling their smoke-saturated houses (even freshly baked bread won't hide the odorous evidence that smokers have lived in the house).

Smokers' contention that "smoking only hurts smokers" is patently untrue. In fact, the economic costs alone should stimulate those smokers reading this chapter to pay close attention to the discussion of quitting at the end of this chapter.

Stopping What You Started

Experts in health behavior contend that before people will discontinue harmful health behaviors, such as tobacco use, they must appreciate fully what they are expecting of themselves. This understanding grows in relationship to the following:

1. *Knowledge* about the health risks associated with tobacco use

2. *Recognition* that these health risks are applicable to all tobacco users
3. *Familiarity* with steps that can be taken to eliminate or reduce these risks
4. *Belief* that the benefits to be gained by no longer using tobacco will outweigh the pleasures gained through the use of tobacco
5. *Certainty* that one can start and maintain the behaviors required to stop or reduce the use of tobacco

These steps combine both knowledge and desire (or motivation). Being knowledgeable about risks, however, will not always stop behaviors that involve varying degrees of psychological and physical dependence. The 75 percent failure rate thought to be common among tobacco-cessation programs suggests that the motivation is not easy to achieve or maintain. In fact, on the basis of information reported by the Hazelden Foundation, for persons who are successful in quitting, approximately 18.6 years elapse between the first attempt to stop and actual quitting. The many health benefits of quitting smoking are shown in Figure 9-3.

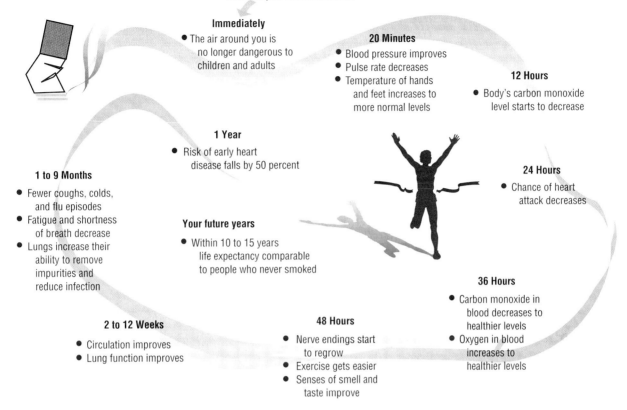

Your first year as a nonsmoker

Immediately
- The air around you is no longer dangerous to children and adults

20 Minutes
- Blood pressure improves
- Pulse rate decreases
- Temperature of hands and feet increases to more normal levels

12 Hours
- Body's carbon monoxide level starts to decrease

1 Year
- Risk of early heart disease falls by 50 percent

24 Hours
- Chance of heart attack decreases

1 to 9 Months
- Fewer coughs, colds, and flu episodes
- Fatigue and shortness of breath decrease
- Lungs increase their ability to remove impurities and reduce infection

Your future years
- Within 10 to 15 years life expectancy comparable to people who never smoked

36 Hours
- Carbon monoxide in blood decreases to healthier levels
- Oxygen in blood increases to healthier levels

2 to 12 Weeks
- Circulation improves
- Lung function improves

48 Hours
- Nerve endings start to regrow
- Exercise gets easier
- Senses of smell and taste improve

Figure 9-3 Benefits of Quitting The health benefits of quitting smoking begin immediately and become more significant the longer you stay smoke-free.

Sources: Adapted from American Cancer Society, "Guide to Quitting Smoking," http://www.cancer.org/docroot/PED/content/PED_10_13X_Guide_for_Quitting_Smoking.asp. October 2006; American Lung Association, "Quit Smoking Benefits." http://www.lungusa.org/site/pp.asp?c=dvLUK900&b=33568, October 2007.

Smoking Cessation Programs

A variety of smoking-cessation programs exist, including those using highly organized formats, with or without the use of prescription or OTC nicotine replacement systems. In past years, most people who managed to quit smoking each year did so by throwing away their cigarettes (going cold turkey) and paying the physical and emotional price of waiting for their bodies to adjust to life without nicotine. Today, however, the use of nicotine replacement products in combination with external smoking cessation approaches, such as those described later in this chapter, or the use of prescription medication is more common. The box "Countdown to Quit Day" highlights strategies to help smokers prepare to quit.

Programs to help people stop their tobacco use are available in a variety of formats, including educational programs, behavior modification, aversive conditioning, hypnosis, acupuncture, and various combinations of these approaches (see the box "Hypnotism" on page 287). Programs are offered in both individual and group settings and are operated by hospitals, universities, health departments, voluntary health agencies, churches, and private practitioners. The better programs will have lim-

ited success rates—20–50 percent as measured over one year (with self-reporting), whereas the remainder will have even poorer results. If results are monitored using the assessment of nicotine breakdown products in the blood, the effectiveness rate of these programs falls even lower, as some "successful" self-reporters are not completely honest in their reporting of cessation. When followed beyond one year, the success of smoking cessation efforts continue to drop, particularly with self-directed efforts (without directed involvement of physicians or group-based leadership), often reaching levels as low as 5 percent.

In a recent meta-analysis of smoking cessation program success involving African Americans, it was found that there is no statistically significant difference between the success of this racial group and others. Of interest, however, was a finding that church-based programs might be more successful for smoking cessation than previously recognized.

Nicotine Substitution Products

Two methods for weaning smokers from cigarettes to a nontobacco source of nicotine are nicotine-containing chewing gum (Nicorette) and transdermal patches, in either prescription or OTC versions (Nicoderm, Nicotrol, Habitrol, Prostep, and others), using either single-strength or step-down formulas. A brief description of both gum and the transdermal patch is provided next, although subtle variations exist between prescription and OTC formulations and between brands.

Nicotine-Containing Chewing Gum Correct use of nicotine-containing chewing gum requires an immediate cessation of smoking, an initial determination of dosage (4 mg or 2 mg of nicotine per piece), knowledge of the appropriate manner of chewing each piece of gum,

the appropriate time to chew each piece, the maximum number of pieces to be chewed each day, and time to begin withdrawal from the therapy. When used in combination with physician guidance or program support provided by the manufacturer, cessation using nicotine-containing gum may have a success rate of 40 percent or more, based on blood evaluation. Nicotine-containing chewing gum therapy costs approximately $100 for a 10- to 12-week treatment cycle.

Transdermal Nicotine Patches The more recently developed transdermal (through the skin) nicotine patches appear to be less effective (25 percent) than does the gum

Hypnotism: A Solution for Smokers?

On at least one occasion each year a "professional" hypnotist visits the community in which we (the authors) live. A large advertisement appears in the local paper a day or two before his visit to identify his location (usually a motel conference room) and the problems (obesity and smoking) that his brand of hypnosis proves effective against. The cost of a one-time session generally ranges between $30 (for one condition) and $50 (for both conditions), with a discount for groups of two or more preregistered persons. Effective rates are generally stated to be 97.5 percent for weight reduction and 98 percent for smoking abatement. The term *effective* is, of course, never defined.

In terms of smoking abatement, what about the services of a clinically trained and hospital-based psychologist who specializes in the use of hypnosis? Does hypnosis of this type have efficacy in smoking abatement—either as a sole treatment modality or in combination with other therapies?

Important insights into this question were gleaned in two studies in 2006. The first study, conducted by researchers at Ohio State University at Lima, undertook an analysis of 12 previous studies in which hypnosis was used to treat nicotine dependence.[*] The authors concluded that women were 1.37 times more likely than men to be helped by the application of hypnosis, delivered in a clinical setting. Further, the authors suggested that a similar gender-specific difference in effectiveness, favoring women over men, was predictable in most all forms of smoking cessation therapy, not just hypnosis.

A second study reported in 2006 was conducted in a Texas hospital setting and involved eight intense hypnosis sessions delivered over a two-month period by clinically qualified hypnotists.[†] Using an initial quitting date of one week following the first session, participants were evaluated at 12 weeks and 26 weeks to see if they were still tobacco-free. The assessment method was blood-based measurement of carbon monoxide. It was reported that 60 percent of the participants were tobacco-free at 12 weeks and 40 percent were tobacco-free at 26 weeks. Unfortunately, no data were available on the percentage of participants who were still tobacco-free at the end of one year.

In light of the declining level of success through the first half-year, the percentage of participants who remained tobacco-free probably would have been still lower at the end of one year. In that case, these hypnosis-based attempts at smoking cessation would be no more (and possibly much less) successful at the end of one year than more traditional cessation techniques using nicotine replacement or medication.

The results of the meta-analysis just described paint a much different picture of the effectiveness of hypnosis in smoking cessation than that claimed by the "motel room" hypnotist.

[*]Green JP, Jay Lynn S, Montgomery GH, A meta-analysis of gender, smoking cessation, and hypnosis: A brief communication, *Int J Clin Exp Hypn,* Vol. 54, No. 2, April 2006, 224–233.
[†]Elkins GR, Rajab MH, Clinical hypnosis for smoking cessation: Preliminary results of a three-session intervention, *Int J. Clin Exp Hypn,* Vol. 54, No. 3, July 2006, 303–315.

just described, but in many ways the patches are more easily used. If a step-down version (21 mg, 14 mg, 7 mg) is employed, determinations must be made as to the appropriate initial dosage (based on number of cigarettes smoked per day and body weight), the length of time at the initial dosage before stepping down, and the manner of withdrawal after a usual 8- to 12-week treatment period. The single-dose (15 mg) version, of course, eliminates the step-down component. Costs associated with transdermal nicotine replacement therapy range from $130 to $160, depending on the type and brand.

Other Nicotine Replacement Products   In addition to the nicotine-replacement therapies already described, a nicotine inhaler and spray have been approved (in prescription form) by the FDA. Because of the large surface area of the lungs and rapid absorption into the blood, inhalation-based delivery of nicotine has become a very attractive alternative to transdermal and oral routes of replacement.

In all delivery forms and formulations, nicotine replacement therapy can be associated with contraindications and adverse reactions, including skin irritation, redness, and irregular heart rates. People who are concerned that nicotine-replacement therapies are simply a "trade-off" of addictions (from cigarettes to gum, patches, or a nasal spray) should remember that while using the therapy

Nicotine patches are one form of nicotine replacement therapy available to help smokers quit.

Table 9.4 How Methods of Smoking Cessation Stack Up

Of the nation's estimated 48 million smokers, 70% want to quit, and 46% try each year. Only 1 in 40 succeeds. Federal guidelines, based on published studies, estimate varied success rates for a number of medications designed to help smokers quit.

Medications	Nicotine gum	Nicotine inhaler	Bupropion SR (Zyban)	Nicotine spray	Nicotine patch	Combination
Number of studies	13	4	2	3	27	3
Five-month quit rate	23.7%	22.8%	30.5%	30.5%	17.7%	28.6%
Advantage	Can be used to offset cravings	Mimics smoking	Nonnicotine, an antidepressant	Higher nicotine levels	Private, one/day	Combines benefits
Disadvantage	Poor taste	Low nicotine levels	Must screen for seizures	Irritation, sneezing	Skin irritation	Not FDA approved
Over the Counter (OTC) or prescription (Rx)	OTC	Rx	Rx	Rx	Both	Both

Source: Vergano, D. As many opinions as treatments in tobacco fight, *USA Today*, June 19, 2001, copyright 2001, reprinted with permission; quit rate data from *Treating Tobacco Use and Dependence*, U.S. Public Health Service: John Hughes, University of Vermont, November 2000.

the former smoker is no longer being exposed to carbon monoxide and carcinogens, and the step-down feature allows for a gradual return to a totally nicotine-free lifestyle. Therefore, a short period of cross-addiction should be viewed simply as the cost of recovery.

Neurotransmitter-Based Prescription Medications

Recently developed prescription medications used in combination with other cessation methods improve the latter's effectiveness rate to somewhat above the 40 percent (perhaps approaching 50 percent) level reported for nicotine-containing chewing gum, according to a blood-based assessment. These drugs affect receptors in the CNS, reducing the pleasurable effects of nicotine and thus decreasing dependency. Among the more recently "discovered" prescription medications for smoking cessation is methoxsalen. Although intended for the treatment of psoriasis, a skin condition, this medication has been found to constructively alter the breakdown of nicotine in persons who have a particular genetic mutation that lessens their need for frequent cigarettes.

Several additional nicotine-free prescription medications to aid smoking cessation have now been approved or are nearing approval. These agents can be used alone or with nicotine replacement therapy. Bupropion (Zyban, Wellbutrin) is an antidepressant drug that increases the production of dopamine, a neurotransmitter. Production of dopamine declines when a smoker quits, creating the craving to smoke. Prozac, the serotonin-reuptake inhibitor antidepressant approved for the treatment of depression, bulimia nervosa, PMS, and obsessive-compulsive disorder, has also shown promise as an adjunct to smoking cessation. See Table 9.4 for a comparison of various cessation approaches that are well established in the marketplace.

Prescription Medications Based on Nicotine Receptor Inhibitors

Several newer medications have been recently approved or are still in controlled trials. One such medication, developed in Europe, is marketed in the United States as Chantix (varenicline).[47] Chantix influences nervous system receptors for nicotine to level out the peaks and valleys normally associated with smoking. This leveling-out aids cessation by diminishing the "highly satisfying" character of the first inhalation following a low-nicotine valley, and by minimizing the discomfort experienced while in a state of nicotine depletion (a valley). Many other smoking cessation medications were initially effective during controlled trials, only to lose their effectiveness when used by the general public. Chantix may well follow this disappointing course.

A second medication, now on the first track for approval, is another European drug, rimonabant, that will be marketed in the United States as Acomplia. This medication initially was developed to aid in weight loss, but it has shown efficacy in aiding smoking cessation.

Anti-Smoking Vaccines

The goal of anti-smoking vaccines is to prevent nicotine from reaching nicotine receptors in the brain by conditioning the immune system to attack the nicotine molecules. Research in vaccine development has begun to bear fruit. Clinical trials are currently under way on a vaccine named NicVAX.[48] In these trials, subjects will receive four or five immunization shots over a period of many weeks. In response, the immune system should eventually begin producing antibodies (see Chapter 12) against nicotine. Most likely the initial role of NicVAX will be the prevention of relapse in persons who have undergone other forms of smoking cessation. At least four other vaccines are in earlier stages of development.

Despite the satisfaction of the dependency that continued smoking brings, approximately 80 percent of adult smokers have, on at least one occasion, expressed a desire to quit, and the majority of these have actually attempted to become nonsmokers. Today, with the over-the-counter availability of transdermal nicotine patches, nicotine-containing gum, prescription medications such as antidepressants, nicotine inhalers, and nicotine receptor inhibitors, the number of smokers making concerted and repeated attempts to stop smoking is up considerably over that seen in the past. It therefore seems apparent that tobacco use is a source of **dissonance.** This dissonance stems from the need to deal emotionally with a behavior that is both highly enjoyable and highly dangerous but known to be difficult to stop. The degree to which this dissonance exists probably varies from user to user.

Tobacco Use: A Question of Rights

For those readers who have found themselves involved (or nearly so) in confrontation situations involving smokers' versus nonsmokers' rights, we hope the following section allows you to see more clearly the positions that you have taken. For those who have somehow remained removed from this discussion, consideration of these issues now may be good preparation for the future. Regardless, consider these two important questions:

1. To what extent should smokers be allowed to pollute the air and endanger the health of nonsmokers?

2. To what extent should nonsmokers be allowed to restrict the personal freedom of smokers, particularly since tobacco products are sold legally?

At this time, answers to these questions are only partially available, but one trend is developing: the tobacco user is being forced to give ground to the nonsmoker. Today, in fact, it is becoming more a matter of where the smoker will be allowed to smoke, rather than a matter of where smoking will be restricted. Smoking is currently becoming less and less tolerated. The health concerns of the majority are prevailing over the dependence needs of the minority.

TALKING POINTS You're having a discussion with a friend about life insurance and mention that you get a 10 percent reduction in your annual premium because you're a nonsmoker. Your friend, who is a smoker, becomes annoyed and says that this is just one example of how smokers are penalized. How would you respond?

Key Terms

dissonance (**dis** son ince) A feeling of uncertainty that occurs when a person believes two equally attractive but opposite ideas.

Taking Charge of Your Health

- Commit yourself to establishing a smoke-free environment in the places where you live, work, study, and recreate.
- Support friends and acquaintances who are trying to become smoke-free.

- Support legislative efforts, at all levels of government, to reduce your exposure to environmental tobacco smoke.
- Be civil toward tobacco users in public spaces, but respond assertively if they infringe on smoke-free spaces.

- Support agencies and organizations committed to reducing tobacco use among young people through education and intervention.

SUMMARY

- The percentage of American adults who smoke is continuing to decline.
- In spite of a reversal on the part of more recent college graduates, cigarette smoking has traditionally been inversely related to the level of formal education.
- A number of demographic variables influence the incidence of tobacco use.
- The tobacco industry continues to aggressively market its products to potential smokers.

- Multiple theories regarding nicotine's role in dependence have been advanced, including a better understanding of the proportional influences of genetics, environment, and personality.
- Nicotine exerts acute effects both within the central nervous system and on a variety of other tissues and organs.
- Tobacco smoke can be divided into gaseous and particulate phases. Each phase has its unique chemical composition.

- Thousands of chemical components and hundreds of carcinogenic agents are found in tobacco smoke.
- Nicotine and carbon monoxide have predictable effects on the function of the cardiovascular system.
- The development of nearly one-third of all cancers can be attributed to tobacco use, and virtually every form of cancer is found more frequently in smokers than in nonsmokers.
- Chronic obstructive lung disease (COLD), also called chronic obstructive pulmonary disease (COPD), is a likely consequence of long-term cigarette smoking, with early symptoms appearing shortly after beginning regular smoking.

- Smoking alters normal structure and function of the body, as seen in a wide variety of noncardiovascular and noncancerous conditions, such as infertility, problem pregnancy, and neonatal health concerns. Additional health concerns include the diminished ability to smell, periodontal disease, vitamin inadequacies, and bone loss leading to osteoporosis.
- The use of smokeless tobacco carries its own health risks, including oral cancer.
- The presence of secondhand smoke results in involuntary (or passive) smoking by those who must share a common air source with smokers.
- Stopping smoking can be undertaken in several ways.

REVIEW QUESTIONS

1. What percentage of the American adult population smoke? In what direction has change been occurring?
2. What is the current direction that adolescent smoking is taking?
3. What was the outcome of the class action suit brought by all states, and what was the effect of the Master Settlement Agreement (1999) on the ability of the tobacco industry to market its products?
4. What are the two principal dimensions of nicotine dependence? What are specific aspects seen within physical dependence?
5. Identify each of the theories of nicotine dependence discussed in the chapter.
6. How do modeling and manipulation explain the development of emotional dependence on tobacco?
7. In the amount consumed by the typical smoker, what is the effect of nicotine on central nervous system function? How does this differ in chain smokers?
8. What effects does nicotine have on the body outside of the central nervous system? How does the influence

of nicotine resemble that associated with the stress response?
9. What is the principal effect of carbon monoxide on cardiac function?
10. What influences does passive smoking have on nonsmoking adult partners of smokers? On their children?
11. How is the federal government attempting to limit the exposure that children and adolescents currently have to tobacco products and tobacco advertisements?
12. In comparison to cigarettes, what health risks are associated with pipe and cigar smoking?
13. How might concerned parents begin to "tobacco proof" their children to keep them from becoming smokers in the future?
14. What prescription and OTC products are now available to assist smokers in quitting?
15. What percentage of smokers are able to quit, and what is the best way to confirm that quitting has occurred?

ANSWERS TO THE "WHAT DO YOU KNOW?" QUIZ

1. True   2. False   3. True   4. False   5. False   6. False   7. True

ENDNOTES

1. State-specific prevalence of current cigarette smoking among adults and second-hand rules and policies in home and workplaces—United States, 2005. *Morbidity and Mortality Weekly Report*, Vol. 55, No. 42, October 27, 1148–1151 (Table 1).
2. State-specific prevalence of current cigarette smoking among adults and second-hand rules and policies in home and workplaces—United States, 2005. 2006. *MMWR*. Oct 27; 55(42):1148–1151. (Table 2).
3. Aldworth J, et al. 2006. *Results from the 2005 National Survey on Drug Use and Health: National Findings*. SAMHSA. Department of Health and Human Services, DHHS Publication No. SMA 06-4194.
4. Youth risk behavior surveillance—United States, 2005, 2006, *MMWR*. June 9; 55(SS-5):1–108. (Table 20).
5. Patterson F, et al. Cigarette smoking practices among American

college students: Review and future directions. *Journal of American College Health*, Vol. 52, No. 5, March–April 2004, 203–210.
6. Tobacco use among adults—United States, 2005. 2006. *MMWR*. Oct 27; 55(42):1145–1148. (Table).
7. Aldworth J, et al. 2006 *Results from the 2005 National Survey on Drug Use and Health: Detailed Tables: Detailed Tables*. SAMHSA. Department of Health and Human Services. (Table 2.81B). (DHHS Publication Number Not Assigned).
8. Aldworth J, et al. 2006 *Results from the 2005 National Survey on Drug Use and Health: Detailed Tables*. SAMHSA. Department of Heath and Human Services. (Table 2.35B). (DHHS Publication Number Not Assigned).
9. QuickStats: Cigarette smoking prevalence among adults aged 18 years who have ever spent 24 hours on the streets, in a shelter, or in a

jail or prison, by sex—United States, 2004. 2006. *MMWR.* March 17; 55(10):287.

10. QuickStats: Percentage of U.S.-born and foreign-born adults aged 18 years reporting selected health risk factors and conditions, 1998–2003. 2006. *MMWR.* March 24; 55(11):313.

11. Wilson, JJ. *Summary of the Attorneys General Master Tobacco Settlement Agreement.* 1999. National Conference of State Legislators. March; pages 1–44. www.academic.idayton.edu/health/syllabi/tobacco/summary.htm.

12. Henriksen L, et al. Industry sponsored anti-smoking ads and adolescent reactance: test of a boomerang effect. *Tobacco Control,* Vol. 15, No. 1, February 2006, 13–18.

13. Shiffman S, Paty J. Smoking patterns and dependence: contrasting chippers and heavy smokers. *Journal of Abnormal Psychology,* Vol. 115, No. 3, August 2006, 509–523.

14. Tong EK, et al. Nondaily smokers should be asked and advised to quit. 2006. *Am J Prev Med.* Jan; 30(1):23–30.

15. Maes HH, et al. A twin study of genetic and environmental influences on tobacco initiation, regular tobacco use, and nicotine dependence. 2004. *Psychol Med.* Oct; 34(7):1251–1261.

16. Wang D, Ma JZ, Li MD. Mapping and verification of susceptibility loci for smoking quantity using permutation linkage analysis. *Pharacogenomics,* Vol. 5, No. 3, 2005, 166–172.

17. Li MD, et al. A genomewide search finds major susceptibility loci for nicotine dependence on chromosome 10 in African Americans. *American Journal of Human Genetics* Vol. 79, No. 4, October 2006, 745–751.

18. Gelernter J, et al. Genomewide linkage scan for nicotine dependence: identification of a chromosome 5 risk loci. 2006. *Biological Psychiatry.* Oct 31. (e-publication ahead of print).

19. Sullivan PF, et al. Candidate genes for nicotine dependence via linkage, epistasis, bioinformatics. 2004. *Med Genet B Neuropsychiatr Genet.* April 1; 126(1): 23–36.

20. Sullivan PF, Kendler KSW. The genetic epidemiology of smoking. 1999. *Nicotine Tob Res, Suppl.* 2:51.

21. DiFranza JR, et al. Development of symptoms of tobacco dependence in youths: 30 month follow up data from the DANDY study, 2002. *Tobacco Control,* Sept; 11(3):228–235.

22. Wheeler KC, et al. Screening adolescents for nicotine dependence: The Hooked On Nicotine Checklist. 2004. *Journal of Adolescent Health.* Sept; 35(3):225–230.

23. Fidler JA, et al. Vulnerability to smoking after trying a single cigarette can lie dormant for three years. 2006. *Tobacco Control,* Jun; 15(3):205–209.

24. Bricker JB, et al. Nine-year prospective relationship between parental smoking cessation and children's daily smoking. 2003. *Addiction.* 98(5):585–593.

25. DiFranza JR, et al. Tobacco Consortium, Center for Child Health Research of the American Academy of Pediatrics. 2006. *Pediatrics.* Jun; 117(6):e1237–1248.

26. Saladin KS. *Anatomy and Physiology: The Unity of Form and Function* (4th ed.). New York: McGraw-Hill. 2007.

27. American Cancer Society. *Cancer Facts and Figures—2006.* Atlanta: American Cancer Society. 2006.

28. American Heart Association/American Stroke Association. *Heart Disease and Stroke Stastistics—2006 Update.*

29. Gray N. The consequences of the unregulated cigarette. 2006. *Tobacco Control,* Oct; 15(5):405–408.

30. Mackay J, Eriksen M, Shafey O. *The Tobacco Atlas* (2nd ed.). 2006. American Cancer Society.

31. Werley MS, Coggins CR, Lee PN. Possible effects on smokers of cigarette mentholation: A review of the evidence relation to key research questions. 2006. *Regul Toxicol Pharmacol.* Nov. (e-publication ahead of print).

32. *Cigars: Health Effects and Trends.* 1998. Cancer Monograph Series (no. 9) National Cancer Institute. (Reviewed March 2000).

33. *The Health Consequences of Using Smokeless Tobacco: A Report of the Advisory Committee to the Surgeon General.* 1986. U.S. Department of Health and Human Services. Public Health Service. NIH Publication No. 86-2874.

34. Koziowski LT, et al. Maximum yields might improve public health—if filter vents were banned: A lesson from the history of vented filters. 2006. *Tobacco Control,* Jun, 15(3):262–266.

35. Habek D, et al. Fetal tobacco syndrome and perinatal outcome. 2002. *Fetal Diagn Ther.* Nov–Dec; 17(6):367–371.

36. DiFranza JR, Aligne CA, Weitzman M. Prenatal and postnatal environmental tobacco smoke exposure: Children's health. 2004. *Pediatrics.* Apr; 113(4 Suppl):1007–1015.

37. Hassa H, et al. Effect of smoking on semen parameters of men attending an infertility clinic. 2006. *Clin Exp Obstet Gynecol.* 33(1): 19–22.

38. Elhanbly S, et al. Erectile dysfunction in smokers: A penile dynamic and vascular study. *J Androl.* 2004. Nov–Dec; 25(6):991–995.

39. Centers for Disease Control and Prevention. Annual smoking-attributed mortality, years of potential life lost, and productivity losses—United States, 1997–2001. 2005. *Morbidity and Mortality Weekly Report,* 2005; 54(25):625–628.

40. *The Health Consequences of Involuntary Exposure to Tobacco Smoke: A Report of the Surgeon General.* U.S. Department of Health and Human Services. 2006. June; www.surgeongeneral.gov/library/secondhandsmoke/.

41. Enstrom JE, Kabat GC. Environmental tobacco smoke and coronary heart disease mortality in the United States—a meta-analysis and critique. 2006. *Inhal Toxicol.* Mar; 18(3):199–210.

42. Wen W, et al. Environmental tobacco smoke and mortality in Chinese women who have never smoked: prospective study. 2006 *BMJ.* Aug; 333(7654):376. (e-publication 2006 Jul 12).

43. Mitchell EA, Milerad J. Smoking and the sudden infant death syndrome. *Review of Environmental Health,* Vol. 21, No. 2, April–June 2006, 81–103.

44. *States and municipalities with 100% smokefree laws in workplaces, restaurants, or bars.* ANRF—American Nonsmokers' Rights Foundation. Oct; 2006. www.asr@no-smoke.org.

45. *List of smoking bans: Bans in public places or bars/restaurants.* (modified Nov. 15, 2006), www.en.wikipedia.org/wiki/List_of_smoking_bans.

46. MMWR-Annual smoking-Attributable mortality, years of potential life lost, and economic costs—United States, 1995–1999. 2002. *MMWR Highlights.* April 12; 51(14); www.cdc.gov/tobacco/research_data/economics/mmwr5114.highlights.htm.

47. Oncken C, et al. Efficacy and safety of the novel selective nicotinic acethycholine receptor partial agonist, varenicline, for smoking cessation. 2006. *Arch Intern Med.* Aug; 166(15):1571–1577.

48. Hatsukami DK, et al. Safety and immunogenicity of a nicotine conjugate vaccine in current smoking. 2005. *Clin Pharmacol Ther.* Nov; 78(5):456–467.

Personal Assessment

A Simple Dependency Test: Your Relationship with Cigarettes

To nonsmokers it must seem that smokers would realize the existence of their dependency on cigarettes; however, such might not be the case. The following Hooked On Nicotine Checklist (HONC) is a simple way to determine whether a cigarette-based dependency exists. If you are a smoker, answer each question asked by the HONC in an honest manner; then give careful consideration to your findings. If you are a nonsmoker, ask a smoker to complete the HONC and share responses to each item with you—a good discussion could ensue.

Nicotine Addiction's 10 Warning Signs: HONC—Hooked On Nicotine Checklist

1. Have you ever tried to quit but couldn't?
2. Do you smoke now because it is really hard to quit?
3. Have you ever felt like you were addicted to tobacco?
4. Do you ever have strong cravings to smoke?
5. Have you ever felt like you really needed a cigarette?
6. Is it hard to keep from smoking in places where you are not supposed to, like school?

In answering the last four questions, when you tried to stop smoking, or when you have not used tobacco for a while . . .

7. Did you find it hard to concentrate?
8. Did you feel more irritable?
9. Did you feel a strong need or urge to smoke?
10. Did you feel nervous, restless, or anxious because you couldn't smoke?

Interpretation

Answering yes to any one of these 10 questions indicates that you may already be hooked on nicotine and are chemically dependent.

TO CARRY THIS FURTHER . . .

Think about it! Your yes answer is your own honest self-assessment that you have already lost the freedom and ability to simply and effortlessly walk away. Two-thirds of all teens whom you see smoking regularly will spend their entire life as slaves to nicotine.

Source: From J. R. DiFranza, J. A. Savageau, K. Fletcher, J. K. Ockene, N. A. Rigotti, A. D. McNeill, M. Coleman, and C. Wood, "Measuring the Loss of Autonomy Over Nicotine Use in Adolescents: The DANDY Development and Assessment of Nicotine Dependence in Youths (DANDY) Study. *Archives of Pediatrics and Adolescent Medicine*, 2002; 156; 397–403. Used with permission by AMA and Dr. J. R. DiFranza, MD.

Preventing Diseases

Part Four consists of four chapters that focus on disease prevention. Each illness you contract or develop can harm your health in each of its dimensions; therefore, prevention should be a high priority. There are many positive personal health choices you can make to reduce your risk of developing many diseases.

1. Physical Dimension

We usually associate illness with pain, fear, discomfort, and limitations. But paradoxically, health problems can also improve the physical dimension of health. For example, exposure to certain infectious diseases may allow your body to develop immunity. Illness can also force you to rest, reduce your workload, and reconsider your health behavior. Weight loss, smoking cessation, improved dietary practices, genetic counseling, or a renewed commitment to fitness may follow your recovery from an illness.

2. Emotional Dimension

Emotionally healthy people feel good about themselves and others and are able to cope with most of life's demands. Being diagnosed with an illness or disease can jeopardize your emotional resources. You may feel anxious, isolated, and vulnerable. Fortunately, many diseases can be prevented or at least managed or treated successfully.

3. Social Dimension

People rarely face an illness or manage a chronic health condition alone. People who have heart disease, cancer, diabetes, or HIV infection often join support groups or establish friendships with others who have the same condition. In addition, you probably interact with people during activities aimed at preventing diseases. For example, you might exercise with a partner or meet people at a weight-loss group.

4. Intellectual Dimension

We can best use our intellect when we are free from health problems. In some cases, diseases or medications can impair our intellectual functioning. However, managing a condition or recovering from an illness can allow you to learn about your body, your personality, and the health care system. Learning how to reduce your risk of certain diseases will also require you to draw on your intellectual resources.

5. Spiritual Dimension

Your ability to serve others can be hindered by an illness or chronic condition. In addition, your faith can be shaken when a family member falls ill or when you are diagnosed with a serious disease. For most people, however, this initial questioning leads to an even stronger faith or spirituality than they had before the experience.

6. Occupational Dimension

Diseases and your efforts to prevent them can have a significant effect on your job performance. If you have an acute illness, you probably will not be able to work temporarily. If you have a chronic condition or disease, you must try to manage it well enough that you are still able to work. Some conditions are so severe that employment becomes impossible. However, your efforts to prevent illness, such as fitness activities, will enhance your job performance.

Enhancing Your Cardiovascular Health

What Do You Know about Keeping Your Heart Healthy?

- About one in every three American adults has some form of cardiovascular disease. True or False?

- There are more cardiovascular disease risk factors that you can change (such as your cholesterol levels) than those you cannot change (such as your age). True or False?

- The risk for a heart attack is the same for a person who smoked a pack a day of cigarettes and quit more than a year ago as for the person who has smoked for 20 years and is continuing to smoke a pack a day. True or False?

- You do not need to have your cholesterol checked until you are 30 years old. True or False?

- Only health care professionals should use an automated external defibrillator (AED) to assist a person experiencing a cardiac arrest. True or False?

- African Americans have a greater risk of stroke than Caucasians. True or False?

- Individuals with diabetes have a greater risk of developing cardiovascular disease than people of the same age without diabetes. True or False?

Check your answers at the end of the chapter.

Great progress has been made with respect to **cardiovascular** disease (CVD), the focus of this chapter. Although heart disease continues to be the top killer overall and the number two killer of Americans under the age of 85 (behind cancer), between 1990 and 2000 the death rates from CVD declined 17 percent.[1] Still, CVD claimed about 871,500 lives in 2004.[1] (By comparison, cancer caused 550,270 deaths, accidents caused 108,694, Alzheimer's disease caused 65,829, and HIV/AIDS caused 12,995.) CVD directly caused 36 percent of all deaths, or 1 out of every 2.8 deaths in 2004; it contributed to another 22 percent of deaths. The prevalence of CVD—the number of Americans currently living with one or more forms of CVD—is even higher, with about 1 in 3 adults affected (Table 10.1).

Today, nearly 2,400 Americans die each day of CVD, an average of 1 death every 36 seconds. Cardiovascular diseases claim more lives each year than the next four leading causes of death combined. If all

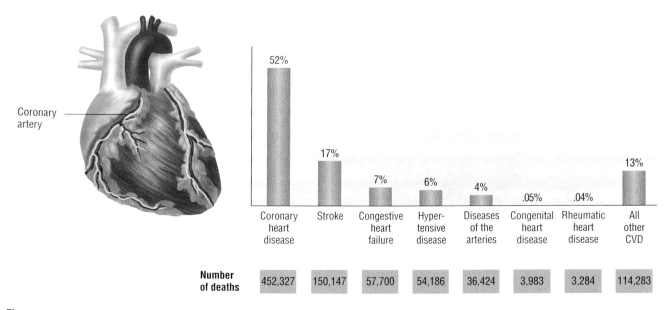

Coronary artery

	Coronary heart disease	Stroke	Congestive heart failure	Hyper-tensive disease	Diseases of the arteries	Congenital heart disease	Rheumatic heart disease	All other CVD
Percentage	52%	17%	7%	6%	4%	.05%	.04%	13%
Number of deaths	452,327	150,147	57,700	54,186	36,424	3,983	3,284	114,283

Figure 10-1 Deaths from Cardiovascular Disease   Of the 872,364 deaths in the United States in 2004* resulting from cardiovascular diseases, nearly half were attributable to heart attack.

The most recent year for which statistics are available.
Source: American Heart Association. Heart Disease and Stroke Statistics—2007 Update, *Circulation* 115: 69–171.

Table 10.1   Estimated Prevalence of Major Cardiovascular Diseases

Hypertension	72,000,000
Coronary heart disease	15,800,000
Stroke	5,700,000
Congestive heart failure	5,200,000
Congenital heart disease*	1,300,000
TOTAL (people)	79,400,000

Note: The sum of the individual estimates exceeds 79,400,000 because so many people have more than one cardiovascular disorder.

*The prevalence of congenital cardiovascular defects is estimated to range from 650,000 to 1.3 million.

Source: American Heart Association, Heart Disease and Stroke Statistics—2007 Update, *Circulation* 115: 69–171.

major forms of CVD were eliminated, life expectancy in the United States would increase by almost seven years. Figure 10-1 shows the number of deaths from major forms of CVD each year; more information on these specific diseases is presented later in this chapter.

Fortunately, there are many concrete steps you can take to reduce your personal risk for cardiovascular disease. In this chapter, we explain how the heart works and help you identify your CVD risk factors. Prevention efforts are most effective when started in childhood, but it is never too late to adopt a wellness lifestyle. Quitting smoking, becoming physically active, following a nutritious diet, and controlling your blood pressure are important ways of reducing your risk of heart disease and improving your overall health.

Normal Cardiovascular Function

The cardiovascular system, also called the *circulatory system,* uses a muscular pump to send a complex fluid on a continuous trip through a closed system of tubes. The pump is the heart, the fluid is blood, and the closed system of tubes is the network of blood vessels.

The Vascular System

The term *vascular system* refers to the body's blood vessels. Although we might be familiar with the arteries (vessels that carry blood away from the heart) and the veins (vessels that carry blood to the heart), arterioles, capillaries, and venules are also part of the vascular system. Arterioles are the smaller-diameter extensions of arteries. These arterioles lead eventually to capillaries, the smallest extensions of the vascular system. At the capillary level, oxygen, food, and waste are exchanged between cells and the blood.

After the blood leaves the capillaries and begins its return to the heart, it drains into small veins, or venules. The blood in the venules flows into increasingly larger vessels called *veins.* Blood pressure is highest in arteries

> **Key Terms**
>
> **cardiovascular** Pertaining to the heart (*cardio*) and blood vessels (*vasculara*).

ENDNOTES

1. American Heart Association. *Heart Disease and Stroke: Statistical Update.* AHA, 2007.
2. Thibodeau GA, Patton KT. *Structure and Function of the Human Body* (11th ed.). St. Louis, MO: Mosby-Year Book, 2000.
3. Brubaker PH, Kaminsky LA, Whaley MH. *Coronary Artery Disease.* Champaign, IL: Human Kinetics, 2002.
4. Centers for Disease Control and Prevention. Facts on high blood pressure, www.cdc.gov/blood pressure/facts.htm.
5. National Center for Health Statistics. Health, United States, 2006, www.cdc.gov/nchs/hus.htm, May 11, 2007.
6. National Health Interview Survey (released December 12, 2006), www.cdc.gov/nchs/about/major/nhis/released200612.htm.
7. Sesso HD, Paffenbarger RS, Lee I. Physical activity and coronary heart disease in men: The Harvard alumni health study. *Circulation,* 2000; Vol. 102, pp. 975–980.
8. Lee I, Sesso HD, Paffenbarger RS. Physical activity and coronary heart disease in men: Does the duration of exercise episodes predict risk? *Circulation,* 2000; Vol. 102, pp. 981–986.
9. American Diabetes Association. Standards of Medical Care in Diabetes 2007. *Diabetes Care,* 2007; 30:S40–S41.
10. National Institutes of Health. *Clinical Guidelines on the Identification, Evaluation, and Treatment of Overweight and Obesity in Adults.* 1998.
11. American Heart Association. Homocyst(e)ine, diet, and cardiovascular diseases. *Circulation,* 1999; Vol. 99, pp. 178–182.
12. American Heart Association. Markers of Inflammation and Cardiovascular Disease. *Circulation,* 2003; Vol. 107, pp. 499–511.
13. National Cholesterol Education Program. The Third Report of the Expert Panel on Detection, Evaluation, and Treatment of High Blood Cholesterol in Adults, NIH Publication No. 02-5215, 2002.
14. American Heart Association/American College of Sports Medicine. Automated external defibrillators in health/fitness facilities. *Circulation,* 2002; Vol. 105, pp. 1147–1150.
15. American Heart Association. Aspirin as a therapeutic agent in cardiovascular disease. *Circulation,* 1997; Vol. 96, 2751–2753.
16. National Heart, Lung, and Blood Institute. *The Seventh Report of the Joint National Committee on* Prevention, Detection, Evaluation, and Treatment of High Blood Pressure (JNC 7). www.nhlbi.nih.gov/guidelines/hypertension/index.htm, July 21, 2003.

Personal Assessment

What is your risk for heart disease?

Coronary Disease Risk Prediction Score Sheet for Men Based on Total Cholesterol Level

For steps 1–6, determine the points for your characteristics and record these in the summary box (step 7). Using the point total determine your risk score in step 8. Step 9 allows you to compare your risk level to that of the average person of your age. (If you are younger than 30 years old, use the 30–34 age group.) Ideally, you want your value to be at or below the "low risk" score.

Step 1

Age	
Years	Points
30–34	−1
35–39	0
40–44	1
45–49	2
50–54	3
55–59	4
60–64	5
65–69	6
70–74	7

Step 2

Total Cholesterol		
(mg/dl)	(mmol/L)	Points
<160	≤4.14	−3
160–199	4.15–5.17	0
200–239	5.18–6.21	1
240–279	6.22–7.24	2
≥280	≥7.25	3

Key	
Color	Risk
green	Very low
white	Low
yellow	Moderate
rose	High
red	Very high

Step 3

HDL Cholesterol		
(mg/dl)	(mmol/L)	Points
<35	≤0.90	2
35–44	0.91–1.16	1
45–49	1.17–1.29	0
50–59	1.30–1.55	0
≥60	≥1.56	−2

Step 4

Blood Pressure					
Systolic (mm Hg)	Diastolic (mm Hg)				
	<80	80–84	85–89	90–99	≥100
<120	0				
120–129		0 pts			
130–139			1		
140–159					
≥160					3 pts

Note: When systolic and diastolic pressures provide different estimates for point scores, use the higher number.

Step 5

Diabetes	
	Points
No	0
Yes	2

Step 6

Smoker	
	Points
No	0
Yes	2

Risk estimates were derived from the experience of the NHLBI's Framingham Heart Study, a predominantly Caucasian population in Massachusetts, USA.

Step 7 (sum from steps 1–6)

Adding Up the Points	
Age	———
Total Cholesterol	———
HDL Cholesterol	———
Blood Pressure	———
Diabetes	———
Smoker	———
Point Total	———

Step 8 (determine CHD risk from point total)

CHD Risk	
Point Total	10 Yr CHD Risk
≤−1	2%
0	3%
1	3%
2	4%
3	5%
4	7%
5	8%
6	10%
7	13%
8	16%
9	20%
10	25%
11	31%
12	37%
13	45%
≥14	≥53%

Step 9 (compare to man of the same age)

Comparative Risk		
Age (years)	Average 10 Yr CHD Risk	Low* 10 Yr CHD Risk
30–34	3%	2%
35–39	5%	3%
40–44	7%	4%
45–49	11%	4%
50–54	14%	6%
55–59	16%	7%
60–64	21%	9%
65–69	25%	11%
70–74	30%	14%

* Low risk was calculated for a man the same age, normal blood pressure, total cholesterol 160–199 mg/dl, HDL cholesterol 45 mg/dl, nonsmoker, no diabetes.

Source: www.nhlbi.nih.gov/about/framingham .risktmen.pdf.

Coronary Disease Risk Prediction Score Sheet for Women Based on Total Cholesterol Level

For steps 1–6, determine the points for your characteristics and record these in the summary box (step 7). Using the point total determine your risk score in step 8. Step 9 allows you to compare your risk level to that of the average person of your age. (If you are younger than 30 years old, use the 30–34 age group.) Ideally, you want your value to be at or below the "low risk" score.

Step 1

Age	
Years	Points
30–34	−9
35–39	−4
40–44	0
45–49	3
50–54	6
55–59	7
60–64	8
65–69	8
70–74	8

Step 2

Total Cholesterol		
(mg/dl)	(mmol/L)	Points
<160	≤4.14	−2
160–199	4.15–5.17	0
200–239	5.18–6.21	1
240–279	6.22–7.24	1
≥280	≥7.25	3

Step 3

HDL Cholesterol		
(mg/dl)	(mmol/L)	Points
<35	≤0.90	5
35–44	0.91–1.16	2
45–49	1.17–1.29	1
50–59	1.30–1.55	0
≥60	≥1.56	−3

Step 4

Blood Pressure					
Systolic	Diastolic (mm Hg)				
(mm Hg)	<80	80–84	85–89	90–99	≥100
<120	−3 pts				
120–129		0 pts			
130–139			0 pts		
140–159				2 pts	
≥160					3 pts

Note: When systolic and diastolic pressures provide different estimates for point scores, use the higher number.

Step 5

Diabetes	
	Points
No	0
Yes	4

Step 6

Smoker	
	Points
No	0
Yes	2

Risk estimates were derived from the experience of the NHLBI's Framingham Heart Study, a predominantly Caucasian population in Massachusetts, USA.

Key	
Color	Risk
green	Very low
white	Low
yellow	Moderate
rose	High
red	Very high

Step 7 (sum from steps 1–6)

Adding Up the Points	
Age	———
Total Cholesterol	———
HDL Cholesterol	———
Blood Pressure	———
Diabetes	———
Smoker	———
Point Total	———

Step 8 (determine CHD risk from point total)

CHD Risk	
Point Total	10 Yr CHD Risk
≤−2	1%
−1	2%
0	2%
1	2%
2	3%
3	3%
4	4%
5	4%
6	5%
7	6%
8	7%
9	8%
10	10%
11	11%
12	13%
13	15%
14	18%
15	20%
16	24%
≥17	≥27%

Step 9 (compare to woman of the same age)

Comparative Risk		
Age (years)	Average 10 Yr CHD Risk	Low* 10 Yr CHD Risk
30–34	1%	<1%
35–39	1%	<1%
40–44	2%	2%
45–49	5%	3%
50–54	8%	5%
55–59	12%	7%
60–64	12%	8%
65–69	13%	8%
70–74	14%	8%

* Low risk was calculated for a woman the same age, normal blood pressure, total cholesterol 160–199 mg/dl, HDL cholesterol 55 mg/dl, nonsmoker, no diabetes.

Source: www.nhlbi.nih.gov/about/framingham.risktwom.pdf

TO CARRY THIS FURTHER . . .

Were you surprised with your score on this assessment? What were the factors that gave you the most points? See how changing those factors would lower your risk of heart disease.

Living with Cancer

What Do You Know about Cancer?

◎ Cancer involves conditions arising from the lack of cellular regulation. True or False?

◎ The incidence of cancer is highest during childhood but declines with age. True or False?

◎ Carcinogens are a class of recently developed cancer-fighting drugs. True or False?

◎ Lung cancer is the leading cause of cancer deaths in both adult males and adult females. True or False?

◎ Clear strategies, based on lifestyle changes, now exist to prevent all cancers. True or False?

◎ No cancers are cured more easily today than a decade ago. True or False?

◎ The "war on cancer" would be won if the use of tobacco products were completely eliminated. True or False?

Check your answers at the end of the chapter.

Most people can attest to the disruptive influence an illness can have on their ability to participate in day-to-day activities. When we are ill, school, employment, and leisure activities are replaced by periods of lessened activity and even periods of bed rest or hospitalization. When an illness is chronic, the effect of being ill may extend over long periods, perhaps even an entire lifetime. People with chronic illness must eventually find a balance between day-to-day function and the continuous presence of their condition. Cancer is usually a chronic illness.

In spite of our understanding of its relationship to human health and our ceaseless attempts to prevent and cure it, progress in the "war on cancer" has been relatively limited. In this regard, cancer is clearly an "expensive" condition, both in terms of its human consequences and its monetary costs. It is estimated that 1,444,920 people developed cancer in 2007. Once diagnosed, approximately 66 percent (adjusted for other causes of death) of this group will be alive 5 years later.[1] This 5-year period, called *relative survivability,* includes "persons who are living 5 years after diagnosis, whether disease free, in remission, or under treatment with evidence of cancer."[1] If one limits 2007's new cases to those forms of cancer

Animal-Based Research on the Causes of Cancer

The news media frequently report that animal-based research is providing insight into the causes and prevention of cancer. However, many people wonder how studying animals can tell us anything about cancer in humans. Focusing on environmental carcinogens, let's briefly explore this use of animal-based research, and its reporting in the news media.

Principal players in the development of cancer are a huge number of chemical compounds found in the environment and known collectively as *environmental carcinogens*. Several hundred of these compounds have been studied in detail. For those compounds that have been studied (and for those not studied directly, but whose chemical makeup is similar to those studied), a classifying system has been established by the International Agency for Research on Cancer, part of the World Health Organization: Group 1: carcinogenic to humans; Group 2: probably carcinogenic to humans; Group 2B: possibly carcinogenic to humans; Group 3: unclassifiable as to carcinogenicity in humans; and Group 4: probably not carcinogenic to humans.

Particularly for those compounds now classified in groups 1, 2, and 2B, initial assessment was most likely carried out in laboratory cell cultures using cells taken from animals that are similar in structure and function to humans. If cancerous changes are noted in cell cultures exposed to a substance, then research is extended to study exposure to that substance in living animals—animal-based research.

Although the laboratory animals used in this research are similar in structure and function to humans, their exposure to suspected cancerous compounds must be carefully controlled so that it can be compared to exposure in humans. Factors such as the animals' age at maturity, life span, body weight, body composition, and diet must be carefully considered when determining exposure rates. Generally, animals are exposed at rates that are *proportionally similar* to

"excessive" levels of exposure for humans. If cancer does develop in the animals, then research using a small number of human subjects might be considered. It is more likely, however, that observation of environmentally exposed humans, rather than laboratory controlled exposure of humans, will be used in determining the nature and extent of human risk. Certainly, this was the course that unfolded in determining the health risks of smoking that were detailed in Chapter 9.

When the news media report on studies of environmental carcinogenic exposure and the development of cancer in laboratory animals, they must be careful not to lead the public to *too quickly assume that causation in animals also suggests causation in humans.* In fact, responsible media will be very careful to emphasize that a particular environmental compound that has proven to be carcinogenic in animal-based research has not yet been investigated in human-based studies. Readers of media reports should also use caution in interpreting results of animal studies; see Chapter 10 for more information on different types of research studies.

On the other hand, the tobacco industry for decades used the contention that "animal-based research is not applicable to humans" as a façade behind which to hide information regarding the harmfulness of tobacco use in human. Recall that only when their own research findings were exposed to the public in conjunction with the Master Tobacco Settlement Agreement of 1999 did they admit their awareness of the relationship of cigarette smoking to human lung cancer.

InfoLinks

www.iarc.fr

ntp.nichs.nih.gov

for which early detection through screening is applicable (breast, colon, rectum, cervix, prostate, oral cavity, and skin), 86 percent will be alive after 5 years. Understandably, the term *cured* is used guardedly, since an initially diagnosed case of cancer can affect survivability beyond the end of the 5-year time period. Regardless of survivability, for those who develop cancer, the physical, emotional, and social costs will be substantial.

The financial cost of cancer to society is also troublesome. The National Institutes of Health (NIH) estimates that in 2006 alone cancer cost the American economy $206.3 billion, including $110.2 billion for loss of productivity due to death, $78.2 billion for direct medical costs, and $17.9 billion for indirect costs due to loss of productivity during treatment and recovery.[1] Not reflected in this total is the sizable amount of money spent on primary cancer prevention, such as school-based programs, public education efforts, and lobbying efforts intended to remove harmful products and pollutants

from the environment. (See the box "Animal-Based Research on the Causes of Cancer" for more information on environmental carcinogens.)

No single explanation can be given for why progress in eliminating cancer has been so limited. It is a combination of factors, including the aging of the population, continued use of tobacco, the high-fat American diet, the continuing urbanization and pollution of our environment, the lack of health insurance for an estimated 53 million Americans to pay for early diagnosis and proper treatment,[2] or simply our delayed recognition of cancer's true role in deaths once ascribed to other causes. Regardless, we continue to be challenged to control this array of abnormal conditions that we collectively call cancer. There is, however, increasing optimism that with a greater understanding of cancer genetics, new pharmacological agents, and the development of vaccines to prevent and treat cancers, real progress will finally be made.

TALKING POINTS A close friend justifies her high cancer-risk lifestyle by saying that "Everyone will die of something." How would you counter this point?

Cancer: A Problem of Cell Regulation

Just as a corporation depends on individuals to staff its various departments, the body depends on its basic units of function, the cells. Cells band together as tissues, such as muscle tissue, to perform a prescribed function. Tissues in turn join to form organs, such as the heart, and organs are assembled into the body's several organ systems, such as the cardiovascular system. Such is the "corporate structure" of the body.

If individuals and cells are the basic units of function for their respective organizations, the failure of either to perform in a prescribed, dependable manner can erode the overall organization to the extent that it might not be able to continue. Cancer, the leading cause of death among adults under 80 years of age,[3] is a condition reflecting cell dysfunction in its most extreme form. In cancer, the normal behavior of cells ceases.

Cell Regulation

Most of the body's tissues lose cells over time. This continual loss requires that replacement cells come from areas of young and less specialized cells. The process of specialization required to turn the less specialized cells into mature cells is controlled by genes within the cells. On becoming specialized, these newest cells copy, or replicate, themselves. These two processes are carefully monitored by the cells' **regulatory genes.** Failure to regulate specialization and replication results in abnormal, or potentially cancerous, cells.

In addition to genes that regulate specialization and replication, cells also have genes designed to repair mistakes in the copying of genetic material (the basis of replication) and genes to suppress the growth of abnormal cells should it occur. Thus, repair genes and tumor suppressor genes, such as the *p53* gene (altered or missing in half of all cancers), can also be considered regulatory genes in place to prevent the development of abnormal cells. Should these genes fail to function properly, resulting in the development of malignant (cancerous) cells, the immune system (see Chapter 13) will ideally recognize their presence and remove them before a clinical (diagnosable) case of cancer can develop.

Because, when they are not working properly, specialization, replication, repair, and suppressor genes can become cancer-causing genes, or **oncogenes,** these four types of genes can also be referred to as **proto-oncogenes,**

or potential oncogenes.[4] Beyond the involvement of the regulatory genes just discussed, nonregulatory genes also may have the potential to become oncogenic, resulting in an even wider array of cancer stimulators. Today nearly 200 different oncogenes have been identified, and this number may well expand significantly in the near future. Currently a $100 million pilot project to further explore the role of genes in human cancers is under way.

How normal genes become oncogenes is a question that cannot be completely answered at this time. Regardless, abnormal cells produce abnormal proteins, and the absence of normal proteins alters the body's ability to function appropriately, from the molecular to the organ system level.

Oncogene Formation

All cells have proto-oncogenes, so what events alter otherwise normal genes, including the critically important regulatory genes, causing them to become cancer-causing genes? Three mechanisms, genetic mutations, viral infections, and carcinogens, have received much attention.

Genetic mutations develop when dividing cells miscopy genetic information. If the gene that is miscopied is a gene that controls specialization, replication, repair, or tumor suppression (a proto-oncogene), the oncogene that results will allow the formation of cancerous cells. A variety of factors, including aging, free radical formation, and radiation, are associated with the miscopying of the complex genetic information that constitutes the genes found within the cell, including those intended to prevent cancer.

In both animals and humans, cancer-producing infectious agents,[5] such as the feline leukemia virus in cats and the human immunodeficiency virus (HIV) and multiple forms of the human papillomavirus (HPV) in humans (see Chapter 13), have been identified. These viruses seek out cells of a particular type, such as cells of the immune system or the lining of the cervix, and substitute some of their genetic material for some of the cells' thus converting them into virus-producing cells. In so doing, they convert proto-oncogenes into oncogenes. Once converted into oncogenes, the altered genes are passed on through cell division.

> **Key Terms**
>
> **regulatory genes** Genes that control cell specialization, replication, DNA repair, and tumor suppression.
>
> **oncogenes** Faulty regulatory genes that are believed to activate the development of cancer.
>
> **proto-oncogenes** (pro toe **on** co genes) Normal regulatory genes that may become oncogenes.

A third possible explanation for the development of oncogenes involves the presence of environmental agents known as *carcinogens*. Over an extended period, carcinogens, such as chemicals found in tobacco smoke, polluted air and water, toxic wastes, and even high-fat foods, may convert proto-oncogenes into oncogenes. These carcinogens, such as those found in tobacco smoke, may work alone or in combination with co-carcinogenic promoters (see Chapter 9, Table 9.3) to alter the genetic material, including regulatory genes, within cells. Thus people might develop lung cancer only if they are exposed to the right combination of carcinogens over an extended period.

You may already see that some of the specific risk factors in each area—such as radiation in the development of mutations, sexually transmitted viruses in cancers of the reproductive tract, and smoking-introduced carcinogens in the development of lung cancer—can be moderated by adopting health-promoting behaviors.

Our understanding of the role of genes in the development of cancer is expanding rapidly. On occasion the public learns the identity of selected oncogenes. Very likely many readers have heard of the *BRCA1* and *BRCA2* genes associated with breast and ovarian cancer, the *RAS* oncogene thought to influence 30 percent of all cancers, and the *p53* suppressor oncogene that may be involved in more cancers than is any other single oncogene. As geneticists continue to build on the base established by the Human Genome Project and in doing so discover additional genetic links to cancer, the possibility of some form of oncogene suppressor technology becomes a more realistic possibility in the war against cancer. That said, some within the scientific community believe that ultimately the etiology (cause) of cancer will prove to be so complex and multifaceted that the role of genetic causation will be more limited than it is currently anticipated to be.[6]

In light of the complexity of cancer, some people in the scientific community believe that cancer can never be truly prevented. Rather, they feel that the ability to stop and then reverse cancerous changes at an early stage of development is more likely than is the prevention of this complex disease process. However, this text addresses the concepts of prevention in the belief that prevention-based practices reflect our personal contribution to the "war on cancer."

The Cancerous Cell

Compared with noncancerous cells, cancer cells function in similar and dissimilar ways. It is the dissimilar aspects that often make them unpredictable and difficult to manage.

Perhaps the most unusual aspect of cancerous cells is their infinite life expectancy. Specifically, it appears that cancerous cells can produce an enzyme, *telomerase,* that blocks the cellular biological clock that informs normal cells that it is time to die.[7] In spite of this ability to

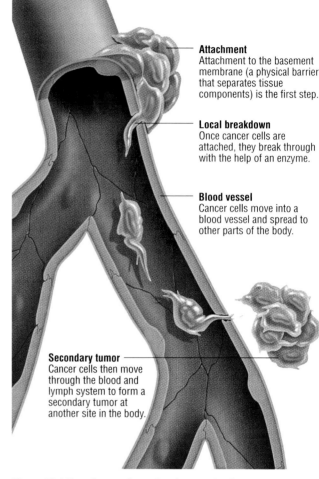

Attachment
Attachment to the basement membrane (a physical barrier that separates tissue components) is the first step.

Local breakdown
Once cancer cells are attached, they break through with the help of an enzyme.

Blood vessel
Cancer cells move into a blood vessel and spread to other parts of the body.

Secondary tumor
Cancer cells then move through the blood and lymph system to form a secondary tumor at another site in the body.

Figure 11-1 How Cancer Spreads Locomotion (movement) is essential to the process of metastasis (spread of cancer). Scientists have identified a protein that causes cancer cells to grow arms, or pseudopodia, enabling them to move to other parts of the body.

Source: National Cancer Institute. *Horizons of Cancer Research*, NIH Pub. No. 89-3011 ©1989.

live forever, cancer cells do not necessarily divide more quickly than normal cells do. In fact, they can divide at the same rate or even on occasion at a slower rate.

In addition, cancerous cells do not possess the *contact inhibition*[8] (a mechanism that influences the number of cells that can occupy a particular space at a particular time) of normal cells. In the absence of this property, cancer cells accumulate, altering the functional capacity of the tissue or organ they occupy. Further, the absence of *cellular cohesiveness*[8] (a property seen in normal cells that "keeps them at home") allows cancer cells to spread through the circulatory or lymphatic system to distant points via **metastasis** (Figure 11-1). Interestingly, once migrating cancer cells arrive at a new area of the body, they "rediscover" their cellular cohesive capabilities. A final unique characteristic of cancerous cells is their ability to command the circulatory system to send them additional blood supply to meet their metabolic needs and to provide additional routes for metastasis. This *angiogenesis*[8] capability of cancer cells makes them extremely hardy compared with noncancerous cells.

Staging Cancer   In light of the interesting capabilities of malignant cells just described, it is critically important in the diagnosis and treatment of cancer that *oncologists* (physicians who have specialized in the care of cancer patients) know not only the type of cancer but also its extent. The latter determination is reflected in the concept of "staging" cancer.

For purposes of effective communication regarding the staging of cancer, the international medical community has adopted the *TNM* staging system.[1] This system first identifies the extent of a malignancy as to the extent of the primary tumor (T), whether it has or has not progressed to regional lymph node involvement (N), and the presence or absence of metastasis (M). On establishing a TNM profile of the tumor, a numerical stage (I, II, III, or IV) is determined. This categorization reflects: (I) *In situ* or "at the point of origin"; (II) *Local*—an invasive cancer confined to the organ of origin; (III) *Regional*—cancer extended into the immediately neighboring tissue or into regional lymph nodes; and (IV) *Distant*—cancer extended to distant parts of the body, either by discontinuous metastasis or through the lymphatic drainage to distant nodes.

On the basis of this system, important decisions regarding treatment, management, and prognosis (survivability) of the cancer are made—information important to all persons involved in the medical care to be received.

Benign Tumors

Noncancerous, or benign, tumors can also form in the body. These tumors are usually enclosed by a membrane and do not spread from their point of origin. Benign tumors can be dangerous when they crowd out normal tissue within a confined space.

Types of Cancer

Again, for the purposes of effective diagnosis and appropriate treatment, cancers can be named or labeled on the basis of their cell type of origin (such as hepatoma) and/or the organ in which they are located (such as the liver). To the medical community, the name of cancers, based on the cell type of origin, is most often used in making determination regarding diagnosis and treatment, whereas for the general public, the labeling of cancer on the basis of the organ of origin is more familiar and understandable. In this section the labeling based on the cell type of origin is given brief consideration, while the body of the chapter describes cancer based on its organ of origin. In some cases labeling may also be extended back to embryonic germ layer of origin, but this is beyond the scope of this textbook.

For the majority of physicians and the patients with whom they must communicate, descriptions of cancer based on the organ of origin are technically adequate and, with explanation to patients, understandable. In the list that follows, several cell- or tissue-based cancers are discussed.

Carcinoma. Found most frequently in the skin, nose, mouth, throat, stomach, intestinal tract, glands, nerves, breasts, urinary and genital structures, lungs, kidneys, and liver; approximately 85 percent of all malignant tumors are classified as carcinomas.

Sarcoma. Formed in the connective tissues of the body; bone, cartilage, and tendons are the sites of sarcoma development; only 2 percent of all malignancies are of this type.

Melanoma. Arises from the melanin-containing cells of skin; found most often in people who have had extensive sun exposure, particularly a deep, penetrating sunburn; although once rare, the amount of this cancer has increased markedly in recent years; remains among the most deadly forms of cancer.

Neuroblastoma. Originates in the immature cells found within the central nervous system; neuroblastomas are rare; usually found in children.

Adenocarcinoma. Derived from cells of the endocrine glands.

Hepatoma. Originates in cells of the liver; although not thought to be directly caused by alcohol use, seen more frequently in people who have experienced sclerotic changes in the liver.

Leukemia. Found in cells of the blood and blood-forming tissues; characterized by abnormal, immature white blood cell formation; several forms are found in children and adults.

Lymphoma. Arises in cells of the lymphatic tissues or other immune system tissues; includes lymphosarcomas and Hodgkin's disease; characterized by abnormal white cell production and decreased resistance.

Key Terms

metastasis (muh **tas** ta sis) The spread of cancerous cells from their site of origin to other areas of the body.

benign Noncancerous localized non-malignant tumors contained within a fibrous membrane.

tumor Mass of cells; may be cancerous (malignant) or noncancerous (benign).

sclerotic changes (skluh **rot** ick) Thickening or hardening of tissues.

Men	Estimated New Cases*	Estimated Deaths
Prostate	218,890	27,050
Lung & bronchus	114,760	89,510
Colon & rectum	79,130	26,000
Urinary bladder	54,040	9,630
Melanoma of the skin	33,910	5,220
Non-Hodgkin's lymphoma	34,200	9,600
Kidney	31,590	8,080
Oral cavity	24,180	5,180
Leukemia	24,800	12,320
Pancreas	18,830	16,840
Esophagus	12,130	10,900
Liver	13,650	11,280
All sites	766,860	289,550

*Excludes basal and squamous cell skin cancers and in situ carcinoma except urinary bladder.

Women	Estimated New Cases*	Estimated Deaths
Breast	178,480	40,460
Lung & bronchus	98,620	70,880
Colon & rectum	74,630	26,180
Uterine corpus	39,080	7,400
Ovary	22,430	15,280
Non-Hodgkin's lymphoma	28,990	9,060
Melanoma of the skin	26,030	2,890
Thyroid	25,480	880
Leukemia	19,440	9,470
Pancreas	18,340	16,530
Urinary bladder	17,120	4,120
Brain	9,330	5,590
Multiple myeloma	8,940	5,240
All sites	678,060	270,100

Figure 11-2 Cancer Cases and Deaths   These 2007 estimates of new cases of cancer and deaths from cancer reveal some significant similarities between men and women. Note that lung cancer is the leading cause of cancer deaths for both sexes.

Source: American Cancer Society. *Cancer Facts and Figures 2007.* Atlanta: American Cancer Society, Inc. Used with permission.

Figure 11-2 presents information about the estimated new cases of cancer and deaths from cancer at various sites in both men and women.[1] Table 11.1 shows that cancer incidence and mortality rates vary among different racial and ethnic groups.

Cancer at Selected Sites in the Body

A second and more familiar way to describe cancer is on the basis of the organ site at which it occurs. The following discussion relates to some of these more familiar sites. A lack of space, in combination with the wide arrays of human cancers, limits the number of specific malignancies that can be described. Remember also that regular screening procedures can lead to early identification of cancer at these sites (see the box "Screening Guidelines for the Early Detection of Cancer in Asymptomatic People" on page 326).

Skin Cancer

In the footnote in Figure 11-2, you will see that the American Cancer Society (ACS) excludes two of the three forms of skin cancer, and reports statistics only for melanoma, the least common form of skin cancer but the most serious of the three forms. However, when all three forms (melanoma, basal cell, and squamous cell) are taken into account, skin cancer is the most common kind of cancer, with an estimated 1 million new cases in 2007. On the basis of this prevalence, this textbook covers skin cancer first.

Thanks largely to our desire for a fashionable tan, many teens and adults have spent more time in the sun (and in tanning booths) than their skin can tolerate. As

Table 11.1 Incidence and Mortality Rates* by Site, Race, and Ethnicity, United States, 1999–2003

Incidence	White	African American	Asian American and Pacific Islander	American Indian and Alaska Native	Hispanic/Latino†
All sites					
Males	555.0	639.8	385.5	359.9	444.1
Females	421.1	383.8	303.3	305.0	327.2
Breast (female)	130.8	111.5	91.2	74.4	92.6
Colon & rectum					
Males	63.7	70.2	52.6	52.7	52.4
Females	45.9	53.5	38.0	41.9	37.3
Kidney & renal pelvis					
Males	18.0	18.5	9.8	20.9	16.9
Females	9.3	9.5	4.9	10.0	9.4
Liver & bile duct					
Males	7.2	11.1	22.1	14.5	14.8
Females	2.7	3.6	8.3	6.5	5.8
Lung & bronchus					
Males	88.8	110.6	56.6	55.5	52.7
Females	56.2	50.3	28.7	33.8	26.7
Prostate	156.0	243.0	104.2	70.7	141.1
Stomach					
Males	9.7	17.4	20.0	21.6	16.1
Females	4.4	9.0	11.4	12.3	9.1
Uterine cervix	8.6	13.0	9.3	7.2	14.7

Mortality	White	African American	Asian American and Pacific Islander	American Indian and Alaska Native	Hispanic/Latino†‡
All sites					
Males	239.2	331.0	144.9	153.4	166.4
Females	163.4	192.4	98.8	111.6	108.8
Breast (female)	25.4	34.4	12.6	13.8	16.3
Colon & rectum					
Males	23.7	33.6	15.3	15.9	17.5
Females	16.4	23.7	10.5	11.1	11.4
Kidney & renal pelvis					
Males	6.2	6.1	2.6	6.8	5.3
Females	2.8	2.8	1.2	3.3	2.4
Liver & bile duct					
Males	6.3	9.6	15.5	7.8	10.7
Females	2.8	3.8	6.7	4.0	5.0
Lung & bronchus					
Males	73.8	98.4	38.8	42.9	37.2
Females	42.0	39.8	18.8	27.0	14.7
Prostate	26.7	65.1	11.8	18.0	22.1
Stomach					
Males	5.4	12.4	11.0	7.1	9.2
Females	2.7	6.0	6.7	3.7	5.2
Uterine cervix	2.4	5.1	2.5	2.6	3.4

*Per 100,000, age-adjusted to the 2000 U.S. standard population.

†Persons of Hispanic/Latino origin may be of any race.

‡Excludes deaths from Minnesota, New Hampshire, and North Dakota due to unreliable data.

Sources: Incidence (except American Indian and Alaska Native): Howe HL, Wu X, Ries LAG, et al. Annual report to the nation on the status of cancer 1975–2003, featuring cancer among U.S. Hispanic/Latino populations. *Cancer.* 2006; 107: 1643–1658. Incidence (American Indian and Alaska Native 1999–2002): Ries LAG, Harkins D, Krapcho M, et al.(eds) SEER Cancer Statistics Review, 1975–2003, National Cancer Institute, Bethesda, MD, www.seer.cancer.gov/csr/1975_2003/,2006. Mortality: SEER Program (www.seer.cancer.gov) SEER*Stat Database: Mortality—All COD, Public-Use With State, Total U.S. (1990–2003), National Cancer Institute, DCCPS, Surveillance Research Program, Cancer Statistics Branch, released April 2006. Underlying mortality data provided by NCHS; American Cancer Society. *Cancer Facts and Figures 2007.* Atlanta: American Cancer Society, Inc. Used with permission.

Screening Guidelines for the Early Detection of Cancer in Asymptomatic People

Site	Recommendation
Breast	• Yearly mammograms are recommended starting at age 40. The age at which screening should be stopped should be individualized by considering the potential risks and benefits of screening in the context of overall health status and longevity. • Clinical breast exams should be part of a periodic health exam about every 3 years for women in their 20s and 30s, and every year for women 40 and older. • Women should know how their breasts normally feel and report any breast change promptly to their health care providers. Breast self-exam is an option for women starting in their 20s. • Women at increased risk (e.g., family history, genetic tendency, past breast cancer) should talk with their doctors about the benefits and limitations of starting mammography screening earlier, having additional tests (i.e., breast ultrasound and MRI), or having more frequent exams.
Colon and rectum	Beginning at age 50, men and women should begin screening with 1 of the examination schedules below: • A fecal occult blood test (FOBT) or fecal immunochemical test (FIT) every year • A flexible sigmoidoscopy (FSIG) every 5 years • Annual FOBT or FIT and flexible sigmoidoscopy every 5 years* • A double-contrast barium enema every 5 years • A colonoscopy every 10 years *Combined testing is preferred over either annual FOBT or FIT, or FSIG every 5 years, alone. People who are at moderate or high risk for colorectal cancer should talk with a doctor about a different testing schedule.*
Prostate	The PSA test and the digital rectal examination should be offered annually, beginning at age 50, to men who have a life expectancy of at least 10 years. Men at high risk (African American men and men with a strong family history of 1 or more first-degree relatives diagnosed with prostate cancer at an early age) should begin testing at age 45. For both men at average risk and high risk, information should be provided about what is known and what is uncertain about the benefits and limitations of early detection and treatment of prostate cancer so that they can make an informed decision about testing.
Uterus	**Cervix:** Screening should begin approximately 3 years after a woman begins having vaginal intercourse, but no later than 21 years of age. Screening should be done every year with regular Pap tests or every 2 years using liquid-based tests. At or after age 30, women who have had 3 normal test results in a row may get screened every 2 to 3 years. Alternatively, cervical cancer screening with HPV DNA testing and conventional or liquid-based cytology could be performed every 3 years. However, doctors may suggest a woman get screened more often if she has certain risk factors, such as HIV infection or a weak immune system. Women ages 70 years and older who have had 3 or more consecutive normal Pap tests in the last 10 years may choose to stop cervical cancer screening. Screening after total hysterectomy (with removal of the cervix) is not necessary unless the surgery was done as a treatment for cervical cancer. **Endometrium:** The American Cancer Society recommends that at the time of menopause all women should be informed about the risks and symptoms of endometrial cancer, and strongly encouraged to report any unexpected bleeding or spotting to their physicians. Annual screening for endometrial cancer with endometrial biopsy beginning at age 35 should be offered to women with or at risk for hereditary nonpolyposis colon cancer (HNPCC).
Cancer-related checkup	For individuals undergoing periodic health examinations, a cancer-related checkup should include health counseling, and depending on a person's age, and gender, might include examinations for cancers of the thyroid, oral cavity, skin, lymph nodes, testes, and ovaries, as well as for some nonmalignant diseases.

American Cancer Society guidelines for early cancer detection are assessed annually in order to identify whether there is new scientific evidence sufficient to warrant a reevaluation of current recommendations. If evidence is sufficiently compelling to consider a change or clarification in a current guideline or the development of a new guideline, a formal procedure is initiated. Guidelines are formally evaluated every 5 years regardless of whether new evidence suggests a change in the existing recommendations. There are 9 steps in this procedure, and these "guidelines for guideline development" were formally established to provide a specific methodology for science and expert judgment to form the underpinnings of specific statements and recommendations from the society. These procedures constitute a deliberate process to ensure that all society recommendations have the same methodological and evidence-based process at their core. This process also employs a system for rating strength and consistency of evidence that is similar to that employed by the Agency for Healthcare Research and Quality (AHRQ) and the U.S. Preventive Services Task Force (USPSTF).

Source: American Cancer Society. *Cancer Facts and Figures 2007.* Atlanta: American Cancer Society, Inc. Used with permission.

Table 11.2 Global Solar UV Index and Risk of Harm from Unprotected UV Exposure

UV Index	Risk Level	Recommended Protection
≥2	Low	Wear sunglasses on bright days. In winter, reflection off snow can nearly double UV strength. If you burn easily, cover up and use sunscreen.
3–5	Moderate	Take precautions, such as covering up, if you will be outside. Stay in shade near midday when the sun is strongest.
6–7	High	Reduce time in the sun between 10 a.m. and 4 p.m. Cover up, wear a wide-brim hat and sunglasses, and use sunscreen with an SPF of at least 15.
8–10	Very high	Take extra precautions; unprotected skin will be damaged and can burn quickly. Minimize sun exposure between 10 a.m. and 4 p.m. Otherwise, seek shade, cover up, wear a wide-brim hat and sunglasses, and use sunscreen with an SPF of at least 15.
11+	Extreme	Take all precautions; unprotected skin can burn in minutes. Avoid sun exposure from 10 a.m. to 4 p.m. Seek shade, cover up, wear a wide-brim hat and sunglasses, and apply sunscreen with an SPF of at least 15 liberally every 2 hours. Beachgoers should know that white sand and other bright surfaces reflect UV and will increase UV exposure.

Source: Environmental Protection Agency, Sunwise Program, "UV Index Scale," www.epa.gov/sunwise1/uvindex2.html.

a result, skin cancer, once common only among people who had to work in the sun, is occurring with alarming frequency. In 2007, more than 1 million Americans developed basal or squamous cell skin cancer, and 59,940 cases of highly dangerous malignant melanoma were diagnosed.[1]

Deaths from skin cancer do occur, with 10,850 estimated in 2007. Approximately 75 percent of these deaths were the result of malignant melanoma.

Risk Factors Severe sunburning during childhood and chronic sun exposure during adolescence and younger adulthood are largely responsible for the "epidemic" of skin cancer being reported. The current emphasis on screening for skin cancer may also be increasing the incidence of early-stage cancer being reported. Progress is being made in deterring people from pursuing the perfect tan. The American Academy of Dermatology reports that the incidence of deliberate tanning is down, and the use of sunscreens has increased. Occupational exposure to some hydrocarbon compounds can also cause skin cancer.

In spite of the progress reported by the American Academy of Dermatology, Americans continue to seek natural sources of sun or tanning salons for cosmetically related tanning, or they find that their exposure cannot be avoided owing to the nature of their jobs. In regard to "purposeful tanning" either outdoors or indoors, recent research has given some creditability to the contention that tanning is emotionally "addictive." Underlying this contention is a small but growing body of evidence that purposeful frequent tanning, using tanning beds, seems to elevate levels of beta-endorphins (a form of biological opiate) in the bloodstream. When frequent tanners have their UV stimulated opioid production blocked, they demonstrate withdrawal-like symptoms. Such is not the case in infrequent and non-tanners.[9]

For those who must or choose to seek extended periods of time in the sun, the most recently established UV (ultraviolet) Index, the Global Solar UV Index, can be found in Table 11.2. This daily index for your ZIP code (in the United States) can be accessed online at www.epa.gov/sunwise/uvindex.html. It is also often given on local television stations or in some local newspapers.

Prevention Prevention of skin cancer should be a high priority for people who enjoy the sun or must work outdoors. The use of sunscreen with a sun protection factor (SPF) of 15 or greater is very important. In addition, parents can help their children prevent skin cancer later in life by restricting their outdoor play from 11 a.m. to 2 p.m., requiring them to wear hats that shade their faces, and applying a sunscreen with an SPF of 15 or higher in generous quantities regardless of skin tone.

In fairness to readers, it must be mentioned that controversy abounds within the scientific community as to the both the effectiveness of sunscreens and the form of sunscreen used (organic versus inorganic).[10] That said, new technologies are under development and the current controversy may eventually be resolved. Regardless, practicing dermatologists continue to recommend their use. However, users are reminded that the level of protection provided is not doubled by simply doubling the SPF—for example, a sunscreen carrying an SPF of 30 does not provide twice the protection provided by a product with an SPF of 15.

A further rationale for preventing the development of skin cancer is the recently described relationship between skin cancer and the heightened probability of developing other forms of cancer later in life. Research suggests that people who have had skin cancer carry a 20–30 percent greater risk of developing other types of cancer than do people who have never developed skin cancer.[11] (The Personal Assessment at the end of the chapter will help you determine your risk of developing this kind of cancer.)

Early Detection Although many doctors do not emphasize this point enough, the key to the successful

Figure 11-3 Normal Mole versus Malignant Melanoma   **A:** Normal mole. This type of lesion is often seen in large numbers on the skin of young adults and can affect any body site. Note its symmetrical shape, regular borders, uniform color, and relatively small size (actual size is about 6 millimeters). **B:** Malignant melanoma. Note its asymmetrical shape, irregular borders, uneven color, and relatively large size (actual size is about 2 centimeters).

treatment of skin cancer is early detection. For basal cell or squamous cell cancer, a pale, waxlike, pearly nodule or red, scaly patch may be the first symptom. Other types of skin cancer may be indicated by a gradual change in the appearance of an existing mole. A physician should be consulted if such a change is noted. Melanoma usually begins as a small, molelike growth that increases progressively in size, changes color, ulcerates, and bleeds easily. To help detect melanoma, the American Cancer Society recommends using the following guidelines:[1]

A is for asymmetry.

B is for border irregularity.

C is for color (change).

D is for a diameter greater than 6 mm.

Figure 11-3 shows a mole that would be considered harmless and one that clearly demonstrates the ABCD characteristics just described. (See the box "Self-Examination for Melanoma" for a description of how to make a regular inspection of the skin.)

Most recently, a relationship between the presence of abnormal moles, called *dysplastic nevi* (flat, irregularly shaped, mottled in color, with irregular edges), and the risk of developing malignant melanoma has been established. By counting these "indicator moles," physicians can judge the relative risk of developing this serious form of skin cancer before it first appears.

Treatment   When nonmelanoma skin cancer is found, an almost 100 percent cure rate can be expected. Treatment of these skin cancers can involve surgical removal by traditional excising or laser vaporization, destruction by burning or freezing, or destruction using x-ray therapy. When the more serious melanomas are found at an early stage, a high cure rate (99 percent) is accomplished using the same techniques. However, when malignant melanomas are more advanced, extensive surgery and chemotherapy are necessary. The 5-year survival rate for regionalized forms of the disease drops to 65 percent, and, unfortunately, long-term disease recovery is uncommon (15 percent).[1]

However, new treatments for malignant melanoma offers a ray of hope to people with the disease. Among the more promising of these is a combination therapy using interleukin-2, an immune system chemical that stimulates various "killer cells" within the immune system and a drug that activates phagocyctic cells within the immune system. Additionally, a vaccine has been developed that stimulates the immune system to attack the melanoma cells more aggressively. This treatment-centered (rather than prevention-centered) vaccine uses components of the patient's own cancer cells to mobilize more white blood cells and produce more antibodies to fight the cancer.

Perhaps because nonmelanoma skin cancers are so common in adults (generally 40 years of age and older) and so successfully treated, we tend not to see these cancers as being a substantial problem. However, the medical management of the 1 million cases diagnosed each year is a substantial cost to our heath care industry, and thus to us as individuals. When treated in a physician's office, the cost of removing a nonmelanoma skin cancer is approximately $500; when removed in an ambulatory (walk-in) clinic the cost increases to nearly $950; and when removed in the hospital the cost exceeds $4,300.[12]

Lung Cancer

Lung cancer is one of the most lethal and frequently diagnosed forms of cancer. Primarily because of the advanced stage of the disease at the time symptoms first appear, only 16 percent of all people with lung cancer (all stages) survive 5 years beyond diagnosis.[1] By the time a person is sufficiently concerned about having a persistent cough, blood-streaked sputum, and chest pain, it is often too late for treatment to be effective. This failure to be able to diagnose lung cancer in its earlier stages could, however, begin to change. Currently, the National Cancer Institute is studying the efficacy of *spiral CT scans* in detecting lung tumors earlier than can be done by conventional chest x-rays. In a study of over 30,000 persons at risk of developing lung cancer, CT scanning found 412 persons with stage I lung cancer. Following surgery, 88 percent of these individuals were still alive after 10 years. At a current cost of $200 to $300, CT scanning

Changing for the Better

Self-Examination for Melanoma

Through a routine physical exam, my brother found out he has melanoma. How should I check myself for this condition?

How to look for melanoma

1. Examine your body front and back in the mirror, then right and left sides with arms raised.

2. Bend your elbows and carefully look at your palms, forearms, and under your upper arms.

3. Look at the backs of your legs and feet, the spaces between your toes, and the soles of your feet.

4. Examine the back of your neck and scalp with a hand mirror. Part your hair for a closer look.

5. Finally, check your back and buttocks with a mirror.

What to look for
Potential signs of malignancy in moles or pigmented spots:

Asymmetry

One half unlike the other half

Irregularity Border

Border irregular or poorly defined

Color

Color varies from one area to another; shades of tan, brown, or black

Diameter

Diameter larger than 6 mm, as a rule (diameter of a pencil eraser)

Source: Courtesy of the American Academy of Dermatology.

technology is rapidly replacing the standard chest x-ray as the primary means of detecting lung cancer.[13]

Risk Factors   Today it is known that genetic predisposition is important in the development of lung cancer. Perhaps, in fact, the majority of people who develop this form of cancer have an inherited "head start." When people who are genetically at risk also smoke, their level of risk for developing lung cancer is significantly greater than it is for nonsmokers. Of particular interest at this time are multiple genes on chromosome 3. Damage to three tumor suppressors on this chromosome is found in virtually every case of small-cell lung cancer and 90 percent of nonsmall-cell lung cancer. Most of the remaining lung cancer cases appear in people who smoke but are not genetically predisposed.

Cigarette smoking is the single most important behavioral factor in the development of lung cancer. For men who smoke, the rate of lung cancer is 23 times higher than it is for men who do not smoke. For women who smoke, the rate is 13 times higher than for women who do not smoke. Smokers account for nearly 87 percent of all cases of lung cancer, and lung cancer itself produces at least 30 percent of all cancer-caused deaths.[1]

Since 1987, lung cancer has exceeded breast cancer as the leading cause of cancer death in women, although more new cases of breast cancer than lung cancer are diagnosed each year. The incidence of lung cancer in men has shown a gradual decline over the last several years that parallels their declining use of tobacco products. In contrast to men, in women the rate of lung cancer development has remained relatively constant over the last several years. Women tend to develop a different form of lung cancer than men, suggesting that they might absorb toxins more completely than men do.[14] Also, among nonsmokers, women are more likely to develop lung

The March 6, 2006, death of Dana Reeve, at the age of 44, from lung cancer shocked the nation and called to our attention the fact that even nonsmokers are susceptible to this highly lethal form of cancer. In August 2005, soon after the death of her husband, Christopher Reeve, Dana Reeve announced her illness and that she had begun a demanding course of treatment in an attempt to recover her health. As she battled, questions abounded as to why nonsmokers who reside with nonsmokers could be victims of lung cancer.

Dana Reeve's illness made us aware that women who are nonsmokers are clearly more susceptible to developing lung cancer than are their male counterparts. Today it is recognized that nearly 20 percent of female lung cancer victims are nonsmokers. Experts speculate that females may be more susceptible than males to environmental carcinogenic agents, including secondhand smoke and radon gas. A second line of reasoning suggests that nonsmoking female lung cancer victims may have a genetic susceptibility to develop lung cancer through noncarcinogenic mechanisms, such as those described earlier in this chapter in the discussion of oncogene formation. Furthermore, the lung cancer that develops in nonsmoking women tends to be of a more aggressive type than that seen in males who are nonsmokers.

cancer, although recent studies have challenged this conclusion.[15] (See the box "Lung Cancer in Nonsmokers" for more information on this group.) The tumor type found in women may also be estrogen-sensitive, as is true for forms of breast cancer, in comparison to the primary type developed by men.[14] One hopes that this decline in new cases of lung cancer in women reflects a continuing decline in tobacco use.

Environmental agents, such as radon, asbestos, beryllium, uranium, and air pollutants, make a smaller contribution to the development of lung cancer. Radon alone may be the principal causative agent in most lung cancer found in nonsmokers.

Prevention The preceding information clearly suggests that not smoking or quitting smoking and avoidance of secondhand smoke (see Chapter 9) are the most important factors in the prevention of lung cancer. In addition, place of residence, particularly as it relates to air pollution, is a long-suspected risk factor for lung cancer. Nonsmokers who are considering living with a smoker or working in a confined area where secondhand smoke is prevalent should carefully consider the risk of developing lung cancer. A recent study does,

however, lessen concern over moderate alcohol use and the risk of developing lung cancer.

Treatment The prognosis for surviving lung cancer remains extremely guarded. Depending on the type of lung cancer, its extent, and factors related to the patient's overall health, various combinations of surgery, radiation, and chemotherapy remain the physicians' primary approach to treatment. Today, for persons with early-stage lung cancer, chemotherapy, following surgery, has increased survivability slightly. Additionally, an experimental vaccine (GVAX) now in the early stages of testing has shown extremely encouraging results in patients with nonsmall-cell lung cancer, the most common form of the disease. GVAX, in both patient-specific and nonspecific forms, are in Phase III clinical trials.[16] Also, a once-promising drug, Iressa, used as a last-resort drug by terminally ill lung cancer patients, now seems far less promising after subsequent study.

Colorectal Cancer

Colorectal cancer—cancer of the colon (the large intestine) and the rectum (the terminal portion of the large

I know I'm supposed to eat more fruits and vegetables, but they don't seem to fit in my usual meals and snacks. What are some convenient ways to eat more fruits and vegetables?

Eating fruits and vegetables of different colors gives your body a wide range of valuable nutrients and other natural substances beneficial for your health. See Chapter 5 for the recommended daily intake of fruits and vegetables for your sex, age, and activity level. Use the following strategies from the National Cancer Institute's "Fruits and Veggies Matter" initiative to help you eat a colorful variety of fruits and vegetables every day:

Breakfast

- Stir low-fat or fat-free granola into a bowl of low-fat or fat-free yogurt. Top with sliced apples or berries.
- Have fruit as a midmorning snack.
- Add berries or bananas to your waffles, pancakes, cereal, oatmeal, or toast.
- Top toasted whole-grain bread with peanut butter and sliced bananas.
- Add vegetables like bell peppers, broccoli, spinach, mushrooms, or tomatoes to your omelet.

Lunch and Dinner

- Place a box of raisins in your child's backpack and pack one for yourself, too.
- Order salads, vegetable soups, or stir-fried vegetables when eating out. Ask for more vegetable toppings (like mushrooms, peppers, and onions) and less cheese on your pizza.
- Choose beans, corn on the cob, or a side salad with low-calorie dressing instead of French fries.
- Add some cooked dry beans to your salad. Or, if you have a sweet tooth, add chopped apples, pears, or raisins.
- Add broccoli, green beans, corn, or peas to a casserole or pasta.
- Have soup. You can stick with the basics like tomato or vegetable soup or mix up some minestrone or veggie chili to cut winter's chill.
- Add lettuce, tomato, onion, and cucumber to sandwiches.
- Try eating at least two vegetables with dinner.

Snacks

- Try hummus and whole-wheat pitas or baked tortilla chips with bean and corn salsa.
- Snack on vegetables like bell pepper strips and broccoli with a low-fat or fat-free dip.
- Stash bags of dried fruit at your desk, and keep a bowl of fruit on your desk or counter.
- Top fat-free or low-fat yogurt with sliced fresh fruit, or blend fruit and yogurt for a smoothie.
- For quick and easy snacks, stock up on fresh, ready-packed, dried, frozen, and canned fruits and vegetables. Encourage your children to choose their own fruit when shopping.
- Store cleaned, cut-up vegetables in the fridge at eye level and keep a low-fat or fat-free dip on hand.

Source: Centers for Disease Control and Prevention, "Fruit and Veggies—More Matters," www.fruitsandveggiesmatter.gov.

---

intestine)—is the third most common kind of new cancer (excluding skin cancers) in both males and females, the second leading cause of cancer deaths in males (behind lung cancer), and the third leading cause of cancer deaths in females (behind lung and breast cancers) (see Figure 11-2).

Colorectal cancer, like many other forms of cancer, has a complex pathology, whose explanation lies beyond the scope of this book. However, classification as to the exact type of tumor and its location of origin within the colon or rectum will provide the oncologist with important information regarding the potential pattern of spread and the nature of treatment. Fortunately, when diagnosed in a localized state, colorectal cancer has a relatively high survival rate (90 percent when localized, and 64 percent for all stages).[1]

Risk Factors   Underlying the development of colorectal cancer are at least two potentially important areas of risk: genetic susceptibility and dietary patterns. Genes have recently been discovered that lead to familial colon cancer and familial polyposis (abnormal tissue growth that occurs before the formation of cancer) and are believed to be responsible for the tendency of colorectal cancer to run in families. Dietary risk factors include diets that are high in saturated fat from red meat and low in fruits and vegetables, which contain antioxidant vitamins and fiber (see the box "Fruits and Vegetables—Eat More for Better Health"). In regard to fiber's ability to prevent colorectal cancer, however, the ability of dietary fiber, when taken in supplement form, is in question.

In addition to familial and dietary links to an increased risk of colorectal cancer, alcohol use and smoking (alone or in combination) also appear related, particularly in terms of age of onset. In persons who regularly drink and/or smoke, colorectal cancer may appear five to seven years earlier than in those people who do not.[17] This pattern was particularly noted in males.

Prevention   Small outpouchings in the lower intestinal tract wall, called *polyps,* are frequently important in the eventual development of colorectal cancer. Prompt

Cancer's Seven Warning Signals

Listed below are the seven warning signs of cancer, which the acronym CAUTION will help you remember:

1. **C**hange in bowel or bladder habits
2. **A** sore that does not heal
3. **U**nusual bleeding or discharge
4. **T**hickening or lump in the breast or elsewhere
5. **I**ndigestion or difficulty in swallowing
6. **O**bvious change in a wart or mole
7. **N**agging cough or hoarseness

If you have a warning signal for more than five days, see your doctor!

removal of polyps has been shown to lower the risk of colorectal cancer. Further, some evidence indicates that the development of colorectal cancer may be prevented or slowed through regular exercise, an increase in dietary calcium intake, and long-term folic acid supplementation. Additionally, oral contraceptive use may be protective for women. Recently, the belief that the consistent use of a low-dose (81 mg) aspirin could reduce polyp formation was strongly disputed by a 20-year study of 83,000 nurses. Little difference in polyp formation was noted between those taking daily aspirin therapy and those who did not.[18]

Again, routine screening for colorectal cancer should be considered a form of prevention, much as PSA testing is for prostate cancer and mammography is for breast cancer.

Early Detection   Symptoms of colorectal cancer include bleeding from the rectum, blood in the stool, and a change in bowel habits (see the box "Cancer's Seven Warning Signals"). In addition, a family history of inflammatory bowel disease, polyp formation, or colorectal cancer should make one more alert to symptoms.[1] In people over age 50, any sudden change in bowel habits that lasts 10 days or longer should be evaluated by a physician. The American Cancer Society's recommendations for colorectal cancer screening, beginning at age 50—including fecal occult blood tests, flexible

sigmoidoscopy examinations, double-contrast barium enema examinations, and colonoscopy examinations—are detailed in the box "Screening Guidelines for the Early Detection of Cancer in Asymptomatic People" on page 326. However, in March 2005, the American College of Gastroenterology proposed that, because of the higher incidence of colorectal cancer in African Americans, routine colonoscopy should begin at age 45 for this group rather than at age 50. On the basis of information gleaned from the study just mentioned, smokers and regular users of alcohol could expect recommendations for earlier screening, beginning at age 45.

Although colonoscopy is currently the "gold standard" in the screening for colorectal cancer, two new forms of colonoscopy have been developed. Neither of them involves inserting the long flexible tube so dreaded by many patients. The most widely publicized of these is the virtual colonoscopy, for which the patient swallows a miniaturized camera that can be followed as it moves through the lower intestinal tract, generating digitized pictures of the entire colon. CT colonography (CTC), which uses serial tomography (a form of CT scan) to visualize the colon, is also well publicized. Both of these alternatives to the traditional colonoscopy are in use today, but should any abnormalities be identified, patients are then likely to be reexamined using the older but highly trusted flexible colonoscopy protocol.

It should be noted that the digital stool-sample test (in which a finger, or "digit," is inserted into the rectum), which is the only stool-sample test used by many doctors and taken during physical examinations, as well as the newer test to find traces of cancer cell DNA in the stool, have both been found to be less effective than previously believed.

Treatment   When one or more of these screening procedures suggests the possibility of disease within the lower intestinal tract, a careful visual evaluation of the entire length of the colon will be undertaken. During colonoscopy, areas of concern can be biopsied and the presence of a malignancy confirmed. Upon diagnosis, a localized and noninvasive malignancy will be removed surgically. When an invasive tumor is identified, supportive treatment with radiation or chemotherapy is necessary. Metastatic cancer requires chemotherapy. New guidelines regarding screening for metastatic tumors arising from a primary colorectal cancer are being formulated. These guidelines are meant to remind physicians that metastatic tumors are unlikely to be found through use of colonoscopy.

Breast Cancer

Surpassed only by lung cancer, breast cancer is the second leading cause of death from cancer in women. It is the third leading cause of cancer deaths overall. Nearly

Key Terms

sigmoidoscopy   Examination of the sigmoid colon (lowest section of the large intestine), using a short, flexible fiberoptic scope.

colonoscopy (co lun **os** ko py)   Examination of the entire length of the colon, using a flexible fiberoptic scope to inspect the structure's inner lining.

Learning from Our Diversity

Breast Cancer: A Rare Diagnosis in Men

With all the attention given to breast cancer in women—in the news, by physicians, and by research foundations—you may be surprised to learn that men are also diagnosed with this condition. For every 100 women who develop breast cancer, however, only one case is reported among men. Estimates for the year 2007 suggest that no more than 2,030 American men will develop breast cancer. When compared to the 178,480 cases anticipated in women during the same year, the rarity of breast cancer in men becomes apparent.

The typical male breast cancer victim is usually older than 60 and often has a family history of the disease. The *BRCA2* tumor suppressor gene mutation is also found within the victim's genetic lineage. In some cases, the male breast cancer victim has the inherited condition of Klinefelter's syndrome, in which a second X (or female) sex chromosome is present. The presence of the extra sex chromosome produces enhanced estrogen within the male body, resulting in adolescent development of prominent breasts and a higher risk of breast cancer later in life. Other conditions, such as various forms of liver disease,

also result in higher levels of estrogen and, eventually, a greater risk of male breast cancer.

In most ways male breast cancer is very similar in type to that seen in women. Infiltrating ductal cancer, ductal carcinoma in situ, and a form of cancer arising from the ducts immediately beneath the nipple (Paget's disease) have been reported. Because of this close similarity to female breast cancer, medical management of male breast cancer closely parallels that seen in women. Surgery (a modified radical mastectomy), chemotherapy, external radiation, and hormonal therapy are used alone or in combination. The latter therapy may include not only drugs to block the influence of estrogen on estrogen-sensitive cancer cells, but removal of testicles as well. As with virtually all forms of cancer, early diagnosis and treatment are of critical importance.

InfoLinks

www.cancernet.nci.nih.gov

---

one in eight women will develop breast cancer in her lifetime, resulting in an estimated 178,480 new invasive cases and 40,460 deaths in 2007.[1] In men, an estimated 2,030 new cases and 450 deaths occurred in 2007[1] (see the box "Breast Cancer: A Rare Diagnosis in Men"). As women age, their risk of developing breast cancer increases. Regardless of age, however, waiting to learn whether a suspicious lump is benign or is a relatively harmless fluid-filled cyst is stressful. Today, 98 percent of women whose breast cancer is localized (confined to the breast) survive more than 5 years.

Most recently it has been reported that the actual rate of new cases of breast cancer has declined. According to data from 2003 (the last year for which actual versus estimated numbers of new cases of various forms of cancer are known), a 7.2 percent decline in new breast cancer cases was reported. Initial interpretation of this dramatic finding relates to a sharp decline in the use of menopause-related hormone therapy.[19]

Risk Factors   Although all women and men are at some risk of developing breast cancer, the following groups of women have a higher risk.

- Women whose menstrual periods began at an early age, or whose menopause occurred late (although the former may be more important than the latter is)

- Women who had no children, had their first child later in life, or did not nurse

- Women who have used hormone replacement therapy (HRT)—particularly combined estrogen and progestin or combined estrogen and testosterone

- Women who have a high degree of breast density (high level of glandular tissues relative to fat) or biopsy-established hyperplasia

- Women whose diets are high in saturated fats, who are sedentary, or who are obese after menopause (particularly central body cavity obesity; see Chapter 6)

- Women who carry the *BRCA1* and/or *BRCA2* mutated tumor suppressor genes, or those with a strong family history of breast cancer

As mentioned, significant concern exists regarding the long-term use of hormone replacement therapy and the development of breast cancer in postmenopausal women. In fact, in a government-sponsored study (Women's Health Initiative Study) the link appeared so strongly and early that the study was terminated much earlier than had been planned. Researchers found that tumor development in women taking HRT versus those on a placebo was more common, that tumors were larger at diagnosis, and that tumors were more often invasive.[20] Many physicians are now advising that HRT be used only on a very short-term basis to relieve the symptoms of menopause, rather than the much longer period of time previously deemed appropriate.

While initial concerns about the risk of breast cancer in postmenopausal women was centered on the use of HRT medication combining estrogen and progesterone, recent attention is being directed to those using HRTs that combine estrogen and testosterone. These medications, often compounded (formulated) by pharmacists on the directions of a physician, may increase the risk of more invasive breast cancer.[21]

The effects of environmental pollutants and regional influences have also been investigated as causative factors in the development of breast cancer. Environmental pollutants vary from region to region and are influenced by a number of factors, including the type of industrial and agricultural activity in a particular area. A wide array of regional factors may be involved, including the genetic background of people in a given area and lifestyle differences involving diet, alcohol consumption, and exercise patterns.

The role of genetic predisposition in the development of breast cancer has also received considerable attention. For example, a small percentage (perhaps 5 percent) of women with breast cancer have inherited or developed mutations in one or both of two tumor suppressor genes (proto-oncogenes), *BRCA1* and *BRCA2*. Discovered in 1994 and 1995, respectively, and currently the focus of extensive research, more than 200 mutations in these genes have been identified. In a study involving 5,000 Ashkenazi Jews (Jews of Central and Eastern European descent) living in the Washington, D.C., area, mutation in the *BRCA1* gene resulted in a 56 percent greater chance of developing breast cancer by age 70 (versus a 13 percent greater risk for people without a mutated version of the gene).[22] In the years since these genes' identification, studies have been ongoing in an attempt to more accurately define the level of risk for developing breast cancer among women who carry one or both *BRCA1* or *BRCA2* mutations. At this time, however, it cannot be definitively determined whether a given carrier of a mutated gene will actually develop cancer. Both of these genes are also associated with increased risk of developing ovarian cancer (see pages 342–343) and, perhaps, prostate cancer in men.

In addition to the much-studied *BRCA1* and *BRCA2* genes discussed earlier, other genetic mutations have been implicated in the development of breast cancer, thus complicating further all aspects of screening, treatment, prevention, and public education. Among these additional mutations is one that influences a protein (MAP kinase) that functions as a "chemical switch" in controlling cell replication. In cancer patients with extra copies of the *HER-2* gene, cancerous cells are less likely to respond to chemotherapy. Yet another involves a portion of a gene (*CYP17*) that plays a role in the synthesis of estrogen, and a fourth mutation results in the malfunction of the important APC tumor suppressor gene.

> **Key Terms**
>
> **prophylactic mastectomy** Surgical removal of the breasts to prevent breast cancer in women who are at high risk of developing the disease.

The Personal Assessment at the end of the chapter may be helpful in determining your relative level of risk of developing breast cancer.

Prevention   As already discussed, a variety of risk factors are thought to be important in the development of most cases of breast cancer. Accordingly, some degree of prevention is possible when factors such as diet; alcohol use; physical activity level; decisions about contraception, pregnancy, and breastfeeding; occupational exposure to toxins; and even place of residence are considered.

For women who have a primary family history of breast cancer (sisters, mother, or grandmothers with the disease) and who have been found to carry one or both of the BRCA genes, an extreme form of prevention is also possible—**prophylactic mastectomy.** In this surgical procedure, both noncancerous breasts are removed, in an attempt to eliminate the possibility of future cancer development. When carefully planned, breast reconstruction surgery can be undertaken immediately, with satisfactory results. Some physicians, however, recommend against the surgery, preferring to monitor susceptible women very carefully and frequently.

One important consideration related to this procedure is that not every person who carries a mutated tumor suppressor gene will develop cancer, making the surgery unnecessary.

At the present time pharmacological prevention represents the newest approach to reducing the incidence of breast cancer. Two medications, raloxifene (Evista), a drug initially intended for the prevention of osteoporosis, and tamoxifen (Nolvadex) are undergoing extensive long-term evaluation to further define their safety and effectiveness in the prevention of breast cancer. The National STAR (Study of Tamoxifen and Raloxifene) Trial is following 20,000 postmenopausal women at high risk for the development of breast cancer. Current assessments of data reveal that these two estrogen-receptor modulatory drugs are equally effective in lowering the expected risk for breast cancer within the study population (both drugs reduced the risk by 50 percent). However, raloxifene accomplished this reduction with fewer side effects. More specifically, in comparison to tamoxifen, raloxifene use resulted in one-third to one-fifth fewer cases of uterine cancer, pulmonary embolisms, deep-vein thrombosis, and cataracts.[23] Tamoxifen, however, is already approved for use with premenopausal women and is less inclined to foster invasive breast tumors.

Early Detection: Breast Self-Examination   For several decades a fundamental component of early detection of breast cancer has been breast self-examination (BSE). Generally recommended for women 20 years of age and older, the procedure was to be performed during the menstrual period or during the day immediately following the end of the menstrual period, when estrogen

Breast Self-Examination

I've never felt confident about doing a breast self-exam. What is the proper technique?

- Lie down and place your right arm behind your head. The exam is done while lying down, not standing up. This is because when you are lying down, your breast tissue spreads evenly over your chest wall and is as thin as possible, making it much easier to feel all the breast tissue.

- Use the finger pads of the three middle fingers on your left hand to feel for lumps in the right breast. Use overlapping, dime-size circular motions of the finger pads to feel the breast tissue.

- Use three different levels of pressure to feel all the breast tissue. Light pressure is needed to feel the tissue closest to the skin; medium pressure to feel a little deeper; and firm pressure to feel the tissue closest to the chest and ribs. A firm ridge in the lower curve of each breast is normal. If you're not sure how hard to press, talk with your doctor or nurse. Use each pressure level to feel the breast tissue before moving on to the next spot.

- Move around the breast in an up and down pattern starting at an imaginary line drawn straight down your side from the underarm and moving across the breast to the middle of the chest bone (sternum or breastbone). Be sure to check the entire breast area, moving downward until you feel only ribs and up to the neck or collarbone (clavicle).

- There is some evidence that the up-and-down pattern (sometimes called the vertical pattern) is the most effective pattern for covering the entire breast without missing any breast tissue.

- Repeat the exam on your left breast, using the finger pads of your right hand.

- While standing in front of a mirror with your hands pressing firmly down on your hips, look at your breasts for any changes of size, shape, contour, dimpling, pulling, or redness or scaliness of the nipple or breast skin. (Pressing your hands down on your hips contracts the chest wall muscles and enhances any breast changes.) Continue to look for changes with your arms down at your sides, and then with your arms raised up over your head with your palms pressed together.

- Examine each underarm while sitting up or standing and with your arm only slightly raised so you can easily feel in this area. Raising your arm straight up tightens the tissue in this area and makes it difficult to examine it.

Source: "How to Perform a Breast Self-Exam" used with the permission of the American Cancer Society, Inc. from www.cancer.org. All rights reserved.

Breast Self Examination
Examine up to the collarbone, out to armpit, in to middle of chest, and down to bottom of rib cage

levels are at their lowest and cystic activity in breast tissue is minimal (or on the same day of each month by post-menopausal women). The box "Breast Self-Examination" illustrates the proper technique. Although breast self-examination is an easily learned technique, today its role as the primary method of detecting breast cancer in its earliest stage has been usurped by clinical breast examination (CBE) performed by a physician during scheduled checkups and by mammography and other imaging technologies. However, clinical breast examination also has been a source of some concern because of the inconsistencies among clinicians in performing the

procedure. Steps have now been taken to correct this, and the American Cancer Society continues to strongly endorses its role in early breast cancer detection. Additionally, during physician visits in which CBE has been done, the ACS recommends that women review, with their clinicians, their own BSE techniques.

Early Detection: Mammography Although researchers once disagreed about the age at which women should begin routine mammography and the extent to which mammography is effective in finding masses in dense breast tissue, today mammograms are physicians' best tool for the early detection of breast cancer. Accordingly, the American Cancer society recommends that mammography begin at age 40.

Whether women begin routine mammography at 40, as advised by the ACS, or earlier particularly for women with previous breast cancer or a family history of breast disease, women should continue these examinations on an annual basis. Recommendations regarding mammography for older women (age 65 and older) are, however, a bit more individually determined and should be discussed annually with physicians. For older women, overall health status and expectations for reaching a normal life expectancy are weighed relative to the lessening cost-effectiveness of mammography.

Because of the important role routine mammography plays in the early identification of breast lesions, the Mammography Quality Standards Act (MQSA) is a valuable step toward ensuring that mammography is performed by experienced technicians, using correctly calibrated equipment, and interpreted by skilled radiologists. Every woman should be certain that her mammography is being performed in a MQSA-certified facility. However, even when interpreted by experienced radiologists, mammograms are at times difficult to interpret, leading to false-positive findings and the likelihood of additional (diagnostic versus screening) mammography, ultrasound, and/or biopsies. Although expensive and emotionally unsettling, the majority of these false-positive findings are eventually found to have been negative. The percentage of false-positive screenings varies with age, but overall, approximately 15 percent of women screened annually will on one occasion have a false positive finding. Of course, there can also be false negatives (indicating no cancer, when in fact cancer is present).[24] These tragic occurrences can result in treatment being seriously delayed and are the basis for the highest percentage of medical malpractice lawsuits.

To secure the highest quality images for interpretation, the soft-tissue film-based mammography of the past is increasingly supplemented by newer technologies, including full-field digital mammography (FFDM), which replaces x-ray film with digital sensors capable of generating digitized images that can viewed, stored, and electronically distributed in a secure fashion for interpretation at off-site locations, thus providing second and third opinions. Computer-aided detection (CAD)-based films, or digital mammography, is also finding its place in screening mammography. This technology feeds film-based or digitally produced images into a massive computerized library of normal breast images and "tags," in a visible manner, any portion of the breast that appears suspicious.

Many other technologies have been developed that could potentially aid in the screening or diagnosis of cancer, now or, most likely, in the future. Those with current applications include ultrasonography (ultrasound),

which provides sound-wave-generated images, and magnetic resonance imaging, which produces an image by magnetically reorienting the molecular structure of human tissue. Both technologies are used, but not routinely, in breast cancer identification. Other technologies, including novel ultrasound, computer-aided detection with MRI, scintimammography, positron emission tomography (PET), and elastography, may be available for use in the future. At the current time they are not yet either FDA approved for general clinical use or FDA approved specifically for screening.[25]

Ideally, these newer approaches will identify tumors in their earliest stages of development and reduce the percentage of false-positive and false-negative results associated with traditional mammography procedures.

Treatment   Regardless of the method of detection, if a lump is found, a breast biopsy can determine whether the lump is cancerous. If the lump is cancerous but localized, treatment is highly effective, with cure rates at nearly 100 percent. The most frequently used treatments are **lumpectomy** combined with radiation, lumpectomy without radiation, and mastectomy. The use of chemotherapy following surgery is strongly advocated as well. Today the injection of a radioactive "tag" before surgery allows identification of the nearest lymph node (the *sentinel node*) to which breast cancer cells may have spread, thus allowing the surgeon to spare noncancerous nodes. When the cancer is invasive or has metastasized, more radical surgery (mastectomy with lymph node removal) combined with chemotherapy and/or various forms of radiation may be the most effective course of treatment.

When drug therapy is deemed desirable in treating breast cancer, oncologists may consider two drugs that have recently become available or whose earlier protocols have been redefined. The first, tamoxifen, discussed earlier in terms of breast cancer prevention, is a hormonelike drug that prevents estrogen from stimulating cancer cell growth. The use of tamoxifen has proven highly effective in women who have the type of breast cancer stimulated by the presence of estrogen. Used for many years for more localized tumors, today the use of tamoxifen has been extended to the treatment of highly metastasized breast cancers. Tamoxifen's ability to stimulate uterine cancer development, blood clots, strokes, and cataracts, however, is a potentially serious side effect of the drug's use and must be closely monitored.

The second drug, trastuzumab (Herceptin), is an antibody-like agent used in combination with other chemotherapeutic drugs in highly advanced breast cancer. This drug interferes with the activity of a protein produced by the *HER-2* oncogene that normally fosters tumor cell division.

As we would expect, additional cancer treatment and prevention drugs are becoming available. Two such drugs, Fermara and Arimidex, which belong to a class

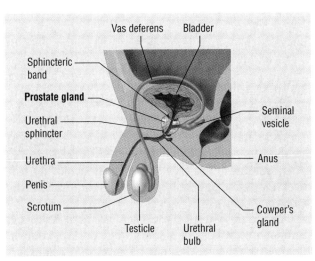

Figure 11-4 Location of the Prostate Gland within the Male Reproductive System

of drugs called *aromatase inhibitors,* reduce or stop the production of estrogen. Currently, researchers are determining the manner in which these drugs will join (or replace) tamoxifen and, perhaps, Herceptin in the treatment of breast cancer.

Prostate Cancer

If the names Bob Dole, General Norman Schwarzkopf, Jerry Lewis, and Colin Powell are familiar, then you know four older men who have been diagnosed with and treated for prostate cancer. In fact, prostate cancer is so common that in 2007 an estimated 218,890 new cases were diagnosed, and 27,050 men died of the disease.[1] Prostate cancer is a leading cause of cancer deaths in American men, exceeded only by lung cancer deaths.

The prostate gland is a walnut-size gland located near the base of the penis (see Figure 11-4). It surrounds the neck of the bladder and the urethra. The prostate secretes a number of components of semen, such as nutrients used to fuel sperm motility.

Risk Factors   Compared with other cancers, the risk factors for prostate cancer are less clearly defined. The most predictable risk factor is age. Currently, 65 percent of all prostate cancer cases are diagnosed in men over 65 years of age; however, cases in men under age 50 are not infrequent. African American men and men with a family history of prostate cancer are at greater risk of developing this form of cancer. This greater incidence of prostate cancer in African American males may be partially explained by the existence of an abnormal gene on chromosome 8 that is associated more commonly with prostate tumors in this racial group than in the general population.[26] A link between prostate cancer and dietary fat intake, including excessive red meat and dairy product

consumption, has also been suggested. With the discovery of the *BRCA1* and *BRCA2* genes related to breast and ovarian cancer, a genetic link with prostate cancer was also established. Men with one of these genetic mutations have an increased risk of developing prostate cancer.

Prevention   Although the American Cancer Society does not specifically address prevention of prostate cancer, prevention is not an unrealistic goal. Clearly, moderation of dietary fat intake is a preventive step. Increased dietary intake levels of vitamin E and the micronutrient selenium have been shown to play a preventive role in prostate cancer. In addition, an ongoing assessment of the drug finasteride (Proscar), used in the treatment of benign prostatic hyperplasia (BPH) (enlargement of the prostate), has indicated that the drug can reduce the incidence of tumors of the prostate. The Prostate Cancer Prevention Trial is expected to produce additional insights into the prevention of prostate cancer.[27]

Early Detection   Possible signs of prostate disease, including prostate cancer, are listed in the box "Symptoms of Prostate Disease." A physician should be consulted if any of these symptoms appear, particularly in men ages 50 or older. Screening for prostate cancer should begin by age 40. This screening consists of an annual rectal examination performed by a physician and a blood test, the **prostate-specific antigen (PSA) test,** administered every 2 years. Although the initial version of the PSA

Key Terms

lumpectomy   A surgical treatment for breast cancer in which a minimal amount of breast tissue is removed; when appropriate, this procedure is an alternative to mastectomy, in which the entire breast and underlying tissue are removed.

prostate-specific antigen (PSA) test   A blood test used to identify prostate-specific antigen, an early indicator that the immune system has recognized and mounted a defense against prostate cancer.

test was very successful in diagnosing prostate cancer, new, age-specific test values are now employed. These new interpretive standards allow increased specificity in determining risk. This said, however, the PSA test continues to deliver both false negative and false positive results. At this time there is considerable uncertainty as to whether screening for prostate cancer using the PSA test should be continued. Because of concern about the "overtreatment" of males who have elevated PSA levels, in combination with little apparent difference in the survival of men with prostate cancer based on whether they had or had not been screened, consensus is building that physicians should explain the limitations of the PSA test, and then allow their male patients to decide whether to be screened.[28] For those males who have a history of PSA screenings, the velocity of a rise (over two consecutive tests) in the PSA levels could be more clinically significant than the absolute level of prostate-specific antigen, although this too is unresolved.[29]

Another version of the PSA test has also been developed. This test can identify the "free" antigen most closely associated with the more aggressive forms of prostate cancer, thus cutting down on the false positives and extensive use of biopsies. In addition, an ultrasound rectal examination is used in men whose PSA scores are abnormally high.

Treatment   Today prostate cancer is treated surgically, or through the use of external radiation or the implantation of radioactive seeds (brachytherapy) into the gland, in combination with relatively short-term use of hormonal therapy. In addition, an experimental vaccine has recently been tested on humans with promising results.[30] Of course, each form of treatment carries the potential for side effects, including an 80 percent chance of impotence over a 10-year period; incontinence with surgery; diarrhea and tiredness with external radiation; some anal discomfort in association with the implantation of radioactive seeds into the prostate with internal radiation; and thinning of bones and some cardiovascular issues in conjunction with longer term hormone therapy.

One form of prostate cancer grows so slowly that men whose cancer is of this type, whose tumors are very localized, and whose life expectancy is less than 10 years at the time of diagnosis, are not treated but are closely monitored for any progression of the cancer. The 5-year survival rate for men with localized prostate cancer is virtually 100 percent! In terms of treatment type, the choice of treatment to be employed can be influenced by the physician being consulted. A recent survey of urologists and radiation oncologists found the urologists (who are surgeons) strongly favor a surgical approach, while radiologists favor radiation. Accordingly, second opinions and/or enrollment in clinical trials are highly recommended.

Testicular Cancer

Cancer of the testicle is among the least common forms of cancer; however, it is the most common solid tumor in men ages 15 to 34. Awareness of this type of cancer was raised in 1996 and 1997, when seven-time winner of the Tour de France Lance Armstrong and champion figure skater Scott Hamilton were diagnosed with testicular cancer. In both men, chronic fatigue and abdominal discomfort were the first symptoms of the disease. The American Cancer Society estimates that in 2007 testicular cancer was diagnosed in 7,920 men and caused the deaths of 380.[1]

Four forms of testicular cancer have been described: seminoma, teratoma, carcinoma, and choriocarcinoma. The most prevalent, seminoma, forms in the seminiferous tubules (where sperm originate) and is generally first observed during testicular self-examination as a small, hard mass on the side (or near the front) of the testicle. Fortunately, this form of testicular cancer is now highly curable.

Risk Factors   Risk factors for testicular cancer are variable, ranging from family history to environmental factors. The disease is more frequently seen in white Americans and in men whose testicles were undescended during childhood. Additional risk factors, such as difficulty during the mother's pregnancy, elevated temperature in the groin, and mumps during childhood, have been reported. The incidence of this cancer has been increasing in recent decades, while a corresponding drop in sperm levels has also been observed. Although no single explanation can be given for these changes, environmental factors such as agricultural pesticide toxicity may be involved. Once pesticides are concentrated in the tissues of the human body, during pregnancy they mimic estrogen. This, in turn, may lead to testicular dysgenesis syndrome, or the failure of the testicles to develop normally. The suspicion that testicular cancer is linked to vasectomies appears to be unfounded.

Prevention   Because risk factors for testicular cancer are so variable, prevention is limited to regular self-examination of the testicles. Symptoms such as fatigue, abdominal discomfort, and enlargement of the testicle should be reported to a physician, since these can be associated with other disease processes. A male infant with one or both testicles in the undescended position (resulting in an empty scrotum) should be seen promptly by a physician so that corrective procedures can be undertaken.

Early Detection   In addition to the fatigue and abdominal distress reported by both Armstrong and Hamilton, other symptoms of testicular cancer include a small, painless lump on the side or near the front of the testicle,

Testicular Self-Examination

I feel unsure about how to perform a testicular self-exam. What is the correct method?

Your best hope for early detection of testicular cancer is a simple three-minute monthly self-examination. The following explains how to do a testicular self-examination. The best time is after a warm bath or shower, when the scrotal skin is most relaxed.

1. Roll each testicle gently between the thumb and fingers of both hands.
2. If you find any hard lumps or nodules, you should see your doctor promptly. They may not be malignant, but only your doctor can make the diagnosis.

After a thorough physical examination, your doctor may perform certain x-ray studies to make the most accurate diagnosis possible.

Monthly testicular self-examinations are as important for men as breast self-examinations are for women.

Source: American Cancer Society.

InfoLinks

www.mskcc.org/document/Wictest.htm

a swollen or enlarged testicle, and a heaviness or dragging sensation in the groin or scrotum. The importance of testicular self-examination, as well as early diagnosis and prompt treatment, cannot be overemphasized for men in the at-risk age group of 15 to 34 years; see the box "Testicular Self-Examination."

Treatment Depending on the type, stage, and degree of localization of the tumor, surgical intervention generally includes removal of the testicle, spermatic cord, and regional lymph nodes. Chemotherapy and radiation might also be used. The highly publicized recovery of Lance Armstrong (and his subsequent accomplishments in professional biking) made the "Einhorn Regiment" (a combination of three chemotherapy agents) one of the chemotherapy protocols most widely recognized by the general public. Today, treatment is very effective, with 96 percent of all testicular cancer patients surviving 5 years and 99.5 percent surviving 5 years when the cancer was localized at the time of diagnosis.[1] It should be noted, however, that concern exists regarding the development of other forms of cancer, such as leukemia, later in life.

Cervical Cancer

In 2007 an estimated 11,150 new cases of cancer of the cervix (the anatomical neck of the uterus) occurred in the United States.[1] Fortunately, the death rate from cervical cancer has dropped greatly since 1950, largely because of the **Pap test.** This test screens for precancerous cellular changes (called *cervical intraepithelial neoplasia,* or *CIN*) and malignant cells. If malignant cells are found, it is hoped that they represent only cancer in situ (at the site of origin), rather than a more advanced invasive stage of the disease. Unfortunately, this simple and relatively inexpensive screening test is still underused, particularly in women over age 60, the group in which cervical cancer is most frequently found.

Refinements in laboratory techniques and the incorporation of computerization have enhanced the diagnostic precision of the Pap test. ThinPrep represents the former, while PAPNET and FocalPoint have enhanced the technologist's ability to identify abnormal cells.

Risk Factors Because of the clear association between sexually transmitted infections and cervical cancer, risk

---

Key Terms

Pap test A cancer-screening procedure in which cells are removed from the cervix and examined for precancerous changes.

Pap test results and their meanings can include:

- **Normal.** The cervical cells are healthy.

- **Unsatisfactory for evaluation.** The slide can't be read. Causes include douching, bleeding, infection, or not enough cells on the slide. The test should probably be repeated in 2–3 months.

- **Benign.** The Pap test showed infection, irritation, or normal cell repair. If you have an infection, you might need medication.

- **Atypical Squamous Cell: Unknown Significance (ASC-US) or ASC-H (High-grade changes).** The Pap test showed some abnormal changes in the cells, but the cause is not clear. Infection is a common cause.

- **Low-grade Squamous Intraepithelial Lesion (LSIL).** You might have been infected with the human papillomavirus (HPV). Some types of the virus are associated with an increased risk for cancer of the cervix. Your health care provider will recommend specific follow-up. This might include another Pap smear or a coloscopy—a look at the cervix with a high-power microscope.

- **High-grade Squamous Intraepithelial Lesion (HSIL).** The cells of the cervix can progress toward cancer, but they aren't cancer yet. Fewer than half of the women with this test will develop cancer. Colposcopy is needed. Biopsy and treatment might be necessary.

- **Squamous Cell Carcinoma.**

TALKING POINTS Three risk factors are associated with HPV-induced cervical cancer: early age of first sexual intercourse, higher-than-average number of partners, and lack of protection against sexually transmitted diseases (for example, condoms). How would you introduce this topic to a teenage daughter, sister, or niece?

Prevention Sexual abstinence is the most effective way of reducing the risk of developing cervical cancer (for example, Catholic nuns have extremely low rates of cervical cancer). However, abstinence is unlikely to be the choice for most women; other alternatives include fewer sexual partners, more careful selection of partners to minimize contact with those at high risk, the use of condoms, and the use of spermicides. In addition, of course, regular medical assessment, including annual Pap tests (and the ThinPrep Pap test), represents prevention through early detection. Of course, the HPV vaccine will further increase prevention.

Early Detection At this time, the importance of women having Pap tests for cervical cancer performed on a regular basis cannot be overemphasized. However, the specific scheduling of cervical screening is undergoing adjustment. For young sexually active women, initial screening using the Pap test (ThinPrep) should be undertaken within 3 years of first exposure. For young women not sexually at risk, or for women who have had a hysterectomy, the initial screening with the Pap test can be determined in consultation with health care providers. Once initiated, however, following three consecutive annual negative tests, the interval between tests may be increased upon discussion with health care providers. The American Cancer Society estimates that cervical cancer claimed the lives of 3,670 women in 2007.

The Pap test is not perfect, however. When tests are read in laboratories highly experienced in interpreting Pap slides, about 7 percent will be false negatives, resulting in a 93 percent accuracy rate. In less-experienced laboratories, false negatives may be as high as 20 percent (see the box "What Pap Test Results Mean"). Unfortunately, not all women whose test results are accurately assessed as abnormal receive adequate follow-up care, nor do they have subsequent Pap tests regularly enough. For many women with an abnormal Pap test, visual assessment (colposcopy) of the cervix will be performed. Traditional technology generates some false negatives. However, a newer technology, the Luma Cervical Imaging System, has enhanced the ability of the clinician to visually identify signs of tissue change.

In addition to changes discovered by a Pap test, symptoms that suggest potential cervical cancer include abnormal vaginal bleeding between periods and frequent spotting.

factors for this form of cancer include early age of first intercourse, large number of sexual partners, history of infertility (which may indicate chronic pelvic inflammatory disease), and clinical evidence of *human papillomavirus* (*HPV*) infections (see pages 405–406 in Chapter 13). For patients with previous HPV infections or whose sexual history suggests a higher risk for HPV, a ThinPrep Pap test has been shown effective in detecting the DNA from four HPVs that are known to be cancer causing, while being as easy to use as the traditionally used Pap test. Today the test is approved only for identifying HPV infection, but it is also capable of detecting both chlamydia and gonorrhea. In 2006 the first effective vaccine against the HPV variants associated with cervical cancer became available. This vaccine and the forms of HPV against which it protects are described in greater detail in Chapter 13 on page 406.

In addition to sexual history, cigarette smoking and socioeconomic factors are also risk factors for cervical cancer. The latter most likely relates to less frequent medical assessment, including infrequent Pap tests. (The Personal Assessment at the end of the chapter will help women evaluate their risk of developing cervical cancer.)

Treatment   Should precancerous cellular changes (CIN) be identified, treatment can include one of several alternatives. Physicians can destroy areas of abnormal cellular change using cryotherapy (freezing), electrocoagulation, laser destruction, or surgical removal of abnormal tissue. More advanced (invasive) cancer of the cervix can be treated with a hysterectomy combined with other established cancer therapies. A combination of radiation and chemotherapy is the most effective treatment for cervical cancer.

Uterine (Endometrial) Cancer

The American Cancer Society estimates that in 2007, 39,080 cases of uterine cancer (cancer within the inner wall of the body of the uterus, rather than within the cervix or neck of the uterus) were diagnosed in American women. In addition, 7,400 women died of the disease.[1] Although African Americans have a lower incidence of uterine cancer than white women do, their death rate is nearly twice as high.

Risk Factors   Unlike cervical cancer, in which a strong viral link has been identified, the principal risk factor related to the development of endometrial cancer is a high estrogen level. Accordingly, the following factors are related to higher levels of estrogen and, thus, to the development of endometrial cancer:

- Early menarche (early onset of menstruation)
- Late menopause
- Lack of ovulation (infertility)
- Never having given birth
- Estrogen replacement therapy (ERT not moderated with progesterone)
- Obesity
- Use of tamoxifen (a drug used in breast cancer therapy)
- History of polycystic ovary syndrome
- Hereditary nonpolyposis colon cancer

To some degree, endometrial cancer is seen more frequently in people who are diabetic, hypertensive, or who have gallbladder disease.

Prevention   The risk factors associated with high levels of estrogen are areas in which prevention might be targeted. In addition, the need for regular gynecological care that includes pelvic examination is a principal factor in minimizing the risk of uterine cancer. Pregnancy and the use of oral contraceptives both provide some protection from endometrial cancer.[1] Some degree of prevention may also be accomplished through a diet high in phytoestrogens that may provide an antiestrogenic effect. Most recently, however, an assessment of circulating enterolactone, the main form of dietary phytoesgtrogens in Westerns diets, failed to show a protective role against uterine cancer in ranges associated with normal dietary intake.[31]

Early Detection   Compared with cervical cancer, which is routinely identified through Pap tests, endometrial cancer is much more likely to be suspected on the basis of symptoms (irregular or postmenopausal bleeding) and confirmed by biopsy. Although more invasive, biopsy is a more effective method than ultrasound to diagnose uterine cancer.

Treatment   The treatment for early or localized endometrial cancer is generally surgical removal of the uterus (hysterectomy). Other therapies, such as radiation, chemotherapy, and hormonal therapy, may then be added to the treatment regimen. However, in terms of hormone replacement therapy (HRT), in which estrogen is combined with a synthetic progesterone, the FDA, The National Institute on Aging, and various medical associations now advise that no woman 65 or older with an intact uterus should take HRT owing to several concerns, including an increased risk for endometrial cancer. For women who are undergoing menopause and experiencing troublesome symptoms such as night sweats and hot flashes, HRT should be used in the smallest doses that provide relief and for the shortest duration of time possible.

Vaginal Cancer

Although rare, cancer of the vagina (the passage leading to the uterus) is of concern to a particular group of women: the daughters of more than 3 million mothers who were given the drug DES (diethylstilbestrol) to prevent miscarriages. Because of the effects of DES on the development of the fetal reproductive system, these daughters face the risk of developing a form of vaginal (and cervical) cancer called *clear cell cancer*. The medical community has been following large groups of daughters to better assess their level of risk. In a longitudinal study that followed such women and a control group of 1,374 unexposed age-mates, the risk of developing vaginal cancer was two to four times higher in the affected group than it was in women whose mothers were not given DES. A recent study looking at the same population of women, who were exposed to DES during inter-uterine development, demonstrated that they were now experiencing an earlier onset of menopause than was found in a group of age-mates who had not been exposed to DES.[32]

Outside this unique group of women, vaginal cancer is relatively rare. The American Cancer Society estimates that in 2007, there were 2,140 new cases diagnosed, and 790 women died as the result of vaginal cancer.[1] Early detection can be accomplished using a Pap test when vaginal wall cell samples are taken. Treatment centers on surgical removal of the vagina and associated lymph nodes. Other supportive therapies may also be included in the treatment regimen.

Ovarian Cancer

Since the death in 1989 of actress Gilda Radner, a star in the early years of *Saturday Night Live,* public awareness of ovarian cancer has increased in the United States. The American Cancer Society estimates that in 2007, there

> **Key Terms**
>
> **prophylactic oophorectomy** Surgical removal of the ovaries to prevent ovarian cancer in women at high risk of developing the disease.

were 22,430 new cases diagnosed, and 15,280 women died of the disease.[1] Most cases develop in women over age 40 who have not had children or began menstruation at an early age. The highest rate is in women over age 60. Today ovarian cancer causes more deaths than does any other form of female reproductive system cancer.

For a relatively small percentage of all women (10 percent), the inheritance of either the *BRCA1* or *BRCA2* suppressor gene mutation (see pages 322 and 334) significantly increases the risk of developing both breast and ovarian cancer. Today it is estimated that about 20 percent of all cases of ovarian cancer stem from these genetic mutations.

Beyond the 20 percent of cases attributed to genetic mutations, what might account for the majority of ovarian cancers? A number of studies, with varying degrees of assurance, suggest that decades of estrogen replacement therapy (ERT) used to counter symptoms of menopause, maintain bone mass, and provide hormonal protection from heart disease could be responsible for the majority of ovarian cancers.[33] As mentioned in conjunction with endometrial cancer, hormone replacement therapy is now used for only the briefest period of time.

Prevention Methods of preventing or lowering the risk of developing ovarian cancer are very similar to those recommended for breast cancer. These include using oral contraceptives, giving birth and breast-feeding (for at least three months), reducing dietary fat intake, abstaining from alcohol use, and performing regular physical activity.

For the small group of women with a strong family history of ovarian cancer, a **prophylactic oophorectomy** should be seriously considered. In this surgical procedure, both ovaries are removed. Carefully monitored hormone replacement therapy is then used to provide the protective advantages of estrogen in maintaining cardiovascular health and bone density.

Early Detection Because of its vague symptoms, ovarian cancer has been referred to as a *silent cancer.* Women in whom ovarian cancer has been diagnosed often report that the only symptoms of their cancer's presence were digestive disturbances, gas, urinary incontinence, stomach distention, and crampy abdominal pain over a few short weeks. The last symptom should be medically evaluated immediately.

Two recently approved and now available screening tests for ovarian cancer and other cancers, the CA125 and CA125 II, detect specific proteins (antigens) produced by malignant cells. Although these tests are available and their use is becoming more common (with women presenting with symptoms of possible ovarian cancer), new tests are being developed. One such test is centered around the detection in the blood of carbohydrates shed from the surface of cancer cells.[34] More routine use of these tests is anticipated.

For women with a strong family history of ovarian cancer (four primary family members who have had breast or ovarian cancer, with two or more cases occurring before age 50) or women of Ashkenazi Jewish descent (see page 334), genetic screening, newly available screening tests, and transvaginal ultrasound screening are likely to be recommended. These women may also be referred for participation in one of several prevention trials now under way.

Treatment   At this time, treatment of ovarian cancer requires surgical removal of the ovary, followed by aggressive use of chemotherapy. Use of the chemotherapeutic drug paclitaxel (Taxol), obtained from the bark and needles of the Pacific yew tree, results in a 50 percent survival rate 19 months after the completion of therapy. Recently, the use of an experimental three-drug combination—cyclophosphamide, paclitaxel, and cisplatin—has resulted in a 70 percent survival rate 22 months after chemotherapy. An even more recent advance in chemotherapy for ovarian cancer involves a two-drug therapy that, when delivered directly into the abdominal cavity, has extended survival rates beyond those associated with intravenous administration of the same agents—65.6 months versus 49.7 months.[35]

Pancreatic Cancer

Pancreatic cancer is one of the most lethal forms of cancer, with a survival rate of only 5 percent 5 years after diagnosis.[1] Because of this gland's important functions in both digestion and metabolic processes related to glucose utilization, its destruction by a malignancy leaves the body in a state incompatible with living.

In 2007 an estimated 37,170 new cases of pancreatic cancer were diagnosed, and 33,370 deaths occurred.[1]

Risk Factors   Pancreatic cancer is more common in men than women, occurs more frequently with age, and develops most often in African American men. Smoking is clearly a risk factor for this form of cancer, with smokers more than twice as likely to develop the disease. Other risk factors have been tentatively suggested, such as chronic inflammation of the pancreas (pancreatitis), diabetes mellitus, alcohol-induced liver deterioration (cirrhosis), obesity, and high-fat diets.[1] Recently a meta-analysis (a restudy of earlier studies) assessed the long-term use of nonsteroidal anti-inflammatory drugs to see if they are a risk factor in the development of pancreatic cancer. No clear link was found between using these medications, including aspirin, and enhanced risk of pancreatic cancer.[36]

Prevention   Not smoking and abstaining from alcohol use are the most effective steps toward preventing this form of cancer. Further, reducing the risk of type 2 diabetes mellitus, through weight loss and exercise, would also make an important contribution to prevention. Annual medical examinations are, of course, associated with overall cancer prevention.

The role of dietary and supplemental vitamin D is currently being assessed. Preliminary findings from a group of studies that included nearly 120,000 men and women suggest a positive role for vitamin D in the prevention of pancreatic cancer.[37] At this time, however, there are no recommendations to increase vitamin D intake as a preventative for pancreatic cancer.

Early Detection   Early detection of this cancer is difficult because of the absence of symptoms until late in its course. Perhaps for people with a history of chronic pancreatitis, physicians might consider routine ultrasound assessment or computerized axial tomography scans (CT scans). Once symptoms appear, a biopsy is performed.

Treatment   At this time there is no effective treatment for pancreatic cancer. Surgical removal of malignant sites within the gland, in addition to radiation and chemotherapy, is usually tried. Certainly, if a particular patient with pancreatic cancer qualifies, enrollment in a clinical trial would be worth consideration.

Lymphatic Cancer

In 1996 sports fans were saddened by the news that National Hockey League great Mario Lemieux had been diagnosed with cancer of the lymphatic system, the basis of the body's immune capabilities. Lemieux's cancer was Hodgkin's disease, a form of lymphoma. Following treatment in 1996, he appears to be in complete remission. In fact, in 2001 he resumed his playing career, but has since retired.

An estimated 71,380 new cases of lymphoma (8,190 cases of Hodgkin's disease and 63,190 cases of non-Hodgkin's lymphoma) were diagnosed in 2007. The number of deaths from both forms of lymphoma was near 19,730.[1] The incidence of Hodgkin's disease has declined over the last 35 years, while the incidence of non-Hodgkin's disease has nearly doubled, but is now holding steady.[1]

Risk Factors   Risk factors for lymphoma are difficult to determine. Some possible factors are a general reduction in immune protection, exposure to toxic environmental chemicals such as pesticides and herbicides, and viral infections. As you will learn in Chapter 13, the virus that causes AIDS (HIV) is a leukemia/lymphoma virus that was initially called HTLV-III (human T-cell leukemia/lymphoma virus-type III). A related leukemia/lymphoma virus, HTLV-I, is also suspected in

The Macrobiotic Diet

As common and potentially serious as cancer is, it is not a condition likely to be treated exclusively with alternative therapies. However, the use of a *macrobiotic diet* has been used by some cancer patients with anecdotal reports of success.

When the macrobiotic diet was introduced into the United States from Asia in the 1960s, it was first viewed as nutritionally deficient in comparison to all recognized forms of dietary intake, including the more restrictive forms of vegan vegetarianism. Central to the diet was the extensive (if not total) reliance on brown rice, seaweed, and a fish-based gruel. It also involved restrictions regarding food preparation, such as the type of cookware to be used.

Today the typical macrobiotic diet has been nutritionally enhanced to derive 50 percent of its calories from whole grains, 25–30 percent from vegetables, 5–10 percent from soups of various types, and 5–10 percent from beans and sea vegetables. It also features highly specific "macrobiotic" lifestyle guidelines, such as when eating is to occur, the rate at which food is to be chewed, hours of sleep required, and restrictions on the types of clothing materials and cosmetics to be used. This complex program must be learned through careful study at an organization such as the Kushi Institute, established by Michio Kushi, who introduced macrobiotics into this country from Japan.

In an attempt to evaluate the merits of the macrobiotic diet, studies of macrobiotic-based cancer treatment plans were funded by the National Center for Complementary and Alternative Medicine (NCCAM) in 1993—one at the University of Minnesota (directed by Michio Kushi's son) and a second at the University of Colorado (Denver). On February 25, 2002, the NCCAM Advisory Committee and researchers met for an initial assessment of the macrobiotic diet study. During the meeting, 9 Best Case Series (BCS) participant reports from an initial group of 18 participants were reviewed, and 6 participants gave personal accounts to the review panel. From these sources of information, serious methodological flaws were noted, including a virtual absence of medical records and x-rays on any of the 9 participants, the variety of ways in which diets were composed and prepared, and the absence of any oncology-based assessment before or during the study period.

In absence of current and more carefully controlled studies on effectiveness of the macrobiotic diet in preventing or curing cancer, a recent meta-analysis of studies involving a variety of nutritional interventions in patients with cancer or precancerous lesions may prove helpful in better understanding cancer-related diets.[*]

Conducted in England, this meta-analysis evaluated 59 individual studies in which dietary alterations (with and without supplementation) were used in an attempt to cure diagnosed cases of cancer or prevent the precancerous conditions from becoming malignancies. Twenty-five of the studies involved active cancer, and 34 involved precancerous conditions. Researchers deemed only 5 studies well designed and carefully controlled. All 59 studies were evaluated on the basis of cancer mortality, disease-free survival, cancer recurrence, and progression of cancerous lesions, and neither benefit nor harm could be found from approaching prevention and cure on the basis of nutritional intervention. It is likely that future studies of the macrobiotic diet will conclude that the macrobiotic diet, like most other dietary approaches, is neither helpful nor harmful in curing cancer or preventing precancerous conditions from becoming malignancies.

[*]Davies AA, et al. Nutritional interventions and outcomes in patients with cancer or pre-invasive lesions: Systematic review. *J Natl Cancer Inst.* 2006. July 19; 98(14):961–973.

InfoLinks

nccam.nih.gov

---

of nutrients. Moderate exercise also stimulates the production of enzymes that remove free radicals.

- *Limit your exposure to the sun.* It is important to heed this message even if you enjoy many outdoor activities. Particularly for people with light complexions, the radiation received through chronic exposure to the sun may foster the development of skin cancer. Of course, the same advice applies to tanning beds, the use of which may lead to skin cancers, including melanoma.

- *Consume alcohol in moderation, if at all.* People who consume a lot of alcohol have an increased prevalence of several types of cancer, including cancer of the oral cavity, larynx, and esophagus. Whether this results directly from the presence of carcinogens in alcohol or is more closely related to the alcohol user's tendency to smoke has not yet been established.

Cancer and Wellness

When you carefully consider the preceding suggestions, you will clearly see that you can do a great deal to prevent or at least minimize the development of cancer. A wellness-oriented lifestyle is the best weapon in your personal "war on cancer." However, all risk factor reduction is relative. Observation and experience tell us that life cannot be totally structured around the desire to achieve maximum longevity or reduce morbidity at all costs. Most people need to strike a balance between life that is emotionally, socially, and spiritually satisfying and life that is structured solely for the purpose of living a long time and minimizing exposure to illness. Regardless of our personal lifestyles, however, we can educate others, provide comfort and support to those who are living with cancer, and support the funding of continuing and innovative new cancer research.

Taking Charge of Your Health

- Stay attuned to media reports about cancer so that you can make informed choices.
- Support agencies devoted to the prevention of cancer.
- Monitor your work, home, and recreational environments to determine whether they are placing you at risk for cancer.
- Perform regular self-examinations for forms of cancer that can be detected through these techniques.
- Undergo the recommended cancer screening procedures for your age and sex.
- If you have cancer, participate actively in your own treatment.

SUMMARY

- Cancer is a condition in which the body is unable to control the specialization, replication, and repair of cells or the suppression of abnormal cell formation.
- A variety of agents, including genetic mutations, viruses, and carcinogens, stimulate the conversion of regulatory genes (proto-oncogenes) into oncogenes.
- Skin cancer prevention requires protection from excessive ultraviolet ray exposure.
- Cigarette smoking and genetic predisposition are both related to the development of lung cancer.
- Mammograms are an important component of breast cancer identification. Drugs capable of preventing breast cancer are available; however, their use is being carefully studied.
- Regular use of Pap tests is related to the early detection of cervical cancer. Sexually transmitted viral infections are strongly suspected of causing cervical cancer.

- Uterine (endometrial) cancer is more common than cervical cancer. High levels of estrogen are strongly associated with this form of cancer.
- The PSA test improves the ability to diagnose prostate cancer. Age, high-fat diets, and inheritance of a mutated suppressor gene are known risk factors.
- Colorectal cancer has a strong familial link and is seen in populations that consume diets high in fat and low in fruits and vegetables. Polyp formation is associated with an increased risk of this form of cancer.
- Early detection based on self-examination and screening is the basis for the identification and successful treatment of many cancers.
- Risk reduction, through living a wellness lifestyle, remains at the heart of cancer prevention.

REVIEW QUESTIONS

1. What is the relationship between regulatory genes and tumor suppressor genes in the development of cancer? Why are regulatory genes called both proto-oncogenes and oncogenes?
2. What properties do cancer cells possess that are lacking in normal cells?
3. What are some of the major types of cancer, based on the tissue from which they originate? What are some of the more familiar cancers based on organ of origin?
4. What signs indicate the possibility that a skin lesion has become cancerous?
5. What are the principal factors that contribute to the development of lung cancer? Of breast cancer?
6. When should regular use of mammography begin, and which women should begin using it earliest?
7. What important information can be obtained with the use of Pap tests? What innovations are associated with the ThinPrep Pap test?
8. How does the PSA test contribute to the early detection of prostate cancer?
9. What are the steps for effective self-examination of the breasts and testicles? What is the current status of breast self-examination?
10. What are the risk reduction activities identified in this chapter?

ANSWERS TO THE "WHAT DO YOU KNOW?" QUIZ

1. True   2. False   3. False   4. True   5. False   6. False   7. False

ENDNOTES

1. *American Cancer Society.* Cancer Facts and Figures 2007. American Cancer Society, 2007.
2. Cohen RA, Martinex ME. *Health Insurance Coverage: Early Release of Estimates from the National Health Interview Survey, January–June 2006.* www.cdc.gov/nchs/nhis.htm.
3. Jemal A, et al. Trends in the leading causes of death in the United States, 1997–2002. 2005. *JAMA.* Sept. 14. 294(10):1255–1259.
4. Saladin KS. *Anatomy and Physiology: The Unity of Form and Function* (4th ed.). New York: McGraw-Hill, 2007.
5. Buonaguro FM, Lewis GK, Pelicci P. Introducing infections agents and cancer. 2006. *Infect Agent Cancer.* Sept. 14.

Personal Assessment—*continued*

Cervical Cancer*

1. Age group
   A. Less than 25 (10)
   B. 25–39 (20)
   C. 40–54 (30)
   D. 55 and over (30)

2. Race/nationality
   A. Asian American (10)
   B. Puerto Rican (20)
   C. African American (20)
   D. White (10)
   E. Mexican American (20)

3. Number of pregnancies
   A. 0 (10)
   B. 1 to 3 (20)
   C. 4 and over (30)

4. Viral infections
   A. Herpes and other viral infections or ulcer formations on the vagina (10)
   B. Never (1)

5. Age at first intercourse
   A. Before 15 (40)
   B. 15–19 (30)
   C. 20–24 (20)
   D. 25 and over (10)

6. Bleeding between periods or after intercourse
   A. Yes (40)
   B. No (1)

YOUR TOTAL POINTS _____

Explanations

1. The highest occurrence is in the 40-and-over age group. The numbers represent the relative rates of cancer for different age groups. A 45-year-old woman has a risk three times higher than that of a 20-year-old.

2. Puerto Ricans, African Americans, and Mexican Americans have higher rates of cervical cancer.
3. Women who have delivered more children have a higher occurrence.
4. Viral infections of the cervix and vagina are associated with cervical cancer.
5. Women with earlier intercourse and with more sexual partners are at a higher risk.
6. Irregular bleeding may be a sign of uterine cancer.

Interpretation

40–69 This is a low-risk group. Ask your doctor for a Pap test. You will be advised how often you should be tested after your first test.

70–99 In this moderate-risk group, more frequent Pap tests may be required.

100 or higher You are in a high-risk group and should have a Pap test (and pelvic examination) as advised by your doctor.

TO CARRY THIS FURTHER . . .

Regardless of score, you should discuss with your physician the desirability of the ThinPrep Pap test (or one similar to it); it is designed to identify the presence of DNA from one or more of the HPV strains associated with cervical cancer.

_____

*Lower portion of uterus. These questions would not apply to a woman who has had a complete hysterectomy.

Source: Adapted from the American Cancer Society.

Managing Chronic Conditions

What Do You Know about Chronic Diseases?

- Chronic conditions most often develop slowly, but once in place they abruptly abate or resolve. True or False?

- When an X-link recessive condition exists, it is the biological mother who is defined as the carrier, while the male child is the afflicted recipient of that condition. True or False?

- Congenital abnormalities, such as a cleft lip or cleft palate, develop shortly after birth. True or False?

- Type 1 diabetes mellitus and type 2 diabetes mellitus are exactly the same condition, except that one form requires the use of insulin (from outside the body), while the other does not. True or False?

- Irritable bowel syndrome becomes defined as irritable bowel disease if more than one year of treatment does not result in significant improvement. True or False?

- Multiple sclerosis (MS) is a chronic condition of the nervous system, although its cause lies in the abnormal functioning of the immune system. True or False?

- Parkinson's disease and Alzheimer's disease are both conditions reflecting changes to the brain's ability to use neurotransmitters in the normal manner. True or False?

Check your answers at the end of the chapter.

Online Learning Center Resources
www.mhhe.com/payne10e

Visit the Online Learning Center for tools to improve your grade and get the most out of your course—chapter objectives, practice quizzes, key terms flashcards, chapter summaries for your digital audio player, Web activities, self-assessments, and many other study aids.

In clinical medicine, thousands of diseases, illnesses, and conditions can be diagnosed and treated. For ease of communication, these diseases and illnesses have been individually named and categorized. We have chosen a set of categories—*genetic/inherited, congenital, metabolic, autoimmune, degenerative, and infectious*—and a sample of conditions that we believe you will be interested in learning about. Knowledge of these conditions will increase your understanding of chronic disease processes and how they differ from infectious diseases. Where appropriate, you will also find useful information about risk factors and lifestyle changes you can make to reduce your risk of developing a chronic condition.* †

---

*Only a clinician can diagnose and treat these conditions. The information contained in this chapter is intended only to inform.
†We have placed each condition into its most appropriate category. However, the characteristics of a given condition may overlap with those in a second group. We will point this out when it occurs.

The young woman that we want you to meet was, not too many years ago, taking a personal health course much you like you are now. She was bright, highly engaged, and eager for the world that awaited her beyond college. However, early in the semester in which she was in this class absences due to illness began to accumulate, a brief period of hospitalization occurred, and by semester's end she had been diagnosed with Crohn's disease. Crohn's disease is characterized by episodes of diarrhea, rectal bleeding, malabsorption of nutrients, and frequent periods of generalized fatigue. Daily scheduled activities are often interrupted by periods of hospitalization and, on a near daily basis, the frequent need for restroom facilities.

The academic year following the diagnosis of Crohn's disease was even more disrupted when the young woman experience initial episodes of cyclic vomiting syndrome, a condition characterized by the unanticipated onset of vomiting (as often as 15 to 20 times per day) shortly after the ingestion of food. Upon extensive evaluation at an internation-ally renowned medical institution, the label "idiopathic gastroparesis" was assigned to her newest problem. As the conditioned worsened, nutritional intake was accomplished by using a catheter surgically implanted into the small intestine through which nutritive dense liquids were introduced—the delivery of 900 calories required up to 12 hours per day. Eventually, a gastric pacemaker was implanted into her abdominal cavity, thus increasing gastric emptying to a level adequate to abandon the use of tube feedings. This latter form of intervention allowed a window of improved health. Unfortunately, however, the effectiveness of the gastric pacemaker proved difficult to maintain, and the use of tube feeding was reinstated.

At this time, the young woman who was so recently in the same personal health course that you are, and still only in her late 20s, has been diagnosed with multiple sclerosis, a disease reflected in the loss of "insulation" around nerves necessary to conduct electrical impulses to skeletal muscles, impeding movement-related activities, including mobility.

In light of this multiplicity of illnesses, daily activities center around taking multiple drugs by mouth, feedings, and injections of an MS disease modifying medication, the use of a "walker" to navigate, and finding someone to drive her to doctor appointments. Her once wide circle of friends has been reduced to a loving spouse and family, home care providers, and a network of devoted cyberfriends—most of whom share some of the same medical conditions.

If this seems to be an unusually severe collection of illnesses for one young person to have, it certainly is. If you're considering that it was in any way "asked for," it wasn't. In fact, this young woman lived a "health enhanced lifestyle" in all of the ways you will learn about in this textbook. Rather, it is yet another example of the unpredictable nature of life's journey. However, in spite of her own inability to ensure a high level of health through healthy living, she would nevertheless encourage you to take your health seriously because "*when it is gone, you'll miss it.*" To see you do any less would be truly distressing to her.

The first five categories of conditions—genetic/ inherited, congenital, metabolic, autoimmune, and **degenerative**—are discussed in the sections that follow. They have in common a slow, gradual course of development and remain a part of people's lives for long periods of time; thus they are said to be **chronic** conditions. Conversely, the infectious diseases are often quickly contracted and, once treatment has begun, stay active for a limited amount of time. These are referred to as the **acute** conditions (although HIV/AIDS is now defined as a chronic condition because of its extended duration). This sixth category, the infectious conditions, comprises illnesses caused by pathogenic organisms often transmitted from person to person. These conditions are discussed separately, in Chapter 13. The worldwide HIV/AIDS epidemic, the increasing threat of infectious diseases such as MRSA, and the comeback of familiar infections that are now resistant to antibiotics make this separate coverage necessary.

Three types of chronic conditions—obesity, cardiovascular disease, and cancer—are also addressed separately (in Chapters 6, 10, and 11, respectively) because of their importance to so many families and to the health of the nation. Many other chronic conditions are addressed in appropriate chapters throughout the book. For example, low-back pain is discussed in Chapter 4, osteoporosis in Chapter 4, and chronic obstructive lung disease in Chapter 9. Even though these conditions are not discussed in this chapter, they too fit into one or more of the categories described and are either chronic or acute in nature.

Chronic Disease Prevention

With the well-deserved emphasis placed on the prevention of heart disease and cancer, you might expect that virtually all diseases are preventable if you follow a wellness lifestyle. While it is true that many conditions are strongly linked to the lifestyle choices you make, we know little about how to prevent most of the chronic diseases described in this chapter (see the box "When It Is Gone, You'll Miss It!"). Learning about these conditions reminds us that even the most carefully tended human body is vulnerable to the effects of aging and the array of diseases that, in many cases, we do not yet understand. Accordingly, we are challenged to move beyond our perception of health as the absence of disease and illness. As we first discussed in Chapter 1, only then can we see that the value of health is not what it prevents, but rather what it makes possible—a life characterized by growth and development through each stage of the life cycle (see the box "Chronic Illness—The End or a Turning Point?").

Genetic/Inherited Conditions

Genetic or inherited conditions can occur in any of three ways: (1) abnormal genetic material (genes) are transmitted from one or both biological parents at conception; (2) abnormal genetic material is formed by mutation of normal genetic material at a very early stage of cellular replication and, subsequently, passed on with each cell doubling; or (3) an abnormal number of chromosomes—more or fewer than the normal number of 46—is inherited or formed. We will present brief descriptions of conditions from this broad category, including Klinefelter's syndrome, Turner's syndrome, cystic fibrosis, and color vision deficiency.

In discussing chronic diseases, other than the more prominent ones such as cardiovascular disease, cancer, and diabetes mellitus, we must note that few requirements for reporting the incidence of such diseases exist (unlike infectious diseases). For example, very few states keep records of autoimmune diseases such as lupus; fewer than 10 monitor developmental disabilities; and fewer than one-half of the states report on asthma. Because of these inadequacies it is likely that many chronic diseases are underestimated, so emerging trends are difficult to determine, and environmental factors associated with their development remain unrecognized.

Abnormal Number of Sex Chromosomes

At the time of conception (fertilization) an ovum (egg) from the biological mother containing 23 chromosomes is penetrated by a sperm from the biological father that also contains 23 chromosomes. This fusion of genetic material results in an initial human cell that contains 46 chromosomes, the number found in virtually every human cell. Of these 46 chromosomes, two are **sex chromosomes** (an X from the biological mother and an X or Y from the biological father). A normal male would thus possess a 44XY (44 nonsex chromosomes plus an X chromosome and a Y chromosome) chromosomal profile, and a normal female would be depicted as 44XX. Occasionally, people are born who possess more or fewer than the normal 46 chromosomes because they have more than or fewer than the normal 2 sex chromosomes.

Klinefelter's Syndrome Klinefelter's syndrome is one condition in which an abnormal number of sex chromosomes is present. It occurs in males and is a relatively rare (1 in 1,000 male births)[1] condition in which a Y sex

Key Terms

degenerative A slow but progressive deterioration of the body's structure or function.

chronic Develops slowly and persists for an extended period of time.

acute Having a sudden onset and a prompt resolution.

sex chromosomes The X and Y chromosomes that determine sex; chromosomes other than the autosomes.

Figure 12-2 An Infant with Cleft Lip and Cleft Palate This common congenital abnormality is repaired before the child is two years old. Surgical correction is usually quite successful, both cosmetically and functionally.

success that characterizes today's medical care of these facial abnormalities.

Patent Foramen Ovale (PFO)

During intrauterine life, blood flow in the fetal heart bypasses the right ventricle, the chamber that normally pumps unoxygenated blood to the lungs for oxygenation (see Chapter 10). The lungs are bypassed because the fetus is in effect "under water" and, thus, cannot use its lungs. A hole (the foramen ovale) in the interatrial septum, the wall that divides the upper right chamber of the heart from the upper left chamber, provides the necessary passageway around the lungs. At the time of birth, however, when the fetus begins to breathe air, this hole is normally closed by a small flap of tissue. The blood is then redirected from the right atrium into the right ventricle to be sent to the lungs.[7]

In about one in five live births, the foramen ovale fails to close completely, without any apparent leakage of blood. In the absence of other cardiac abnormalities, this patent foramen ovale does not cause any problems, is rarely identified, and, thus, prompts no medical attention. In some infants or children, however, a patent foramen ovale may leak, allowing unoxygenated blood to flow into the left atrium and then into the left ventricle of the heart and out into the general circulation.[7] This leakage may result in some **cyanosis** and cause a heart murmur to develop.

Key Terms

cyanosis Blue coloration of the lips, skin, and nail beds caused by inadequate oxygenation of the blood.

Patent foramen ovale is usually diagnosed by the child's primary care physician. No treatment is needed unless other heart abnormalities exist or the volume of unoxygenated blood reaching the left side of the heart is too great.

The possible worsening of the leakage of PFO (both diagnosed and undiagnosed) in adults who regularly scuba dive has caused concern. Researchers speculate that inappropriate decompression techniques, resulting in dangerous ambient pressures and the formation of nitrogen bubbles, in combination with a small patent foramen ovale, may increase the risk of decompression illness as small nitrogen bubbles are distributed throughout the body by the arterial blood flow.[8] Experts disagree somewhat about whether scuba divers should undergo an echocardiogram to test for the presence of a patent foramen ovale. If you are concerned, discuss the issue with your physician.

The patent foramen ovale congenital abnormality is associated with a risk of stroke and migraine headache. Physicians are now more inclined to suggest undertaking surgical repair of these cardiovascular abnormalities years after their initial discovery as a preventive measure against midlife stroke.[9] In regard to migraine headaches, it has been established that a high percentage of persons with this abnormality also have debilitating migraine headaches, and that many found relief after surgical repair.[10]

Scoliosis

Most cases of scoliosis (abnormal lateral spinal curvatures) have no known cause and are thus classified as *idiopathic*. For a small percentage, particularly when present at birth, a genetic basis is thought to exist. In general, curvatures that are less than 10 degrees (or 20 degrees and nonprogressive) are considered postural malalignments and do not require treatment.

Most spinal curvatures begin as a lateral deviation of the spine (curvature to the side) in either the thoracic (upper back) or lumbar (lower back) region (Figure 12-3). The normally aligned spine above or below the initial curvature then begins to curve in the opposite direction to offset the original curvature. This eventually gives the spine an "S" shape. If it is not corrected, the increasing curvature of the spine causes the vertebrae that form the spinal column to rotate. As the vertebrae rotate forward, the ribs follow accordingly, eventually altering the entire architecture of the chest cavity. This causes noticeable postural problems, including uneven positioning of the shoulder blades and a "rib hump" deformity. In addition, the changing shape of the chest compresses the heart, lungs, and related structures that pass through the middle of the chest. Increasing disfiguration and discomfort accompany each degree of additional curvature and rotation.

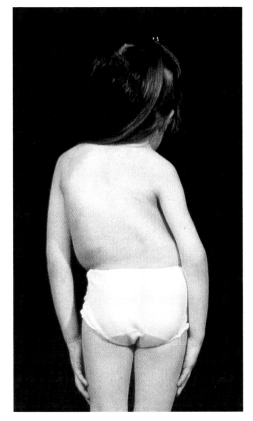

Figure 12-3 Scoliosis Evidence of scoliosis is commonly noted in late childhood or early adolescence.

For most people with scoliosis, the curvature that initially develops during the preteen years progressively worsens until the spine stops growing after puberty (see the box "Recognizing Signs of Scoliosis"). Since treatment is the key to preventing these problems, most American elementary schools screen students between the 4th and 6th grades to identify children who need additional evaluation. Children should be screened every 6 to 9 months until growth of the spine slows and then stops. Curvatures of 20 degrees but less than 30 degrees when initially diagnosed may require treatment but will generally not progress after skeletal growth stops. Curvatures greater than 30 degrees will, however, usually continue to increase well after skeletal growth has stopped and into adulthood unless effective treatment is undertaken.

In this country, scoliosis is treated by orthopedic surgeons. Once the spine has been radiographically evaluated and the precise nature of the condition determined, one of the following three treatment options is chosen:

- *Do nothing.* Depending on the patient's age and the degree of curvature, it may be appropriate to do nothing and simply monitor the condition to see whether further change occurs.
- *Use a brace.* In children and adolescents, a curve in the mild range (between 25 and 35 degrees) is most effectively treated by bracing the back with a specially fitted metal brace for 23 hours per day. This treatment continues until the spine has moved into acceptable alignment.
- *Undergo surgery.* When a curvature in a preteen or adolescent is near or beyond 45 degrees, the treatment of choice may well be surgical realignment of several vertebrae within and beyond the curvature.

Only about 2 percent of females and 1 percent of males have scoliosis. For those who do, however, new options regarding treatment will hopefully be forthcoming.

Metabolic Disorders

The third category of chronic conditions is metabolic. Metabolic disorders are caused by the body's inability to control chemical processes that regulate the building up (anabolism) and tearing down (catabolism) of tissue. Diabetes mellitus type 2 and diabetes mellitus type 1 are, perhaps, the most familiar of the metabolic disorders.

Congenital abnormalities, which you learned about in the last section, are caused by abnormal structure that leads to abnormal function. The metabolic disorders, on the other hand, are caused directly by abnormal function. The body is unable to normally utilize various nutrients in the growth and repair of tissues and in the regulation

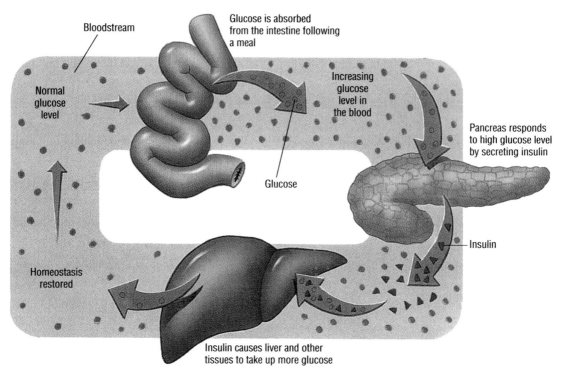

Figure 12-4 Normal Blood Glucose Regulation   The secretion of insulin is regulated by a mechanism that tends to reverse any deviation from normal. Thus an increase in blood glucose level triggers secretion of insulin. Since insulin promotes glucose uptake by cells, blood glucose level is restored to its lower, normal level.

Within the figure (labels):
- Bloodstream
- Glucose is absorbed from the intestine following a meal
- Normal glucose level
- Increasing glucose level in the blood
- Pancreas responds to high glucose level by secreting insulin
- Glucose
- Insulin
- Homeostasis restored
- Insulin causes liver and other tissues to take up more glucose

of body processes. The conditions described in this section have clear metabolic components. They may also have some characteristics that overlap with other categories of conditions. For example, a genetic predisposition is associated with type 2 diabetes mellitus and an autoimmune response with type 1 diabetes.

Diabetes Mellitus

News headlines tell us that American youth are at high risk for developing type 2 diabetes mellitus and its associated heart disease and other health problems. We used to believe that type 2 diabetes was a disease of middle age. The CDC launched SEARCH for Diabetes in Youth,[11] a campaign intended to find children and adolescents with a set of prediabetes markers, referred to as metabolic syndrome, likely resulting from a childhood of poor diet and gross inactivity, in combination with a genetic predisposition for diabetes (see Chapter 10 for more on metabolic syndrome). Certainly those younger persons who had already progressed to clinical levels

of insulin resistance were also sought out by this CDC-sponsored program.

Additionally, the American Diabetes Association issued new guidelines (in *Diabetes Care*) to hone the diagnostic criteria and the pharmacological treatment for children, adolescents, and young adults with previously unrecognised type 2 diabetes mellitus.[12]

Type 2 Diabetes   In people who do not have diabetes mellitus, the body's need for energy is met through the "burning" of glucose (blood sugar) within the cells. Glucose is absorbed from the digestive tract and carried to the cells by the blood or stored in the liver as glycogen for later conversion back to glucose.[7] Glucose passes into the cell through a transport system that moves the glucose molecule across the cell's membrane. Activation of this glucose transport mechanism requires the hormone **insulin** (Figure 12-4). Specific receptor sites for insulin can be found on the cell membrane. Insulin is also required for the conversion of glucose into glycogen in the liver and for the formation of fatty acids in adipose cells. Insulin is produced in the islet cells of the pancreas. The release of insulin from the pancreas corresponds to the changing levels of glucose within the blood.[7]

In adults, and tragically in an increasing percentage of children and adolescents, with a genetic predisposition for developing type 2 diabetes, trigger mechanisms (most likely obesity and inactivity) begin a process through which the body cells become increasingly less sensitive

---

Key Terms

insulin A hormone produced by the islet cells of the pancreas that is necessary for the normal utilization of glucose.

A Wellness Plan for Preventing Type 2 Diabetes Mellitus

I've recently been diagnosed with type 2 diabetes. How can I live well with this condition?

The rate at which Americans develop type 2 diabetes mellitus is on the rise, partly because the population is aging. The disease typically affects older people and thus is sometimes called *adult-onset diabetes.* African Americans, Hispanic Americans, and Native Americans are at greater risk than are members of other ethnic groups, but anyone can develop the disease. There is no foolproof way to prevent diabetes, but you can take steps to lower your risk.

- *Obesity and Overweight*
  Not all obese people become diabetic, but 90 percent of people with diabetes are overweight. In addition, body fat distribution is important—those who are heavy around the middle ("apple shaped") are more susceptible to the disease than those whose fat is stored in the buttocks and thighs ("pear shaped"). Evidence indicates that both men and women who gain weight in adulthood increase their risk of diabetes. A recent study conducted at Harvard University showed that women who had gained 11 to 17 pounds since age 18 doubled their risk of diabetes; those who had gained between 18 and 24 pounds tripled their risk.

  If diabetes runs in your family and you are overweight, you are four times as likely to become diabetic as a person with neither risk factor and twice as likely as a person with only one of these risk factors. Whatever your family history, staying within a healthy weight range and losing weight if you are overweight (see Chapter 6) will lower your risk of diabetes. If you tend to weight-cycle (repeatedly lose weight and then gain it back), keep trying. It is not true, as was once believed, that weight-cycling (yo-yo dieting) is in itself harmful to health.

- *Genetics*
  Some progress has been made in identifying the genes that predispose a person to become obese or develop diabetes, but many more years of research will undoubtedly be required before this knowledge is of any practical use. As already mentioned, a family history of diabetes puts you at increased risk. This does not mean that people with a family history are certain to develop diabetes. But if the disease runs in your family, you should try to reduce other risk factors.

- *Diet*
  Following a sound diet is a worthwhile step toward preventing diabetes. A semivegetarian diet (see Chapter 5) is known to lower the risk of heart disease and cancer and may also lower the risk of diabetes. It is low in fat, especially animal fat, and rich in fruits, grains, vegetables, and low-fat or non-fat dairy products. Such a diet is unlikely to promote weight gain and often promotes weight loss. It also provides the vitamins, minerals, and other nutrients you need to help prevent chronic diseases.

- *Exercise*
  Direct evidence shows that regular physical activity helps prevent diabetes. In one study, researchers from the University of California at Berkeley and Stanford University found that men who were very active—expending 3,500 calories in exercise per week—were only half as likely to develop diabetes as men who were sedentary, expending less than 500 calories per week in leisure-time activity. In fact, those who benefited most from exercise were those at highest risk for diabetes.

  Other strong evidence indicates that vigorous exercise has a protective effect against diabetes in both women and men. This is not just because exercise can promote weight loss—physical activity lowers blood sugar whether or not you lose weight.

- *Vitamin and Mineral Supplements*
  There is no evidence that any supplement can prevent diabetes, despite manufacturers' claims for chromium and other supplements. People with diabetes are often deficient in some vitamins and minerals, such as vitamin E, zinc, magnesium, and occasionally chromium. But these deficiencies may be caused in part by a reduced ability to absorb and utilize these nutrients. Thus they may be a result of the disease, not the cause.

- *Smoking*
  Smoking boosts your risk of diabetes and exacerbates the disease if you already have it. If you are a smoker, do whatever it takes to quit (see Chapter 9). Diabetes is just one of the many serious threats to your health that will be greatly reduced if you stop smoking now.

- *Stress*
  Stress negatively influences type 2 diabetes mellitus in two ways. First, with regard to physiological function, the body's natural response to stress (see Chapter 3) increases the level of glucose and free fatty acids in the blood, thus placing greater than normal demands on the diabetic's already compromised insulin response. Second, during periods of stress people with diabetes may not maintain the level of control over their condition that is normally in place. This can occur in different ways. For example, while stressed, they may be too occupied to monitor blood glucose levels on a regular basis, they may alter their dietary patterns in a less than healthful manner, or they may decrease their level of physical activity and thus lower their level of insulin sensitivity.

  When taken in combination, the detrimental influence of stress and the control of type 2 diabetes mellitus demand advanced coping capabilities on the part of the person with this form of diabetes. Chapter 3 discusses at length ways in which persons can increase their ability to prevent stress, moderate its intensity, or expend the high blood glucose levels found in association with the stress response.

Source: © Health Letter Associates, 1996, 1997, www.wellnessletter.com. Used with permission.

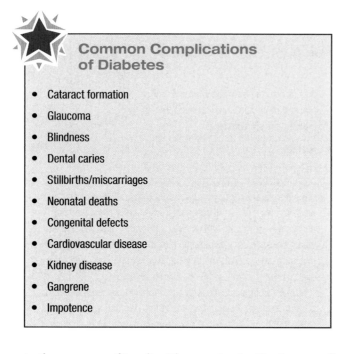

Common Complications of Diabetes

- Cataract formation
- Glaucoma
- Blindness
- Dental caries
- Stillbirths/miscarriages
- Neonatal deaths
- Congenital defects
- Cardiovascular disease
- Kidney disease
- Gangrene
- Impotence

to the presence of insulin. The growing ineffectiveness of insulin in moving glucose into cells causes the buildup of glucose in the blood. Elevated levels of glucose in the blood give rise to **hyperglycemia,** a hallmark symptom of type 2 diabetes mellitus.

In response to this buildup, the kidneys begin the process of filtering glucose from the blood. Excess glucose then spills over into the urine resulting in frequent urination. This removal of glucose in the urine is a second important symptom of type 2 diabetes. Increased thirst, a third symptom of developing diabetes, occurs in response to the movement of fluid from extracellular spaces into the circulatory system to maintain homeostasis.

For many adults with type 2 diabetes or with a prediabetic status often referred to as "glucose intolerance" or "lowered insulin sensitivity," dietary modification (with an emphasis on monitoring total carbohydrate intake, not just sugar), weight loss, and regular exercise, is the only treatment required to maintain an acceptable level of glucose. Weight loss improves the condition by "releasing" more insulin receptors, and exercise increases the actual number of receptor sites. With better insulin recognition, the person can return to a more normal state of functioning.

For people whose condition is more advanced, dietary modification, increased activity, and weight loss alone will not be effective in managing the condition, and oral drugs that stimulate insulin output, called hypoglycemic agents, will be required. Increasingly, very aggressive management, including both hypoglycemic agents and insulin, is successfully reducing risks associated with the disease. Many persons, however, have difficulty controlling blood sugar levels even with the use of insulin.

In addition to genetic predisposition and obesity as important factors in type 2 diabetes mellitus, unresolved stress appears to play a role in the development of

hyperglycemic states (see the box "A Wellness Plan for Preventing Type 2 Diabetes Mellitus" on page 361). Although stress alone probably cannot produce a diabetic condition, it is likely that stress can induce a series of endocrine changes that can lead to a state of hyperglycemia. Depression too can elevate blood glucose levels and thus increase the risk of expressing type 2 diabetes.

Diabetes in both of its principal forms can cause serious damage to virtually all of the body's organ systems, but particularly the cardiovascular, nervous, and renal systems (see the box "Common Complications of Diabetes").

For the 20.8 million Americans with diagnosed diabetes, the estimated 6.2 million not yet diagnosed, as well as the 68 million who are afflicted with dimensions of metabolic syndrome,[13] their future health will be determined by prompt diagnosis and treatment, subsequent daily monitoring, and compliance with suggested lifestyle adjustments. Perhaps no single group of Americans is more susceptible for rapid decline in the direction of type 2 diabetes mellitus than Hispanic Americans of Mexican descent.

As mentioned previously, self-monitoring of glucose levels is a critical component of diabetes prevention. To this end, the American Diabetes Association has fine-tuned its recommendations regarding self-monitoring.[14] When using plasma glucose (finger prick) monitoring (glucometer), the following levels are applicable for the general adult population:

- 90 mg/dl to 130 mg/dl before meals and 110 mg/dl to 150 mg/dl at bedtime
- Less than 180 mg/dl one to two hours after meals

Modified values are assigned by the ADA for use in monitoring plasma glucose levels in children and in pregnant women. Modification levels for children are related to the nervous system's need for blood glucose during development; pregnant women need to monitor themselves for the development of a transitory form of diabetes know as gestational diabetes.

A second index now measured is a hemoglobin faction (HbA1c) that provides a sensitive reflection of longer term blood glucose utilization (over a two- to three-month period). The current target level is less than 7 percent. Plasma glucose levels maintained at 180 mg/dl should facilitate reaching and maintaining an A1c level at or below the 7 percent level.[15]

A third important biomedical index to maintain, in addition to hemoglobin faction and blood glucose, in the prevention of type 2 diabetes is that of blood pressure. Today, for persons of susceptibility, it is now advised that blood pressure readings be 135 or less over 80 or less.

Type 1 Diabetes A second type of diabetes mellitus is type 1 diabetes mellitus. The onset of this type of diabetes usually occurs before age 35, most often during child-

Differences between Types of Diabetes Mellitus

Type 1 Diabetes Mellitus
(These symptoms usually develop rapidly; the body produces no insulin.)

- Extreme hunger
- Extreme thirst
- Frequent urination
- Extreme weight loss
- Irritability
- Weakness and fatigue
- Nausea and vomiting

Type 2 Diabetes Mellitus
(These symptoms usually develop gradually; the body is insensitive to insulin.)

- Any of the symptoms for type 1 diabetes
- Blurred vision or a change in sight
- Itchy skin
- Tingling or numbness in the limbs

If you notice these symptoms occurring, bring them to the attention of your physician.

---

hood. In contrast to type 2 diabetes, in which insulin is produced but is ineffective because of insensitivity, in type 1 diabetes the body produces no insulin at all (see the box "Differences between Types of Diabetes Mellitus"). Destruction of the insulin-producing cells of the pancreas by the immune system (possibly in search of a viral infection within the islet cells of the pancreas) accounts for this sudden and irreversible loss of insulin production.

In most ways the two forms of diabetes are similar, with the important exception that type 1 always requires the use of insulin from an outside source, whereas many people with type 2 diabetes mellitus will not require supplemental insulin, though some might need to take insulin to adequately overcome the insulin insensitivity that is the hallmark of type 2 diabetes. Today insulin is taken by injection (one to four times per day) or through the use of an insulin pump, which provides a constant supply of insulin. Delivery of insulin by inhalation has recently been introduced. Transdermal delivery of insulin (by a patch) is also an option. Development of the glucometer, a highly accurate device for measuring the amount of glucose in the blood, allows better management of this condition. Progress toward development of an immunization for type 1 diabetes mellitus and in vitro pancreas cell transplantation also has occurred.

An even more recently introduced variation of a transplant-based treatment (or cure) of type 1 diabetes is the use of cadaver islet cells. These cells are harvested from the pancreas of a nondiabetic deceased donor and implanted into the pancreas of a person with type 1 diabetes. This experimental procedure is under refinement.

With both forms of diabetes mellitus, sound dietary practices, physical activity, and control of stress are important for keeping blood glucose levels within a normal range. When diabetes mellitus is not properly managed, several serious problems can result, including blindness, gangrene, kidney disease, and heart attack. People who cannot establish good control of the disease are likely to die prematurely.

Double-Diabetes or Type 3 Diabetes Most recently a "third" form of diabetes mellitus has appeared in the medical literature. This form is seen in children with type 1 diabetes, who usually have normal insulin receptors but must take exogenous insulin. In these children, most likely because of their metabolic syndrome, their body loses the ability to recognize exogenous insulin, leading to the development of type 2 diabetes mellitus. When both forms of diabetes mellitus coexist in a person, that condition is called *double diabetes* or *type 3 diabetes mellitus.*[16]

Hypoglycemia

When people with type 1 diabetes do not eat enough, exercise too much, or take too much insulin, they may develop excessively low levels of blood sugar (blood glucose), resulting in a state of classic **hypoglycemia.** In nondiabetic people, difficulty maintaining high enough blood glucose levels may also be associated with drug use, liver damage, partial removal of the stomach, fasting, pancreatic tumors, and rare forms of adrenal and breast tumors, or as a prediabetic symptom.[17] People who have classic hypoglycemia experience headaches, mild confusion, low energy levels, anxiety, sweating, and tremors. They may look pale and behave somewhat abnormally. The form of hypoglycemia just described is the form seen routinely by medical personnel and on occasion by classroom teachers, coaches, and the parents of children with type 1 diabetes.

A rare form of hypoglycemia called *reactive hypoglycemia* is seen in people who are hypersensitive to the presence of sugar in the blood. In these people, a meal that is high in simple carbohydrates (sugars) stimulates excessive insulin production. This insulin removes blood

---

Key Terms

hyperglycemia The condition of having an abnormally high blood glucose level.

hypoglycemia The condition of having an abnormally low blood glucose level.

sugar too quickly, leading to a state of hypoglycemia. People with reactive hypoglycemia have the same symptoms seen in hypoglycemia caused by other factors.

Before reactive hypoglycemia can be definitively diagnosed, the many other causes of low blood sugar (including diabetes mellitus) must first be ruled out. Treatment of reactive hypoglycemia involves dietary modification centered on the consumption of frequent, small meals that contain high levels of complex carbohydrates and few simple carbohydrates. These dietary modifications make the movement of glucose into the bloodstream more gradual, thus eliminating high glucose loads. This "spacing out" of glucose delivery to the blood reduces the body's tendency to overproduce insulin.

In the 1970s the diagnosis of hypoglycemia was made by some physicians to placate patients who complained of vague symptoms of anxiety, moodiness, fatigue, and a loss of interest in normal activities. Once clinical conditions such as depression were ruled out, patients were told that they "must be experiencing hypoglycemia." Patients were then put on a special diet and assured that they would begin to feel better "now that the problem was known." In many cases, patients reported dramatic improvement. Thus hypoglycemia was, for the better part of a decade, much more "common" than it is now believed to be. Today, this less frequently seen, yet still controversial, hypoglycemia is referred to as *functional hypoglycemia* by some. Central to its clear substantiation is a normal blood glucose reading at the time of symptoms (which can be difficult to obtain) and suggestions of a psychiatric illness on a valid mental health inventory.

Autoimmune/Hypersensitivity Disorders

In Chapter 13 you'll learn more about the immune system. Until that time, the immune system can be described as an integrated collection of tissues, organs, and specific areas of endocrine (ductless) cells working to protect the body from foreign protein. On occasion, however, the immune system fails to recognize the body's own protein as being familiar (self) and mistakenly identifies its own protein as foreign (other) and begins attacking it in an attempt to "protect" the body. When this begins, an autoimmune disorder has begun. In this section of the chapter, examples of the autoimmune response will be described.

Key Terms

autoimmune disorders Disorders caused by the immune system's failure to recognize the body as "self"; thus the body mounts an attack against its own cells and tissues.

Figure 12-5 Tenderpoint Locations   Persons with fibromyalgia experience tenderness in at least 11 of the 18 tenderpoint locations.

Fibromyalgia

Fibromyalgia syndrome (FMS) is a chronic condition with symptoms that are so complex an affected person might never be diagnosed and treated despite years of discomfort. For the 2 percent of the adult population believed to have FMS, intermittent periods of morning stiffness, muscle pain, fatigue, numbness and tingling, poor sleep, chronic headaches, jaw discomfort, and many other problems are often seen simply as signs of aging or stress. To trained physicians (often rheumatologists), however, these symptoms may indicate FMS. Accordingly, this syndrome can be diagnosed and effectively treated. Of course, other chronic conditions can coexist with FMS.

The cause of fibromyalgia is unclear at this time. Theories focus on immune system dysfunction (autoimmunity), altered neurotransmitter regulation, hormonal abnormalities (cortisol and HGH), and subtle brain dysfunction. Additionally, certain trigger events—infections, emotional stress, physical trauma, thyroid dysfunction, and connective tissue disorders—may cause FMS.

The diagnosis of FMS is based on medical history and the assessment of discomfort in 18 so-called *tenderpoint locations* (see Figure 12-5). For research purposes, people who experience pain in at least 11 of the 18 tenderpoints are diagnosed with FMS. A lower number of "hits" is considered to be diagnostic in a nonresearch setting. Most people with chronic discomfort will be found to have several tenderpoints during the examination. People who lack tender points and morning stiffness, but, as in fibromyalgia, have chronic widespread pain, may have one or more co-morbid conditions, including depression, anxiety, irritable bowel syndrome, chronic fatigue syndrome, systemic lupus erythematosus, or rheumatoid arthritis.[18]

Figure 12-6 Common Asthma Triggers   If you have asthma, do you know which triggers are troublesome for you?

The treatment of fibromyalgia centers on improving sleep and reducing pain. Physicians can prescribe medications to enhance the effectiveness of sleep-inducing neurotransmitters (such as serotonin and norepinephrine). Nonsteroidal anti-inflammatory drugs (NSAIDs), such as ibuprofen, are used for pain relief. Mild sedatives and muscle relaxants are also employed. Other therapies include synthetic narcotics or transdermal patches for pain relief, acupuncture, and therapeutic massage. Treatments for fibromyalgia also include nonmedication-based approaches, such as exercise, acupuncture, cognitive-behavioral therapy, and relaxation therapy. Research on the effectiveness of these treatments is limited. However, there is some evidence that aerobic exercise may be the most efficacious.[19]

The prognosis for people with FMS is unclear, since few long-term studies have been carried out. For most patients, the condition will remain chronic, with periods of remission and active discomfort occurring intermittently. Whether daily functioning will be significantly impaired later in life remains to be seen.

Asthma

Bronchial asthma is a chronic respiratory disease characterized by acute attacks of breathlessness and wheezing caused by chronic airway inflammation with episodes of narrowing of the bronchioles. Although the mechanisms associated with asthmatic attacks are understood, the reason that some people develop a high level of immune system hypersensitivity is not fully known. The identification of a gene (which may be one of several) related to asthma suggests a genetic predisposition that is expressed during exposure to one or more triggering agents, or allergens.

Two main types of asthma have been identified: extrinsic and intrinsic. In extrinsic asthma, allergens such as pollen, urban air pollutants, dust mites, mold spores, animal fur or dander, and feathers produce sudden and severe bronchoconstriction that narrows the airways. Increased sputum production further narrows the bronchioles and restricts the passage of air. This narrowing fosters the development of chronic inflammation of the airways, which is the most damaging aspect of asthma. Wheezing is most pronounced when the person attempts to exhale air through the narrowed air passages. For many people with asthma, exercise, cigarette smoke, and certain foods or drugs can cause an asthma attack (Figure 12-6). Physicians once suspected that immunizations (for measles, mumps, and rubella) predisposed people to extrinsic asthmatic attacks by hypersensitizing the immune system, but this view currently finds lessened support.

The incidence of extrinsic asthma increased within the general population and particularly among children during the 1980s and 1990s. Today that increase has leveled. That said, however, asthmatic attacks account for nearly one-fifth of the pediatric emergency room visits in this country. Minority children, in particular, are most at risk of developing asthma and dying from its complications. Underlying this increased risk for asthma among minority children is a combination of factors. Among the environmental factors potentially causing this increase are the diminished quality of both outdoor and indoor urban air quality (acidic particles), high levels of urban violence (stress), and overexposure to ozone in high-density traffic areas. However, genetic predisposition may also play an important role in this increase; studies comparing asthma levels among children of different races who share the same environment consistently find higher rates among minority children than their non-minority classmates. A final environmental factor that may account for some of the reported increase is the more complete reporting of acute asthmatic attacks and deaths (by hospital ERs) without, unfortunately, the much-needed increase in initial diagnosis and medical management that would have prevented the acute attacks and death.

Intrinsic asthma, the less common form, has similar symptoms but is most closely related to obesity, stress, frequent respiratory tract infections, hormone replacement therapy (for perimenopausal and postmenopausal women),[20] or possibly by the aftereffects of maternal antibiotics taken during pregnancy. Allergens play a lesser role in this form of asthma, which may be more strongly influenced by genetic predisposition for a hypersensitive immune response to foreign protein (allergens).

Prevention or effective management of asthma is often possible using a combination of approaches. Most important, of course, is the maintenance of high-level wellness through a healthful lifestyle that includes a sound diet, regular exercise, and effective stress management. Each person who has asthma should work with his or her physician to develop a sound, individually tailored management plan. If you have asthma, complete the Personal Assessment at the end of the chapter to determine whether you are doing all you can to manage your condition effectively.

A number of components can be included in an asthma management plan. Exercises that are well tolerated, such as swimming, can help maintain a more normal level of respiratory function. Immunotherapy, in which the patient with extrinsic asthma is desensitized through injections of weakened allergens, is often attempted. In addition, the careful use of corticosteroid drugs several times per day by inhalation reduces inflammation. However, in early 2006 the FDA raised concerns about the use of other asthma-related medications, often in combination with these widely use corticosteroids. "Black box" warnings could be added to the labels of these medications to call attention to the possibility of fatal interactions.

Additional drugs have recently been introduced. Among these are *antileukotrienes* that reduce the immune system's ability to foster inflammation,[21] a new class of engineered antibodies that bind to natural antibodies, thus preventing the activation of mast cells that trigger the asthmatic response,[21] and others that reduce the effects of exercise and cold air that frequently trigger asthma attacks.

Bronchial thermoplasty is a newly developed surgical approach to the treatments of asthma. In this procedure, a transmitter-tipped catheter is passed through the trachea and into the main airway leading to each lung. Once the catheter is in place, high-frequency radio waves are sent through the catheter to destroy a portion of the smooth muscle layer of airway wall, thus reducing the amount of narrowing of the airway that can occur.[22] Each year in this country, several thousand people die as the result of asthma attacks. Some experts believe that this number could be reduced if physicians were more aggressive in their treatment of the bronchial inflammation component of the condition.

People with exercise-induced asthma (EIA), a common type of extrinsic asthma, should take several important steps when attempting to exercise (see the box "Tips for Controlling Exercise-Induced Asthma").

For the 1.5 million Americans (many of them children) with extreme hypersensitivity to peanut-based allergens, which can lead to potentially fatal asthmatic attacks (50 to 100 per year), the development of a peanut-allergy drug was much anticipated. However, development of the medication has been curtailed due to

Considering Complementary Care

Symptomatic Irritable Bowel Syndrome

Gastrointestinal disorders in general, and irritable bowel syndrome (IBS) specifically, are treated through a wide array of conventional therapies. Recently, however, a less conventional therapy, hypnotherapy, was used with adequate success in a number of different studies.

In a recent meta-analysis of studies in which hypnosis was employed as the principal treatment for irritable bowel syndrome (IBS), 15 studies reported in the medical literature between 1970 and 2005 were reevaluated as to their study design and reported findings.

Meta-analysis showed improvement in gut health, a reduction in extracolonic symptoms, lowered levels of anxiety, and an improved sense of quality of life. Signs associated with depression were also reduced.

On the basis of these studies, and of earlier anecdotal reports also suggesting positive results, hypnotherapy appears to be moving slowly in gaining acceptance as a treatment for the symptomatic relief of IBS.

Source: Gholamrezaei A, Ardestani SK, Emami MH. Where does hypnotherapy stand in the management of irritable bowel syndrome? A systematic review. 2006. *J Altern Complement Med.* July-Aug; 12(6):517–527.

safety concerns that arose during early stages of human trials.

Irritable Bowel Syndrome (IBS) and Inflammatory Bowel Disease (IBD)

Although these conditions have strikingly similar labels, they are different in several important ways. IBS is a *syndrome*—the presence of an array of symptoms in the absence of a single definable disease. IBD involves more definitive pathological processes that give rise to more discernible conditions. IBS and IBD both are significantly more common in females than in males, and both can coexist in the same person.

Irritable bowel syndrome (IBS) is characterized by highly uncomfortable episodes of spasticity-based pain, diarrhea, or constipation that are localized to the colon, or large intestine. Even for persons who are only occasionally afflicted with constipation or diarrhea, the mere thought of having to deal frequently with unpredictable pain, diarrhea, and constipation should elicit feelings of compassion for those with IBS. *Spastic colon* is also an antiquated term used frequently by the general public to describe this condition. For some diagnosed with IBS, the drug Zelnorm has proven effective in reducing the frequency and duration of symptoms by helping coordinate nerve and muscle activity of the colon, although currently the safety of this drug is in question. As distressing as this condition can be, it is important to remember that IBS is nonprogressive and localized to the colon, causes no damage to the colon, and, though painful, can be controlled with noninvasive measures, and is never fatal. Diet, stress management, and medication can help control the alienating and embarrassing issues associated with IBS. The box "Symptomatic Irritable Bowel Syndrome" discusses research into the use of hypnosis to relieve IBS symptoms.

In comparison to IBS, inflammatory bowel disease (IBD) is a more highly defined pathological progress that involves invasive, inflammatory changes to the gastrointestinal tract. Two recognizable diseases that fall under the label IBD are ulcerative colitis (UC) and Crohn's disease (CD).

Treatments for ulcerative colitis depend on the severity and duration of symptoms, but they focus on promptness of diagnosis and initiation of treatment, minimization of complications (such as anemia and malabsorption), maintenance of normal growth (when dealing with young children), and establishing remission, in which symptoms and disease progression are significantly minimized. Treatment options include dietary changes, enteral (tube) feeding, "gut rest," antidiarrheal medications, and the use of corticosteroids when symptoms have been present for a longer duration. The box "Managing Inflammatory Bowel Disease" provides suggestions for reducing the occurrence of this syndrome. Inflammation is identified through abnormal bloodwork results or visual changes seen through a colonoscopy. A class of nonsteroidal anti-inflammatory drugs, the aminosalicylates, may be used to sustain periods of remission. During very active periods of disease, immunomodulator drugs may be used to suppress inflammation,[23] but these drugs compromise immune system function and their use must be carefully monitored.[24] Removal of the colon, known as a colectomy, may be the only "cure" for this condition. Patients with ulcerative colitis have a significantly elevated risk of colon cancer.

Unlike ulcerative colitis, Crohn's disease can occur anywhere along the course of the gastrointestinal tract ("from tip to tail"), from the mouth and lips to the anus. This condition involves clear pathological changes within the gastrointestinal tract and, unlike ulcerative colitis, is the only form of IBD that can penetrate the wall of the gastrointestinal tract. At times, persons with Crohn's disease can develop **fistulas,** open pathways between the gastrointestinal wall and neighboring structures, such as the vagina and urinary bladder.

Crohn's disease is increasingly treated with immunosuppressive drugs. These drugs produce antibodies, aimed principally against tumor necrosis factor (TNF), and are intended to counter the immune system's inappropriate destruction of elements within the intestinal wall (see Chapter 13 for additional information on immune system function). Because they suppress the immune system, these powerful drugs must be monitored carefully and patients should take extra caution to avoid exposure to colds, flu, and other opportunistic infections.[24] Surgery is often needed to remove the colon and parts of the small intestine when inflammation does not respond to treatment with diet and drugs. Unfortunately, Crohn's disease often "reappears" near the site where the bowel was removed or in other areas of the GI tract. Therefore, many Crohn's patients develop "short-gut syndrome" and issues of gross malnutrition when they lose significant amounts of intestine in areas where nutrients are absorbed.

Along with the inflammatory changes that happen to the GI tract in a person with IBD, there are "extraintestinal manifestations," involving the eyes, skin, and joints. There might also be side effects related to the medications.

Though there is no known "cure," neither IBS nor IBD is generally considered to be fatal. One complication from IBD, known as toxic megacolon, is the most likely possible exception to that contention. Toxic megacolon, in which extensive inflammation of the colon wall occurs, must be addressed immediately and aggressively. It can arise from excessive inflammatory or bowel obstruction from either ulcerative colitis or Crohn's disease and can cause the colon to perforate. Usually treatment for this involves removal of the entire colon.

Although the etiology of IBD is not completely known, there are strong indications that genetic mutations underlie its development, leading to the establishment of an autoimmune reaction to proteins within the gastrointestinal wall. It has also been found that there are family patterns of both IBS and IBD, further suggesting that genetically based etiologies are in play.

Systemic Lupus Erythematosus (SLE)

Systemic lupus erythematosus, or simply *lupus,* is one of the most familiar autoimmune disorders or connective tissue disorders. These conditions are caused by an extensive and inappropriate attack by the body's immune system on its own tissues, which then serve as **self-antigens.** (See Chapter 13 for a discussion of the immune response.)

The word **systemic** refers to the widespread destruction of fibrous connective tissue and other tissues. *Erythematosus* (*erythema*- means "red") refers to the reddish rash that imparts a characteristic "mask" to the face of a person with SLE. The disease is seen in women 25 times more often than in men, and it first appears during young adulthood, although it is now known that autoantibodies may first appear in the blood as much as a decade before the first observable symptoms of SLE appear (see the box "Lupus—Different in Women and Men?"). Specificity was added to this time estimate in a second study. In this study of 130 lupus patients, it was found that in about one-fifth of patients eventually diagnosed with SLE, antibodies were present in the blood, on average, about three years prior to their definitive diagnosis.[25] All persons in the study were initially tested upon the appearance of their earliest symptom of probable lupus.

Particularly interesting in most large studies is the gender inequity reported among African American women and women of Hispanic and Asian origin than among other women.

The course of systemic lupus erythematosus is gradual, with intermittent periods of inflammation, stiffness, fatigue, pleurisy (chest pain), and discomfort over wide

Learning from Our Diversity

Lupus—Different in Women and Men?

From a purely statistical point of view, systemic lupus erythomatosis (SLE) is much more common in women. In fact, 90 percent of all cases are seen in women, with the age of onset generally in young adulthood. In light of the preponderance of SLE in younger (premenopausal) women, a high level of estrogen seems very likely to be a principal factor in the development of the condition in women who are genetically predisposed to the condition. Conversely, high levels of androgenic hormones (principally testosterone) provide a protective influence against the development of SLE in men. When SLE is seen in younger men, however, androgenic hormone levels are generally found to be lower than normal. Not surprisingly, SLE is more often initially diagnosed in older men, when testosterone levels have fallen with age. Understandably, after menopause, when estrogen levels have fallen drastically, women are only twice as likely as men to develop SLE.

As noted in the text discussion of SLE, a wide array of organ systems are negatively influenced by SLE. However, when the condition is found in younger men, the degree of kidney damage is greater than that seen in younger women. Because of this damage to the urinary system, younger male SLE victims are more vulnerable than are their female counterparts to life-shortening effects of renal failure. However, because pregnancy is unique to women, the pregnancy/childbirth complications brought about by SLE (increased incidence of miscarriages, premature births, and preeclampsia) distinguish women with SLE from those without SLE.

Beyond the gender-specific aspects of SLE just mentioned, the condition generally appears in a fairly similar fashion in both sexes. For each, prompt diagnosis and appropriate treatment are the keys to a longer and healthier life.

---

areas of the body, including muscles, joints, and skin. Similar changes may take place in the tissues of the nervous system, kidneys, and heart.[2]

Researchers do not know why the immune system attacks the body in such an extensive and aggressive way. It is likely, however, that a combination of genetic predisposition, hormones (estrogen), chronic emotional stress (see Chapter 3), ultraviolet radiation (including sunlight), and an earlier viral infection may be involved in its development.

A physician may suspect lupus based on the patient's description of her symptoms and make a diagnosis using a number of laboratory tests, including the identification of an SLE factor in the blood. A skin biopsy may be taken to confirm structural changes in the connective tissue layer below the skin.

Management of lupus generally involves the occasional or long-term use of nonsteroidal anti-inflammatory drugs (NSAIDs), malarial drugs for the skin rash, and a low dose of prednisone (a corticosteroid) to reduce fever, treat episodes of pleurisy, and minimize certain neurological symptoms. The immune system itself may be medically suppressed as well. These treatments must be carefully monitored because they have serious side effects.

Management of lupus centers on the prevention of episodes of the disease called *flares*. These periods of active lupus are often triggered by exposure to the sun, periods of fatigue, or an infectious disease, all of which should be avoided as much as possible.

TALKING POINTS You learn that two young women who are your coworkers have recently been diagnosed with lupus and Crohn's disease, respectively. How can you be supportive of them? What would you say to them about their conditions, particularly on days when it is obvious that they are not feeling well?

Multiple Sclerosis (MS)

For proper nerve conduction to occur within portions of the brain and the spinal cord, an insulating sheath of myelin must surround the neurons (nerve cells). In the progressive disease multiple sclerosis (MS), the cells that produce myelin are destroyed, myelin production ceases, and the underlying nerves are badly damaged. Neurological functioning eventually becomes so disrupted that vital functions are significantly impaired. The cause of MS is not known. Research continues to focus on virus-induced autoimmune mechanisms in which T cells attack viral-infected myelin-producing cells. At this time a large number of viruses have been discovered in the cerebrospinal fluid (CSF) of persons with MS and other neurological disorders. These viruses generally are not found in persons who do not have these conditions. Among the most actively accessed viruses are herpes simplex virus 1 (HSV-1), herpes simplex virus 2 (HSV-2), Epstein-Barr virus (EBV), varicella zoster virus (VZV), human cytomegalovirus (HCMV), human herpes virus 6 (HHV-6), and the JC virus (JCV). Patients with different forms of MS will have different collections of viruses. However, the virus most commonly found in the spinal fluid of persons with MS (regardless of type) and others with neurological disorders is the varicella zoster virus

Key Terms

fistula A fissure, break, or hole in the wall of an organ.

self-antigens The cells and tissues that stimulate the immune system's autoimmune response.

systemic (sis **tem** ic) Distributed or occurring throughout the entire body system.

(VZV), making it a chief suspect in the etiology of multiple sclerosis.[26] Some immune system evidence of this virus can be found in about 90 percent of all Americans, but not at the levels associated with MS.

Multiple sclerosis usually appears for the first time during the young adult years. It may take one of four forms, depending on the interplay of periods of stabilization (remitting), renewed deterioration (relapsing), continuous deterioration (progressive), and combinations of the above. The initial symptoms of the condition are often visual impairment, prickling and burning in the extremities, and an altered gait. In its most advanced stages, movement is greatly impaired, and mental deterioration may be present. It should be noted, however, that MS may be a "silent epidemic" among children, including those younger than 10 years of age. To facilitate a more timely diagnosis of MS, children showing mild tremors or reporting intermittent dimming of vision should be seen by a pediatric neurologist. It is currently estimated that over 20,000 American children may have early-onset MS.

The definitive diagnosis of MS is made through MRI scans for lesions (areas of myelin erosion) in the spinal nerves or the brain. Additionally, a newly developed blood test can assist p hysicians in determining at what point in time assertive medical management of patients should begin following the initial presentation of symptoms.

Treatment of MS is aimed at reducing the severity of symptoms and extending the periods of remission. Today a variety of therapies are used, including immune system–targeted drugs, steroid drugs, drugs to relieve muscle spasms, a medication to fight fatigue, injections of nerve blockers, and physical therapy.

At the heart of modern treatment of MS are several drugs, all of which were developed since 1993, some as recently as 2006. Among these are five *immunomodulating drugs*—Avonex, Betaseron, and Rebif (all versions of interferon beta and taken by injection), and Copaxon and Tysabri (which use different avenues to modify the activity of the immune system and are taken by injection and infusion, respectively); and an *immunosuppressant drug*, Novantrone (initially developed for the treatment of cancer, taken four times per year by infusion).[27] The goals of these therapies are to reduce the frequency of attacks, reduce the accumulation of lesions within the spinal cord and brain, and slow the accumulation of disabilities. Research continues into other therapies, including the use of stem cells.

Additional medications are available to address complications of MS, such as spasticity and the use of statins (cholesterol-lowering drugs) in MS-developing laboratory mice. To date, this represents the closest approximation of "prevention" that has been obtained in the field of MS treatment.

Psychotherapy is an important adjunct to the treatment of MS. Profound periods of depression often accompany the initial diagnosis of this condition.

Emotional support is helpful in dealing with the progressive impairment associated with the condition; see the box "Support Is Just a Click Away" for more information.

Degenerative Diseases

A fifth category of chronic conditions is that of degenerative diseases. Conditions within this category are among the most debilitating of all chronic conditions in that they generally appear late in life, in conjunction with the overall frailty of advanced age, and thus put great demand on caregivers. Eventually, expensive institutional care is required when the level of debilitation prevents the afflicted persons from meeting the activities of daily living (ADL) or even maintaining a sense of self and of the world in which they live. Paramount among these degenerative conditions are Parkinson's disease and Alzheimer's disease.

Parkinson's Disease

Once called "shaking palsy," Parkinson's disease is now recognized as a specific neurological disorder belonging to a family of conditions called *motor system disorders*. Parkinson's disease involves the chronic progressive loss of dopamine production within specific areas of the brain. These areas, called the substantia nigra and striatum, transmit signals required to produce purposeful muscle activity that leads to more highly coordinated movement. The four primary signs of the disease reflect this loss of muscular coordination: (1) tremor or trembling in the hands, arms, legs, jaw, and face; (2) rigidity or stiffness of the limbs or trunk; (3) slowness of movement; and (4) postural instability and impaired balance. As these symptoms worsen, people with Parkinson's disease become progressively less able to talk, walk, and perform simple tasks associated with daily living.

As is true for Alzheimer's disease, Parkinson's disease can be staged using one or both of the following systems.[28] The most basic way to classify a person's progression in Parkinson's disease is in terms of early, moderate, or advanced stage. The advanced stage is characterized by loss of independence in terms of activities of daily living, limited efficacy of medications being used, significant changes in posture, limited speech, and frequent changes in movement.

The more complex system for staging uses Stage I through Stage V. In Stage V, persons are almost totally confined to bed or to a chair; while in Stage IV both sides of the body are affected, the person needs substantial help in standing or walking, and tasks of daily living are difficult to impossible to accomplish without assistance.

Parkinson's-like symptoms are associated with other conditions, such as head injury, tumors, prolonged use

Support Is Just a Click Away

Support groups are composed of people who come together to help one another through the demands of a chronic health condition. These groups have traditionally been organized by institutions in the local health care community, such as hospitals, by the local affiliates of national organizations, such as the American Cancer Society, or by citizens who have the same chronic condition. Today, however, more and more support group members are connected not by physical proximity but by the Internet.

Health self-help groups on the Internet develop in one of two ways. The first occurs when a brick-and-mortar organization, such as a national agency or health care institution, develops a support group for its homepage. The second way is for a person with the condition (or a family member of that person) to organize an online group.

You can find a health support group simply by surfing the Net. Or you can be referred to a site by a health care professional, friend, family member, colleague, or someone with a similar condition. You can also go to the home page of a medical institution or a national agency to find out if it provides a support group link.

For someone with a newly diagnosed chronic condition, the initial contact with a support group may be made to get information about the condition and its treatment. For others, it is a way of connecting with other people who have the condition. Web support groups provide windows to the outside world, particularly for those whose conditions limit their mobility and social contacts. The Internet support group transcends the restrictions of various diseases to make new connections possible.

Note that online support groups' members are rarely physicians or other highly trained health professionals, so you shouldn't rely on this source for specific technical information. Instead, your main sources of information about medical management of a chronic condition should be your health care providers. Seasoned members of support groups need to remind themselves that newly diagnosed members are inexperienced and vulnerable. It will take them time to adjust to the frankness and clinical sophistication demonstrated by some group members in addressing their health problems.

Some hospitals provide notebook computers to patients so they can maintain contact with their support groups. In this way, health care institutions are encouraging patients to support their efforts and, perhaps, helping them recover more quickly. Additionally, with the increased affordability of notebook computers and the increased availability of wireless Internet, being connected with one's support group is increasingly less restricted.

---

of tranquilizers, and manganese and carbon monoxide poisoning. The labels *Parkinson's syndrome* and *atypical Parkinson's* are used to describe these conditions. It is believed that as many as one in five elderly Americans shows some Parkinsonian signs.

About 500,000 Americans have been diagnosed with primary Parkinson's disease, and about 50,000 new cases are diagnosed annually. The exact number of people with this condition has always been difficult to establish with certainty, since some people assume that these changes are the result of aging and thus do not seek medical evaluation. The incidence of Parkinson's disease is the same in men and women. The condition is usually first seen in people over age 50, with 60 being the average age at first diagnosis. Compared with African Americans and Asian Americans, whites are more likely to be diagnosed with Parkinson's disease. A relatively small percentage of people develop the disease as early as age 40. Slightly fewer cases of Parkinson's disease are seen among smokers than among nonsmokers (the risks of smoking, however, greatly outweigh the slightly lower risk of Parkinson's disease among smokers).

Three explanations of the cause of Parkinson's disease have been proposed. The first involves the formation of highly excited unstable chemical compounds known as *free radicals*. With aging, the formation of these highly unstable free radicals increases, and they accumulate within a large variety of body tissues. These free radicals seek stability by physically altering the chemical structure of tissues with which they have contact, including the cells of the substantia nigra. Once damaged, the cells of the substantia nigra and striatum die; thus their dopamine production is lost and the symptoms of Parkinson's appear.

The second possible explanation relates to environmental toxins that are suspected to produce Parkinson's-like symptoms in humans. However, no widely occurring environmental toxins of this nature have been discovered that could account for the large number of cases of Parkinson's disease in this country and around the world. This theory was, however, given support by a follow-up on responses from over 140,000 persons initially surveyed in 2001 as part of the Cancer Prevention Study II Nutrition Cohort. From this large study population, nearly 6 percent had substantial exposure to pesticides as farmers, ranchers, or fishermen. These individuals had a 70 percent higher incidence of Parkinson's disease than a matched group from within the population who had no substantial exposure to pesticides.[29] At this point, however, pesticide exposure alone could not account for the high incidence of the disease reported worldwide.

The third theory about the cause of Parkinson's disease suggests an inherited predisposition associated with genetic material found within the mitochondria of cells. Mitochondria are cell structures in which energy is

Actor Michael J. Fox has Parkinson's disease and actively supports research for a cure.

produced to fuel specific cellular tasks, such as the production of dopamine. Currently, however, a genetic basis for Parkinson's is thought most likely only in those cases of the disease that occur in persons considerably younger than typical victims and often with a substantial family history of the condition—perhaps 10 percent of all cases of Parkinson's disease.

Parkinson's disease is usually diagnosed by a neurologist after the patient is referred by a primary care physician. Although there is no single test for diagnosing Parkinson's disease, medical imaging, such as CT scans and MRI scans, may be helpful in ruling out conditions that mimic the disease.

Several medications are used to delay the progression of the disease. Each of these medications functions in one of two ways. The dopamine enhancers, best represented by levodopa, are chemically converted into dopamine, thus sustaining an adequate level of dopamine needed for coordinating motor control. Still a valuable contributor in the treatment of Parkinson's, the use of levodopa is now being delayed until the patient has undergone initial treatment with a second class of drugs, the dopamine agonists.

The dopamine agonist drugs, unlike levodopa, do not increase the amount of dopamine within selected brain areas; instead they influence dopamine receptors in the brain to better recognize the diminished dopamine still being produced in the brain. Administering this second class of medications during the earliest stage of the disease makes it possible to delay the use of levodopa until later in the disease's progression, while avoiding certain problems associated with the early use of levodopa.[30]

As helpful as these medications are, however, their influence is temporary and at best only slows the progress of the disease.

Although only in the earliest stage of human trials, a compound derived from glial cells, called GDNF, has shown a clear ability to increase dopamine production while at the same time reducing the limitations in the loss of motor control initially present. Considerable research and development remains to be done on this new treatment approach; currently, this research remains in tissue culture and animal stages.

Pharmacological treatment of Parkinson's disease can also be combined with the surgical implantation of a deep brain stimulation (DBS) unit. When implanted, this device delivers controlled electrical impulses, via electrodes, to targeted areas of the brain (principally the thalamus) in order to complete the electrical transportation of information once based on the availability of dopamine. This technology is most often used in later stages of the disease. DBS is not a cure for Parkinson's disease, nor does it structurally alter or destroy brain tissue.

The use of stem cells to generate new dopamine-producing neurons has been a much anticipated "cure" for Parkinson's disease. To date, the use of stem cells in the United States has been limited, partly due to the controversy surrounding their collection (see the box "Stem Cells"). Even farther into the future, it might become possible to implant entire neurons, thereby eliminating the time required for implanted stem cells to undergo the specialization and replication necessary to be effective therapies for Parkinson's.

At this time a radically different form of treatment for Parkinson's disease is under refinement. A xenotransplant-based technique has been developed through which fetal pig cells are transplanted into the brains of Parkinson's patients for the purpose of reestablishing functional dopamine-producing cells in the areas of the brain deprived of this ability by the disease. In the limited number of persons having had this procedure, levels of success are sufficiently high enough to encourage continued study, in spite of some ethical and safety (animal-to-human virus transmission) concerns regarding the use of animal tissues.

 TALKING POINTS Your grandmother seems increasingly frustrated by your grandfather's "clumsiness" and has complained that he is becoming increasingly unsteady and nervous. What might you say to her about his condition? What would you suggest she say to him?

Alzheimer's Disease (AD)

Although it affects only 1–2 percent of elderly people, organic brain syndrome, in either its acute or chronic

The potential use of stem cells to treat chronic diseases such as Parkinson's disease, diabetes, and Alzheimer's disease has been the focus of much recent research, media attention, and controversy. Stem cells are undifferentiated pluripotent cells, meaning they have the ability to divide and renew themselves for long periods and to differentiate into many specialized types of cells, including nerve, muscle, and blood cells. The hope is that stem cells can be used to replace a specific type of diseased cell with healthy cells—for example, stem cells might be introduced into a person with Parkinson's disease and directed to develop into healthy dopamine-producing cells, thereby treating the underlying cause of Parkinson's disease.

The primary controversy in the study of stem cells is their source. Most pluripotent stem cells come from human embryos that have been fertilized outside the body in the same process used for *in vitro* fertilization; the embryos are destroyed in the process. Stem cells from other sources may be less flexible in terms of the number of cell types they can develop into. Stem cells can be derived from the following sources:

Human embryos. Cells are removed from the blastocyst, a ball of cells that forms during the first week of embryonic development; these stem cells are then grown in the laboratory to produce sufficient numbers of cells to be used for transplantation.

A related method of producing stem cells is so-called therapeutic cloning, in which the nucleus of an adult body cell is placed in an egg from which the nucleus has been removed. The egg is allowed to develop in the lab into a blastocyst, and the resulting stem cells are removed. The same technique can potentially be used for reproductive cloning if the resulting embryo is implanted into a surrogate and develops into a fetus; it is this technique that produced Dolly the sheep and other cloned animals, which are genetically identical to the adult from which the original body cell nucleus was taken. See Chapter 17 for more on therapeutic and reproductive cloning.

Amniotic fluid. Stem cells can be harvested from the fluid that surrounds the developing embryo within the amniotic sac. Aspiration of these cells from within the uterus does not harm the embryo, as they are sloughed off on a regular basis. This process

may reduce the concerns associated with the use of embryos for stem cell research.

Cord blood. At birth, fetal blood cells can be obtained from the umbilical cord when it is cut and then grown in the laboratory. Today, stem cells from cord blood are being "banked" in case the child, later in life, needs access to a source of highly compatible pluripotent cells.

Adult cells. Relatively pluripotent cells (adult stem cells) can be found in tissues throughout the human body, where they serve for tissue growth and repair. To date, adult stem cells have been harvested from bone marrow, the nasal lining, skin, and even the retina of the eye. Many researchers believe that these cells are overly specialized and thus not comparable to more pluripotent stem cells taken from embryos, amniotic fluid, or cord blood.

The extent to which stem cell therapy becomes a standard approach to treating chronic illnesses in this country will reflect the interplay of scientific, political, and ethical issues not yet fully resolved.

Infolinks

stemcells.nih.gov

---

form, is a collection of incapacitating, heart-rending, and costly afflictions. **Alzheimer's disease** is the best known of these conditions, affecting approximately 5 million adults in this country and perhaps as many as 12 million worldwide. Today, more than ever before, it is *the* disease associated with aging.

The initial signs of Alzheimer's disease are often subtle and may be confused with mild depression or frontotemporal dementia (FTD), a collection of degenerative brain disorders. At this stage of the disease process, however, the person might have some difficulty answering questions like these:

- Where are we now?
- What month is it?
- What is today's date?
- When is your birthday?
- Who is the president?

During the ensuing months, people with this condition experience greater memory loss, confusion, and **dementia.** In the most advanced stage, people with Alzheimer's disease are incontinent (unable to control bladder and bowel function), display infantile behavior, and finally become totally incapacitated as a result of the destruction of brain tissue. Patients with advanced Alzheimer's disease usually must be institutionalized.

Several theories have been advanced about the cause of Alzheimer's disease. Increasing evidence indicates that genetic mutations on chromosomes 1, 14, 19, or 21 may encourage the development of the disease.[31] Other theories suggest links between Alzheimer's disease and

Key Terms

xenotransplant A transplant of tissue from an animal, such as a pig, to a human recipient.

Alzheimer's disease Adult-onset form of dementia resulting from loss of acetylcholine production within specific areas of the brain.

dementia The loss of cognitive abilities, including memory and reason.

abnormal protein development, deficiencies in acetylcholine (a neurotransmitter) production, loss of nicotine receptors in specific areas of the brain, abnormal blood flow, or exposure to infectious agents or toxins.

In the current classification system for AD, two principal categories are used, *early-onset AD* (before age 65) and *late-onset AD* (after age 65). Early-onset AD, encompassing types 1, 3, and 4, accounts for approximately 25 percent of all AD patients and is clearly an inherited form of the disease. Chromosomes 1 (*PSEN2* gene), 14 (*PSEN1* gene), and 21 (*APP* gene) have been identified as factors in this form of the disease. Late-onset AD, designated as type 2, the most prevalent form of the disease, is less clearly understood from a genetic point of view, although chromosome 19 (*APOE* gene) is believed to be involved. The *APOE* gene on chromosome 19 comes in three versions E2, E3, and E4; the *E4* form is associated with heightened risk for Alzheimer's disease.

In addition to chromosomes 1, 14, 19, and 21, chromosomes 9, 10, and 12 are also of interest. It has been suggested that perhaps as many as 20 specific genes involved in the development of AD are located on these and other chromosomes. Of these genes, strong interest exists in the *SORL1* gene, which plays a role in amyloid beta protein production.[32]

The precise diagnosis of Alzheimer's disease and similar disorders is difficult to make before the patient dies. Only during an autopsy can the characteristic signs of the disease—*neurofibrillary tangles* (twisted strands of neuronal material) and *senile plaque* (compressed masses of cellular material, badly damaged nerve fibers, and a core composed of *amyloid beta protein*)—be identified to confirm the diagnosis. Before death, all other conditions capable of causing dementia must be individually ruled out. Thus, tentative or probable diagnosis of Alzheimer's disease is made by a process of elimination. Newer medical imaging technologies, such as MRIs and PET scans, have become so refined that it is now *nearly* possible to confirm the diagnosis of Alzheimer's disease before death. Today these technologies have been combined with the application of selected memory tests allowing clinicians to clearly view subtle signs of diminished functional activity in specific areas of the brain. Using this approach, the ability to predict the development of Alzheimer's disease, particularly in persons with a known genetic marker for the condition, may be at hand.

Effective drugs to treat Alzheimer's disease have not yet been developed. That said, four drugs (Razadyne [galantamine], Exelon [rivastigmine], Aricept [donepezil], and Cognex [tacrine]) provide temporary improvement in intellectual function in mild to moderate AD by inhibiting the enzyme that breaks down the neurotransmitter *acetylcholine,* whose diminished availability is the basis of Alzheimer's disease.[33] The drug Cognex remains on the market, but its use has become minimal. A fifth medication, Namenda (menantine), used in moderate to severe AD, functions by blocking glutamate, a substance capable of damaging neurons. Many additional drugs are in various stages of development, including Flurizan, a slightly modified version of an NSAID initially developed for use in treating arthritis that is thought capable of preventing the actual formation of amyloid beta proteins.[34]

At this time, a wide array of studies attempting to link behavioral patterns to the prevention of cognitive diseases that occur with aging and decline, including the development of AD, are under way. Among these are studies assessing the role of fatty acids (particularly n-3 omega fatty acid) in preventing cognitive decline, the role of exercise (particularly walking) in improving cognitive capabilities in aging adults, and the contributions of regular light alcohol consumption in protecting against Alzheimer's-like conditions. Additional studies in the same vein include those related to the effectiveness of NSAIDs (nonsteroidal anti-inflammatory drugs) in preventing cognitive decline, as well as their interactions with other AD-approved medications, the ability of antioxidant vitamins (carotenes, vitamin C, and vitamin E) to prevent dementia, and the role of high-dose HRT in the cause or exacerbation of cognitive decline, including AD. Current studies in prevention-oriented research are investigating the role of the Mediterranean diet (see Chapter 5) reductions in dietary fats, and steps needed to reduce the growing incidence of metabolic syndrome (prediabetes) that is developing at alarming rates in this country and around the world.

In addition to the speculative preventive approaches just described, vaccines for the prevention of Alzheimer's disease are now in clinical trials. These vaccines utilize a synthetic version of the beta-amyloid protein to stimulate an immune response against the beta-amyloid that occurs in conjunction with the disease. On the basis of the initial human trials, immunizations appear safe, but their effectiveness requires continuing study.[35]

In addition to the vaccine research just mentioned, new delivery systems for Alzheimer's medications are under development. Among these new delivery techniques are skin patches, similar to those used in nicotine dependency and birth control, and implantable rods, similar to those used to deliver contraceptive medications.

A Final Thought about Health and Chronic Conditions

In this chapter we have addressed different types of chronic conditions, many of which have their onset in younger adulthood. Recall the definitions of health, both traditionally and developmentally oriented, that were introduced in Chapter 1. For persons diagnosed with any of the illnesses presented here, the traditional definitions of health could easily label them as being "sick," "ill," or "unhealthy." From a developmental perspective, however, these persons almost certainly hold aspirations of living the fullest life possible, in light of the limitations imposed by their medical conditions. To do this, they must reassess the aspirations held for them by society and the life experiences they envisioned for themselves. Once having made these reassessments, and not always easily, they begin applying resources less dependent on the structure and function of the body, but more in tune with the resources of the mind, intellect, spirit, and the supportive presence of other people. As these alternative centers of resourcefulness become more easily recognizable and skillfully and comfortably called on, the ability to engage more and more fully in life increases. Thus, these people experience an increasing number of "good days" and a greater sense of being healthy—even though the body (and perhaps society) may disagree.

Taking Charge of Your Health

- Stay attuned to media reports about chronic conditions so that you can make informed choices.
- Support agencies devoted to the prevention of chronic health conditions.
- Monitor your work, home, and recreational environments to determine whether they are enhancing your risk for developing a chronic health condition.
- Undergo the recommended screening procedures and other preventive procedures related to chronic conditions for your age and sex.
- If you have a chronic condition, participate actively in your own treatment.

SUMMARY

- Chronic conditions can be classified into several categories: genetic/inherited, congenital, metabolic, autoimmune, and degenerative.
- Klinefelter's syndrome and Turner's syndrome are conditions reflecting an abnormal number of sex chromosomes.
- Cystic fibrosis and sickle-cell trait and disease are conditions reflecting the inheritance of one or more recessive genetic traits.
- Color vision deficiency and fragile X syndrome are sex-linked inherited recessive conditions reflecting recessive traits carried on the X chromosome. Males exhibit the symptoms, while females are carriers.
- Cleft lip, cleft palate, and patent foramen ovale (PFO) are congenital abnormalities, reflecting developmental errors in the formation of the face and heart, respectively, that occur during the embryonic stage of interuterine life. Scoliosis likely begins during interuterine development, but may progress postnatally.
- Type 2 and type 1 diabetes mellitus are metabolic disorders reflecting insulin-based difficulties in the production of insulin or its recognition, thus depriving the body of its normal ability to utilize blood glucose. Type 3 diabetes reflects a combination of types 1 and 2 in the same individual.
- Fibromyagia, systemic lupus erythematosus (SLE), and asthma are chronic conditions reflecting immune system dysfunction by either overresponding to allergens or by attempting to destroy the body's own proteins.
- Irritable bowel syndrome and inflammatory bowel disease reflect gastrointestinal system conditions, primarily seen in females, related to hypersensitivity or autoimmune responses. Multiple sclerosis (MS) is caused by an attack by the immune system on cells that produce myelin, the insulation critical to nervous system function in the brain and spinal cord.
- Parkinson's disease is characterized by loss of fine muscular control caused by the gradual cessation of dopamine production within the brain.
- Alzheimer's disease is a form of dementia (or loss of cognitive ability) caused by the gradual loss of the brain's ability to produce acetylcholine, a neurotransmitter essential for normal mental functioning.

REVIEW QUESTIONS

1. Identify and describe the five categories of chronic conditions presented in this chapter.
2. What is the genetic basis of Turner's syndrome? Klinefelter's syndrome? What physical features characterize persons with Turner's syndrome and Klinefelter's syndrome?
3. Cystic fibrosis is a *recessive genetic disorder;* explain this term. What functional difficulties are experienced by people with cystic fibrosis? What is the condition's long-term prognosis?
4. What complex protein structure is present in an abnormal form in people with sickle-cell disease? What shape are the red blood cells in people with this condition? Why are genetic screening and counseling considered important for sickle-cell disease and trait?

soil. The spores of the tetanus bacterium, for example, can survive in soil for up to 50 years, entering the human body in a puncture wound.

Portal of Exit   For pathogenic agents to cause diseases and illnesses in others, they must leave their reservoirs. Thus the third link in the chain of infection is the *portal of exit*, or the point at which agents leave their reservoirs.

The principal portals of exit are familiar—the digestive system, urinary system, respiratory system, reproductive system, and the blood, especially with infectious diseases that infect humans.

Mode of Transmission   The fourth link in the chain of infection is the *mode of transmission*, or the way in which pathogens move from reservoirs to susceptible hosts. Two principal methods are direct transmission and indirect transmission.

We see three types of direct transmission in human-to-human transmission. These include contact between body surfaces (such as kissing, touching, and sexual intercourse), droplet spread (inhalation of contaminated air droplets), and fecal-oral spread (feces on the host's hands are brought into contact with the new host's mouth), as could occur when changing the diaper of an infected infant.

Indirect transmission between infected and uninfected people occurs when infectious agents travel by means of nonhuman materials. Vehicles of transmission include inanimate objects (known as *fomites*), such as water, food, soil, towels, clothing, and eating utensils.

Infectious agents can also be indirectly transmitted through vectors. The term *vector* describes living things, such as insects, birds, and other animals, that carry diseases from human to human. An example of a vector is the deer tick, which transmits Lyme disease.

Airborne indirect transmission includes the inhalation of infected particles that have been suspended in an air source for an extended time. Unlike droplet transmission, in which both infected and uninfected people must be in close physical proximity, noninfected people can become infected through airborne transmission by sharing air with infected people who were in the same room hours earlier. Viral infections such as German measles can be spread this way.

Portal of Entry   The fifth link in the chain of infection is the *portal of entry*. As with the portals of exit, portals of entry have three primary methods that allow pathogenic agents to enter the bodies of uninfected people. These are through the digestive system, respiratory system, and reproductive system. In addition, a break in the skin provides another portal of entry. In most infectious conditions, the portals of entry are the same systems that served as the portals of exit from the infected people. In HIV, however, we see cross-system transmission. Oral

and anal sex allow infectious agents to pass between the warm, moist tissues of the reproductive and digestive systems.

The New Host   All people are, in theory, at risk for contracting infectious diseases and thus could be called susceptible hosts. In practice, however, factors such as overall health, acquired immunity, health care services, and health-related behavior can affect susceptibility to infectious diseases (see the box "Infectious Disease: A Challenge for Older Adults").

Stages of Infection

When a pathogenic agent assaults a new host, a reasonably predictable sequence of events begins. That is, the disease moves through five distinctive stages.[1] You may be able to recognize these stages of infection each time you catch a cold.

1. *The incubation stage.* This stage lasts from the time a pathogen enters the body until it multiplies enough to produce signs and symptoms of the disease. The duration of this stage can vary from a few hours to many months, depending on the virulence of the organisms, the concentration of organisms, the host's level of immune responsiveness, and other health problems. This stage has been called a *silent stage.* The pathogen can be transmitted to a new host during this stage, but this is not likely. A host may be infected during this stage but not be infectious. HIV infection is an exception to this rule.

2. *The prodromal stage.* After the incubation stage, the host may experience a variety of general signs and symptoms, including watery eyes, runny nose, slight fever, and overall tiredness for a brief time. These symptoms are nonspecific and may not be severe enough to force the host to rest. During this stage the pathogenic agent continues to multiply. Now the host is capable of transferring pathogens to a new host, but this is not yet the most infectious stage of an infectious disease. One should practice self-imposed isolation during this stage to protect others. Again, HIV infection is different in this stage.

3. *The clinical stage.* This stage, also called the *acme* or *acute stage,* is often the most unpleasant stage for the host. At this time the disease reaches its highest point of development. Laboratory tests can identify or analyze all of the clinical (observable) signs and symptoms of the particular disease. The likelihood of transmitting the disease to others is highest during this peak stage; all of our available defense mechanisms are in the process of resisting further damage from the pathogen.

4. *The decline stage.* The first signs of recovery appear during this stage. The infection is ending or, in

Learning from Our Diversity

Infectious Disease: A Challenge for Older Adults

It's not always easy for young adults in excellent health to recover quickly and completely from some infectious diseases. Later in life the recovery often becomes much more difficult and in some cases impossible. For a variety of reasons older adults do not respond to infectious conditions with the same resiliency as they once did.

Central to this issue is the gradual degradation of the immune system over time. For reasons not fully understood, the immune system loses both its ability to recognize the presence of pathogens that have entered the body and its ability to mount an effective response against them. Particularly important in this regard are the decreased prevalence of active immune system cells and the inability of existing immune cells to respond effectively. Whether this reduced level of immune protection is a "programmed" aspect of aging (all human life does end at some point in time) or whether it reflects a process that is preventable (perhaps through lifestyle modifications) remains hotly debated. Perhaps no group of older adults is at greater risk because of a compromised immune system than are those with AIDS. The nearly 80,000 persons over age 50 with this immune-system-destroying disease have a decreased ability to resist all infectious conditions, even when their HIV levels are suppressed through drug therapy.

In addition to the normal aging of their immune systems, older adults are generally afflicted with a variety of chronic conditions. The presence of multiple chronic illnesses (known as comorbidity) places the body under great stress, which also undermines the immune system. The combined effects of these conditions result in damage to different organ systems of the body—most importantly, the cardiovascular system, the respiratory system, and the renal system. Any time these systems are compromised by the effects of illness, either chronic or acute, the body becomes particularly vulnerable to infectious agents that routinely exist in our environment.

Compounding this situation is the inability of many older adults to understand the potential seriousness of infections at this stage of their lives. They may even have a false sense of confidence that their bodies are just as "good" at warding off infections as they once were. In addition, a lack of social support, isolation from health care facilities, and the inability to afford expensive prescription medication together make important medical care less available at a time when it could be effective.

When these factors are combined, as they are for many older adults, serious and even fatal infectious conditions become a reality. Therefore, anyone who is responsible for the health and well-being of older persons needs to understand their susceptibility to infectious conditions and recognize the fact that timely and competent care is of critical importance.

---

some cases, falling to a subclinical level. People may suffer a relapse if they overextend themselves.

5. *The recovery stage.* Also called the *convalescence stage,* this stage is characterized by apparent recovery from the invading agent. The disease can be transmitted during this stage, but this is not probable. Until the host's overall health has been strengthened, he or she may be especially susceptible to another (perhaps different) disease pathogen. Fortunately, after the recovery stage, further susceptibility to the pathogenic agent is typically lower because the body has built up immunity. This buildup of immunity is not always permanent; for example, many sexually transmitted diseases can be contracted repeatedly.

We will discuss HIV/AIDS later in the chapter; for now, however, we need to note that this critically important pandemic infectious disease does not easily fit into the five-step model of infectious diseases just presented. In individuals infected with HIV there is an initial asymptomatic *incubation stage,* followed by a *prodromal stage* characterized by generalized signs of immune system inadequacy. However, once the level of specific protective cells of the immune system declines to the point that the body cannot be protected from opportunistic diseases, and the label AIDS is assigned, the five-stage model becomes less easily applied.

Body Defenses: Mechanical and Cellular-Chemical Immune Systems

Much as a series of defensive alignments protect a military installation, so too is the body protected by sets of defenses. These defenses can be classified as either mechanical or cellular-chemical (Figure 13-2). Mechanical defenses are first-line defenses, because they physically separate the internal body from the external environment. Examples include the skin, the mucous membranes of the respiratory and gastrointestinal tracts, earwax, the hairs and cilia that filter incoming air, and even tears. These defenses serve primarily as a shield against foreign materials that may contain pathogenic agents. These defenses can, however, be disarmed, such as when tobacco smoke kills the cilia that protect the airway, resulting in chronic bronchitis, or when contact lenses reduce tearing, leading to irritation and eye infection.

The second component of the body's protective defenses is the cellular-chemical system or, more commonly, the **immune system.** The immune system is far

> **Key Terms**
>
> **immune system** The system of cellular and chemical elements that protects the body from pathogens, abnormal cells, and foreign protein.

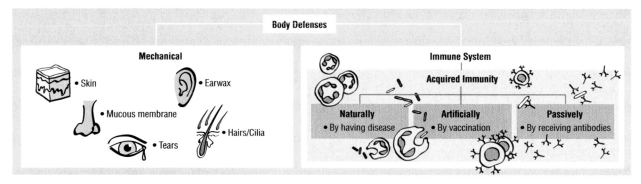

Figure 13-2 Body Defenses against Invading Organisms Mechanical defenses are the first line of protection, since they separate the internal body from the external environment. The immune system defenses include chemicals and specialized cells that provide protection from a vast array of antigens.

more specific than the mechanical defenses. Its primary mission is to eliminate microorganisms, foreign protein, and abnormal cells from the body. A wellness-oriented lifestyle, including sound nutrition, effective stress management, and regular exercise, supports this important division of the immune system. The microorganisms, foreign proteins, or abnormal cells that activate this cellular component are collectively called *antigens*.[2]

Divisions of the Immune System

Closer examination of the immune system, or cellular-chemical defenses, reveals two separate but highly cooperative groups of cells. One group of cells originates in the fetal thymus gland and has become known as *T cell–mediated immunity*, or simply **cell-mediated immunity.** The second group of cells that makes up cellular immunity are the B cells (bursa of Fabricius), which are the working units of **humoral immunity.** [3] Cellular elements of both cell-mediated and humoral immunity are found within the bloodstream, the lymphatic tissues of the body (including that within the gastrointestinal system), and the fluid that surrounds body cells.

Although we are born with the structural elements of both cell-mediated and humoral immunity, developing an immune response requires that components of these cellular systems encounter and successfully defend against specific antigens. When the immune system has done this once, it is, in most cases, primed to respond quickly and effectively if the same antigens appear again. This confrontation produces a state of **acquired immunity (AI).** [1] Acquired immunity develops in different ways, as shown in Figure 13-2.

- **Naturally acquired immunity (NAI)** develops when the body is exposed to infectious agents. Thus when we catch an infectious disease, we fight the infection and in the process become immune (protected) from developing that illness if we encounter these agents

again. For example, when a child catches chicken pox and recovers, it is unlikely that the child will develop a subsequent case of chicken pox. Before the advent of immunizations, this was the only way of developing immunity.

- **Artificially acquired immunity (AAI)** occurs when the body is exposed to weakened or killed infectious agents introduced through vaccination or immunization. As in NAI, the body fights the infectious agents and records the method of fighting the agents. Young children, older adults, and adults in high-risk occupations should consult their physicians about immunizations.

- **Passively acquired immunity (PAI),** a third form of immunity, results when antibodies are introduced into the body. These extrinsic antibodies are for a variety of specific infections, and they are produced outside the body (either in animals or by the genetic manipulation of microorganisms). When introduced into the human body, they provide immediate protection until the body can develop a more natural form of immunity. This form of short-term but immediate protection is provided when the emergency room staff administers a tetanus-toxoid "booster." Note that in PAI no actual pathogenic agents are introduced into the body—only the antibodies against various forms of disease-causing agents.

Regardless of how infectious agents are acquired, either through naturally acquired immunity (NAI) or through artificially acquired immunity (AAI), the result is an "arming" of the body's own immune system. This process is frequently labeled as *active immunity*. This contrasts to passively acquired immunity (PAI) in which the body "borrows" another's immune elements without actual involvement of the body's own immune system. The latter case is called *passive immunity*.[4]

In addition to the forms of immunity just described, unborn infants are also provided with a period of

Figure 13-3 The Immune Response Cellular and chemical elements act together to destroy pathogens and guard against repeat infections.

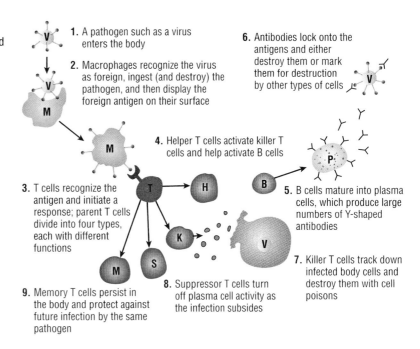

1. A pathogen such as a virus enters the body

2. Macrophages recognize the virus as foreign, ingest (and destroy) the pathogen, and then display the foreign antigen on their surface

3. T cells recognize the antigen and initiate a response; parent T cells divide into four types, each with different functions

4. Helper T cells activate killer T cells and help activate B cells

5. B cells mature into plasma cells, which produce large numbers of Y-shaped antibodies

6. Antibodies lock onto the antigens and either destroy them or mark them for destruction by other types of cells

7. Killer T cells track down infected body cells and destroy them with cell poisons

8. Suppressor T cells turn off plasma cell activity as the infection subsides

9. Memory T cells persist in the body and protect against future infection by the same pathogen

short-term immunity via the biological mother's immune system elements crossing the placental barrier (see Chapter 17) and then following birth via breast milk. This *maternal immunity,* however, gradually deteriorates but is concurrently being replaced by the child's own increasingly functional immune system.

Collectively, these forms of immunity can provide important protection against infectious disease.

The Immune Response

Fully understanding the function of the immune system requires a substantial understanding of human biology and is beyond the scope of this text. Figure 13-3 presents a simplified view of the immune response.

When antigens (whether microorganisms, foreign protein, or abnormal cells) are discovered within the body, various types of white blood cells confront and destroy some of these antigens. Principal among these blood cells are the *macrophages* (very large white blood cells) that begin ingesting antigens as they are encountered. In conjunction with this "eating" of antigens, macrophages display segments of the antigen's unique protein coat on their outer surface. Now in the form of macrophage/antigen complexes, macrophages transport their captured antigen identifiers to awaiting T cells, whose recognition of the antigen will initiate the full cell-mediated immune response. This involves the specialization of "basic" T cells into four forms: helper T cells, killer T cells, suppressor T cells, and memory T cells.

Once helper T cells have been derived from "parent" T cells by the presence of the macrophage/antigen complex, they notify a second component of cellular immunity, the killer T cells. Killer T cells produce powerful chemical messengers that activate specific white blood cells that destroy antigens through the production of caustic chemicals called cytotoxins, or "cell poisons." In addition to the helper T cells' activation of killer T cells, helper T cells also play a critical role in the activation of B cells, principal players in the expression of humoral immunity.

Key Terms

cell-mediated immunity Also called *T cell–mediated immunity;* is principally provided by the immune system's T cells, both working alone and in combination with highly specialized B cells.

humoral immunity Also called *B cell–mediated immunity;* is responsible for the production of critically important immune system elements known as *antibodies.*

acquired immunity (AI) A form of immunity resulting from exposure to foreign protein (most often wild, weakened, or killed pathogenic organisms).

naturally acquired immunity (NAI) A type of acquired immunity resulting from the body's response to naturally occurring pathogens.

artificially acquired immunity (AAI) A type of acquired immunity resulting from the body's response to pathogens introduced into the body through immunizations.

passively acquired immunity (PAI) Temporary immunity achieved by providing extrinsic antibodies to a person exposed to a particular pathogen.

Activation of the humoral immunity component of the overall immune response involves the helper T cells' ability to construct a working relationship among themselves, the macrophage/antigen complexes (mentioned earlier), and the small B cells. Once these three elements have been constituted into working units, the B cells are transformed into *plasma cells.* Plasma cells then utilize the information about the antigen's identity to produce massive numbers of **antibodies.** On release from the plasma cells, these antibodies then circulate throughout the body and capture free antigens in the form of *antigen/antibody complexes.*[4] The "captured" antigens are now highly susceptible to a variety of white blood cells that ingest or chemically destroy these infectious agents.

To assure that the response to the presence of the antigen can be appropriately controlled, a third group of T cells, the suppressor T cells, have been formed by the activation of parent T cells. These suppressor T cells monitor the outcome of the humoral response (antibody formation) and, when comfortable with the number of antibodies produced, turn off further plasma cell activity. The fourth group of specialized T cells, the memory T cells, record this game plan for fighting the antigen invasion so that any subsequent similar invasion will be quickly fought.

An additional group of cells that operates independently from the T cell/B cell interplay just described are the *natural killer (NK) cells.* These immune cells continuously patrol the blood and intracellular fluids looking for abnormal cells, including cancer cells and viral-infected cells. When these are found, the NK cells attack them with destructive cytotoxins in a process called *lysing.*[4] (Can you think of a popular household sanitizing product that uses a version of *lysing* in its brand name?)

Clearly, without a normal immune system employing both cellular and humoral elements, we would quickly fall victim to serious and life-shortening infections and malignancies. As you will see later, this is exactly what occurs in many people infected with HIV.

Emerging medical technology holds promise for repairing damaged immune systems. Perhaps in the not too distant future, *adult stem cells* can be harvested from other areas of the body of a person whose immune system has been compromised, or from the body of a carefully matched donor, and used to return a damaged immune system to a normal level of functioning. A second form of immune system repair involves harvesting *cord blood (stem) cells* taken from the umbilical cord blood collected and "banked" at birth.[5] After careful matching, these cells can be transplanted into a recipient in anticipation that they will specialize into the cell type needed by the damaged or diseased immune system. The virtual absence of any specialization in stem cells at the time of harvesting provides an opportunity for the highly generic stem cells to develop into immune system cells once transplanted into the recipient's body. Perhaps the most interesting use of this technology first occurred in October 2000, when a young cancer victim's immune system was restarted via a stem cell transplant obtained from the cord blood of her newborn brother, who was conceived for the purpose of being a stem cell donor. It should be noted, however, that this was a highly unusual procedure. Considerable controversy now surrounds the use of stem cells obtained from embryonic or fetal tissue sources. Even though these are considered to be the "best" stem cells, restrictions by the federal government (and several states) on their collection and use have forced clinicians to use stem cells from the sources mentioned earlier, as well as from cadavers. This situation could change, however, with the new alignment of the Congress following the midterm elections of 2006.

Immunizations

Although the incidence of several childhood communicable diseases is at or near the lowest level ever, we are risking a resurgence of diseases such as measles, polio, diphtheria, and rubella. The possible increase in childhood infectious illnesses is based on the disturbing finding that only 81 percent of American preschoolers are adequately immunized, which is principally due to the failure of many parents to complete their children's immunization programs. Today health professionals are attempting to raise the level of immunization to 90 percent of all children under the age of 2 years.

Vaccinations against several potentially serious infectious conditions are available and should be given. These include the following:

- *Diphtheria.* A potentially fatal illness that leads to inflammation of the membranes that line the throat, to swollen lymph nodes, and to heart and kidney failure
- *Whooping cough.* A bacterial infection of the airways and lungs that results in deep, noisy breathing and coughing
- *Hepatitis B.* A viral infection that can be transmitted sexually or through the exchange of blood or bodily fluids; seriously damages the liver
- *Hepatitis A.* A viral infection contracted from fecal contamination of food or water

---

Key Terms

antibodies Chemical compounds produced by the body's immune system to destroy antigens and their toxins.

- *Haemophilus influenzae type B.* A bacterial infection that can damage the heart and brain, resulting in meningitis, and can produce profound hearing loss
- *Tetanus.* A fatal infection that damages the central nervous system; caused by bacteria found in the soil
- *Rubella (German measles).* A viral infection of the upper respiratory tract that can cause damage to a developing fetus when the mother contracts the infection during the first trimester of pregnancy
- *Measles (red measles).* A highly contagious viral infection leading to a rash, high fever, and upper respiratory tract symptoms
- *Polio.* A viral infection capable of causing paralysis of the large muscles of the extremities
- *Mumps.* A viral infection of the salivary glands
- *Chicken pox.* A varicella zoster virus spread by airborne droplets, leading to a sore throat, rash, and fluid-filled blisters
- *Meningococcus.* A viral infection of the membranes covering the brain; symptoms are flulike
- *Pneumococcal infection.* A bacterium capable of causing infections, including pneumonia, heart, kidney, and middle ear infections
- *Childhood diarrhea.* Caused by a rotavirus, this form of diarrhea is responsible for 55,000 to 70,000 hospitalizations, and 20 to 60 deaths, annually of infants and young children
- *Human papillomavirus infections.* Sexually transmitted viruses, some forms of which are directly related to the development of cervical cancers. Vaccinations are approved for use with females 9 to 26 years of age
- *Shingles.* Varicella zoster virus exacerbation resulting in painful episodes of inflammation of sensory nerve endings. Vaccinations are approved for use with adults beginning at 60 years of age, particularly for those who had chickenpox during childhood

Parents of newborns should take their infants to their family-care physicians, pediatricians, or well-baby clinics operated by county health departments to begin the immunization process. The Children's Immunization Schedule shown on the Online Learning Center is recommended by the American Academy of Pediatrics, the American Academy of Family Physicians, and the Centers for Disease Control and Prevention. As children quickly discover, and parents already know, most of today's immunizations are administered by injection. To improve compliance with the immunization schedule (some parents have a fear of "shots" resulting from early childhood experiences and thus avoid completing the schedule), researchers are attempting to develop a single immunization that would combine many individual vaccines. In addition, research is being conducted on new delivery systems, including a skin patch, nasal spray, and vaccine-enriched foods, such as potatoes.

In recent years concern has arisen regarding the role of childhood immunizations in the development of other serious childhood physical and emotional health problems, such as type 1 diabetes mellitus, asthma, autism, and sudden infant death syndrome (SIDS). At this time studies investigating the possible relationship between recommended immunizations and the conditions mentioned previously have found no demonstrable cause-and-effect relationships. Persons interested in more in-depth information regarding adverse affects and contraindications associated with immunizations, the Vaccine Adverse Events Reporting System (VAERS), administered by the Food and Drug Administration (FDA) and the CDC, is in the public domain. Like other reporting systems, the VAERS has limitations; however, information from a wide array of research studies can be readily obtained through the system.[6]

Although immunization is universally viewed as important for infants and children, adults have immunization needs that can be unmet. Accordingly, the CDC's National Immunization Program now provides an immunization schedule for adults. Figure 13-4 lists the immunizations that should be updated or initially received by adults. Adults are particularly underprotected in regard to diphtheria and tetanus.

 TALKING POINTS Through community service work, you meet a couple who say that they have not had their children immunized and don't see the reason for doing so. How would you explain the importance of having this done?

Causes and Management of Selected Infectious Diseases

This section focuses on some of the common infectious diseases and some diseases that are less common but serious. You can use this information as a basis for judging your own disease susceptibility.

Nosocomial Infections

Although the classroom, residence hall, home, worksite, and virtually any place where people gather in large numbers and in close proximity would seem "ideal" places to contract an infectious disease, a better place might come as a surprise—any place where nosocomial infectious agents call "home." Nosocomial infections are infections spread in conjunction with the delivery of health care services—most often from providers to patients or from patients to other patients. Persons who are

Fighting the Common Cold

Everyone, at one time or another, thinks about how to prevent a cold or how to recover from one. For many people the use of herbal or homeopathic products seems worthy of consideration. Four such products are routinely suggested as being effective in the prevention and/or recovery from colds (and in some cases the flu).

Echinacea, a dietary supplement derived from the roots of the purple coneflower (*Echinacea purpurea*), is purported to be effective in strengthening the immune system and in so doing reducing the number of colds typically contracted during the course of a year. However, in an article appearing in the *New England Journal of Medicine* (July 2005), researchers at the University of Virginia reported that echinacea was ineffective in the prevention of colds.

Elderberry, in extract form, represents a second herbal product whose ability to prevent the development of colds and influenza has been reported. Additionally, elderberry extract has been reported to be effective in reducing the duration of flu-related symptoms from the usual six days to as few as two days. Mild gastrointestinal complications have also been reported in conjunction with elderberry extract use if taken without food in the stomach.

Goldenseal, an herbal product, is generally taken in combination with echinacea. It is believed that goldenseal has some antibacterial

efficacy, as well as the ability to stimulate the production of mucus within the respiratory track. To date no antiviral capabilities have been demonstrated with goldenseal, so a direct influence on cold and flu agents seems unlikely. Herbalists suggest that goldenseal detoxifies the body in some fashion.

Oscillococcinum, a nonherbal homeopathic flu medication popular in Europe, contains small quantities of duck liver (see the discussion of homeopathic medication in Chapter 18). Underlying the purported effectiveness of oscillococcinum is its vaccinelike protection resulting from a heightened immune system response to the minuscule amount of flu virus contained in the infected duck liver.

Remember that neither dietary supplements nor homeopathic medications must undergo the rigorous clinical trials required by the FDA for prescription medications. Nor do they need to meet the standards for safety and effectiveness required by the FDA for OTC products. Anecdotal information and studies conducted in other countries are the primary basis for the claims made for these products.

---

shortness of breath, coughing up rust-colored mucus, or persistent sore throat or hoarseness, you should contact a physician. Because we now consider colds to be transmitted most readily by hand contact, you should wash your hands frequently (see the box "How to Wash Your Hands").

Two factors seem predictable in terms of "preventing" colds. The first involves the less than average number of colds seen in children between 6 and 11 years of age who had attended larger preschool programs (more than six other children).[7] The second factor involved a lower than average number of colds in adults who exercised at vigorous levels of intensity.[8] A third factor, the use of large doses of vitamin C supplements to prevent colds or shorten their duration, is far less predictable than long thought. In a 2004 meta-analysis of 29 studies involving 11,077 persons using vitamin C supplementation of 200 mg or more (up to 4 g) daily, upon onset of symptoms, showed no significant benefit over placebo users in regard to criteria for duration and severity.[9]

Influenza

Influenza is also an acute contagious disease caused by viruses. Some influenza outbreaks have killed thousands and even millions of people, such as the influenza pandemics of 1889–1890, 1918–1919, 1957, and 2003–2004.

The viral strains that produce this infectious disease have the potential for more severe complications than the viral strains that produce the common cold. The viral strain for a particular form of influenza enters the body through the respiratory tract. After brief incubation and prodromal stages, the host develops signs and symptoms not just in the upper respiratory tract but throughout the entire body. These symptoms include fever, chills, cough, sore throat, headache, gastrointestinal disturbances, and muscular pain (see Table 13.2).

Antibiotics are generally not prescribed for people with influenza, except when the patient has a possible secondary bacterial infection. Physicians may recommend only aspirin, fluids, and rest. Parents are reminded not to give aspirin to children because of the danger of Reye's syndrome. Reye's syndrome is an aspirin-enhanced complication of influenza in which central nervous system changes can occur, including brain swelling. For a person hoping to avoid the debilitating symptoms of flu, five antiviral vaccines are currently available; two are intended for influenza virus type A and three for both virus types A and B.

Most young adults can cope with the milder strains of influenza that appear each winter or spring. However, pregnant women and older people—especially older people with additional health complications, such as heart disease, kidney disease, emphysema, and chronic bronchitis—are not as capable of handling this viral

The manner in which the hands are washed is as important as frequency is. Because of the preventive role of effective hand washing in the prevention of cold and influenza transmission, the CDC has formulated guidelines for hand washing.

1. Hands transmit infectious agents when they touch the eyes, nose, or mouth.
2. Hands should be washed (with hot water and soap):
   - Before, during, and after you prepare food.
   - Before you eat and after you use the bathroom.
   - After handling animals or animal waste.
   - When your hands are dirty.
   - More frequently when someone in your home is sick.
   - Immediately following a period of frequent hand shaking.
3. Effective hand washing involves the following steps:
   - First wet your hands and apply liquid soap or clean bar soap (place bar soap back on rack, thus allowing bar to dry).
   - Next, rub your hands vigorously together and scrub all hand surfaces.
   - Continue for 10–15 seconds.
   - Rinse well and dry with clean towel.

Source: Centers for Disease Control and Prevention. National Center for Infectious Disease. *Hand Washing: An Ounce of Prevention Keeps the Germs Away.* 2000. www.cdc.gov/ncidod/op/handwashing.htm.

Washing your hands often is the best way to prevent the common cold.

attack. People who regularly come into contact with the general public, such as teachers, should also consider annual flu shots.

Today nearly 100 million Americans receive annual "flu shots." In past years, these annual immunizations, tailored to work against the flu viruses anticipated for the coming flu season, were principally received by adults over 50 years of age and others with special needs. During the flu epidemic of 2003–2004, younger adults moved into the recipient population. The nation's supply of 115 million doses of vaccine for the 2006–2007 flu season proved to be adequate, as, again, thousands of people from within the eligible pool chose not to be immunized. The box "Who Should Get Inactivated Influenza Vaccine" identifies the people who should receive an annual immunization against influenza.

In the near future, the term *flu shot* may be less frequently heard. In June 2003, the FDA approved the sale of Flumist, a nasal spray inhalation delivery system for influenza vaccine. Its use is approved for people ages 2 to 49. Its use is not, at this time, recommended for persons most in need of the highest level of protection.

The flu season generally runs from November through February, with nearly 115,000 persons developing clear symptoms of influenza, and 36,000 dying from its complications.

Avian (Bird) Influenza

As noted earlier in the chapter, countries are interconnected to such an extent that emerging infections can be spread globally in a matter of days, if not hours. Because of this, the probability of future pandemics—including one of *avian (bird) flu*—is nearing certainty. Based on extrapolations from the 1918 influenza pandemic and taking into account improvements in health care, the most conservative estimates of deaths if (some experts confidently say "when") avian flu reaches pandemic levels are 1 billion people ill, with 2 to 7 million deaths. Experts in infectious disease epidemiology have predicted that one-quarter to one-third of the world's population would become ill and 180 million deaths would result. The financial costs would be $1.25 trillion or more.[10] See the box "Recent Timeline of Avian Flu" on page 393.

number of states are requiring that health care providers provide clearly stated information regarding the value of meningococcal meningitis immunization. Some people, however, have questioned the cost-effectiveness of immunizing all entering college students.

Meningococcal meningitis is a bacterial infection of the thin membranous coverings of the brain. In its earliest stages, this disease can easily be confused with the flu. Symptoms usually include a high fever, severe headache, stiff neck, nausea with vomiting, extreme tiredness, and the formation of a progressive rash. For about 10 percent of people who develop this condition, the infection is fatal, often within 24 hours. Therefore the mere presence of the symptoms described above signals the need for immediate medical evaluation. If done promptly, treatment is highly effective.

Lyme Disease

Lyme disease is an infectious disease that has become a significant health problem in eastern, southeastern, upper midwestern, and west coast states, with 19,931 cases in 2006 (23,305 in 2005). The significant increase in the number of cases of Lyme disease since 1992 (when 9,909 cases were reported) most likely reflects widening geographical distribution of the disease, a greater awareness of its symptoms by the general public, and more consistent reporting by physicians. This bacterial disease results when infected blacklegged ticks (also called deer ticks), usually in the nymph (immature) stage, attach to the skin and inject the infectious agent as they feed on a host's blood. The deer ticks become infected by feeding, as larvae, on infected white-footed mice.

The symptoms of Lyme disease vary but typically appear within 30 days as small red bumps surrounded by a circular red rash at the site of bites. The red rash has been described as being like a "bull's eye" in appearance—a pale center surrounded by a reddish margin. However, in some persons this characteristic rash does not appear, thus other symptoms must be recognized so that diagnosis is not delayed. Flulike symptoms, including chills, headaches, muscle and joint aches, and low-grade fever, may accompany this acute phase. A chronic phase develops in about 20 percent of untreated infected persons. This phase may produce disorders of the nervous system,

Key Terms

Lyme disease A bacterial infection transmitted by deer ticks.

toxic shock syndrome (TSS) A potentially fatal condition caused by the proliferation of certain bacteria in the vagina whose toxins enter the general blood circulation.

heart, or joints. Fortunately, Lyme disease can be treated with antibiotics. Unfortunately, however, no immunity develops, so infection can recur. Some physicians order tests and begin antibiotic therapy too quickly. The basis of treatment should be the appearance of clinical symptoms, not simply the reporting of a tick bite. Lyme disease may be more difficult to diagnose in children than in adults.

With much anticipation on the part of the medical community, outdoor enthusiasts, and people living in Lyme-disease-intense areas, an immunization (Lymerix) entered the market in 1998. Although it was effective in approximately 80 percent of recipients, it had side effects similar to the symptoms of Lyme disease. Therefore demand was low, and the vaccine was withdrawn by its manufacturer in 2002. Today, second-generation versions of the Lymerix technology are under development. However, until an effective and safe vaccine is developed, prevention is in the hands of the individual.

People who live in tick-prone areas, including near small urban/suburban wood lots, and participate in outdoor activities can encounter the nearly invisible tick nymphs. These people should check themselves frequently to be sure that they are tick-free. They should tuck shirts into pants, tuck pants into socks, and wear gloves and hat when possible. They should shower after coming inside from outdoors and check clothing for evidence of ticks. Pets, particularly dogs who enjoy outdoor play and then return indoors, can carry infected ticks into the house. If you find ticks, carefully remove them from the skin with tweezers and wash the affected area. There is no vaccine available for humans, so prevention is very important. Repellants containing DEET or permethrin are effective in repelling ticks; they should be used according to directions on the label. A form of "natural" prevention seems to occur in conjunction with frequent noninfected tick exposure in the past, but this should not discourage persons from using preventive measures.

As a final aside on Lyme disease, in July 2006 the FDA issued a news release to inform the public of adverse reactions, including a death, to Lyme disease medication bismacine, or chromacine.[16] This untested and thus unapproved compound contains bismuth, a heavy metal that can seriously damage the cardiovascular and renal systems. Bismacine is compounded as an injection by some local druggists, under the auspices of "alternative" practitioners.

Hantavirus Pulmonary Syndrome

Since 1993 a small but rapidly growing number of people have been dying of extreme pulmonary distress caused by the leakage of plasma into the lungs. In the initial cases, the people lived in the Southwest, had been well until they began developing flulike symptoms over one or two days, then quickly experienced difficulty breathing, and died only hours later. Epidemiologists quickly suspected a viral agent such as the *hantavirus,* known to exist in Asia and, to a lesser degree, in Europe. Exhaustive laboratory work led to the culturing of the virus and confirmed that all of these patients had been infected with an American version of the hantavirus. Researchers identified this latest infectious condition as *hantavirus pulmonary syndrome.*

Today hantavirus pulmonary syndrome has been reported in areas beyond the Southwest, including most of the western states and some of the eastern states. The common denominator in all these areas is the presence of deer mice. It is now known that this common rodent serves as the reservoir for the virus. In fact, so common is the mouse that in 2000 the National Park Service began warning hikers, campers, and off-road bikers that hantavirus probably existed in every national park and that caution should be taken to avoid high-risk sites. As recently as 2006, 9 new cases were reported in 5 southwestern states, resulting in 5 deaths.[17]

The virus moves from deer mice to humans when people inhale dust contaminated with dried virus-rich rodent urine or saliva-contaminated materials, such as nests. If you must remove rodent nests from a house, born, or shed, wear rubber gloves, pour a disinfectant or bleach on the nests and soak them thoroughly, and finally, pick up the nests with a shovel and burn them or bury them in holes that are several feet deep. This said, prevention is a better alternative to removing nests and can be accomplished by sealing up holes in structures, trapping and disposing of deer mice in an effective manner, and cleaning up sources of food that would otherwise attract mice.

Because there is no vaccine for hantavirus pulmonary syndrome, people who likely have been exposed to the infected excrement of deer mice should seek early evaluation of flulike symptoms.

West Nile Virus

First detected in New York City in 1999, *West Nile virus* was, by the summer of 2000, identified in 6 eastern states. By the end of 2002, the West Nile virus had spread westward to include 34 states. By the end of 2003, the West Nile virus had been found in all but 2 of the 48 contiguous U.S. states. By the end of 2006, the most recent year for which data are available, the virus had been identified in all of the contiguous states, with human cases reported in all but 5 states.[18] During 2006, 4,219 persons were infected, 1,433 developed symptoms of neurological involvement (the most problematic form of infection), and 161 died.[19]

This vector-borne infectious virus is transmitted from a reservoir, most often birds, by mosquitoes that in turn infect humans.[1] Human-to-human transmission (via mosquitoes) apparently does not occur, although the

West Nile virus is transmitted to humans via the bite of a mosquito.

CDC has reported at least four cases of virus transmission in conjunction with infected transplanted tissue.[20] West Nile virus infection involves flulike symptoms, including fever, headache, muscle ache, fatigue, and joint pain. In young children, persons with immune systems weakened by HIV, and older adults, West Nile virus infection may involve encephalitis, a potentially fatal inflammation of the brain. Physicians recommend that any unusual neurological symptoms be considered as a possible West Nile infection. The West Nile virus deaths that have occurred since the infection's initial appearance in 1999 have been the result of encephalitis.

In an attempt to determine the extent of the West Nile virus range, public health officials throughout the United States have tested mosquitoes, sentinel chickens, crows, other birds, cows, and other animals, including humans. Additionally, mosquito habitats are being treated in an attempt to reduce the vector population. Public service announcements focusing on protection against mosquito bites are routinely made in high-risk areas. Additionally, a newly developed immunization that protects birds is being field tested; a horse vaccine is available.

Additional aspects of the disease have been reported to the CDC, including the presence of the virus in blood transfusions. (Today, clinically recovered patients cannot give blood for 60 days following release from the hospital.) The West Nile virus has also been isolated from breast milk, and cases of prenatal transmission have been confirmed. Also, a new test to accurately screen for infected blood has been developed, as has a new diagnostic test that significantly reduces the time needed to obtain confirmation of the West Nile virus.

Tampon-Related Toxic Shock Syndrome

Toxic shock syndrome (TSS) made front-page headlines in 1980, when the CDC reported a connection

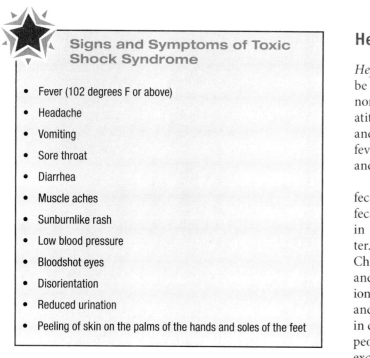

Signs and Symptoms of Toxic Shock Syndrome

- Fever (102 degrees F or above)
- Headache
- Vomiting
- Sore throat
- Diarrhea
- Muscle aches
- Sunburnlike rash
- Low blood pressure
- Bloodshot eyes
- Disorientation
- Reduced urination
- Peeling of skin on the palms of the hands and soles of the feet

between TSS and the presence of a specific bacterial agent (*Staphylococcus aureus*) in the vagina associated with the use of tampons.

Superabsorbent tampons can irritate the vaginal lining three times more quickly than regular tampons do. This vaginal irritation is aggravated when the tampon remains in the vagina for a long time (more than five hours). When this irritation begins, the staphylococcal bacteria (which are usually present in the vagina) have relatively easy access to the bloodstream. When these bacteria proliferate in the circulatory system, their resultant toxins produce a massive T cell response (see pages 384–386). These immune system products exacerbate the effects of the bacterial toxin on body tissues; see the box "Signs and Symptoms of Toxic Shock Syndrome." A woman with TSS can die, usually as a result of cardiovascular failure, if left untreated. Fortunately, less than 10 percent of women diagnosed as having TSS die.

To minimize the risk of TSS, all premenopausal women, particularly those new to use of tampons, should consider these recommendations for safe tampon use: (1) tampons should not be the sole form of sanitary protection used, and (2) tampons should not remain in place for too long. Women should change tampons every few hours and intermittently use sanitary napkins. Tampons should not be used during sleep. Some physicians recommend that tampons not be used at all if a woman wants to be extraordinarily safe from TSS.

 TALKING POINTS As a parent you are preparing yourself to discuss menstruation with your rapidly maturing daughter. What would you say regarding the safe use of tampons?

Hepatitis

Hepatitis is an inflammatory process in the liver that can be caused by several viruses. Types A, B, C (once called non-A and non-B), D, and E have been recognized. Hepatitis can also be caused indirectly from abuse of alcohol and other drugs. General symptoms of hepatitis include fever, nausea, loss of appetite, abdominal pain, fatigue, and jaundice (yellowing of the skin and eyes).[1]

Type A hepatitis is often associated with consuming fecal-contaminated food, such as raw shellfish raised in fecal-contaminated water, raw vegetables field-washed in contaminated water, or contaminated drinking water. As an example, in November 2003, 520 patrons of a Chi-Chi's Mexican restaurant near Pittsburgh became ill and 3 died as a result of eating contaminated green onions. Poor sanitation, particularly in the handling of food and diaper-changing activities, has produced outbreaks in child care centers. Experts estimate that up to 200,000 people per year experience this infection. This number far exceeds the reported 26,000 to 27,000 cases per year, suggesting that a very large reservoir exists among children who are routinely asymptomatic before 6 years of age. In 2005 it was recommended that all children between 1 and 2 years of age be immunized against hepatitis A. Today that recommendation is in place, with the first immunization given at 12 months and the second by 18 months of age. Persons who contract hepatitis A generally develop acquired immunity, thus preventing a recurrence.[21]

Type B hepatitis (HBV) is spread in various ways, including sexual contact, intravenous drug use, tattooing, body piercing, and even sharing electric razors. On the basis of these modes of transmission, college students should be aware of their potential risk for HBV infection. Beyond the risk factors just identified, medical and dental procedures are also a potential means of transmitting the virus, including patient to practitioner, and practitioner to patient transmission. Chronic HBV infection has been associated with liver cirrhosis and is the principal cause of liver cancer. An effective immunization for hepatitis B is now available; thus, the incidence of HBV in children and adolescents has dropped by one-fifth since 1999. However, an increase has been noted in people over 19 years of age. Although it is given during childhood, it should be seriously considered for older unvaccinated people and college students. In 2002 the American Academy of Pediatrics recommended that all newborns be immunized before leaving the hospital. Adults should seriously consider being immunized against hepatitis B, particularly if they are likely to have multiple sex partners, have sex partners from high-risk groups, or are a caregiver to an infected person. For those who are infected, six medications are now available for use in treating hepatitis B.

Hepatitis C is contracted in ways similar to hepatitis B (sexual contact, tainted blood, in association with

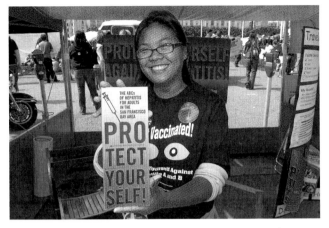

Effective vaccines are available for both hepatitis A and hepatitis B.

tattooing and piercings, and shared needles). In the absence of immunization, the pool of infected people is in excess of 4.1 million, and the death rate is expected to climb. Currently a dual-drug therapy for HCV involving multiple forms of interferon in combination with the drug ribavirin is the treatment of choice. Many infected persons remain asymptomatic for decades, and many persons infected with HCV recover from this liver-threatening infection. People in the latter group appear to have a genetically based ability to stimulate a high level of natural killer cells (NK cells) within the immune system.[22] In a recent study, a two-drug combination treatment resulted in a virus-free state for nearly 60 percent of a large group of infected persons treated for 1 year. In spite of encouraging news such as this, recovery from HCV infection seems less likely the case for infected African Americans, a phenomenon that cannot currently be explained.

The newly identified type D (delta) hepatitis is very difficult to treat and is found almost exclusively in people already suffering from type B hepatitis, since the hepatitis D virus requires the presence of the hepatitis B virus in order to gain full pathogenicity. This virus, like type B hepatitis and HIV, makes unprotected sexual contact, including anal and oral sex, very risky. Hepatitis E, associated with water contamination, is rarely seen in this country other than in people returning from hepatitis E virus–endemic areas of the world.

AIDS

AIDS (acquired immunodeficiency syndrome) has become the most devastating infectious disease in recent history and it is virtually certain to be among the most devastating diseases in history unless a cure is forthcoming. Setting aside for the present the international scope of the HIV/AIDS epidemic, statistics for the United States alone paint a distressing picture. On the basis of data reported through December 2005, a total of 984,155 Americans have been diagnosed with AIDS, and 550,394 have died from its effects (or 55.9 percent of all cases).[23] Table 13.3 shows the estimated number of persons living with HIV/AIDS at the end of 2005, by race/ethnicity, sex, and transmission category in 33 confidential name-based reporting areas. Note that for adolescents and adults, male-to-male homosexual contact, female heterosexual contact, and male injection drug use are the leading means of transmission. When HIV/AIDS data are viewed in terms of race and ethnicity, it will be noticed that there is a disproportionate distribution of cases for African Americans and Latinos, in comparison to other groups. Based on the decadal census of 2000, Whites compose 69.1 percent of the American population but were 33.8 percent of the U.S. persons living with HIV/AIDS at the end of 2005. Latinos constitute 12.5 percent of the U.S. population but 17.1 percent of the HIV/AIDS cases, while African Americans constitute 12.1 percent of the population but 47.3 percent of the HIV/AIDS cases. As reported for 2005, Asian Americans, at 3.7 percent of the population, have only 0.6 percent of the cases, while Native Americans and Alaska Natives compose 0.7 percent of the population and 0.4 percent of the HIV/AIDS cases.[23, 24] There is no easy explanation for the discrepancies seen in these data.

In addition to the human tragedy suggested by these statistics, the financial cost of treating the HIV/AIDS epidemic is sizable. Today it is estimated that annual medical care costs (including medications) for an infected individual are approximately $20,000, and that over $13 billion is expended annually by the public and third-party funding sources. Although these costs appear to be falling gradually owing to the effectiveness of newer medications, the buying power of AIDS advocacy groups, the movement of older medications into generic status, and efforts on the part of the pharmaceutical industry to lower costs, the financial burden that AIDS places on the health care system makes the disease demanding for all Americans.

Cause of AIDS   AIDS is the disease caused by HIV, a virus that attacks the helper T cells of the immune system (see pages 385–386). When HIV attacks helper T cells, people lose the ability to fight off a variety of infections that would normally be easily controlled. Because these infections develop while people are vulnerable, they are collectively called *opportunistic infections.* HIV-infected (HIV-positive) patients become increasingly vulnerable to infection by bacteria, protozoa, fungi, and several viruses. A variety of malignancies also develop during this period of immune-system vulnerability.

HIV positive with AIDS was originally diagnosed based on the presence of specific conditions. Among these were *Pneumocystis carinii* pneumonia and Kaposi's sarcoma, a rare but deadly form of skin cancer. Gradually, experts recognized that additional conditions were associated with advancing deterioration of the immune

Figure 13-7 A Human Papillomavirus Infection (Genital Warts)

11, while viral forms 16, 18, 31, 33, and 35 foster changes in other areas (Figure 13-7). Found most commonly on the penis, scrotum, labia, cervix, and around the anus, these lesions represent the most common symptomatic viral STD in this country. Although most genital wart colonies are small, they may become very large and block the anus or birth canal during pregnancy.

Treatment for HPV, including genital warts, may include patient-applied gels or creams or physician-administered cryotherapy, topical medication, or surgery. Regardless of treatment, however, the viral colonies will probably return. One should use condoms to attempt to prevent transmission of HPV.

As noted in Chapter 11, in conjunction with cervical cancer, a vaccine effective for HPV 6 and 11 (genital warts) and 16 and 18 (cervical cancer) has been approved for use by the FDA. The current recommendation calling for the inoculation of young women between the ages 9 to 26 years, and older if just beginning sexual activity, is being strongly encouraged by the health care community. In states that are considering mandatory inoculation as a part of required school-based immunizations, controversy abounds. With approximately 7 percent of children sexually active by age 13, and nearly 25 percent by age 15, when is young too young? Some experts suggest that when young women clearly display signs of sexual maturation, including the onset of menstruation, then the inoculation is appropriate. The need for an eventual booster has not yet been determined.

Additional vaccines are under development, some intended for use in newly infected patients, some for long-established infections but before clear changes in the cervical lining cells occur, and others for more advanced cervical cancer. Most of the last two classes of vaccines are for treatment rather than prevention of HPV infections.

Gonorrhea

Another extremely common (339,593 cases reported in 2005) STD, *gonorrhea* is caused by a bacterium (*N. gonorrhoea*).[31] The incidence of gonorrhea rose 18 percent between 1997 and 2001, perhaps, in part, because of decreasing fear of HIV/AIDS brought about by the effectiveness of the protease inhibitors being widely reported at that time. However, since 2001 the reported cases of gonorrhea have declined; however, 2005 marked a slight upturn over 2003 and 2004.[31] In men this bacterial agent can produce a milky-white discharge from the penis, accompanied by painful urination. About 80 percent of men who contract gonorrhea report varying degrees of these symptoms. This figure is approximately reversed for women: only about 20 percent of women are symptomatic and thus report varying degrees of frequent, painful urination, with a slimy yellow-green discharge from the vagina or urethra. Oral sex with an infected partner can produce a gonorrheal infection of the throat (pharyngeal gonorrhea). Gonorrhea can also be transmitted to the rectal areas of both men and women.

An interesting finding relative to gonorrhea in adolescents suggests that the incidence of gonorrhea within the adolescent population correlated closely with the consumption of beer, suggesting that alcohol consumption fosters a higher level of high-risk sexual behavior, including earlier onset of sexual activity, an increased number of partners, and less selectivity in choosing those partners. With heavy consumption of beer on many college campuses, this finding does not bode well for the highly asymptomatic female population.

Physicians diagnose gonorrhea by culturing the bacteria. The only class of drugs recommended by the CDC for treatment of gonorrhea is the cephalosporins. Although prevalent in other areas of the world, drug-resistant strains are not extensive in the United States. However, a clear increase in drug-resistant strains has been reported along the West Coast, in various Pacific areas, such as Hawaii, other Pacific Islands, and Asia. Infected persons who might have contracted the disease while in these areas should report this information to their physicians. An alternative treatment plan for persons with drug-resistant strains of gonorrhea appears in the Online Learning Center. For the latest updates on treatments for gonorrhea, see the CDC website, www.cdc.gov/std.

Testing for gonorrhea is included as a part of prenatal care so that infections in mothers can be treated before they give birth. If the birth canal is infected, newborns can easily contract the infection in the mucous membranes of the eye.

Herpes Simplex

Public health officials think that the sexually transmitted genital herpes virus infection rivals chlamydia as the most prevalent STD. To date about 45 million Americans have been diagnosed, although the asymptomatic (thus undiagnosed) population could increase this figure substantially. *Herpes* is really a family of more than 50 viruses, some of which produce recognized diseases in humans (chicken pox, **shingles,** mononucleosis, and others). One subgroup, called herpes simplex 1 virus (HSV-1), produces an infection called *labial herpes* (oral or lip herpes). Labial herpes produces common fever blisters or cold sores around the lips and oral cavity. Herpes simplex 2 virus (HSV-2) is a different strain that produces similar clumps of blisterlike lesions in the genital region (Figure 13-8). Laypeople call this second type of herpes the STD type, but both types produce identical clinical pictures. About 5 to 30 percent of cases are caused by HSV-1. Oral-genital sexual practices most likely account for this crossover infection.

Herpes appears as a single sore or as a small cluster of blisterlike sores. These sores burn, itch, and (for some) become very painful. The infected person might also report swollen lymph glands, muscular aches and pains, and fever. Some patients feel weak and sleepy when they have blisters. The lesions may last from a few days to a few weeks. Viral shedding lasts a week on average; then the blisters begin scabbing, and new skin is formed. Even when the patient has become asymptomatic, viral transmission is still possible.

Herpes is an interesting virus for several reasons. It can lie dormant for long periods. For reasons not well understood but perhaps related to stress, diet, or overall health, the viral particles can be stimulated to travel along the nerve pathways to the skin and then create an active infection. Thus herpes can be considered a recurrent infection. Fortunately for most people, recurrent infections are less severe than the initial episode and do not last as long. Because herpes may occur at intervals following initial treatment with antivirals, two choices exist. One is to treat each recurrence as it arises (episodic recurrent treatment), and the second is to attempt to suppress recurrence through continuous use of medication (daily suppressive therapy). Additionally, physicians may recommend other medications for relief of various symptoms. Visit the Online Learning Center for more information about treatment. Genital herpes is almost always diagnosed through a clinical examination.

At this time a much anticipated Phase III trial is under way testing new vaccines manufactured by Glaxo-Smith Kline Biologicals. Earlier, but in much smaller

Figure 13-8 A Severe Herpes Infection

trials, it was found that the vaccine was effective in providing protection for about 70 percent of the female subjects but was almost completely ineffective for males. The current trial, still ongoing, involves two versions of the vaccine, one version intended to be a prophylactic (preventive) vaccine and the other a therapeutic (treatment) vaccine.[32] Most likely the vaccine technology will employ genetically altered viruses in which genes controlling replication will have been removed or altered in a manner preventing viral replication.

Currently, the best method of preventing herpes infection is to avoid all direct contact with a person who has an active infection. Do not kiss someone with a fever blister—or let them kiss you (or your children) if they have an active lesion. Do not share drinking glasses or eating utensils. Check your partner's genitals. Do not have intimate sexual contact with someone who displays the blisterlike clusters or rash. Condoms are only marginally helpful and cannot protect against lesions on the female

> **Key Terms**
>
> **shingles** Painful fluid-filled skin eruptions along underlying sensory nerve pathways—caused by reactivation of once-sequestered herpes zoster (chicken pox) virus.

vulva or the lower abdominal area of men. Be careful not to infect yourself by touching a blister and then touching any other part of your body.

Although there is currently no cure for HSV-2, antiviral medication can be effectively employed. Intended as prophylactic medications (to be taken daily), these antiviral medications do reduce the number and duration of viral shedding episodes. Certainly, the sexual partners of persons infected with HSV-2 need to be fully aware and involved in the management of this sexually transmitted infection. The box "Talking with Your Partner about Herpes" provides helpful suggestions in enhancing communication and cooperation among partners.

Newborn babies are especially susceptible to the virus if they come into contact with an active lesion during birth. Newborns have not developed the defense capabilities to resist the invasion. They can quickly develop a systemic (general) infection (neonatal herpes) that is often fatal or local infections that produce permanent brain damage or blindness. Fortunately, most of these problems can be prevented through proper prenatal care. A cesarean delivery can be performed if viral particles might be present at birth, although this is done less often today than in the past.

Syphilis

Like gonorrhea, *syphilis* is caused by a bacterium (*Treponema pallidum*) and is transmitted almost exclusively by sexual intercourse. The incidence of syphilis, a CDC-reportable disease, is far lower than that of gonorrhea. In 1950 a record 217,558 cases of syphilis were reported in this country. The number of cases then fell steadily to fewer than 80,000 cases in 1980. From 1980 through 1990 the incidence climbed, reaching nearly 140,000 cases in 1990. Another decline then began, and in 1993 the number of cases dropped to 101,259. In 2000 the CDC reported that syphilis had fallen to the lowest level (5,972) in 42 years. By 2005, however, reported cases of primary syphilis had risen to 8,724.[33]

Whether the upward trend in the number of reported cases of primary syphilis continues remains to be seen. As has been true for most of the last decades a high percentage of cases have been associated with HIV infections, largely among gay men in several larger cities. (See the box "Syphilis" for more information on this disease.) Observers have noted an alarming increase in infant syphilis in children born to mothers who use drugs and support their habit through sexual activity. For specific information on the antibiotics used in the treatment of syphilis, visit the Online Learning Center.

Pubic Lice

Three types of lice infect humans: the head louse, the body louse, and the pubic louse all feed on the blood of the host. Except for the relatively uncommon body louse, these tiny insects do not carry diseases. They are, however, very annoying.

Pubic lice, also called *crabs*, attach themselves to the base of the pubic hairs, where they live and lay their eggs (nits). These eggs move into a larval stage after one week; after two more weeks, they develop into mature adult crab lice. People usually notice they have a pubic lice infestation when they suffer intense itching in the genital region. Prescription and OTC creams, lotions, and shampoos are usually effective in killing both the lice and their eggs, although some reports suggest that lice are becoming resistant to OTC treatments.

Lice are not transmitted exclusively through sexual contact but also by contact with contaminated bedsheets and clothes. If you develop a pubic lice infestation, you must thoroughly treat yourself, your clothes, your sheets, and your furniture. Listed following are specific steps to be taken to eradicate pubic lice:[34]

- Wash the infested area; towel dry.
- Follow label directions in using lice medications. Dry with clean towel.
- Following application of lice medications, remove nits from hair shaft with fingernails.

Syphilis

Syphilis is a serious disease that, left untreated, can cause death. The chance of contracting syphilis during a single sexual encounter with an infected partner is now about 30 percent. Syphilis takes a well-established course after it is contracted.

Infection

The syphilis bacterium, *Treponema pallidum*, is a spirochete. It is transmitted from an infected person to a new host through intimate contact. Moist, warm tissue, such as that lining the reproductive, urinary, and digestive tracts, offers an ideal environment for the agent.

Incubation

Syphilis incubates without symptoms for 10 to 90 days, followed by the characteristic primary stage of the disease.

Primary Stage

The primary stage of syphilis lasts 1 to 5 weeks. A small, raised, painless sore called a *chancre* forms at this time. This highly infectious lesion is not easily identified in 90 percent of women and 50 percent of men; thus these people generally do not seek treatment. The chancre heals in 4 to 8 weeks.

Secondary Stage

The extremely contagious secondary stage of the disease occurs 6 to 12 weeks after initial infection. The infectious agents are now systemic, so symptoms may include a generalized body rash, a sore throat, or a patchy loss of hair. A blood test (VDRL) will be positive, and treatment can be effectively administered. If untreated, the second stage subsides within 2 to 6 weeks. A pregnant woman can easily transmit syphilis to her fetus during this stage. Congenital syphilis often results in stillbirth or an infant born with a variety of life-threatening complications. Early treatment of infected pregnant women can prevent congenital syphilis.

Latent Stage

After the secondary stage subsides, an extended period of noninfectiousness occurs. The infectious agents remain dormant within the body cells, and the infected person displays few clinical signs during this state.

Late Stage

Syphilis can recur for a third time 15 to 25 years after initial contact. In late-stage syphilis, tissue damage is profound and irreversible. The person suffers damage to the cardiovascular system, central nervous system, eyes, and skin, and death from the effects of the disease is likely.

- Put on clean underwear and clothing after treatment.
- Machine wash all clothing and bedding used by the infected person during the 2–3 days before treatment (use the hot wash cycle for at least 20 minutes).
- Dry-clean clothing that is not washable.
- Inform sexual partners that they are at risk of infestation.
- Do not have sex until treatment is completed.
- Repeat treatment in 7–10 days if lice are still found.

Vaginal Infections

Three common pathogens produce uncomfortable *vaginal infections*. The first is the yeast or fungus pathogen *Candida (Monilia) albicans*, which produces the yeast infection often called *thrush*. These organisms, commonly found in the vagina, seem to multiply rapidly when some unusual stressor (pregnancy, use of birth control pills or antibiotics, diabetes) affects a woman's body. This infection, now called *vulvovaginal candidiasis (VVC)*, is signaled by a white- or cream-colored vaginal discharge that resembles cottage cheese. Vaginal itching and vulvar swelling are also commonly reported. Current treatment is based on the use of one of several prescription and OTC azole drugs. For women who have recurrent VVC, some degree of prophylactic suppression of candidiasis seems possible. As has been recommended for all STDs discussed here, the Online Learning Center provides an extensive listing of recommended and alternative prescription-based medications now used in the treatment of STDs. When OTC medications exist for use in treating sexually transmitted infections, such as those used with vaginal infections, they too are listed.

Men rarely report this monilial infection, although some may report mildly painful urination or a barely noticeable discharge at the urethral opening or beneath the foreskin of the penis.

A second type of sexually transmitted vaginal infection is somewhat less easily described in terms of a clearly defined pathogenic agent. Rather, *bacterial vaginosis (BV)* reflects an imbalance in the normal relationships among all vaginal flora, leading to some bacterial forms gaining a level of pathogenicity sufficient enough to allow the formation of abnormal symptoms. Included among these signs of microbial imbalance are abnormal vaginal discharge, a strong fishlike odor (most often following intercourse), burning during urination, and clinical indicators that can be ascertained by visual inspection by a physician and laboratory test results.[35]

BV has been labeled an STD because it is rarely seen in women who are celibate or who have had a very limited number of sexual partners. Increased risk is associated with having a new sexual partner, having had multiple sexual partners, having used an intrauterine device (IUD), and frequent douching. Directly or indirectly, having BV seems to increase the risk of contracting HIV, contracting other STDs, and developing pelvic inflammatory disease (PID). Bacterial vaginosis is usually treated with antibiotics (see the Online Learning Center). In some cases, the condition resolves itself with changes in sexual practices.

The protozoan *Trichomonas vaginalis,* a third STD-related pathogenic agent, also produces a vaginal infection. This parasite can be transmitted through sexual intercourse or by contact with contaminated (often damp) objects, such as towels, clothing, or toilet seats, that may contain some vaginal discharge. In women, this infection, called *trichomoniasis,* or "trich," produces a foamy, yellow-green, foul-smelling discharge that may be accompanied by itching, swelling, and painful urination. Although topically applied treatments with limited effectiveness for trichomoniasis are available, only one highly effective oral medication is currently on the market. Men infrequently contract trichomoniasis but may harbor the organisms without realizing it. They also should be treated to minimize reinfection of partners.

The vagina is warm, dark, and moist, an ideal breeding environment for a variety of organisms. Unfortunately, some highly promoted commercial products seem to increase the incidence of vaginal infections. Among these are tight panty hose (without cotton panels), which tend to increase the vaginal temperature, and commercial vaginal douches, which can alter the acidic level of the vagina. Both of these products might promote infections. Avoiding public bathrooms when possible is also a good practice. Of course, if you notice any unusual discharge from the vagina, you should report this to your physician.

Cystitis and Urethritis

Cystitis, an infection of the urinary bladder, and urethritis, an infection of the urethra, occasionally can be caused by a sexually transmitted organism. Such infections can also be caused by the organisms that cause vaginitis and organisms found in the intestinal tract. A culture is required to identify the specific pathogen associated with a particular case of cystitis or urethritis. The symptoms are pain when urinating, the need to urinate frequently, a dull aching pain above the pubic bone, and the passing of blood-streaked urine.

Physicians can easily treat cystitis and urethritis with antibiotics when the specific organism has been identified. The drug Monurol, which requires only a single dose, has proved effective. Few complications result from infections that are treated promptly. If cystitis

or urethritis is left untreated, the infectious agent could move upward in the urinary system and infect the ureters and kidneys. These upper-urinary-tract infections are more serious and require more extensive evaluation and aggressive treatment. Therefore one should obtain medical care immediately upon noticing symptoms.

Urinary tract infections in men, not related to the gonorrhea bacterium, are extremely common. Theses cases of nongonococcal urethritis (NGU) are sexually transmitted in predictable ways, with a discharge from the penis and pain on urination being the symptoms that bring men into treatment. Recently it was established that NGU is also transmitted in conjunction with oral sex, when the recipient's penis is exposed to infectious agents from his partner.[36]

A study involving urinary tract infections in mice, whose urinary tract infections are virtually indentical to those in humans, demonstrated that the bacteria involved often avoid complete antibiotic elimination. This occurs when the bacteria clump into pods that are then covered by a "bio-film" produced by the organisms. The film retards further antibody effectiveness, allowing the infection to be re-established when antibiotics have been cleared from the body.

Preventing cystitis and urethritis depends to some degree on the source of the infectious agent. One can generally reduce the incidence of infection by urinating completely (to fully empty the urinary bladder), particularly following intercourse, and by drinking ample fluids to flush the urinary tract. Drinking cranberry juice has been found to reduce urinary tract infections. Prevention of urinary tract infections cannot be disregarded, from both medical and cost perspectives. As noted, untreated cystitis and urethritis can be the basis of serious damage to the kidneys. These two infections combined are the second greatest cause of antibiotic use—which is both costly and increasingly losing effectiveness.

 TALKING POINTS Honesty regarding past sexual experiences is a critical issue in the decision to introduce sexual intimacy into a new relationship. What questions would you feel comfortable being asked by another person, and what questions would you be prepared to ask that person?

Taking Charge of Your Health

- Since microorganisms develop resistance to antibiotics, continue taking all such medications until gone, even when the symptoms of the infection have subsided.
- Check your current immunization status to make sure you are protected against preventable infectious diseases.

- If you are a parent, take your children to receive their recommended immunizations as necessary.
- Because of the possibility of contracting HIV/AIDS and sexually transmitted diseases, incorporate disease prevention into all of your sexual activities.

- Use the Personal Assessment at the end of this chapter to determine your risk of contracting a sexually transmitted disease.
- If you have ever engaged in high-risk sexual behavior, get tested for HIV.

SUMMARY

- A variety of pathogenic agents are responsible for infectious conditions.
- A chain of infection with six potential links characterizes every infectious condition.
- One can acquire immunity for some diseases through both natural and artificial means. Children and adults should be immunized according to a schedule.
- The immune system's response to infection relies on cellular, chemical, and humoral elements.
- Nosocomial infections are infections that develop in conjunction with the delivery of health care services, most often in hospitals and nursing homes.
- The common cold and influenza produce many similar symptoms but differ in their infectious agents, incubation period, prevention, and treatment. Avian (bird) flu may be the basis of the next influenza pandemic.
- Tuberculosis and pneumonia are potentially fatal infections of the respiratory system.

- Bacterial meningitis, a potentially fatal infection of the linings that cover the brain, is of increasing concern on college campuses.
- Hantavirus pulmonary syndrome is caused by a virus carried by ticks; human-to-human transmission has also been reported.
- Hepatitis B (serum hepatitis) is a bloodborne infectious condition that produces serious liver damage. Other varieties are hepatitis A, C, D, and E.
- HIV/AIDS is a widespread, incurable viral disease transmitted through sexual activity, through intravenous drug use, in infected blood products, or across the placenta during pregnancy.
- There are a variety of sexually transmitted conditions, many of which do not produce symptoms in most infected women and many infected men.

REVIEW QUESTIONS

1. Describe the six links in the chain of infection.
2. What are the two principal cellular/chemical components of the immune system, and how do they cooperate to protect the body from infectious agents, foreign protein, and abnormal cells?
3. What is a nosocomial infection, and in what settings are nosocomial infections most likely to develop?
4. How are the common cold and influenza similar? How do they differ in their causative agents, incubation period, prevention, and treatment?
5. Why is bacterial meningitis of greater concern on the college campus than elsewhere?
6. Why is outdoor activity a risk factor for contracting Lyme disease?

7. What role do birds play in the transmission of the West Nile virus? What insect is the vector?
8. How is hepatitis B transmitted, and which occupational group is at greatest risk of contracting this infection? How do forms A, C, D, and E compare with hepatitis B?
9. How is HIV transmitted? How are HIV/AIDS currently treated, and how effective is the treatment? In what areas of the world does the HIV/AIDS epidemic seem virtually unchecked?
10. Why are women more often asymptomatic for STDs than men?

ANSWERS TO THE "WHAT DO YOU KNOW?" QUIZ

1. True   2. False   3. False   4. False   5. False   6. True   7. True

As We Go To Press

Insurance Coverage and Immunization Status

The percentage of American children who have been fully immunized at the appropriate point in time is below that recommended by infectious disease specialists. To reach to the desirable level of 90 percent of children fully protected, nearly 10 percent more children need to receive their immunizations. The identify of these "missing children" may surprise you.

According to recently reported data, the children of fully insured families and those of uninsured families are the most likely to have completed all of their scheduled immunizations. The population segment that is least likely to have been immunized is children of parents who are employed but underinsured. These parents most

likely fall into the demographic group often referred to as the "working poor." They earn too much money to qualify for public assistance, including Medicaid health care coverage of childhood and adult immunizations, but they work in jobs that provide only a bare minimum of health insurance. Congress recently passed legislation to fund more complete health care coverage for these children. However, politics, not the existence of need, resulted in a presidential veto of the SCHIP funding bill intended to extend adequate health care to children of the underinsured.

Personal Assessment—*continued*

Interpretation

5–8	Your risk is well below average
9–13	Your risk is below average
14–17	Your risk is at or near average
18–21	Your risk is moderately high
22+	Your risk is high

TO CARRY THIS FURTHER . . .

Having taken this Personal Assessment, were you surprised at your level of risk? What is the primary reason for this level? How concerned are you and your classmates and friends about contracting an STD?

Source: Centers for Disease Control and Prevention.

part five

Sexuality and Reproduction

Sexuality is an important part of our being. It colors the way we interact with the world around us and affects our goals, relationships, and roles in society.

1. **Physical Dimension**
   Sexuality is closely related to the physical dimension of health. For example, our bodies mature at puberty, we respond to sexual arousal, we make choices about contraception and pregnancy, and we adjust our sexual behavior as we age. Sexual experiences and relationships can be very complex and demanding because they are fueled by energy and time. They are enhanced when the body is well maintained, rested, and relatively free from illness.

2. **Emotional Dimension**
   One of the most stressful aspects of life is sexual intimacy. Feelings about your own sexual behavior can range from exhilaration to ambivalence to depression. Being comfortable with your sexuality comes from being guided by your core values, knowing how to express your sexual feelings openly, being able to set limits when appropriate, and understanding how to communicate effectively with your partner.

3. **Social Dimension**
   Because sexuality often involves interaction with others, the development of social skills in this area is imperative. For many, dating is an excellent arena in which to establish specific social skills. As a relationship becomes more serious, communication skills will grow. These skills are important factors in the process of mate selection and marriage for those who choose this path.

4. **Intellectual Dimension**
   As a relationship matures, opportunities abound for contemplation, analysis, and reflection. You may have to sort through your feelings, examine your values, and use lessons from past experiences as you take part in this process of introspection. You will also draw on your intellectual resources as you learn about reproductive anatomy, fertility, sexual response, contraception, and birth.

5. **Spiritual Dimension**
   As an intimate relationship progresses, you may have to explore your feelings about your sense of morality, the appropriateness of premarital sex, or the value of fidelity in a marriage or other long-term committed relationship. Dating, courtship, and particularly marriage offer opportunities to enhance your spirituality by extending sympathy, support, and love to another person. Some people even find the sexual act itself to be a way of expressing their spirituality.

6. **Occupational Dimension**
   Decisions about reproduction can have a significant effect on your occupational dimension of health. Women who are pregnant may have to work even when they are not feeling well. Then they must decide how much time to take off work after the child is born. They and their partners must also make difficult choices about long-term child care arrangements. The decisions they make will affect their occupational satisfaction and sense of fulfillment.

Exploring the Origins of Sexuality

What Do You Know about the Origins of Sexuality?

◉ A fertilized ovum with the sex chromosomes XX is a biological male. True or False?

◉ One's sexuality is based upon both biological and psychosocial factors. True or False?

◉ Both women and men have seminal vesicles. True or False?

◉ Most women experience very similar menstrual cycles. True or False?

◉ The release of luteinizing hormone (LH) causes ovulation to take place. True or False?

◉ Hormone replacement therapy (HRT) reduces cardiovascular risks. True or False?

◉ PMS tends to occur in women in the days just before menstruation. True or False?

Check your answers at the end of the chapter.

Online Learning Center Resources
www.mhhe.com/payne10e

Visit the Online Learning Center for tools to improve your grade and get the most out of your course—chapter objectives, practice quizzes, key terms flashcards, chapter summaries for your digital audio player, Web activities, self-assessments, and many other study aids.

Early in this new millennium, we have reached a better understanding of both the biological and psychosocial factors that contribute to the complex expression of our sexuality. As a society, we are now inclined to view human behavior in terms of a complex script written on the basis of both biology and conditioning.

Reflecting this understanding is the way in which we use the words *male* and *female* to refer to the biological roots of our sexuality and the words *man* and *woman* to refer to the psychosocial roots of our sexuality. In this chapter, we explore human sexuality as it relates to the dynamic interplay of the biological and psychosocial bases that form our masculinity or femininity.

Biological Bases of Human Sexuality

Within a few seconds after the birth of a baby, someone (a doctor, nurse, or parent) emphatically labels the child: "It's a boy," or "It's a girl." For the parents and society as a whole, the child's biological sexuality is being displayed and identified. Another female or male enters the world.

Genetic Basis

At the moment of conception, a Y-bearing or an X-bearing sperm cell joins with the X-bearing ovum to establish the true basis of biological sexuality.[1] A fertilized ovum with sex chromosomes XX is biologically female, whereas a fertilized ovum bearing the XY sex chromosomes is biologically male. Genetics forms the most basic level of an individual's biological sexuality.

Gonadal Basis

The gonadal basis for biological sexuality refers to the growing embryo's development of *gonads*.[2] Male embryos develop testes about the seventh week after conception, and female embryos develop ovaries about the twelfth week after conception.

Structural Development

The development of male or female reproductive structures is initially determined by the presence or absence of hormones produced by the developing testes—androgens and müllerian inhibiting substance (MIS). With these hormones present, the male embryo starts to develop male reproductive structures (penis, scrotum, vas deferens, seminal vesicles, prostate gland, and Cowper's glands).

Because the female embryo is not exposed to these male hormones, it develops the characteristic female reproductive structures: uterus, fallopian tubes, vagina, labia, and clitoris.

Biological Sexuality and the Childhood Years

The growth and the development of the child in terms of reproductive organs and physiological processes have traditionally been thought to be "latent" during the childhood years. However, a gradual degree of growth occurs in both girls and boys. The reproductive organs, however, undergo faster growth at the onset of puberty and achieve their adult size and capabilities shortly thereafter.

Puberty

The entry into puberty is a gradual maturing process for young girls and boys. For young girls, the onset of menstruation, called *menarche,* occurs at about age 12 or 13 but may come somewhat earlier or later.[3] Early menstrual cycles tend to be anovulatory (ovulation does not occur). Menarche is usually preceded by a growth spurt that includes the budding of breasts and the growth of pubic and underarm hair.[4]

Young males follow a similar pattern of maturation, including a growth spurt followed by a gradual sexual maturity. However, this process takes place about 2 years later than it does in young females. Genital enlargement, underarm and pubic hair growth, and a lowering of the voice commonly occur. The male's first ejaculation is generally experienced by the age of 14, most commonly through **nocturnal emission** or masturbation. For many young boys, fully mature sperm do not develop until about age 15.

Reproductive capability declines only gradually over the course of the adult years. In the woman, however, the onset of **menopause** signals a more direct turning off of the reproductive system than is the case for the male adult. By the early to mid-50s, virtually all women have entered a postmenopausal period, but for men, relatively high-level **spermatogenesis** may continue for a decade or two.[4]

The story of sexual maturation and reproductive maturity cannot, however, be solely focused on the changes that take place in the body. Now we will discuss the psychosocial processes that accompany the biological changes.

 TALKING POINTS Your 12-year-old son comes to you and says that all of his male friends are starting to grow facial hair. He is worried that his own beard will never begin. What could you say to him that could ease his fears?

Psychosocial Bases of Human Sexuality

If you visualized growth and development of sexuality as a ladder (Figure 14-1), one vertical rail of the ladder would represent our biological sexuality. Arising at

> **Key Terms**
>
> **nocturnal emission** Ejaculation that occurs during sleep; "wet dream."
>
> **menopause** Decline and eventual cessation of hormone production by the female reproductive system.
>
> **spermatogenesis** (sper **mat** oh **jen** uh sis) The process of sperm production.

Figure 14-1 Growth and Development of Sexuality   Our sexuality develops through biological and psychosocial stages.

(Labels on the figure, left side:)
Late adolescence
Pubescence
Preadolescence
Childhood
Early childhood
Intrauterine

(Labels on the ladder rungs, top to bottom:)
Initial Adult Gender Identification
Gender adoption
Structural maturation
Gender adoption
Gender preference
Gender identity
Structural development
Gonadal sexuality
Genetic sexuality

(Ladder rails:)
Biological sexuality
Psychosocial sexuality

various points along this rail would be rungs representing the sequential unfolding of the genetic, gonadal, and structural components. These biological bases of our sexuality can be considered the "hard-wired" parts of our sexuality. They are rooted in the linkages of our parents' genetic backgrounds. These are the parts of our sexuality over which we have little control.

Because humans, more so than any other life form, can rise above a life centered on reproduction, we have a second dimension or rail to our sexuality—our **psychosocial sexuality.** The reason we possess the ability to be more than reproductive beings is a question for the

Key Terms

psychosocial sexuality Masculine and feminine aspects of sexuality.

gender General term reflecting a biological basis of sexuality; the male gender or the female gender.

gender identity Recognition of one's gender.

gender preference Emotional and intellectual acceptance of one's own gender.

gender adoption The long process of learning the behavior that is traditional for one's gender.

gender identification Achievement of a personally satisfying interpretation of one's masculinity or femininity.

theologian or the philosopher. We are considerably more complex than the hard-wired functions determined by biology. The process that transforms a male into a man and a female into a woman begins at birth and continues to influence us throughout the course of our lives.

It is during this transformation into a man or woman that we humans have some ability to influence our gender development. Here is where we occasionally are able to make decisions that influence both the way we view ourselves as men or women and the way we are viewed as men or women by others. This is the part of our sexuality that is not completely hard-wired by our genetic background.

Gender Identity

Although expectant parents may prefer to have a child of a particular **gender,** they frequently must wait until the birth of the baby to have their question answered. External genitals "cast the die," and femininity or masculinity begins to receive its traditional reinforcement by the parents and society in general. By the eighteenth month, typical children have both the language and the insight to correctly identify their gender. They have established a **gender identity.** [5] The first rung rising from the psychosocial rail of the ladder has been climbed.

Gender Preference

During the preschool years, children receive the second component of the scripting required for the full development of psychosocial sexuality— **gender preference.** Gender preference refers to the emotional and intellectual acceptance of one's birth gender. Reaching this rung on the psychosocial rail of the ladder takes place during the preschool years, when nearly every boy prefers being a boy and nearly every girl prefers being a girl.

During the preschool years, parents typically begin to control the child's exposure to experiences traditionally reserved for children of the opposite gender. This is particularly true for boys; parents often stop a boy's play activities if they perceive them as being too feminine. (Note: The concept of gender preference is not to be confused with sexual preference. Sexual preference refers to a sexual and/or emotional attraction to sexual partners. Sexual preference is discussed in Chapter 15 in a section entitled "Sexual Orientation.")

Attitudes toward gender roles have become more flexible in recent years. Many parents now allow their children to pursue the activities they enjoy, regardless of whether the activities were once considered strictly masculine, such as playing baseball or building a model airplane, or feminine, such as growing flowers or cooking.

Parents should not become alarmed if their children or teenagers experiment with their gender identity through their appearance or activities. Such experimentation is natural and a part of finding the gender identity

Music Video Portrayals of Men and Women

Back in the 1950s, many American adults were shocked to see the early rock-and-roll performers (like Elvis Presley) shaking their hips as they gyrated to a strange new music form. Half a century later, song writers and music performers continue to shock today's adults. Just ask for a middle-aged adult's comments after watching music videos on TV for 30 minutes.

Not surprisingly, today's young adults seem less concerned than their parents and mentors about the impact that music lyrics and music videos might have. College students we talk to seem to pass them off as "mere entertainment"—a temporary escape from their classes and busy lives. Just fun. Harmless.

But have you stopped to think how these lyrics and videos tend to portray men and women? Have you thought about how they might show a skewed look at the gender roles of men and women? Aren't the men in music videos generally the ones in control of everything? And aren't women generally seen as less in control and more manipulative? Many women in music videos must use their beauty and their sexuality (not their brains) to "trap" the powerful man.

Some would argue that the lyrics in many of the songs don't help portray how a healthy relationship between two people might take place. Lyrics in some songs speak openly about sexual manipulation, lies and deceit, sexual prowess, revenge, power, dominance, and physical and emotional pain. Critics of today's music and videos are especially concerned that young children and adolescents will learn inappropriate ways to deal with interpersonal relationships.

What do you think about this? Are the critics just complaining about something that should be viewed simply as an "escape?" In other words, are people making a mountain about of the proverbial molehill?

And what about you personally? Do you think much about the messages in the music you listen to or the videos you watch? Do you believe that music lyrics and videos have influenced the way you see yourself as a man or woman? Have you tried to apply something you learned in a song or saw in a music video to your personal life? Do you believe that the relationships depicted in music videos generally reflect "reality" or a world of fiction? If you see these media products as forms of escapism, should they even try to portray reality? How do you think your friends would answer these questions?

One thing is for sure: this controversy won't end anytime soon.

that best fits them. Such children often become very secure in their gender identity as adults.

With the recent acceleration in the importance of competitive sports for women, many of the skills and experiences once reserved for boys are now being fostered in young girls. What effect, if any, this movement will have on the speed at which gender preference is reached will be a topic for further research.

Gender Adoption

The process of reaching an initial adult gender identification requires a considerable period of time. The specific knowledge, attitudes, and behavior characteristic of adults must be observed, analyzed, and practiced. The process of acquiring and personalizing these "insights" about how men and women think, feel, and act is reflected by the term **gender adoption,** the first and third rungs below the initial adult gender identification rail of the ladder in Figure 14-1. This process is influenced by many cultural and social factors; see the box "Music Video Portrayals of Men and Women."

In addition to constructing a personalized version of an adult sexual identity, the child and particularly the adolescent must construct a gender schema for a member of the opposite gender. Clearly, the world of adulthood, with its involvement with intimacy, parenting, and employment, requires that men know women and women

know men. Gender adoption provides an opportunity to begin constructing the equally valuable "pictures" of what the genders are like.

Initial Adult Gender Identification

By the time young people have climbed all of the rungs of the sexuality ladder, they have arrived at the chronological point in the life cycle when they need to construct an initial adult **gender identification.** You might notice that this label seems remarkably similar to the terminology used to describe one of the developmental tasks being used in this textbook. In fact, the task of forming an initial adult identity is closely related to developing an initial adult image of oneself as a man or a woman. Although most of us currently support the concept of "person" in many gender-neutral contexts (for some very valid reasons), we still must identify ourselves as either a man or a woman.

Androgyny: Sharing the Pluses

Our society has increasingly accepted an image of a person who possesses both masculine and feminine qualities. This accepted image has taken years to develop because our society traditionally has reinforced rigid masculine roles for men and rigid feminine roles for women.

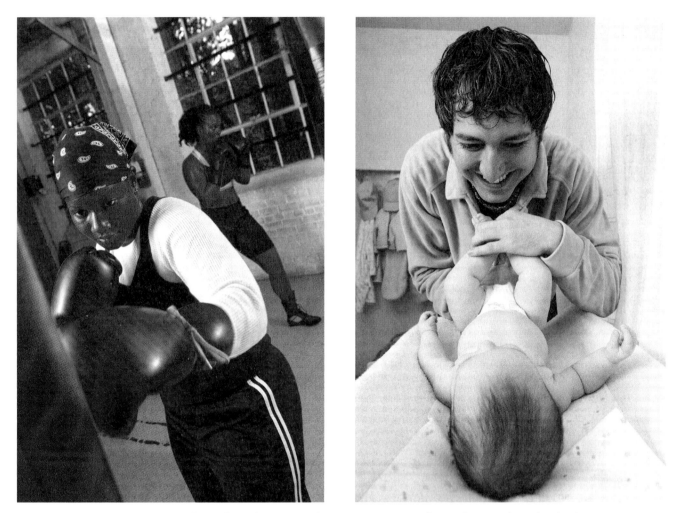

Just as women have broken into traditionally male careers and activities, many men have taken on jobs and tasks that were once considered women's exclusive domain.

In the past, from the time a child was born, we assigned and reinforced only those roles and traits that were thought to be directly related to his or her biological gender. Boys were not allowed to cry, play with dolls, or help in the kitchen. Girls were not encouraged to become involved in sports; they were told to learn to sew, cook, and baby-sit. Men were encouraged to be strong, expressive, dominant, aggressive, and career oriented, whereas women were encouraged to be weak, shy, submissive, passive, and home oriented.

These traditional biases have resulted in some interesting phenomena related to career opportunities. Women were denied jobs requiring above-average physical strength, admittance into professional schools requiring high intellectual capacities, such as law, medicine, and business, and entry into most levels of military participation. Likewise, men were not encouraged to enter traditionally feminine careers, such as nursing, clerical work, and elementary school teaching.

For a variety of reasons, the traditional picture has changed. **Androgyny,** or the blending of both feminine and masculine qualities, is more clearly evident in our society now than ever before. Today it is quite common to see men involved in raising children (including changing diapers) and doing routine housework. It is also quite common to see women entering the workplace in jobs traditionally managed by men and participating in sports traditionally played by men. Men are not scoffed at when they are seen crying after a touching movie. Women are not laughed at when they choose to assert themselves. The disposal of many sexual stereotypes has benefited our society immensely by relieving people of the pressure to be 100 percent "womanly" or 100 percent "macho."

Research data suggest that androgynous people are more flexible and independent, have greater self-esteem, have more positive attitudes toward sexuality, and show more social skills and motivation to achieve.[5] (Complete

Figure 14-2 The Male Reproductive System **A:** Side view, **B:** Front view.

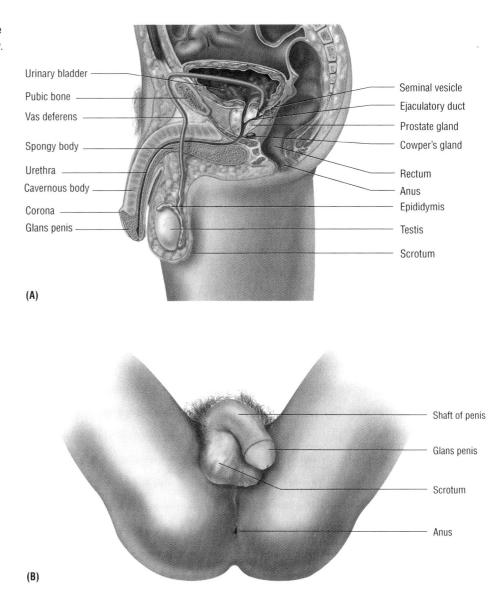

Urinary bladder
Pubic bone
Vas deferens
Spongy body
Urethra
Cavernous body
Corona
Glans penis

Seminal vesicle
Ejaculatory duct
Prostate gland
Cowper's gland
Rectum
Anus
Epididymis
Testis
Scrotum

(A)

Shaft of penis
Glans penis
Scrotum
Anus

(B)

the Personal Assessment at the end of this chapter to explore your own attitudes about sexuality and sex roles.)

 TALKING POINTS How could you demonstrate to your grandmother that the blending of gender roles is a positive development?

Reproductive Systems

The most familiar aspects of biological sexuality are the structures that comprise the reproductive systems. Each structure contributes in unique ways to the reproductive process. Thus, with these structures, males have the ability to impregnate. Females have the ability to become pregnant, give birth, and nourish infants through breast-feeding. In addition, many of these structures are associated with nonreproductive sexual behavior.

Male Reproductive System

The male reproductive system consists of external structures of genitals (the penis and scrotum) and internal structures (the testes, various passageways or ducts, seminal vesicles, the prostate gland, and the Cowper's glands) (Figure 14-2a).

The Testes The *testes* (also called *gonads* or *testicles*) are two egg-shaped bodies that lie within a saclike structure called the *scrotum*. During most of fetal development, the testes lie within the abdominal cavity. They descend into the scrotum during the last two months of fetal life.

> **Key Terms**
>
> **androgyny** (an **droj** en ee) The blending of both masculine and feminine qualities.

The testes are housed in the scrotum because a temperature lower than the body core temperature is required for adequate sperm development. The walls of the scrotum are composed of contractile tissue and can draw the testes closer to the body during cold temperatures (and sexual arousal) and relax during warm temperatures. Scrotal contraction and relaxation allow a constant, productive temperature to be maintained in the testes (Figure 14-2b).

A cross-sectional view of a single testis reveals an intricate network of structures called *seminiferous tubules.* Within these 300 or so seminiferous tubules, the process of sperm production (spermatogenesis) takes place. Sperm cell development starts at about age 11 in boys and is influenced by the release of the hormone ICSH (interstitial cell-stimulating hormone) from the pituitary gland. ICSH does primarily what its name suggests: it stimulates specific cells (called *interstitial cells*) within the testes to begin producing the male sex hormone *testosterone.* Testosterone in turn is primarily responsible for the gradual development of the male secondary sex characteristics at the onset of puberty. By the time a boy is approximately 15 years old, sufficient levels of testosterone exist so that the testes become capable of full spermatogenesis.

Before the age of about 15 most of the sperm cells produced in the testes are incapable of fertilization. The production of fully mature sperm (*spermatozoa*) is triggered by another hormone secreted by the brain's pituitary gland—FSH (follicle-stimulating hormone). FSH influences the seminiferous tubules to begin producing spermatozoa capable of fertilization.

Ducts Spermatogenesis takes place around the clock, with hundreds of millions of sperm cells produced daily. The sperm cells do not stay in the seminiferous tubules but rather are transferred through a system of *ducts* that lead into the *epididymis.* The epididymis is a tubular coil that attaches to the back side of each testicle. These collecting structures house the maturing sperm cells for two to three weeks. During this period the sperm finally become capable of motion, but they remain inactive until they mix with the secretions from the accessory glands (the seminal vesicles, prostate gland, and Cowper's glands).

Each epididymis leads into an 18-inch passageway known as the *vas deferens.* Sperm, moved along by the action of hairlike projections called *cilia,* can also remain in the vas deferens for an extended time without losing their ability to fertilize an egg.

Seminal Vesicles The two vasa deferens extend into the abdominal cavity, where each meets with a *seminal vesicle*—the first of the three accessory structures or glands. Each seminal vesicle contributes a clear, alkaline fluid that nourishes the sperm cells with fructose and permits the sperm cells to be suspended in a movable medium. The fusion of a vas deferens with the seminal vesicle results in the formation of a passageway called the *ejaculatory duct.* Each ejaculatory duct is only about one inch long and empties into the final passageway for the sperm—the urethra.

Prostate Gland The ejaculatory duct is located within the second accessory gland—the *prostate gland* (see Figure 14-2). The prostate gland secretes a milky fluid containing a variety of substances, including proteins, cholesterol, citric acid, calcium, buffering salts, and various enzymes. The prostate secretions further nourish the sperm cells and also raise the pH level, making the mixture quite alkaline. The alkalinity permits the sperm to have greater longevity as they are transported during ejaculation through the urethra, out of the penis, and into the highly acidic vagina.

Cowper's Glands The third accessory gland, the *Cowper's glands,* serves primarily to lubricate the urethra with a clear, viscous mucus. These paired glands empty their small amounts of preejaculatory fluid during the arousal stage of the sexual response cycle. Alkaline in nature, this fluid also neutralizes the acidic level of the urethra. Viable sperm cells can be suspended in this fluid and can enter the female reproductive tract before full ejaculation by the male.[6] This may account for many of the failures of the "withdrawal" method of contraception.

The sperm cells, when combined with secretions from the seminal vesicles and the prostate gland, form a sticky substance called semen.[7] Interestingly, the microscopic sperm actually makes up less than 5 percent of the seminal fluid discharged at ejaculation. Contrary to popular belief, the paired seminal vesicles contribute about 60 percent of the semen volume, and the prostate gland adds about 30 percent.[1] Thus the fear of some men that a vasectomy will destroy their ability to ejaculate is completely unfounded (see Chapter 16).

During *emission* (the gathering of semen in the upper part of the urethra), a sphincter muscle at the base of the bladder contracts and inhibits semen from being pushed into the bladder and urine from being deposited into the urethra.[8] Thus semen and urine rarely intermingle, even though they leave the body through the same passageway.

Penis Ejaculation takes place when the semen is forced out of the *penis* through the urethral opening. The involuntary, rhythmic muscle contractions that control ejaculation result in a series of pleasurable sensations known as *orgasm.*

The urethra lies on the underside of the penis and extends through the three cylindrical chambers of erectile tissue (two *cavernous bodies* and one *spongy body*). Each of these three chambers provides the vascular space required for sufficient erection of the penis. When a male becomes sexually aroused, the areas become congested

DHEA: The Fountain of Youth?

DHEA (dehydroepiandrosterone) is a steroid hormone produced mainly by the adrenal glands. This hormone is the most abundant hormone in the human body. DHEA is converted by the body into other hormones, especially estrogen and testosterone. This hormone peaks in the bloodstream by age 25 and then gradually declines until about age 70, when levels of DHEA may be more than 80 percent lower than they once were.[*]

Recently, researchers have speculated that DHEA may be helpful in treating a variety of ailments. In fact, advocates of DHEA believe that this powerful hormone can reverse the aging process and bring back sexual vigor. Some claim that DHEA can fight off aging by boosting your sex drive, helping you lose weight,[*] improving your immune system, warding off cancer, combating depression,[†] and improving your mood, energy, and memory. DHEA might also be useful in combating chronic fatigue syndrome. However, few large experimental trials of DHEA's effect have been undertaken, so many health professionals remain cautious about the benefits (and risks) of taking DHEA. Some physicians are true supporters of DHEA, while some remain skeptical.

Before you purchase DHEA supplements at your local health food store or on the Internet, speak with your physician about his or her understanding of DHEA's risks and benefits. Be cautious since DHEA is not regulated by the FDA. Since it is clear that DHEA triggers additional hormone production in the body, you will want to avoid DHEA if you have a hormone-related cancer, such as breast, cervical, uterine, ovarian, or prostate cancer. If you are pregnant or breast-feeding, you should not take this supplement. Finally, be prepared for some of the same body changes that take place when people take steroids, including mood changes, facial hair growth, acne, oily skin, and a lowering of the voice in women and breast enlargement in men who take high doses.

[*]Broyles S. Hormone protects against diseases of aging, http://mywebmd .com/content/article/96/103935.htm.

[†]Hitti M. DHEA may help midlife depression, http://mywebmd.com/content/ article/100/105716.htm.

---

with blood (*vasocongestion*). After ejaculation or when a male is no longer sexually stimulated, these chambers release the blood into the general circulation and the penis returns to a **flaccid** state.

The *shaft* of the penis is covered by a thin layer of skin that is an extension of the skin that covers the scrotum. This loose layer of skin is sensitive to sexual stimulation and extends over the head of the penis, except in males who have been circumcised. The *glans* (or head) of the penis is the most sexually sensitive (to tactile stimulation) part of the male body. Nerve receptor sites are especially prominent along the *corona* (the ridge of the glans) and the *frenulum* (the thin tissue at the base of the glans).

Age-Related Hormone Changes   Later in life, men begin to experience some changes in their reproductive system. The level of androgens, or male hormones, decreases with age, and the size of the prostate gland often increases. A deficiency of androgens has been found to cause health concerns in older men, including a lack of strength and energy, changes in mood, lower interest in sex, decreased bone density, and a decrease in muscle mass.[9] Some are calling this the male menopause, or **andropause.** [10]

As a result, researchers are studying the benefits and risks of androgen replacement therapy in older men, similar to the hormone replacement therapy given to women. The benefits are an increase in bone and muscle mass, improved muscular and cardiovascular function, improved sexual function, and an overall better sense of well-being. The possible risks include an increased incidence

of prostate disease, cardiovascular disease, and liver disease.[9] Androgen replacement therapy is available through prescription injections, transdermal patches, oral pills, and most recently through a gel applied daily to the upper arm, shoulders, or abdomen.[11]

Another steroid hormone, DHEA, is believed by some to reverse the aging process and revitalize sexual function; see the box "DHEA: The Fountain of Youth?"

Key Terms

ICSH (interstitial cell-stimulating hormone) (in ter **stish** ul) A gonadotropic hormone of the male required for the production of testosterone.

FSH (follicle-stimulating hormone) A gonadotropic hormone required for the initial development of ova (in the female) and sperm (in the male).

semen A secretion containing sperm and nutrients discharged from the urethra at ejaculation.

vasectomy A surgical procedure in which the vasa deferens are cut to prevent the passage of sperm from the testicles; the most common form of male sterilization.

flaccid (**fla** sid) Nonerect; the state of erectile tissue when vasocongestion is not occurring.

andropause Significant decrease in androgenic hormone production in aging men; also called male menopause.

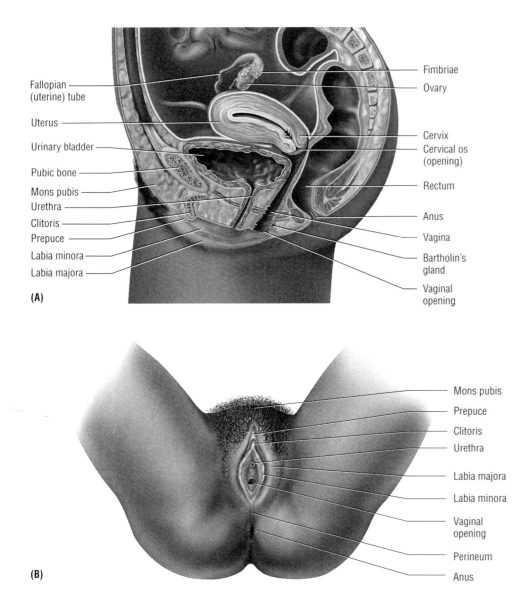

Fallopian (uterine) tube

Uterus

Urinary bladder

Pubic bone

Mons pubis

Urethra

Clitoris

Prepuce

Labia minora

Labia majora

(A)

Fimbriae

Ovary

Cervix

Cervical os (opening)

Rectum

Anus

Vagina

Bartholin's gland

Vaginal opening

Mons pubis

Prepuce

Clitoris

Urethra

Labia majora

Labia minora

Vaginal opening

Perineum

Anus

(B)

Figure 14-3 The Female Reproductive System A: Side view, **B:** Front view.

Female Reproductive System

The external structures (genitals) of the female reproductive system consist of the mons pubis, labia majora, labia minora, clitoris, and vestibule (Figure 14-3). Collectively these structures form the *vulva* or vulval area.

Mons Pubis The *mons pubis* is the fatty covering over the pubic bone. The mons pubis (or mons veneris, "mound of Venus") is covered by pubic hair and is quite sensitive to sexual stimulation.

Labia Majora and Labia Minora The *labia majora* are large longitudinal skin folds that cover the entrance to the vagina, whereas the *labia minora* are the smaller longitudinal skin folds that lie within the labia majora. These hairless skin folds of the labia minora join at the top to form the *prepuce.* The prepuce covers the glans of

the *clitoris,* which is the most sexually sensitive part of the female body.

Clitoris In terms of its tactile sensitivity, the *clitoris* is the most sensitive part of the female genitals. It contains a glans and a shaft, although the shaft is below the skin surface. It is composed of erectile tissue that can become engorged with blood. It is covered by skin folds (the clitoral prepuce) and can collect **smegma** beneath these tissue folds.[5]

Vestibule The *vestibule* is the region enclosed by the labia minora. Evident here are the urethral opening and the entrance to the vagina (vaginal orifice). Also located at the vaginal opening are the *Bartholin's glands,* which secrete a minute amount of lubricating fluid during sexual excitement.

Although sometimes referred to as female circumcision, the practice of surgically altering a young girl's vulva is more appropriately called female genital cutting (FGC) or female genital mutilation (FGM). This procedure is practiced in 28 African countries, several countries in the Middle East, and among some Muslims in Indonesia and Malaysia.[*] And even in the United States. In November 2006 in Lawrenceville, Georgia, an Ethiopian immigrant was convicted of aggravated battery and cruelty to children in a trial in which he was accused of using scissors to remove his 2-year-old daughter's clitoris in 2001. He was sentenced to 10 years in prison. This was thought to be the first criminal case in the United States that involved FGM.[†]

Typically, the procedure takes one of three forms: the removal of the clitoral hood (circumcision), the removal of the clitoris and perhaps the labia minora (clitoridectomy), and the drastic removal of the clitoris, inner lips, and part of the outer lips (infibulation).

For people from Western cultures, these practices may seem barbaric. Indeed, numerous international treaties, conventions, and relief organizations (World Health Organization, United Nations, CARE, United Nations Children's Fund) have developed policy statements that condemn these practices.[‡,§] Often performed by native women with crude instruments in unsanitary conditions, FGM takes place without the use of anesthetics. Female infants or young girls are subjected to this ritualistic cutting. Obvious dangers include severe bleeding, infection, and the formation of scar tissue.

Infibulation is sometimes extended to incorporate the sewing together of the remaining parts of the labia majora. This is thought to ensure virginity in a woman, but poses major risks when a newlywed husband tries to force his penis through the sewn area. Sometimes a midwife must first cut through the scar tissue to open the entrance to the vagina. Years after FGC, women face the possibility of serious complications with childbirth.

It is estimated that FGC and FGM have been performed on over 130 million women worldwide.[§] At face value, these procedures may seem gruesome to us in the West, yet we must pause to consider imposing our values on other cultures . . . cultures that readily accept these acts as important to the foundations of their belief systems. To many of us, these procedures represent a sexist devaluation of women. Yet this is normative behavior for groups of people who believe in carrying traditional values for their society. FGC and FGM pose real ethical dilemmas for those of us in Western cultures. What are your thoughts on this?

[*] Hyde JS, DeLamater JD. *Understanding Human Sexuality*, 9th ed. New York: McGraw-Hill, 2006.
[†] *"Jury Convicts Father in Genital Mutilation of Girl,"* MSNBC.com., November 1, 2006, www.msnbc.msn.com/id/15515179/.
[‡] *"Female Genital Mutilation,"* World Health Organization, www.who.int/mediacentre/factsheets/fs241.
[§] *"Female Genital Mutilation/Cutting,"* United Nations Children's Fund, www.unicef.org.

The *hymen* is a thin layer of tissue that stretches across the opening of the vagina. Once thought to be the only indication of virginity, the intact hymen rarely covers the vaginal opening entirely. Openings in the hymen are necessary for the discharge of menstrual fluid and vaginal secretions. Many hymens are stretched or torn to full opening by adolescent physical activity or by the insertion of tampons. In women whose hymens are not fully ruptured, the first act of sexual intercourse will generally accomplish this. Pain may accompany first intercourse in females with relatively intact hymens.

The internal reproductive structures of the female include the vagina, uterus, fallopian tubes, and ovaries.

Vagina   The *vagina* is the structure that forms a canal from the orifice, through the vestibule, to the uterine cervix. Normally the walls of the vagina are collapsed, except during sexual stimulation, when the vaginal walls widen and elongate to accommodate the erect penis. Only the outer third of the vagina is especially sensitive to sexual stimulation. In this location, vaginal tissues swell considerably to form the **orgasmic platform.**[7] This platform constricts the vaginal opening and in effect "grips" the penis (or other inserted object)—regardless of its size. Thus the belief that a woman receives considerably more sexual pleasure from men with large penises is not supported from an anatomical standpoint.

Uterus   The *uterus* (or *womb*) is approximately the size and shape of a small pear. This highly muscular organ is capable of undergoing a wide range of physical changes, as evidenced by its enlargement during pregnancy, its contraction during menstruation and labor, and its movement during the orgasmic phase of the female sexual response cycle. The primary function of the uterus is to provide a suitable environment for the possible implantation of a fertilized ovum, or egg. This implantation, should it occur, takes place in the innermost lining of the uterus—the *endometrium*. In the mature female,

---

Key Terms

smegma   Cellular discharge that can accumulate beneath the clitoral hood or the foreskin of an uncircumcised penis.

orgasmic platform   Expanded outer third of the vagina, which grips the penis during sexual intercourse.

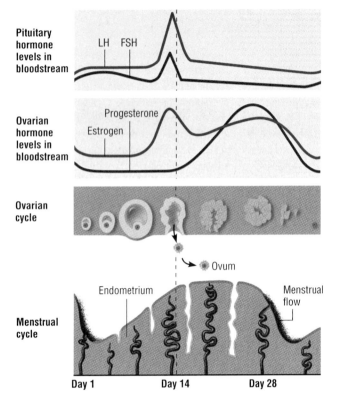

Pituitary hormone levels in bloodstream

LH   FSH

Ovarian hormone levels in bloodstream

Progesterone
Estrogen

Ovarian cycle

Ovum

Menstrual cycle

Endometrium

Menstrual flow

Day 1   Day 14   Day 28

Figure 14-4 Menstrual Cycle   The menstrual cycle involves the development and release of an ovum, supported by hormones from the pituitary, and the buildup of the endometrium, supported by hormones from the ovary, for the purpose of establishing a pregnancy.

the endometrium undergoes cyclic changes as it prepares a new lining on a near-monthly basis.

The lower third of the uterus is called the *cervix.* The cervix extends slightly into the vagina. Sperm can enter the uterus through the cervical opening, or *cervical os.* Mucous glands in the cervix secrete a fluid that is thin and watery near the time of ovulation. Mucus of this consistency apparently facilitates sperm passage into the uterus and deeper structures. However, cervical mucus is much thicker during portions of the menstrual cycle when pregnancy is improbable, and during pregnancy, to protect against bacterial agents and other substances that are especially dangerous to the developing fetus.

The upper two-thirds of the uterus is called the *corpus* or *body.* This is where the fertilized ovum generally implants into the uterus.

Fallopian Tubes   The upper portion of the uterus opens into *two fallopian tubes,* sometimes called *oviducts* or *uterine tubes,* each about four inches long. The fallopian tubes are each directed toward an ovary. They serve as a passageway for the ovum in its weeklong voyage toward the uterus. In most cases, conception takes place in the upper third of the fallopian tubes.

Ovaries   The *ovaries* are analogous to the testes in the male. Their function is to produce the ovum, or egg. Usually, one ovary produces and releases just one egg each month. Approximately the size and shape of an unshelled almond, an ovary produces viable ova in the process known as *oogenesis.*

The ovaries also produce the female sex hormones through the efforts of specific structures within the ovaries. These hormones play multiple roles in the development of female secondary sex characteristics, but their primary function is to prepare the endometrium of the uterus for possible implantation of a fertilized ovum. In the average healthy female, this preparation takes place about 13 times a year for a period of about 35 years. At menopause, the ovaries shrink considerably and stop nearly all hormonal production.

Menstrual Cycle   Each month or so, the inner wall of the uterus prepares for a possible pregnancy. When a pregnancy does not occur (as is the case throughout most months of a woman's fertile years), this lining must be released and a new one prepared. The breakdown of this endometrial wall and the resultant discharge of blood and endometrial tissue is known as *menstruation* (or *menses*) (Figure 14-4). The cyclic timing of this is controlled by a woman's hormones.

Girls generally have their first menstrual cycle, the onset of which is called *menarche,* around age 12 or 13. However, menarche ranges widely, from about age 9 to 17 years.[4] Over the past few decades, the age of menarche has been dropping gradually. This drop appears to be related to heredity, improved overall health, better childhood nutrition, and increased caloric intake. These factors in combination produce the increased body weight evident today in many young adolescent girls that seems to trigger an earlier menarche.

After a girl first menstruates, her cycles may be anovulatory for a year or longer before a viable ovum is released during her cycle. She will then continue this cyclic activity until age 45 to 55.

This text refers to a menstrual cycle that lasts 28 days. Be assured that few women display absolutely perfect 28-day cycles. Most women fluctuate by a few days to a week or more around this 28-day pattern.

It is not uncommon for some women to experience irregular cycles (cycles that differ in length) and even occasional mid-cycle spotting (small amounts of reddish discharge). These events are most likely to occur in young women who are just establishing their cycles, women who are approaching or moving through menopause, and women who are just starting to use hormone-based contraceptive methods. Major life changes, certain illnesses and medications, and unresolved stress can also affect the length of a woman's cycle. Any woman who experiences a significant, dramatic change from her usual pattern should contact her physician or health care practitioner.[5]

Your knowledge about the menstrual cycle is critical for your understanding of pregnancy, contraception, menopause, and issues related to the overall health and comfort of women; see the box "Endometriosis." Although seemingly complicated, each segment of the cycle can be studied separately for better understanding.

The menstrual cycle can be thought of as occurring in three segments or phases: the menstrual phase (lasting about one week), the preovulation phase (also lasting about one week), and the postovulation phase (lasting about two weeks). Day 1 of this cycle starts with the first day of bleeding, or menstrual flow.

Menstrual Phase The *menstrual phase* signals the woman that a pregnancy has not taken place and that her uterine lining is being sloughed off. During a five- to seven-day period, a woman will discharge about one-fourth to one-half cup of blood and tissue. (Only about one ounce of the menstrual flow is blood.) The menstrual flow is heaviest during the first days of this phase. Because the muscular uterus must contract to accomplish this tissue removal, some women have uncomfortable cramping during menstruation. Most women, however, report more pain and discomfort during the few days before the first day of menstrual flow; see the box "Dealing with Menstrual Pain."

Today's methods of absorbing menstrual flow include the use of internal tampons and external pads. Caution must be exercised by the user of tampons to prevent the possibility of toxic shock syndrome (TSS) (see Chapter 13). Because menstrual flow is a positive sign of good health, women are encouraged to be normally active during menstruation.

Preovulation Phase The *preovulation phase* of the menstrual cycle starts about the time menstruation stops. Lasting about one week, this phase is first influenced by the release of follicle-stimulating hormone (FSH) from the pituitary gland. FSH circulates in the bloodstream and directs the ovaries to start the process of maturing approximately 20 primary ovarian *follicles.* Thousands of primary egg follicles are present in each ovary at birth. These follicles resemble shells that house immature ova. As these follicles ripen under FSH influence, they release the hormone *estrogen.* Estrogen's primary function is to direct the endometrium to start the development of a thick, highly vascular wall. As FSH secretions are reduced, the pituitary gland prepares for the surge of the luteinizing hormone (LH) required to accomplish ovulation.[12]

In the days immediately before ovulation, one of the primary follicles (called the *graafian follicle*) matures fully. The other primary follicles degenerate and are absorbed by the body. The graafian follicle moves toward the surface of the ovary. When LH is released in massive

Endometriosis

Endometriosis is a condition in which endometrial tissue that normally lines the uterus is found growing within the pelvic cavity. Because the tissue remains sensitive to circulating hormones, it is the source of pain and discomfort during the latter half of the menstrual cycle. Endometriosis is most commonly found in younger women and is sometimes related to infertility in women with severe cases.

In addition to painful cramping before and during menstruation, the symptoms of endometriosis include low-back pain, pain during intercourse, painful bowel movements, heavy menstrual flow, and difficulty becoming pregnant. Many women with endometriosis, however, experience no symptoms.*

Treatment of endometriosis largely depends on its extent. Drugs to suppress ovulation, including birth control pills, may be helpful in mild cases. For more severe cases, surgical removal of the tissue or a hysterectomy may be necessary. For some women, endometriosis is suppressed during pregnancy and does not return after pregnancy.

Health Guide A–Z: Endometriosis. WebMDHealth. www.my.webmd.com/hw/endometriosis/hw103000.asp, September 5, 2005.

quantities on about day 14, the graafian follicle bursts to release the fully mature ovum. The release of the ovum is called ovulation. Regardless of the overall length of a woman's cycle, ovulation occurs 14 days before her first day of menstrual flow.

The ovum is quickly captured by the fingerlike projections (*fimbriae*) of the fallopian tubes. In the upper third of the fallopian tubes, the ovum is capable of being fertilized in a 24- to 36-hour period. If the ovum is not fertilized by a sperm cell, it will begin to degenerate and eventually be absorbed by the body.

Postovulation Phase After ovulation, the *postovulation phase* of the menstrual cycle starts when the remnants of the graafian follicle restructure themselves into a corpus luteum. The corpus luteum remains inside the ovary, secreting estrogen and a fourth hormone called *progesterone.* Progesterone, which literally means "for pregnancy," continues to direct the endometrial buildup.

Key Terms

luteinizing hormone (LH) (**loo** ten eye zing) A gonadotropic hormone of the female required for fullest development and release of ova; ovulating hormone.

ovulation The release of a mature egg from the ovary.

corpus luteum (kore pus **loo** tee um) Cellular remnant of the graafian follicle after the release of an ovum.

Dealing with Menstrual Pain

I am a 24-year-old woman who has a great amount of menstrual pain. What can I do to lessen this pain?

The medical term is *dysmenorrhea*, but most women know it as menstrual cramps, and most women suffer from it at one time or another. Fortunately, the medical profession seems to be paying more attention to this problem, and various treatments are being studied. Currently, the most popular treatments still seem to be exercise and prostaglandin inhibitors.

The periodic cramps can occur before and during the menstrual phase, when the uterus must contract to remove the uterine lining. These contractions are produced by prostaglandin hormones normally found in the body. The problem occurs when the body produces an excess of one of the prostaglandin hormones, and the result is excessive cramping and pain. Thus prostaglandin-inhibiting medications can be used to reduce the body's production of prostaglandins and thereby reduce the intensity of cramping. Antiprostaglandin medications include ibuprofen, aspirin, and some prescription medications.

Before beginning treatment, however, the first step is to see a physician to rule out other causes of the dysmenorrhea. If other underlying causes are eliminated, consider the following treatment suggestions:

- Consume a well-balanced diet, with limited salt and sugar intake. Reduce spicy foods, and drink six to eight glasses of water per day.

- Consider taking aspirin, ibuprofen, other over-the-counter medications, or prescription medications, with your physician's guidance. Do not take aspirin if you are allergic to aspirin or have anemia, ulcers, or intestinal bleeding.
- Try taking a warm bath or placing a hot water bottle on your abdomen.

Try the following exercise routine that targets menstrual cramping.

- Lie face up with the legs and knees bent; perform abdominal breathing about 10 times. Feel the abdomen slowly inflate and then slowly fall.
- Stand and hold the back of a chair; lift one heel off the floor, then the other. Repeat 20 times.
- Lie on your back; lift and bring your knees to your chin; repeat 10 times.

Other treatments currently being explored include herbal remedies, acupuncture, transcutaneous electrical nerve stimulation, and microwave diathermy.

If pregnancy occurs, the corpus luteum monitors progesterone and estrogen levels throughout the pregnancy. If pregnancy does not occur, high levels of progesterone signal the pituitary to stop the release of LH and the corpus luteum starts to disintegrate on about day 24. When estrogen and progesterone levels diminish significantly by day 28, the endometrium is discharged from the uterus and out the vagina. The postovulation phase ends, and the cycle is complete.

Related Conditions

Premenstrual Syndrome (PMS) PMS is a collection of physical and psychological symptoms that occur in the days just before menstruation in many women of childbearing age. The physical symptoms may include weight gain, breast tenderness, fatigue, headaches, backaches, and abdominal cramps. The psychological symptoms can include irritability, tension, anxiety, mood swings, depression, difficulty concentrating, and aggressiveness. These symptoms vary from woman to woman and from one menstrual cycle to the next. It has been estimated that 85 percent of women experience at least some of these symptoms on a regular basis.[13]

The specific cause of PMS is unknown, but it is likely related to the changing levels of estrogen and progesterone as a woman's body prepares for menstruation. Treating the symptoms of PMS often starts with a healthy diet—reducing one's intake of caffeine, salt, and simple sugar, and increasing one's intake of complex carbohydrates by eating more fresh fruits and vegetables. A simple, daily vitamin/mineral combination pill might also be helpful. Physical exercise is highly recommended to reduce PMS symptoms and elevate one's mood. Over-the-counter nonsteroidal anti-inflammatory drugs (NSAIDs), such as ibuprofen and naproxen, and over-the-counter diuretics can help alleviate uncomfortable physical symptoms. For severe cases of PMS, a physician can prescribe medications. These might include certain antidepressants and prescription diuretics. Although in the past progesterone therapy or combined estrogen-progesterone birth control pills were prescribed for relief from PMS, recent research indicates that these approaches are generally ineffective.[14]

Premenstrual Dysphoric Disorder (PMDD) Premenstrual dysphoric disorder (PMDD) is a severe form of PMS and occurs in about 2–10 percent of menstruating women.[15] As with PMS, PMDD expresses itself in the latter half of the menstrual cycle in the days before menstruation begins. The symptoms of PMDD are similar to those of PMS, but they are so severe that they cause major disruptions in a woman's personal relationships, social activities, and employment. With PMDD, the mood swings, tension, irritability, depression, anger, appetite changes, sleep problems, loss of control, difficulties concentrating, and physical symptoms are magnified far beyond that seen in women with PMS.

To make a diagnosis of PMDD, a physician will likely give a woman a thorough medical examination, including a review and analysis of her symptoms and medical history. He or she will want to rule out emotional problems (such as depression) as possible causes of the symptoms, as well as medical or gynecological concerns (such as endometriosis, menopause, or fibroid tumors) that could also account for the symptoms.

The cause of PMDD appears to be a connection between hormonal fluctuations and a lowered level of serotonin, a neurotransmitter that helps transmit nerve signals. Methods of treatment of PMDD focus on many of the same strategies used to manage PMS: good nutrition, regular aerobic exercise, psychological counseling (to develop coping strategies), and the use of over-the-counter pain relievers and diuretics. Additionally, the FDA has approved the use of three prescription antidepressants to help relieve the symptoms of PMDD. Some physicians prescribe birth control pills or other hormonal drugs to women coping with PMDD, although their effectiveness remains uncertain.[15]

Fibrocystic Breast Condition In some women, particularly those who have never been pregnant, stimulation of the breast tissues by estrogen and progesterone during the menstrual cycle results in an unusually high degree of secretory activity by the cells lining the ducts. The fluid released by the secretory lining finds its way into the fibrous connective tissue areas in the lower half of the breast, where in pocketlike cysts the fluid presses against neighboring tissues. Excessive secretory activity produces in many women a benign fibrocystic breast condition characterized by swollen, firm, or hardened tender breast tissue before menstruation.

Researchers have begun to describe the importance of a healthy diet in preventing fibrocystic breast condition, in particular a low-fat, low-salt, low-red-meat diet that is rich in whole grains, fish, and chicken. The reduction or elimination of caffeine found in coffee, tea, soft drinks, and chocolate might also help reduce these benign breast changes. In some cases, vitamin E and vitamin B-complex supplementation have helped.[5] Women with more extensive fibrocystic conditions can be treated with drugs that have a "calming" effect on progesterone production. Occasional draining of cysts can bring relief.

Amenorrhea **Amenorrhea** is a condition characterized by the absence of menstruation. The lack of menstruation, if not caused by aging or pregnancy, is categorized as either primary or secondary amenorrhea.[8] *Primary amenorrhea* occurs when girls have passed the age of 16 and have never menstruated. Perhaps these girls have not yet reached a critical body weight (with the increased

ratio of body fat) to trigger the menstrual cycle to begin. Additionally, some girls may have inherited a familial tendency to mature later than most of their peers. At an appropriate time for their bodies, these girls will start to menstruate. However, in cases where the primary amenorrhea is determined to be caused by hormonal deficiencies or abnormal body structure, hormone therapy can be quite useful.

Secondary amenorrhea occurs when a previously menstruating woman ceases to menstruate. Likely reasons for secondary amenorrhea include pregnancy, breastfeeding, or the use of hormonal contraceptives. Less common reasons could be linked to unresolved stress, a reduction in body fat, hormonal irregularities, or serious athletic training. Other causes could be anorexia (see Chapter 6) or the female athlete syndrome (see Chapter 4). If a woman has not menstruated in six months and is not pregnant, not breast-feeding, and not using hormonal contraceptives, she should consult with her physician or medical care professional.[8]

Menopause For the vast majority of women in their late 40s through their mid-50s, a gradual decline in reproductive system function, called *menopause,* occurs. Menopause is a normal physiological process, not a disease process. It can, however, become a health concern for some middle-aged women who have unpleasant side effects resulting from this natural ending of ovum production and menstruation.

As ovarian function and hormone production diminish, the hypothalamus, ovaries, uterus, and other estrogen-sensitive tissues must adjust. The extent of menopause as a health problem is determined by the degree to which hot flashes, night sweats, insomnia, vaginal wall dryness, depression and melancholy, breast changes, and the uncertainty of fertility are seen as problems.

Many of today's midlife women are likely to find menopause to be a relatively positive experience. The end of fertility, combined with children leaving home, makes the middle years a period of personal rediscovery for many women; see the box "No Fear of 50."

For women who are troubled by the changes brought about by menopause, physicians may prescribe **hormone replacement therapy (HRT).** This can relieve

Key Terms
amenorrhea The absence of menstruation.
hot flashes Unpleasant, temporary feelings of warmth experienced by women during and after menopause, caused by blood vessel dilation.
hormone replacement therapy (HRT) Medically administered hormones to replace hormones lost as the result of menopause.

Chapter Fourteen Exploring the Origins of Sexuality **429**

many symptoms and offer benefits to help reduce the incidence of osteoporosis (see Chapters 4 and 5). However, HRT has recently been found to increase the risk of breast cancer and cardiovascular problems.[16, 17] These concerns have caused many women to reconsider their use of HRT. See the box "Alternatives to Hormone Replacement Therapy" for more information.

Additional Aspects of Human Sexuality

Earlier in this chapter, we identified the biological and psychosocial bases of our sexuality. In this section we explore three additional aspects of our sexuality—reproductive, genital, and expressionistic—around which many of our important decisions in life are made.* With these new perspectives in mind, you will be better able to see the complexity associated with our development as productive and satisfied beings.

* We cite no specific source for the terms *reproductive sexuality, genital sexuality,* and *expressionistic sexuality.* They are labels we and our colleagues use in instructional units associated with human sexuality.

Reproductive Sexuality

Of these three aspects of sexuality, *reproductive sexuality* reflects the most basic level of sexuality over which the adult must exercise discretion and display insight. Simply stated, reproductive sexuality is related to your knowledge of, desire for, and ability to participate in the act of *procreation*. Pregnancy, delivery, natural childbirth, breast-feeding, fertility control, and pregnancy termination are terms related to this dimension of sexuality. Demographic data indicate that most (but not all) of you will choose to be active in this dimension of your sexuality by becoming parents.

Genital Sexuality

Genital sexuality refers to the nonreproductive use of the reproductive organs. In comparison with the concept of reproductive sexuality, genital sexuality implies recreation and communication rather than procreation. The behaviors and meanings associated with the terms *orgasm, having sex, making love, oral-genital sex,* and *sexual responsiveness* are genital in their orientation.

In the most positive sense, sexual experiences that are genitally oriented should be sensual, erotic, and stimulating and should give the individual a sense of release.

Recall from Chapter 10 that recent studies now question the benefits of hormone replacement therapy (HRT) for women. For the past few decades, it was thought that HRT not only helped women find relief from the uncomfortable symptoms of menopause (hot flashes, night sweats, vaginal dryness, mood swings, and insomnia) but that HRT also helped protect women from osteoporosis, and most importantly, cardiovascular disease.

However, in the largest study of its kind to examine the impact of HRT (specifically the most popular estrogen-progestin combination) on women's health, the National Heart, Lung, and Blood Institute found that HRT actually *increased* the incidence of breast cancer, heart attacks, blood clots, and strokes. Although the increase was not large (for example, women taking hormones were less than one-tenth of 1 percent more likely to have a heart attack), it was enough to have this aspect of the Women's Health Initiative stopped in 2002, three years before completion of the study.[*]

Since the 2002 report,[*] many women have stopped taking the combined estrogen-progesterone pills for menopausal symptoms. For women who still want this form of HRT,

physicians generally recommend they take the lowest dosage for the least amount of time. Thus, women might think in terms of taking HRT for two to five years, not for a lifetime.

Another consequence of the recent concern is the increased interest in alternative approaches to HRT. For concerns about osteoporosis, there are alternative prescription drugs that can be helpful including alendronate (Fosamax) or raloxifene (Evista). A diet that adds calcium-rich foods (dairy products, leafy green vegetables, and sardines) in combination with Vitamin D promotes bone density. Weight-bearing exercise, such as walking and weight lifting, encourages bone growth as well.

Hot flashes and night sweats result from changing estrogen levels and are, perhaps, the most challenging acute symptoms to control. However, reducing the intake of spicy foods, caffeine, and alcohol may help. Vitamin E and soy products help some women, and the use of certain herbs (especially black cohosh) is being studied. For some women, the use of a prescription antidepressant (such as Prozac or Paxil) may reduce hot flashes.

Vaginal dryness can be helped by the use of over-the-counter lubricants and

moisturizers, vaginal estrogen creams, and regular sexual activity. Insomnia can be countered with the use of good sleeping patterns (consistent bedtime hour; a small glass of warm milk; reduced caffeine, alcohol, and food intake before bed). Cardiovascular concerns at menopause can be reduced by a healthy lifestyle that includes not smoking, consuming healthy foods, monitoring blood cholesterol levels, and getting regular exercise.

Interestingly, physical activity cuts across most of the issues related to menopause. Physical activity has been demonstrated to help sleep patterns, provide emotional balance, encourage mental acuity, and bolster cardiovascular functioning. Physical activity also makes many people feel better about their bodies and, thus, become potentially more interested in sexual activity that can help maintain vaginal lubrication.

[*]Writing Group for the Women's Health Initiative Investigators. Risks and benefits of estrogen plus progestin in healthy postmenopausal women: principal results from the Women's Health Initiative Randomized Controlled Trial. *Journal of the American Medical Association*, Vol 288: No 3 (July 17, 2002), 321–333.

Genital sexuality reflects our gift to ourselves and to our partners as well. However, many forms of genital sexuality may not be condoned by certain groups of people or religions.

For some, genital sexuality can be a volatile experience. Far too frequently a genitally centered sexual experience results in an unanticipated and unwanted pregnancy. In such circumstances the couple, or more often the female acting alone, is forced to make decisions that could significantly affect the future. An unexpected pregnancy, even for a relatively mature college person, may result in a series of compromises. In addition, the close association between genital sexuality and sexually transmitted diseases (including HIV infection) makes some sexual activities potentially dangerous.

For some people, genital sexuality becomes the mode of communication with which they feel most comfortable. In such cases, partners may know each other only in a very limited way. Growth in sexual technique may readily occur within the context of a genitally centered relationship, but a fully developed relationship will not

be formed. Genitally based relationships are rarely elevated to a much higher level.

Expressionistic Sexuality

Expressionistic sexuality represents the most broadly based dimension of yourself as a man or woman; see the box "Sexuality as a Means of Spiritual Discovery." As the name implies, this is your expression of your current gender schema. Cognitively, *affectively,* and behaviorally, you are playing out your initial adult gender identification. The way you dress, the occupation you pursue, and the leisure activities you develop are all aspects of this dimension of your sexuality.

Expressionistic sexuality encompasses the reproductive and genital dimensions of your sexuality, but it is more. It is the sexuality that will serve you most fully for the rest of your life. Most adults probably are conventional in their patterns of expressionistic sexuality, yet many people also express a variety of additional patterns (see Chapter 15).

Sexuality as a Means of Spiritual Discovery

Few would argue that many of our expressions of sexuality are truly wonderful. For example, the enjoyment we can receive from a warm caress or an intimate kiss can be stimulating beyond imagination. The fact that our biological anatomy can function in ways that make us feel pleasure can be viewed as one of life's most rewarding gifts.

However, expressions of sexuality can extend beyond merely "feeling good." One's sexuality is an experience that encompasses the whole individual. It is much more than a biological act, a means of procreation, or an orgasmic release. While sexuality is all of these things, it also is a means of conveying intimacy to another person. Ultimately, sexuality is a form of intimate communication between two people. Through sexual expressions, one can convey feelings of love, devotion, caring, individuality, and openness. Of course, these feelings can also be communicated in nonsexual ways, but the depth of feelings that comes with sexual intimacy is especially powerful, and it is perhaps driven and enhanced by strong biological forces.

When sexuality is considered from this broader perspective, it can be viewed as a journey into personal understanding. This can evolve into a lifelong spiritual journey that constantly challenges one's values and stances on a variety of sexuality issues. In this spiritual journey, the brain, the body's most powerful sex organ, plays key roles. The brain helps one analyze feelings, moral and religious issues, relationship possibilities, and value stances. The brain also serves to help one learn about sexual communication, sexual technique, and sexual pleasure.

As you read the sexuality material in this unit, you will see that sexuality encompasses the whole person, in a variety of ways and in a variety of circumstances. Sexual expression is much more than just "doing it." For those who think otherwise, remember that "people who are only interested in sex are probably not very interesting people." Look for the ways in which your sexuality is connected to other aspects of your life.

Taking Charge of Your Health

- Take the Personal Assessment at the end of this chapter to determine how traditional or nontraditional your attitudes are toward sexuality.

- If you wish to become more flexible and expand your social skills, identify ways in which you can increase your androgynous behavior. For example, learn to cook, expand your assertiveness skills, do volunteer work with children, join a club sports team, or learn how to invest in the stock market.

- Most college sexuality textbooks encourage readers to become familiar with their external reproductive "body parts." If you believe that this is important, study the illustrations in this chapter, find a handheld mirror, undress, and identify these structures as best you can.

- If you are a woman who has a significant amount of menstrual pain, try some of the treatment suggestions in this chapter.

- If you are a man who is essentially "clueless" about the menstrual cycle and would like to understand it much better, study the information in this chapter. If you have a very close female friend and you wish to validate some of this information, ask her (diplomatically, of course) if you could get her "impressions" of this natural phenomenon.

SUMMARY

- The biological basis of human sexuality includes genetic, gonadal, and structural components.
- The structural basis of sexuality begins as the male and female reproductive structures develop in the growing embryo and fetus. Structural sexuality changes as one moves through adolescence and later life.
- The psychosocial basis of human sexuality includes gender identity, gender preference, gender adoption, and initial adult gender identification.
- Androgyny is the blending of feminine and masculine qualities.
- The male and female reproductive structures are external and internal. The complex functioning of these structures is controlled by hormones.

- The menstrual cycle's primary functions are to produce ova and to develop a supportive environment for the fetus in the uterus.
- Endometriosis is a condition in which endometrial tissue that normally lines the uterus grows within the pelvic cavity, causing pain before and during menstruation and can lead to infertility.
- Fibrocystic breast condition is characterized by swollen, firm, or hardened tender breast tissue before menstruation.
- Postmenopausal hormone therapy has benefits in treating the symptoms of menopause but may carry risks for some women.
- Sexuality can be viewed from reproductive, genital, and expressionistic perspectives.

REVIEW QUESTIONS

1. Describe the following foundations of our biological sexuality: the genetic basis, the gonadal basis, and structural development.
2. Define and explain the following terms: gender identity, gender preference, gender adoption, and initial adult gender identification.
3. Define androgyny and explain its advantages.
4. Identify the major components of the male reproductive system. Trace the passageway for sperm.
5. Identify the major components of the female reproductive system. Trace the passageway for ova.
6. Identify and describe the four main hormones that control the menstrual cycle.
7. What are some of the nondrug techniques for reducing the symptoms of PMS?
8. What are the symptoms of fibrocystic breast condition and endometriosis?
9. Describe the difference between primary and secondary amenorrhea.
10. Name two circumstances in which postmenopausal hormone therapy might be prescribed for women.

ANSWERS TO THE "WHAT DO YOU KNOW?" QUIZ

1. False   2. True   3. False   4. False   5. True   6. False   7. True

ENDNOTES

1. Thibodeau GA, Patton KT. *Anatomy and Physiology* (6th ed.). St. Louis: Mosby, 2006.
2. Sherwood L. *Human Physiology: From Cells to Systems* (5th ed.). Belmont, CA: Brooks/Cole, 2004.
3. Hyde JS, DeLamater JD. *Understanding Human Sexuality* (9th ed.). New York: McGraw-Hill, 2006.
4. Allgeier ER, Allgeier AR. *Sexual Interactions* (5th ed.). New York: Houghton Mifflin, 2000.
5. Crooks R, Baur K. *Our Sexuality* (9th ed.). Belmont, CA: Wadsworth, 2004.
6. Kelly GF. *Sexuality Today: The Human Perspective* (8th ed.). New York: McGraw-Hill, 2006.
7. Carroll JL. *Sexuality Now: Embracing Diversity* (2nd ed.). Belmont, CA: Thomson Higher Learning, 2007.
8. Strong B, DeVault C, Sayad BW, Yarber WL. *Human Sexuality: Diversity in Contemporary America* (5th ed.). New York: McGraw-Hill, 2005.
9. Barclay L. Unisex Hormones? WebMD Medical News Archive, May 4, 2001, www.webmd.com/content/article/32/1728_79051.htm.
10. Schieszer J. Male Menopause Out of the Closet. MSNBC Interactive, October 1, 2006. www.msnbc.msn.com/id/3543479/.
11. Manos A. FDA Approves Gel to Treat Low Testosterone Levels, WebMD Medical News Archive. March 2, 2000. www.mywebmd.com/content/article/22/1728_55404.htm.
12. Hatcher RA, et al. *Contraceptive Technology* (18th ed.). New York: Ardent Media, 2004.
13. Shuman T. Sexual Health: Your Guide to Premenstrual Syndrome, WebMD Content Article, February 2006. www.webmd.com/content/Article/10/2953_497.htm.
14. Premenstrual Syndrome (PMS): Medications, WebMD Original Article. www.webmd.com/hw/womens_conditions/hw139629.asp.
15. Shuman T. Sexual Health: Your Guide to Premenstrual Dysphoric Disorder, WebMD Content Article, February 2006. www.webmd.com/content/Article/10/2953_498.htm.
16. Writing Group for the Women's Health Initiative Investigation. Risks and benefits of estrogen plus progestin in healthy postmenopausal women: Principal results from the Women's Health Initiative Randomized Controlled Trial. *JAMA* 288 (3) (July 17, 2002): 321–333.
17. Hormone therapy is no heart helper. *Harvard Heart Letter*, 13 (2) (October 2002): 2–4.

generally support relationships that are heterosexual in nature. However, this may soon be changing. (See page 452 for information regarding same-sex marriage.)

Homosexuality

Homosexuality (or homosexual orientation) refers to an attraction to same-gender partners. The term *homosexuality* comes from the Greek word *homos,* meaning "the same." The term *gay* can refer to males or females, whereas the word *lesbian* is used only in reference to females.[5]

The distinctions among the categories of sexual orientation are much less clear than their definitions might suggest. Most people probably fall somewhere along a continuum between exclusive heterosexuality and exclusive homosexuality. Kinsey in 1948 presented just such a continuum.[6]

Students often wonder, "What makes a person gay?" This question has no simple answer. (College sexuality textbooks devote entire chapters to this topic.) Some research has pointed to differences in the sizes of certain brain structures as a possible biological or anatomical basis for homosexuality.[7] Other research proposes possible genetic, environmental, hormonal, or other foundations.

Two studies published in 2006 in the *Proceedings of the National Academy of Sciences* support the biological basis for sexual orientation. One study identified different neural pathways that lesbians and nonlesbians use to process pheromone-like stimuli in the hypothalamic region of the brain.[8] The other study examined four groups of Canadian men (944 subjects) and discovered that men with at least several older brothers were more likely to be gay than were men without older brothers or with just one or two older brothers. This effect was seen only in those men whose older brothers had the same biological mother. The effect was not seen in men whose older brothers were stepbrothers or adopted brothers. The lead researcher theorized that there was some unknown prenatal mechanism (perhaps a mother's increasing immune response to male fetuses, a "maternal memory" for male gestations) that caused her to develop anti-male antibodies that altered the brain chemistry and development of her subsequent male fetuses.[9]

However, for sexual orientation in general, no single theory has emerged that fully explains this complex developmental process. The consensus of scientific opinion is that people do not choose their sexual orientation. Thus, being straight or being gay is something that "just happens." Most gays and lesbians report that no specific event "triggered" them into being gay. Many also indicate that they knew that their orientations were different from those of other children as far back as their prepuberty years.

Given the many challenges of being gay in a straight world, it would seem logical that gays and lesbians do not make conscious efforts to become gay. It is also highly unlikely that heterosexual persons actually choose to be straight. Sexual orientation is something that just unfolds. (See the box "Coming Out—Then What?" on page 442 for insight into some of the issues that gays and lesbians need to face.)

Although operational definitions of sexual orientation may vary from researcher to researcher, Kinsey estimated that about 2 percent of American females and 4 percent of American males were exclusively homosexual.[6, 10] More recent estimates place the overall combined figure at about 10 percent of the population. Clearly the expression of same-gender attraction is not uncommon.

The Ultimate Aphrodisiac?

For centuries, people have searched for the ultimate aphrodisiac, a substance that "arouses sexual desire or increases a person's capacity for sexual activities." Cleopatra reportedly used a mixture of honey and almonds to tempt her lovers, Casanova relied on oysters to boost his sexual prowess, and Josephine Bonaparte tried the aroma of violet to improve her seductive powers. Whether these supposed aphrodisiacs actually worked is a matter of speculation.

Almost any food that resembles external male genitals has been thought, at one time or another, to have aphrodisiac properties. Thus, oysters, bananas, celery, potatoes, and tomatoes have been used as aphrodisiacs,* as have raw turtle eggs, goat testicles, and rhubarb.† Some of the more unusual aphrodisiacs include "Spanish fly" (made from the ground-up remains of insects), "Rocky Mountain oysters" (bull testicles), and ground-up rhinoceros or reindeer horns. (Incidentally, ground-up animal horns are the origin of the word *horny*, a slang term that implies a state of elevated sexual arousal.)

There is no research that proves any of these substances actually works as an aphrodisiac. Although there may be some anecdotal reports that these substances (and other natural products, such as ginseng) help humans, there are no valid studies to substantiate any physiological, biochemical benefit to human sexual arousal or performance.†

If any substance seems to help someone sexually, this is probably because the person has high expectations that it will help. The human mind can play powerful games and, in effect, manipulate a person in ways that are not easily explained. If a person thinks a product will work as an aphrodisiac, then it just might. So, if you think it helps your sexual performance, then keep on eating those carrots and cucumbers and enjoying that extra banana on your cold cereal. Even if these fruits and vegetables ultimately don't improve your sex drive or performance, they are nutritious and quite low in calories, and that's good for your health!

Perhaps aphrodisiacs can be viewed in a totally different way. Maybe the ultimate aphrodisiac can be found through the process of creating an environment that is conducive to sexual arousal. For you and your partner, a romantic dinner at a nice restaurant might boost your libidos. (A bouquet of fresh-cut flowers is always appreciated and is a turn-on for many individuals.) Some couples get excited through physical activity or exercise. Perhaps taking a warm bath with someone special, lighting candles by the bedside, or staying in an out-of-town hotel room will recharge your sexual batteries. Even if you never find your ultimate aphrodisiac, you are likely to have a great time searching for it.

*Crooks RL, Baur K. *Our Sexuality*, 9th ed. Belmont, CA: Wadsworth, 2005.
†McAnulty RD, Burnette MM. *Exploring Human Sexuality: Making Healthy Decisions*, 2nd ed. Boston: Allyn and Bacon, 2004.

TALKING POINTS How would you react if a close family member told you that he or she was gay? Could you be supportive or at least communicate your feelings without anger or criticism?

Bisexuality

People who have the ability to be attracted to either gender are referred to as *bisexuals*. Bisexuals may fall into one of three groups: those who are (1) genuinely attracted to both genders, (2) gay but also feel the need to behave heterosexually, or (3) aroused physically by the same gender but attracted emotionally to the opposite gender. Some people participate in a bisexual lifestyle for extended periods, whereas others move quickly to a more exclusive orientation. The size of the bisexual population is not accurately known.[11] (See the box "Challenges for Bisexuals" on page 443 for more information on bisexual men and women.)

Gender Identity Issues

Gender identity refers to the recognition of oneself as a male or female. As noted in Chapter 14, this recognition initially takes place within about 18 months after birth. Most people then move through their lives, adopting many or all of the traditional gender roles for their biological sex. Most feel reasonably comfortable with who they are as a man or a woman.

However, this typical pattern does not occur for everyone: (a) Some individuals are not comfortable with their biological sex. They struggle with the issue of transsexualism. (b) Transgendered people prefer not conforming to society's traditional expectations for their sex. (c) Other individuals are comfortable with their gender identity but find sexual pleasure from dressing in clothes that are more culturally "appropriate" for the opposite gender. These persons engage in transvestism.

Transsexualism

Transsexualism is an uncommon sexual variation in which a person rejects his or her biological sexuality.

> **Key Terms**
>
> **transsexualism** A sexual variation in which a person rejects his or her biological sexuality.

The male transsexual believes that he truly is a "woman trapped in a man's body." He desires to be the woman who he knows he is. Likewise, the female transsexual believes that she is a male existing in a woman's body. She desires to be the man who she knows she is. (Note that sex therapists and psychiatrists do not view transsexuals as homosexual in their sexual orientation.)

For transsexuals, the periods of gender preference and gender adoption (see Chapter 14) are perplexing as they attempt, often with little success, to resolve the conflict between what their mind tells them is true and what their body displays. Adolescent and young adult transsexuals may cross-dress, undertake gay or lesbian relationships (which they view as heterosexual relationships), and experiment with hormone replacement therapy. Sometimes, transsexuals actively pursue a sex reassignment operation. Thousands of these surgeries have been performed at some of the leading medical centers in the United States. For more detailed information about transsexualism, including theories about the origins of transsexualism, you could consult a textbook used in college human sexuality courses or search the Internet for pertinent websites.

Transgenderism

People who are **transgendered** present appearances and personas that do not conform to the gender role expectations that society has established for their sex. Thus, transgendered persons tend to be nonconformists to

traditional sex roles.[12] Transgendered women take on characteristics and mannerisms of men, and transgendered men take on characteristics and mannerisms of women. They might cross-dress on a full- or part-time basis, although they usually do not do this for sexual arousal purposes (as transvestites typically do).

Do transgendered persons differ from transsexuals? Yes, they are two different categories, according to sexuality experts.[12] The main distinction is that transgendered persons do not feel the need to surgically change their bodies to achieve the physical structures of the other sex. Transsexuals feel trapped in an opposite-sex body, and many would like to have their genitals and body appearance be consistent with the "sex they know themselves to be." However, transgendered individuals know and accept the sex to which they were born; yet they prefer to take on and display mannerisms of the other sex.

Transvestism

Public figures such as Dennis Rodman, Eddie Izzard, Harvey Fierstein, and RuPaul have turned a spotlight on cross-dressing, or transvestism. The term **transvestism** is typically used to describe a heterosexual male who, from time to time, dresses as a woman. (Some gay men and women enjoy cross-dressing on occasion.) The practice of transvestism can range from simple sexual gratification from the wearing of feminine clothing, to the expression of the feminine side of the individual's

Learning from Our Diversity

Challenges for Bisexuals

People whose sexual orientation is toward both men and women are termed *bisexuals*. This can be a confusing label, however. For example, if a man has had one sexual experience with a man, but all of his other sexual experiences are with women, does this mean he is a bisexual? And what about the woman who has sequential relationships with men, followed by an occasional relationship with a woman? Is she bisexual? What about people who are sexually attracted to one gender, but are emotionally more attracted to the other gender? The labels can get confusing and can make one wonder about the value of any label describing sexual orientation. This is just one of the many challenges facing bisexual people.

Some experts suggest that bisexuals (those who have had at least one sexual experience with a man and one with a woman) probably outnumber exclusive homosexuals (those who have had sexual experience *only* with persons of their own gender).[*] One might think that this larger group would be better understood by society, but that seems not to be the case. Bisexuals may have a larger field of potential partners, but this benefit may be offset by the difficulty of "fitting" into society.

Heterosexual people, gay males, and lesbians may not view bisexuality as acceptable, believing that the bisexual person is just incapable of making the decision to go one way or the other.[†] They may accuse the bisexual person of wanting the best of both worlds, as if "having it all" (in terms of sexual possibilities and experiences) is an inappropriate,

bad thing. Then there is the issue of telling a new dating partner that you are attracted to both men and women. Some new partners may find this reality a distinct "turnoff."

For these reasons, numerous college and university counseling centers are expanding their outreach programs to include programs for bisexual students. If you are interested, you might check into the offerings of your campus counseling center to see if they provide educational information, support groups, or specialized counseling for bisexual students. Many campuses also have student groups that focus on gay, lesbian, bisexual, and transgendered students.

Interestingly, it appears that more and more bisexual students are "coming out" despite the challenges they may face. Perhaps this has been encouraged by the public pronouncements of bisexuality by well-known movie stars, such as Drew Barrymore.[‡] In the near future, we may find more public acceptance for people who are bisexual. Would you consider increased public acceptance of bisexuality to be a good or bad thing?

[*]Hyde JS, DeLamater JD. *Understanding Human Sexuality*, 9th ed. New York: McGraw-Hill, 2006.
[†]Kelly GF. *Sexuality Today: the Human Perspective*, 8th ed. New York: McGraw-Hill, 2006.
[‡]Celebrity news. *Drew Barrymore*: "*I am bisexual*," http://us.imdb.com/wn?20030717#6, July 23, 2003.

---

personality. Although many transvestites wish to express the feminine aspects of their personality, most are satisfied with their gender role and their biological gender. Many are married and may or may not have shared this aspect of their personality with their partner.

One large study found that typical cross-dressers are virtually indistinguishable from non-cross-dressing men in their personality traits, sexuality, and measures of psychological wellness.[13]

Years ago, psychologists attempted to cure cross-dressers, but today most have recognized that cross-dressing is lifelong and that they can obtain better results by teaching the cross-dresser to accept his feminine side.

It is rare for a female to be a transvestite, perhaps because the norms for women's clothing are far less restrictive than those for men. For example, while it might be quite normal to see your grandmother wearing a flannel shirt and blue jeans around the house, it would be surprising for you to see your grandfather watching NFL football wearing a frilly negligee.

Some people do not conform to the gender-role expectations that society has established for their sex.

Key Terms

transgendered Refers to persons whose appearance and behaviors do not conform to society's traditional gender role expectations.

transvestism A typical behavior in which a person derives sexual pleasure from dressing in the clothes of the opposite gender.

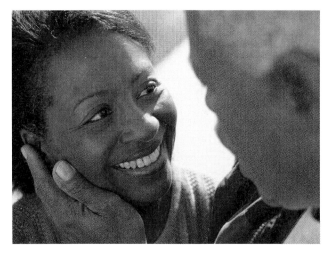

Any sensual contact can be a form of communication and sexual expression between partners.

Patterns of Sexual Behavior

Although sex researchers may see sexual behavior in terms of the human sexual response pattern described earlier, most people are more interested in the observable dimensions of sexual behavior.

Celibacy

Celibacy can be defined as the self-imposed avoidance of sexual intimacy. Celibacy is synonymous with sexual abstinence. People could choose not to have a sexually intimate relationship for many reasons. For some, celibacy is part of a religious doctrine. Others might be afraid of contracting a sexually transmitted disease. For most, however, celibacy is preferred simply because it seems appropriate for them. Celibate people can certainly have deep, intimate relationships with other people—just not sexual relationships. Celibacy may be short term or last a lifetime, and no identified physical or psychological complications appear to result from a celibate lifestyle.

 TALKING POINTS You have decided to remain celibate until you are ready to make a lifetime commitment to someone. How would you explain this to the person you are now dating?

Masturbation

Throughout recorded history, **masturbation** has been a primary method of achieving sexual pleasure. Through masturbation, people can explore their sexual response patterns. Traditionally, some societies and religious groups have condemned this behavior based on the belief that intercourse is the only "right" sexual behavior. With sufficient lubrication, masturbation cannot do physical harm. Today masturbation is considered by most sex therapists and researchers to be a normal source of self-pleasure.

Fantasy and Erotic Dreams

The brain is the most sensual organ in the body. In fact, many sexuality experts classify **sexual fantasies** and **erotic dreams** as forms of sexual behavior. Particularly for people whose verbal ability is highly developed, the ability to create imaginary scenes enriches other forms of sexual behavior.

Sexual fantasies are generally found in association with some second type of sexual behavior. When occurring before intercourse or masturbation, fantasies prepare a person for the behavior that will follow. As an example, fantasies experienced while reading a book may focus your attention on sexual activity that will occur later in the day.

When fantasies occur with another form of sexual behavior, the second behavior may be greatly enhanced by the supportive fantasy. Both women and men fantasize during foreplay and intercourse. Masturbation and fantasizing are inseparable activities.

Erotic dreams occur during sleep in both men and women. The association between these dreams and ejaculation resulting in a nocturnal emission (wet dream) is readily recognized in men. In women, erotic dreams can lead not only to vaginal lubrication but to orgasm as well.

Shared Touching

Virtually the entire body can be an erogenous zone when sensual contact between partners is involved. A soft, light touch, a slight application of pressure, the brushing back of a partner's hair, and gentle massage are all forms of communication that heighten sexual arousal.

Genital Contact

Two important purposes can be identified for the practice of stimulating a partner's genitals. The first is the tactile component of **foreplay.** Genital contact, in the form of holding, rubbing, or caressing, heightens arousal to a level that allows for progression into intercourse.

The second role of genital contact is that of *mutual masturbation to orgasm.* Stimulation of the genitals so that both partners have orgasm is a form of sexual behavior practiced by many people, as well as by couples during the late stage of a pregnancy. For couples not desiring pregnancy, the risk of conception is virtually eliminated when this becomes the form of sexual intimacy practiced.

As is the case in other aspects of intimacy, genital stimulation is best enhanced when partners can talk about their needs, expectations, and reservations. Practice and communication can shape this form of contact into a pleasure-giving approach to sexual intimacy.

Oral-Genital Stimulation

Oral-genital stimulation brings together two of the body's most erogenous areas: the genitalia and the mouth. Couples who engage in oral sex consistently report that this form of intimacy is highly satisfactory. Some people have experimented with oral sex and found it unacceptable, and some have never experienced this form of sexual intimacy. Some couples prefer not to participate in oral sex because they consider it immoral (according to religious doctrine), illegal (which it is in some states), or unhygienic (because of a partner's unclean genitals). Some couples may refrain because of the mistaken belief that oral sex is only for gays and lesbians. Regardless of the reason, a person who does not consider oral sex to be pleasurable should not be coerced into this behavior.

Because oral-genital stimulation can involve an exchange of body fluids, the risk of disease transmission is real. Small tears in mouth or genital tissue may allow transmission of disease-causing pathogens. Only couples who are absolutely certain that they are free from all sexually transmitted diseases (including HIV infection) can practice unprotected oral sex. Couples in doubt should refrain from oral-genital sex or carefully use a condom (on the male) or a latex square to cover the female's vulval area. Increasingly, latex squares (dental dams) can be obtained from drugstores or pharmacies. (Dentists may also provide you with dental dams, or you can make your own latex square by cutting a condom into an appropriate shape.)

Three basic forms of oral-genital stimulation are practiced by both heterosexual and homosexual couples.[12] **Fellatio,** in which the penis is kissed, licked, or sucked by the partner, is the most common of the three. **Cunnilingus,** in which the vulva of the female is kissed, licked, or penetrated by the partner's tongue, is only slightly less frequently practiced.

Mutual oral-genital stimulation, the third form of oral-genital stimulation, combines both fellatio and cunnilingus. When practiced by a heterosexual couple, the female partner performs fellatio on her partner while her male partner performs cunnilingus on her. Gay couples can practice mutual fellatio or cunnilingus.

Intercourse

Sexual intercourse (coitus) refers to the act of inserting the penis into the vagina. Intercourse is the sexual behavior that is most directly associated with **procreation.** For some, intercourse is the only natural and appropriate form of sexual intimacy.

The incidence and frequency of sexual intercourse is a much-studied topic. Information concerning the percentages of people who have engaged in intercourse is readily available in textbooks used in sexuality courses. Data concerning sexual intercourse among college students may be changing somewhat because of concerns about HIV infection and other STDs, but a reasonable estimate of the percentage of college students who have engaged in sexual intercourse is 60–75 percent.

These percentages reflect two important concepts about the sexual activity of college students. The first is that most college students are having intercourse. The second concept is that a large percentage (25–40 percent) of students are choosing to refrain from intercourse. Indeed, the belief that "everyone is doing it" may be a bit shortsighted. From a public health standpoint, we believe it is important to provide accurate health information to protect those who choose to have intercourse and to actively support a person's right to choose not to have intercourse.

Sexually active couples need to share their expectations concerning techniques and the desired frequency of intercourse. Even the "performance" factors, such as depth of penetration, nature of body movements, tempo of activity, and timing of orgasm are increasingly important to many couples. Issues concerning sexually transmitted diseases (including HIV infection) are also critically important for couples who are contemplating intercourse. These factors also need to be explored through open communication.

A variety of books (including textbooks) provide written and visually explicit information on intercourse positions. Four basic positions for intercourse—*man above, woman above, side by side*, and *rear entry*—each offer relative advantages and disadvantages.

Anal Sexual Activity

Some couples practice **anal intercourse,** in which the penis is inserted into the rectum of a partner. Anal

> ### Key Terms
>
> **masturbation** Self-stimulation of the genitals.
>
> **sexual fantasies** Fantasies with sexual themes; sexual daydreams or imaginary events.
>
> **erotic dreams** Dreams whose contents elicit a sexual response.
>
> **foreplay** Activities, often involving touching and caressing, that prepare individuals for sexual intercourse.
>
> **fellatio** (feh **lay** she oh) Oral stimulation of the penis.
>
> **cunnilingus** (cun uh **ling** gus) Oral stimulation of the vulva or clitoris.
>
> **procreation** Reproduction.
>
> **anal intercourse** A sexual act in which the erect penis is inserted into the rectum of a partner.

intercourse can be performed by both heterosexual couples and gay men. According to a recent report in the journal *Archives of Sexual Behavior,* about 20–25 percent of college students have experienced anal intercourse.[14] The anal sphincter muscles contract tightly and tend to resist entry. Thus, couples who engage in anal intercourse must do so slowly, gently, and with adequate amounts of water-based lubricants. Because of the danger of tearing tissues in the rectal area, HIV transmission risk is increased if the inserting male is infected.[3] Unless it is absolutely certain that both partners are uninfected, the inserting male should always wear a condom. Even with a condom, disease transmission is possible, since during anal intercourse, condoms are more likely to tear than during penis-vaginal intercourse. Couples practicing anal sex must not follow anal insertion with insertion into the mouth or vagina because of the likelihood of transmitting infectious agents.

For many people, anal intercourse is not only unpleasant, but simply unnatural for humans. For others, the anal area is just another part of the human body that is especially sensitive to stimulation, and they enjoy the pleasurable sensations that come from intercourse or the insertion of a well-lubricated finger or sex toy. Some people enjoy kissing ("rimming") or touching in the anal area, but this should occur only when the anal area has been fully cleansed or covered with a sheet of protective plastic wrap. As with all sexual behavior, couples need to communicate clearly their feelings about any activity. If one partner is uncomfortable about an activity and wants to stop, his or her feelings must be supported by the other person. A desire for a particular sexual activity must not turn into sexual coercion or a sexual assault.

Until recently, thirteen states had laws on the books that banned **sodomy** (another term for anal sex as well as certain other sexual practices). However, a U.S. Supreme Court ruling (*Lawrence and Garner v. Texas*) in June 2003 invalidated a Texas law that banned private consensual sex (in this case, sodomy) between adults of the same sex. This Texas ruling invalidated the laws of the 12 other states that banned sodomy in one form or another.[3]

Secondary Virginity

Some individuals who have previously engaged in sexual intercourse have chosen to refrain from further sexual

---

Key Terms
sodomy Generally refers to anal or oral sex; a legal term whose definition varies from state to state.
secondary virginity The discontinuation of sexual intercourse after initial exploration.

---

intercourse. They are said to be practicing **secondary virginity.** The practice of secondary virginity reflects a conscious choice for persons to wait until a time when they feel it's all right to resume intercourse.

The decision to be a secondary virgin can be made for a number of reasons. Some prefer to return to abstinence for moral or religious reasons, while others wish to wait until there is more commitment in the relationship. Some come to the realization that they are not yet physically or emotionally ready for intercourse. Others do not want to risk pregnancy or the possibility of contracting a sexually transmitted disease. Some do not have the time or energy needed to become involved in a sexual relationship.

Those who choose secondary virginity are quick to point out its advantages. They no longer worry about certain risks, such as pregnancy or developing an STD. They no longer have to worry about the expense of contraception or the side effects from certain forms of birth control. Some feel great relief knowing that they are successfully following their own moral compass or religious beliefs. By pursuing secondary virginity, they can focus a great deal more time and energy on other important aspects of their relationship.

Sexuality and Aging

Students are often curious about how aging affects sexuality. This is understandable because we live in a society that idolizes youth and demands performance. Many younger people become anxious about growing older because of what they think will happen to their ability to express their sexuality. Interestingly, young adults are willing to accept other physical changes of aging (such as the slowing down of basal metabolism, reduced lung capacity, and even wrinkles) but not those changes related to sexuality.

Research shows that, although sexual activity does decline with age, the capacity to enjoy sex is not altered, and a significant proportion of older adults remain sexually active.[4]

As with other aspects of aging, certain anatomical and physiological changes will be evident, but these changes do not necessarily reduce the ability to enjoy sexual activity. Most experts in sexuality report that many older people remain interested in sexual activity. Furthermore, those who are exposed to regular sexual activity throughout a lifetime report being most satisfied with their sex lives as older adults.[12]

As people age, the likelihood of alterations in the male and female sexual response patterns increases. In the postmenopausal woman, vaginal lubrication commonly begins more slowly, and the amount of lubrication usually diminishes. However, clitoral sensitivity and nipple erection remain the same as in earlier years. The female capacity for multiple orgasms remains the same, although the number of contractions that occur at orgasm typically is reduced.

In the older man, physical changes are also evident. This is thought to be caused by the decrease in the production of testosterone between the ages of 20 and 60 years. After age 60 or so, testosterone levels remain relatively steady. Thus many men, despite a decrease in sperm production, remain fertile into their 80s.[12] Older men typically take longer to achieve an erection (however, they are able to maintain their erection longer before ejaculation), have fewer muscular contractions at orgasm, and ejaculate less forcefully than they once did. The volume of seminal fluid ejaculated is typically less than in earlier years, and its consistency is somewhat thinner. The resolution phase is usually longer in older men. In spite of these gradual changes, some elderly men engage in sexual intercourse with the same frequency as do much younger men.

Bonds between People

As people develop their relationships, they often form bonds that start with friendship and dating activities and then move toward intimacy and love. Let's explore these stepping stones.

Friendship

One of the exciting aspects of college life is that you will probably meet many new people, some of whom will become your best friends. Because of your common experiences, it is likely that you will keep in contact with a few of these friends for a lifetime. Close attachments to other people can have an important influence on all of the dimensions of your health.

What is it that draws friends together? With the exception of physical intimacy, many of the same growth experiences seen in dating and mate selection are also seen in the development of friendships. Think about how you and your best friend developed the relationship you now have. You probably became friends when you shared similar interests and experiences. Your friendship progressed (and even faltered at times) through personal gains or losses. In all likelihood, you cared about each other and learned to share your deepest beliefs and feelings. You cemented your bond by turning your beliefs into behaviors. You resolved conflicts (see the box "Resolving Conflict through Better Communication").

Throughout the development of a deep friendship, the qualities of trust, tolerance, empathy, and support must be demonstrated. Otherwise the friendship can fall apart. You will soon note that the qualities seen in a friendship are very similar to the qualities noted in the upcoming description of companionate love (page 448). In both cases, people develop deep attachments through extensive familiarity and understanding.

Resolving Conflict through Better Communication

Every relationship presents challenges to the individuals involved. Therapists would argue that couples who can learn to resolve conflict effectively have the best chance of maintaining long-term relationships. The hallmark of effective conflict resolution is that each person ends up feeling respected by his or her partner. Not surprisingly, this process is built on effective communication.

Here are some successful ways to communicate better to manage conflict:

- Show mutual respect. Remain calm.
- Identify and resolve the real issue.
- Be a good listener.
- Seek areas of agreement.
- Do not interrupt.
- Mutually participate in decision making.
- Be cooperative and specific.
- Focus on the present and future—not the past.
- Don't try to assign blame.
- Say what you are thinking and feeling.
- When talking, use sentences that begin with "I."
- Avoid using sentences that start with "You" or "Why."
- Set a time limit for discussing problems.
- Accept responsibility.
- Do something fun together.

Dating

A half-century ago, the events involved in a dating relationship were somewhat predictable. People met each other through their daily activities or groups of friends, and a formal request for a date was made. Ninety-nine times out of a hundred, the requestor was male and the invitee was female. After a period of formal and informal dates, the two made a commitment to steady dating or decided to "date around." If the relationship progressed, further commitments were made (for example, letter jackets, class rings, or other jewelry items were exchanged). After months or years of a committed relationship, the couple decided to get married. The man invariably asked for the woman's "hand" (after first receiving permission from her parents), and plans for a wedding ceremony were made.

Does this form of dating and mate selection exist now in the new millennium? For some couples, yes. The traditional way of dating and selecting a life partner works well for them. However, many young and midlife adults prefer a more flexible, less predictable format for

Passive-Congenial Marriage Passive means a low level of commitment or involvement, and the word *congenial* suggests warmth and friendliness. When these two words are combined as they are in *passive-congenial marriage,* they describe perfectly the type of marital relationship sought by some couples.

For some of today's young professionals, the passive-congenial marriage offers a safe harbor from the rigors encountered in the competitive world of corporate business. Children may not be valued "commodities" in the passive-congenial marriage. The added financial and personal stressors related to child rearing could compromise an established lifestyle. You may be able to construct an image of a passive-congenial couple if you can picture two people meeting after work for a quiet dinner at a small restaurant, talking in muffled tones about their corporate battles, and planning their winter cruise.

Maintaining a passive-congenial marriage requires less time and energy than do other forms of marriage. For two people who feel certain that their major contributions to society will be made through their efforts in the workplace, this marriage may be ideal. Certainly you may know many couples who are choosing this increasingly popular form of marriage.

Total Marriage In the *total marriage,* little remains of the unique identities the two people had before their marriage took place. For reasons that are probably lost to the subconscious mind, two people possessing individual personalities use marriage to fuse their identities into one identity—the total pair.

The total marriage requires that the individual partners set aside all aspirations for individual growth and development. Decisions are not made with "me" or even "you" as the center of attention. Rather, energies are directed toward what is best for "us." Life outside the marital relationship and partner's presence does not exist, at least figuratively speaking. Eventually outsiders, when speaking about these individuals, can no longer truly speak about the man or the woman but are limited to speaking about the couple.

Vital Marriage The *vital marriage* is intended to serve as an arena for the growth of both the individuals and the pair. The partners focus on "my growth," "your growth," and "our growth." In a vital marriage, personal goals may at times be subordinated for the good of the partner or the paired relationship. Yet both the partners (and the children) know that those once-subordinated goals will assume top priority when this becomes possible and desirable. The relationship has equality of opportunity.

In describing the vital marriage, we must point out that this type of marital relationship is not perfect, nor is it appropriate for all couples. In today's complex society, the vital marriage may be especially difficult to maintain.

Divorce

Marriages, like many other kinds of interpersonal relationships, can end. Today, marriages—relationships begun with the intent of permanence "until death do us part"—end through divorce nearly as frequently as not.

Why should approximately half of marital relationships end? Unfortunately, marriage experts cannot provide one clear answer to this question. Rather, they suggest that divorce is a reflection of unfulfilled expectations for marriage on the part of one or both partners, including the following:

- The belief that marriage will ease your need to deal with your own faults and that your failures can be shared by your partner
- The belief that marriage will change faults that you know exist in your partner
- The belief that the high level of romance of your dating and courtship period will be continued through marriage
- The belief that marriage can provide you with an arena for the development of your personal power, and that once married, you will not need to compromise with your partner
- The belief that your marital partner will be successful in meeting all of your needs

If these expectations seem to be ones you anticipate through marriage, then you may find that disappointments will abound. To varying degrees, marriage is a partnership that requires much cooperation and compromise. Marriage can be complicated. Because of the high expectations that many people hold for marriage, the termination of marriage can be an emotionally difficult process to undertake (see the box "Coping with a Breakup").

The American attitude toward divorce swung like a pendulum during the last century. Divorce has gone from being an embarrassing, painful ordeal, to a common, relatively simple legal procedure. More recently, some observers have begun to question the wisdom of no-fault divorce.

Our society is concerned about the well-being of children whose parents divorce. Different factors, however, influence the extent to which divorce affects children. Included among these factors are the gender and age of the children, custody arrangements, financial support, and the remarriage of one or both parents. Many children must adjust to accept their new status as a member of a blended family.

Singlehood

For many people, being single is a lifestyle that affords the potential for pursuing intimacy, if desired, and provides an uncluttered path for independence and self-directedness. Other people, however, are single because of divorce, separation, death, or the absence of an opportunity to establish a partnership. The U.S. Census Bureau indicates that 43 percent of women and 40 percent of men over the age of 18 are currently single.[18]

Single people can have many different living arrangements. Some single people live alone and choose not to share a household. Other arrangements for singles include cohabitation, periodic cohabitation, singlehood during the week and cohabitation on the weekends or during vacations, or the platonic sharing of a household with others. For young adults, large percentages of single men and women live with their parents.

Like living arrangements, the sexual intimacy patterns of singles are individually tailored. Some singles practice celibacy, others pursue intimate relationships in a **monogamous** pattern, and others have multiple partners. As in all interpersonal relationships, including marriage, the levels of commitment are as variable as the people involved.

Cohabitation

Cohabitation, or the sharing of living quarters by unmarried people, represents yet another alternative to marriage. According to the U.S. Census Bureau, the number of unmarried, opposite-gender couples living together totals over 4.9 million couples.[18] The number of

reported same gender couples totaled over 700,000 in the year 2003.

Although cohabitation may seem to imply a vision of sexual intimacy between male and female roommates, several forms of shared living arrangements can be viewed as cohabitation. For some couples, cohabitation is only a part-time arrangement for weekends, during summer vacation, or on a variable schedule. In addition, **platonic** cohabitation can exist when a couple shares living quarters but does so without establishing an intimate relationship. Close friends, people of retirement age, and gay couples might all be included in a group called cohabitants.

How well do cohabitation arrangements fare against marriage partnerships in terms of long-term stability? A recent report prepared by the CDC's National Center for Health Statistics[21] indicated that unmarried

---

Key Terms

monogamous (mo **nog** a mus) Paired relationship with one partner.

cohabitation Sharing of a residence by unrelated, unmarried people; living together.

platonic Close association between two people that does not include a sexual relationship.

---

cohabitations are generally less stable than marriages. The probability of a first marriage ending in separation or divorce within 5 years was found to be 20 percent, but the probability of a premarital cohabitation breaking up within 5 years was 49 percent. After 10 years, the probability of a first marriage ending was 33 percent, compared to 62 percent for cohabitations.

Single Parenthood

Unmarried young women continue to become pregnant and then become single parents in this country. In 2004, unmarried mothers accounted for 36 percent of all newborn births in the United States.[22] There is also a significantly different form of single parenthood: the planned entry into single parenthood by older, better educated people, the vast majority of whom are women.

In contrast to the teenaged girl who becomes a single parent through an unwed pregnancy, the more mature woman who desires single parenting has usually planned carefully for the experience. She has explored several important concerns, including questions regarding how she will become pregnant (with or without the knowledge of a male partner or through artificial insemination), the need for a father figure for the child, the effect of single parenting on her social life, and, of course, its effect on her career development. When these questions have been resolved, no legal barriers stand in the way of her becoming a single parent.

A very large number of women and a growing number of men are actively participating in single parenthood as a result of a divorce settlement or separation agreement involving sole or joint custody of children. Increasing numbers of single persons are now adopting children. In the year 2004, single women headed up 8.2 million households with children under the age of 18. In contrast, single men headed up 1.9 million households in the year 2004 with children under the age of 18.[18]

Taking Charge of Your Health

- Take the Personal Assessment at the end of this chapter to learn how compatible you and your partner are.

- If being around someone whose sexual orientation is different from yours makes you feel uncomfortable, focus on getting to know that person better as an individual.

- If you are in an unhealthy relationship, take the first step toward getting out of it through professional counseling or group support.

- If you are in a sexual relationship, communicate your sexual needs to your partner clearly. Encourage him or her to do the same so that you can have a satisfying sex life.

- Consider whether your lifetime plan will include singlehood, marriage, cohabitation, single parenthood, or a gay partnership. Evaluate your current plan in relation to that plan.

SUMMARY

- Men and women share the four stages of sexual response: excitement, plateau, orgasm, and resolution.
- Direct stimulation of the penis and direct or indirect stimulation of the clitoris are the principle avenues toward orgasm.
- The three sexual orientations are heterosexuality, homosexuality, and bisexuality.
- Most sex therapists and researchers consider masturbation to be a normal source of self-pleasure.
- Shared touching, genital contact, oral-genital stimulation, and intercourse are common forms of sexual intimacy.
- Physiological changes may alter the way in which some older people perform sexually.

- Passionate love is gradually replaced by companionate love, which is characterized by deep affection and attachment.
- Although the legality of gay and lesbian marriages continues to be debated, committed relationships between members of the same sex often mimic the dynamics of heterosexual marriages.
- Although most people marry at some time in their lives, other relationships and lifestyles exist, including singlehood, cohabitation, and single parenthood.
- Most relationships can be improved through better communication.

REVIEW QUESTIONS

1. What similarities and differences exist between the sexual response patterns of males and females? Do both women and men experience vasocongestion and myotonia?

2. Explain the differences between heterosexuality, homosexuality, and bisexuality. How common is each of these sexual orientations in our society?

3. What is the general distinction between a transsexual person and a transgendered person?
4. Define celibacy, masturbation, sexual fantasies, erotic dreams, shared touching, genital contact, oral-genital stimulation, and sexual intercourse.
5. What precautions must be considered if a couple decides to engage in anal sexual activity?
6. Identify the physiological changes that occur in men and women as they get older.

7. Identify and describe the five forms of marriage presented in this chapter.
8. What is meant by serial monogamy? What is meant by secondary virginity?
9. What are some differences between passionate love and companionate love?
10. In what ways do gay and lesbian partnerships differ from heterosexual partnerships?

ANSWERS TO THE "WHAT DO YOU KNOW?" QUIZ

1. True   2. False   3. False   4. True   5. False   6. True   7. True

ENDNOTES

1. Masters WH, Johnson VE. *Human Sexual Response.* Philadelphia: Lippincott, Williams & Wilkins, 1966.
2. Strong B, DeVault C, Sayad BW, Yarber WL. *Human Sexuality: Diversity in Contemporary America* (5th ed.). New York: McGraw-Hill, 2005.
3. Hyde JS, DeLamater JD. *Understanding Human Sexuality* (9th ed.). New York: McGraw-Hill, 2006.
4. Carroll JL. *Sexuality Now: Embracing Diversity* (2nd ed.). Belmont, CA: Thomson Higher Education, 2007.
5. Kelly GF. *Sexuality Today: The Human Perspective* (8th ed.). New York: McGraw-Hill, 2006.
6. Kinsey AC, Pomeroy WB, Martin CE. *Sexual Behavior in the Human Male* (reprint). Bloomington: Indiana University Press, 1998.
7. Allen LS, Gorski RA. Sexual orientation and the size of the anterior commisure in the human brain. *Pract Nat Acad Sci USA* 89 (15): 7199–7202. 1992.
8. Berglund H, Lindstrom P, Savic I. Brain response to putative pheromones in lesbian women. *Proceedings of the National Academy of Sciences* 103 (21): 8269–8274. 2006.
9. Bogaert AF. Biological versus nonbiological older brothers and men's sexual orientation. *Proceedings of the National Academy of Sciences* 103 (28): 10771–10774. 2006.
10. Kinsey AC, et al. *Sexual Behavior in the Human Female* (reprint). Bloomington: Indiana University Press, 1998.
11. Masters WH, Johnson VE, Kolodny RC. *Human Sexuality* (5th ed.). Upper Saddle River, NJ: Addison-Wesley, 1997.
12. Crooks RL, Baur K. *Our Sexuality* (9th ed.). Belmont, CA: Wadsworth, 2005.
13. Brown GR, et al. Personality characteristics and sexual functioning of 188 crossdressing men. *J Nervous Mental Dis* 185 (5): 265–273. 1996.
14. Baldwin JI, Baldwin JD. Heterosexual anal intercourse: An understudied, high-risk sexual behavior. *Archives of Sexual Behavior* 29 (4): 357–373. 2000.
15. Health Services at Columbia University. Healthy vs. unhealthy relationships. www.goaskalice.columbia.edu.
16. Health Services at Columbia University. Breaking up can be hard to do. www.goaskalice.columbia.edu.
17. U.S. Census Bureau. Table MS-2: Estimated Median Age at First Marriage, by Sex: 1890 to the Present. *Current Population Survey, March and Annual Social and Economic Supplements, 2005 and earlier.* www.census.gov.
18. U.S. Census Bureau. *Statistical Abstract of the United States: 2006* (125th ed.). Washington DC: U.S. Department of Commerce, 2005.
19. CNN.com. Massachusetts same-sex marriage ban advances. www.cnn.com/2007/POLITICS/01/02/samesex.marriage.ap/index.html.
20. Cuber J, Harroff P. *Sex and the Significant Americans.* New York: Penguin Books, 1965.
21. Bramlett MD, Mosher WD. *Cohabitation, Marriage, Divorce, and Remarriage in the United States.* U.S. Centers for Disease Control and Prevention, National Center for Health Statistics, Vital Health Statistics, 23 (22), 2002.
22. National Center for Health Statistics. Table 10: Nonmarital childbearing by detailed race and Hispanic origin of mother, and maternal age: United States, selected years 1970–2004, *Health: United States, 2006* (PDF, p. 145). www.cdc.gov/nchs/hus.htm.

There's More to Sex Than You Thought

Are you ready for sex? If you're not sure, take time to think it over. If you start having sex before you're ready, you might feel guilty. You might feel bad because you realize this step isn't right for you now. Or your religious upbringing may make you feel as though you're doing something wrong. You also may not be ready for the emotional aspects of a sexual relationship. Most important, you will probably have difficulty handling the complexities of an unplanned pregnancy or a sexually transmitted disease.

If you do feel ready for sex, you still have a choice. Sex may be okay for you now. It may be personally fulfilling, something that enhances your self-esteem. Alternatively, you can choose to abstain from sex until later—another way of enhancing your self-esteem. You'll feel empowered by making the decision for yourself, rather than doing what is expected. Being strong enough to say "no" can also make you feel good about yourself. For some, making this decison may reflect a renewed commitment to spiritual or religious concerns.

If you're married, sex is a good way of connecting as a couple. It's something that the two of you alone share. It's a time to give special attention to each other—taking a break from the kids, your jobs, and your other responsibilities. It's a way of saying: "This relationship is important—it's something I value."

Going through a pregnancy together is another opportunity for closeness. From the moment you know that you're going to be parents, you're connected in a new way. Your focus becomes the expected child. You'll watch the fetus grow on ultrasound, go to parenting and Lamaze classes together, visit the doctor together, mark the various milestones, and share new emotions. When your child is born, you'll be connected as never before.

Whether you're thinking about starting to have sex, making the decision to wait, or examining the sexual life you have now, you can't ignore the possibilities and the consequences. Is the time right for you? Are you doing this for yourself or for someone else? What do you think you will gain from waiting? Do you expect your future partner to also have made the decision to wait? What do you expect to get from a sexual relationship—pleasure, intimacy, love? What do you expect to give? Do you want an emotional commitment? Do you view sex and love as inseparable? Do you understand how sex can enhance your spirituality? Taking time to consider these questions can make you feel good about yourself—no matter what you decide.

Birth Control versus Contraception

Any discussion about the control of your **fertility** should start with an explanation of the subtle differences between the terms **birth control** and **contraception.** These terms reflect different perspectives about fertility control. *Birth control* is an umbrella term that refers to all the procedures you might use to prevent the birth of a child. Birth control includes all available contraceptive measures, as well as sterilization and abortion procedures.

Contraception is a much more specific term for any procedure used to prevent the fertilization of an ovum. Contraceptive measures vary widely in the mechanisms they use to accomplish this task. They also vary considerably in their method of use and their rate of success in preventing conception. A few examples of contraceptives are condoms, hormonal contraceptives, spermicides, and diaphragms.

Beyond the methods mentioned, certain forms of sexual behavior not involving intercourse could be considered forms of contraception. For example, mutual masturbation by couples virtually eliminates the possibility of pregnancy. This practice, as well as additional forms of sexual expression other than intercourse (such as kissing, touching, and massage), has been given the generic term **outercourse.** Outercourse protects against unplanned pregnancy and may also significantly reduce the transmission of sexually transmitted diseases,

including HIV infection (see the box "There's More to Sex Than You Thought").

Reasons for Choosing to Use Birth Control

People use birth control for many reasons. Many career-minded individuals carefully plan the timing and spacing of children to best provide for their children's financial support without sacrificing their job status. Others choose methods of birth control to ensure that they will never have children. Some use birth control methods to permit safe participation in a wide variety of sexual behaviors. Fear of contracting a sexually transmitted disease prompts some people to use particular forms of birth control (see the box "Discussing Birth Control with Your Partner").

Financial and legal considerations can be significant factors in the choice of certain birth control methods. Many people must of necessity take the cost of a method into account when selecting appropriate birth control. The cost of sterilization and abortion can prohibit some low-income people from choosing these alternatives, especially because federal funds do not support such procedures. A number of states have established statutes and policies that make contraceptive information and medical services relatively difficult to obtain.

Discussing Birth Control with Your Partner

I have a new girlfriend and I think we are moving closer and closer to having sex. I know we should talk about birth control and disease prevention, but I don't know how to start. What should I do?

If you believe there is even a chance you will engage in any kind of sex, or if you think your partner may pursue sex with you, you should be prepared and discuss the possibility before being swept along by the heat of an encounter. In addition, you and your partner will feel more comfortable about your relationship and your sexual activity if you first discuss your feelings about contraception, disease prevention, and pregnancy. Consider the following topics:

- First, the fact that you are discussing contraception together does not necessarily mean that you will engage in sex. In addition, you can discuss abstinence as a very effective form of contraception.
- Discussing contraception and disease prevention with your partner is not rude. It is simply common sense.
- Talking about contraception is a way of sharing responsibility and intimacy. It can bring you closer.
- Which type(s) of contraception will you use? See the section "Selecting Your Contraceptive Method" for help in making your choices.

- If you feel unsure about how to broach the subject or are undecided about any of the issues, consider discussing the subject with a counselor or physician before you talk with your partner.
- Sort out your own feelings and understand all the alternatives, including their advantages and disadvantages, before you open the discussion.
- Pick the right occasion. Don't wait until you have begun sexual activity.
- Both partners have dignity and worth, and should be treated with dignity. If you and your boyfriend or girlfriend are discussing contraception and you have different views, you each have the right to your opinions. If necessary, you can agree to disagree.
- Listen carefully and ask questions. Speak honestly about your own feelings and beliefs.
- Who will pay for the contraceptive method? Will both partners share the cost?
- What will both of you do if the female partner becomes pregnant?

Have you discussed these issues in the past before initiating sex with a partner? Do you plan to discuss these issues in the future?

Another important consideration in the use of birth control methods is the availability of professional services. An example of the effect of this factor may be the selection of birth control methods by college students. Some colleges and universities provide contraceptive services through their student health centers. Students enrolled in these schools have easy access to low-cost, comprehensive contraceptive services. Students enrolled in colleges that do not provide such complete services may find that access to accurate information and clinical services is difficult to obtain and that private professional services are expensive.

For many people, religious doctrine will be a factor in their selection of a birth control method. One example is the opposition of the Roman Catholic Church and other religious groups to the use of contraception other than periodic abstinence.

Theoretical Effectiveness versus Use Effectiveness

People considering the use of a contraceptive method need to understand the difference between the two effectiveness rates given for each form of contraception. *Theoretical effectiveness* is a measure of a contraceptive method's ability to prevent a pregnancy when the method is used precisely as directed during every act of intercourse. *Use effectiveness,* however, refers to the effectiveness of a method in preventing conception when used by the general public. Use effectiveness rates take into account factors that lower effectiveness below that based on "perfect" use. Failure to follow proper instructions, illness of the user, forgetfulness, physician (or pharmacist) error, and a subconscious desire to experience risk or even pregnancy are a few of the factors that can lower the effectiveness of even the most theoretically effective contraceptive technique.

Effectiveness rates are often expressed as the percentage of women users of childbearing age who do not become pregnant while using the method for one year. For some methods the theoretical-effectiveness and

---

Key Terms

fertility The ability to reproduce.

birth control All the methods and procedures that can prevent the birth of a child.

contraception Any method or procedure that prevents fertilization.

outercourse Sexual activity that does not involve intercourse.

Table 16.1 Effectiveness Rates of Birth Control for 100 Women during the First Year of Use

Method	Estimated Effectiveness		Advantages	Disadvantages
	Theoretical	Use		
No method (chance)	15%	15%	Inexpensive	Totally ineffective
Withdrawal	96%	73%	No supplies or advance preparation needed; no side effects; men share responsibility for family planning	Interferes with coitus; very difficult to use effectively; women must trust men to withdraw as orgasm approaches
Periodic abstinence	91%–99%	75%	No supplies needed; no side effects; men share responsibility for family planning; women learn about their bodies	Difficult to use, especially if menstrual cycles are irregular, as is common in women; abstinence may be necessary for long periods; lengthy instruction and ongoing counseling may be needed
Spermicide (gel, foam, suppository, film)	82%	71%	No health risks; can be used with condoms to increase effectiveness considerably	Must be inserted 5 to 30 minutes before coitus; effective for only 30 to 60 minutes; some concern about nonoxynol-9
Diaphragm	94%	84%	No major health risks, easily carried in purse, can be used during breast-feeding, no impact on a woman's hormones, usually cannot be felt by either partner	Cannot be used during menstruation; must be left in place for at least 6 hours after coitus; must be fitted by clinician; some women may find it awkward or embarrassing to use; some concern about nonoxynol-9
FemCap (no previous births) (previous births)	? ?	86% 71%	No major health risks, easily carried in purse, can be used during breast-feeding, no impact on a woman's hormones, usually cannot be felt by either partner	Similar to diaphragm disadvantages above
Lea's Shield	?	85%	No major health risks, easily carried in purse, can be used during breast-feeding, no impact on a woman's hormones, usually cannot be felt by either partner	Similar to diaphragm disadvantages above; must be left in place at least 8 hours after last intercourse
Sponge (no previous births) (previous births)	91% 80%	84% 68%	Easy to use; not messy; protection is good for 24 hours and multiple acts of intercourse; no prescription required	Not reusable; contraceptive protection is reduced for women with previous births; some concern about nonoxynol-9
Male condom	98%	85%	Easy to use; inexpensive and easy to obtain; no health risks; very effective protection against some STDs; men share responsibility for family planning	Must be put on just before coitus; some men and women complain of decreased sensation; some concern about nonoxynol-9
Male condom with spermicide	99%	95%		
Female condom	95%	79%	Relatively easy to use; no prescription required; polyurethane is stronger than latex; provides some STD protection; silicone-based lubrication provided; useful when male will not use a condom	Contraceptive effectiveness and STD protection not as high as with male condom; couples may be unfamiliar with a device that extends outside the vagina; more expensive than male condoms

continued

use-effectiveness rates are vastly different; the theoretical rate is always higher than the use rate. Table 16.1 presents data concerning estimated effectiveness rates, advantages, and disadvantages of many birth control methods.

Selecting Your Contraceptive Method

In this section, we discuss some of the many factors that should be important to you as you consider selecting a contraceptive method. Completing the Personal Assessment at the end of this chapter will help you to make this decision.

Those who wish to exercise a large measure of control over their fertility can consider the following:

- It should be safe.
- It should be effective.
- It should be reliable.
- It should be reversible.
- It should be affordable.
- It should be easy to use.
- It should not interfere with sexual expression.

Table 16.1 Continued

| Method | Estimated Effectiveness | | Advantages | Disadvantages |
	Theoretical	Use		
IUD ParaGard (copper T) Mirena (progestin)	99%+ 99%+	99%+ 99%+	Easy to use; highly effective in preventing pregnancy; does not interfere with coitus; repeated action not needed	May increase risk of pelvic infection and infertility in a very small percentage of women; not usually recommended for women who have never had a child; must be inserted by health care personnel; may cause heavy bleeding and pain in some women
Combined pill (estrogen + progestin) Minipill (progestin only)	99%+ 99%+	92%+ 92%+	Easy to use; highly effective in preventing pregnancy; does not interfere with coitus; regulates menstrual cycle; reduces heavy bleeding and menstrual pain; helps protect against ovarian and endometrial cancer	Must be taken every day; requires medical examination and prescription; minor side effects such as nausea or menstrual spotting; possibility of cardiovascular problems in a small percentage of users
Contraceptive ring (estrogen + progestin)	99%+	92%+	Easy to use after learning how to insert; remains in place 3 weeks	Like other hormonal methods, does not protect against STDs; requires physician prescription; possibility of cardiovascular problems in a small percentage of users
Contraceptive patch (estrogen + progestin)	99%+	92%+	Easy to apply; must change weekly for 3 weeks	No STD protection; requires physician prescription; possibility of cardiovascular problems in a small percentage of users
Depo-Provera	99%+	97%+	Easy to use; highly effective for 3-month period; continued use prevents menstruation	Requires supervision by a physician; administered by injection; some women experience irregular menstrual spotting in early months of use
Contraceptive implant	(99%+ estimated)	?	Easy to use; protection is good for 3 years; progestin only; can be used while breast-feeding; no medicine to take daily	No STD protection; requires physician to insert or remove; may cause temporary irregular bleeding; possibility of cardiovascular problems in a small percentage of users
Tubal ligation	99%+	99%+	Permanent; removes fear of pregnancy	Surgery-related risks; generally considered irreversible
Vasectomy	99%+	99%+	Permanent; removes fear of pregnancy	Generally considered irreversible

Source: Adapted from Hatcher RA, et al. *Contraceptive Technology*, 18th ed. New York: Ardent Media, 2004; and Planned Parenthood Federation of America. *Birth Control.* www.plannedparenthood.org.

TALKING POINTS The method of birth control your partner prefers doesn't allow for spontaneous sex. How would you explain that this decreases your enjoyment?

Behavioral Contraceptive Methods

The first contraceptives we'll discuss are those that are based on the sexual behavior of a couple. As with all approaches to contraception, a clear understanding of each method can help you make decisions about sexual activity and birth control that are right for you. For guidelines on locating accurate information on the Web, see the box "Information Online—Birth Control and Sexuality."

Abstinence

Abstinence as a form of birth control has gained attention recently on college campuses. This method is as close to 100 percent effective as possible. There have been isolated reports in medical literature of pregnancy without sexual intercourse, usually involving ejaculation by the male near the woman's vagina. Avoiding this situation should raise the effectiveness of abstinence to 100 percent.

Abstinence as a form of birth control has additional advantages in that it gives nearly 100 percent protection from sexually transmitted diseases, it is free, and it does not require a visit to a physician.

However, some concerns exist about the effectiveness of educational programs that encourage abstinence. In a study of 12,000 adolescents published in 2005, Yale and Columbia University researchers found that teenagers who "pledged virginity until marriage" were more likely to participate in oral sex and anal sex than were nonpledging teens who had not had sexual intercourse. (Both oral and anal sex carry risks of STD transmission.) Additionally, the researchers found that teens who pledged abstinence were less likely to use condoms during their first sexual intercourse and less likely to be tested for STDs than were nonpledging teens.[1] Abstinence works effectively only when it is broadly defined (to include many sexual behaviors) and used correctly and consistently. Abstinence is a challenging proposition for many adolescents and young adults.

Withdrawal

Withdrawal, or **coitus interruptus,** is the contraceptive practice in which the erect penis is removed from the vagina just before ejaculation of semen. Theoretically, this procedure prevents sperm from entering the deeper structures of the female reproductive system. The use effectiveness of this method, however, reflects how unsuccessful the method is in practice (see Table 16.1).

Strong evidence suggests that the clear preejaculate fluid that helps neutralize and lubricate the male urethra can contain *viable* (capable of fertilization) sperm.[2] This sperm can be deposited near the cervical opening before withdrawal, which explains the relatively low effectiveness of this method. Furthermore, withdrawal does not protect users from the transmission of sexually transmitted diseases (STDs). It should never be considered a reliable contraceptive approach.

Periodic Abstinence

Five approaches are included in the birth control strategy called **periodic abstinence:** (1) the calendar method, (2) the Standard Days method, (3) the basal body temperature (BBT) method, (4) the Billings cervical mucus method, and (5) the symptothermal method.[3] All five methods attempt to determine the time a woman ovulates. Figure 16-1 shows a day-to-day fertility calendar that reflects a woman's fertile period. Most research indicates that an ovum is viable for only about 24–36 hours after its release from the ovary. (After they are inside the female reproductive tract, some sperm can survive up to a week.) When a woman can accurately determine when she ovulates, she must refrain from intercourse long enough for the ovum to begin to disintegrate. Fertility awareness, rhythm, natural birth control, and natural family planning are other terms for periodic abstinence. Remember that periodic abstinence methods *do not*

Figure 16-1 Periodic Abstinence These methods try to pinpoint when a woman is most likely to ovulate. Remember that most women's cycles are not consistently perfect 28-day cycles like those shown in most illustrations.

In the figure, the days of the menstrual cycle (1–28) are labeled along the left side, with the following annotations:

- Menstruation—relatively safe for sexual intercourse
- Sperm deposited during these days may remain viable at ovulation
- Unprotected intercourse should not occur
- Ovulation
- Unprotected intercourse should not occur
- Ovum may remain viable through this point
- Relatively safe for unprotected intercourse

Label on far left: Days of menstrual cycle

provide protection against the spread of STDs, including HIV infection.

Periodic abstinence is the only contraceptive method endorsed by the Roman Catholic Church. For some people who have deep concerns for the spiritual dimension of their health, selecting a method other than periodic abstinence may entail a serious compromise of beliefs.

The **calendar method** requires close examination of a woman's menstrual cycle for the last 6–12 cycles. Records are kept of the length (in days) of each cycle. A *cycle* is defined as the number of days from the first day of bleeding of one cycle to the first day of bleeding of the next cycle.

To determine the days she should abstain from intercourse, a woman should subtract 18 from her shortest cycle; this is the first day she should abstain from intercourse. Then she should subtract 11 from her longest cycle; this is the last day she must abstain from intercourse (see the box "Determining Your Cycle").[4]

The *basal body temperature method* requires a woman (for about three or four successive months) to take her body temperature every morning before she rises from bed. A finely calibrated thermometer, available in many drugstores, is used for this purpose. The theory behind this method is that there is a distinct correlation between body temperature and the process of ovulation. Around the time of ovulation, the body temperature rises at least

0.4 degrees F and remains elevated until the start of menstruation. The woman is instructed to refrain from intercourse during the interval when the temperature change takes place.

Drawbacks of this procedure include the need for consistent, accurate temperature readings and the realization that all women's bodies are different. Some women may not fit the temperature pattern projection because of biochemical differences in their bodies. In addition, body temperature can fluctuate. Temperature kits cost about $5–$8 in drugstores.

The newest periodic abstinence approach is called the *Standard Days method*. This method is appropriate only for women who have menstrual cycles that are consistently between 26 and 32 days long. It is not to be used by women who have variable cycles that are shorter than 26 days or longer than 32 days. Having had just one

Key Terms

withdrawal (coitus interruptus) (co ih tus in ter **rup** tus) A contraceptive practice in which the erect penis is removed from the vagina before ejaculation.

periodic abstinence Birth control methods that rely on a couple's avoidance of intercourse during the ovulatory phase of a woman's menstrual cycle; also called *fertility awareness* or *natural family planning*.

calendar method A form of periodic abstinence in which the variable lengths of a woman's menstrual cycle are used to calculate her fertile period.

cycle in the past year shorter than 26 days or longer than 32 days should encourage a woman NOT to use the Standard Days method. She should meet with her health care provider and discuss an alternative method.

To use this method, women must count the days of their menstrual cycle, with day 1 as the first day of menstrual bleeding. Women can have intercourse on days 1–7. On days 8–19, women should refrain from penis/vaginal intercourse or use a barrier method of contraception. Days 8–19 are the fertile days. From day 20 until the end of the cycle, unprotected intercourse can take place.[4] Keep in mind that the Standard Days method does not protect against the transmission of STDs.

The *Billings cervical mucus method* is another periodic abstinence technique. Generally used with other periodic abstinence techniques, this method requires a woman to evaluate the daily mucus discharge from her cervix. Users of this method become familiar with the changes in both appearance (from clear to cloudy) and consistency (from watery to thick) of their cervical mucus throughout their cycles. Women are taught that the unsafe days are when the mucus becomes clear and is the consistency of raw egg whites. Such a technique of ovulation determination must be learned from a physician or family planning professional.

The *symptothermal method* of periodic abstinence combines the use of the BBT method and the cervical mucus method.[4] Thus, some family planning professionals consider the symptothermal method a combination of all of the periodic abstinence approaches.

Those who wish to practice one of these periodic abstinence methods should consult a professional to learn how to chart their menstrual cycle and detect the physical signs that help predict the "unsafe" days. Besides the lack of protection against STDs, the periodic abstinence methods have the following potential problems:

- Partner may be uncooperative.
- Couple may take risks during "unsafe" days.
- Record-keeping may be poor.
- Illness and lack of sleep can affect body temperature.
- Vaginal infections and douches change mucus.
- Method cannot be used if the woman has irregular periods or temperature patterns.

Over-the-Counter Contraceptive Methods

OTC methods are ones that couples can choose easily because they do not require a physician's prescription, they are readily available in supermarkets or drugstores,

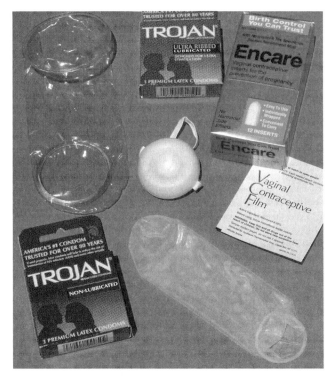

Over-the-counter methods of contraception are widely available in drugstores and supermarkets. They include male and female condoms, spermicides, and the contraceptive sponge.

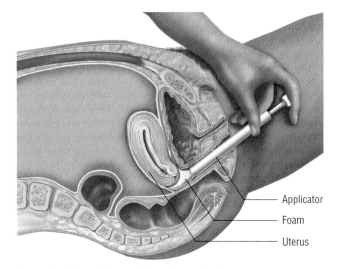

Figure 16-2 Use of Spermicide Spermicidal foams and suppositories are placed deep into the vagina in the region of the cervix no longer than 30 minutes before intercourse.

and they are approved by the U.S. Food and Drug Administration (FDA). They all work by providing some kind of obstacle or mechanism that prevents the sperm from joining with an ovum.

Spermicides

Spermicides are agents that are capable of killing sperm. When used alone, they offer a moderately effective form of contraception for the woman who is sexually active on an infrequent basis. Modern spermicides are generally safe (but see the following precaution), reversible forms of contraception that can be obtained without a physician's prescription in most drugstores and supermarkets. They are available in foams, creams, jellies, film, or suppositories. Spermicides are relatively inexpensive. Applicator kits cost about $8, and refills cost around $4–$8 (see Figure 16-2). Suppositories and film are also priced in this range (see the box "Vaginal Contraceptive Film").

Spermicides are made of water-soluble bases with a sperm-killing agent in the base. Frequently spermicides are used with other contraceptives, such as diaphragms, shields, caps, and condoms. Spermicides do not protect users from contracting pathogens that cause various STDs. In fact, people who use nonoxynol-9 many times each day are more likely to transmit infections, including HIV.[5] This is due to an increase in skin irritations and abrasions, which provide the avenue for passage of pathogens into the bloodstream.

Couples should realize that condoms, when used consistently and correctly, provide much better disease protection and contraceptive effect than spermicides used alone. In fact, the small amount of nonoxynol-9 that is added to the lubricant with some condoms is not sufficient to serve as an effective backup contraceptive if the condom breaks. Thus, some health centers and family planning agencies have stopped distributing condoms coated with a spermicide.[6] If you and/or your partner have concerns about your use of spermicides, you should seek advice from your health care provider.

Condoms

Colored or natural, smooth or textured, straight or shaped, plain or reservoir-tipped, dry or lubricated—the latex condom is approaching an art form. Nevertheless, the familiar **condom** remains a safe, effective, reversible contraceptive device. All condoms manufactured in the United States must be approved by the FDA.[7]

Key Terms

spermicides Chemicals capable of killing sperm.

condom A latex shield designed to cover the erect penis and retain semen upon ejaculation; "rubber."

For couples who are highly motivated in their desire to prevent a pregnancy, the effectiveness of a condom can approach that of an oral contraceptive. A condom can be nearly 100 percent effective when used with contraceptive foam. For couples who are less motivated, the condom can be considerably less effective. Condoms cost from 25¢ to $2.50 each.

> **Key Terms**
>
> **contraceptive sponge** A small, pillow-shaped contraceptive device that contains a spermicide; placed deep in the vagina to cover the cervical opening.
>
> **diaphragm** A soft rubber cup designed to cover the cervix.

The condom offers a measure of protection against sexually transmitted diseases. For both the man and the woman, chlamydial infections, gonorrhea, HIV infection, and other STDs are less likely to be acquired when the condom is used correctly (see the box "Maximizing the Effectiveness of Condoms"). Some lubricated condoms also contain a spermicide, yet the small amount of spermicide present in the condom's lubricant is not enough to consistently prevent conception if the condom should break. Current recommendations are to use dry condoms or lubricated condoms without spermicide. Also, any additional lubricants used should be water-based lubricants.

The FDA has approved two types of nonlatex condoms. The polyurethane male condom and the polyurethane female condom are available as one-time-use condoms (see the box "The Female Condom" on page 470).[3] These condoms are good alternatives for people who have an allergic sensitivity to latex, estimated to be up to 7 percent of the population.[8] Also, they are thinner and stronger than latex condoms and can be used with oil-based lubricants. Currently, these condoms are believed to provide a level of protection against STDs that is close to that of latex condoms. The contraceptive effectiveness of the polyurethane condoms remains somewhat less than that of the male latex condom.[9, 5]

Contraceptive Sponge

The **contraceptive sponge** is a small, pillow-shaped polyurethane device containing nonoxynol-9 spermicide. The sponge is dampened with tap water and inserted deep into the vagina to cover the cervical opening. This device provides contraceptive protection for up to 24 hours, regardless of the number of times intercourse occurs. After the last act of intercourse, the device must be left in place for at least 6 hours. Once removed, the sponge must be discarded. The sponge must not be left in place for longer than 24 or 30 hours because of the risk of toxic shock syndrome. Used alone, the sponge does not provide reliable protection against STDs and HIV infection. Consult your physician if you are concerned about the use of nonoxynol-9 spermicide. In women who have not given birth to children, the contraceptive effectiveness of the sponge is similar to that of the diaphragm. The sponge is less effective in women who have given birth.

The sponge has an interesting history. Before its removal from the market in 1995, the sponge was the most popular female over-the-counter contraceptive in the United States. The sponge came off the market because the manufacturer decided it was too expensive to retool the manufacturing plant to meet governmental safety regulations. The removal of the sponge prompted the TV sitcom show *Seinfeld* to develop an episode in which the character Elaine Benes purchased as many sponges as she could before they disappeared from the New York City marketplace. She then used her sponges sparingly and only with men she judged to be "spongeworthy."[10]

After reapproval in 2005, the sponge became available in the United States. Sponges cost between $2.50 and $3.00 each and come in packs of three.[10]

Prescription Contraceptive Methods

Many approaches to contraception require a physician's prescription. Generally, these methods have higher effectiveness rates, but they also come with possible risks and side effects to the user. Some devices require careful fitting or placement. Some prescription methods use devices that require the user to follow careful instructions. Some approaches use hormones that can have dangerous consequences for a very small percentage of users. It is for these reasons that these products or approaches are not available on an over-the-counter basis.

Diaphragm

The **diaphragm** is a soft rubber cup with a springlike metal rim that rests in the top of the vagina. The diaphragm covers the cervical opening (Figure 16-3). During intercourse the diaphragm stays in place quite well and cannot usually be felt by either partner.

(A) (B) (C)

Figure 16-3 Use of a Diaphragm **A:** Spermicidal cream or jelly is placed into the diaphragm. **B:** The diaphragm is folded lengthwise and inserted into the vagina. **C:** The diaphragm is then placed against the cervix so that the cup portion with the spermicide is facing the cervix. The outline of the cervix should be felt through the central part of the diaphragm.

The diaphragm is always used with a spermicidal cream or jelly placed inside the cup and around the rim. When used properly with a spermicide, the diaphragm is a relatively effective contraceptive, and when combined with the man's use of a condom, its effectiveness is even greater. The diaphragm must be inserted before intercourse. It should provide effective protection for 6 hours. If this time interval extends beyond 6 hours, some clinicians recommend that additional spermicide be placed in the vagina.

Use of additional spermicide with multiple acts of intercourse is optional. After intercourse, the diaphragm must be left in place for at least 6 hours before it is removed. Because of the risk of toxic shock syndrome (TSS), the diaphragm must not remain in the vagina longer than 24 hours.[4] Women should avoid using diaphragms, caps, and shields during any kind of vaginal bleeding, including menstruation.[5] It is always best to ask a health care provider for specific instructions.

Diaphragms must always be fitted and prescribed by a physician.[11] The cost of obtaining a diaphragm and keeping a supply of spermicide may be higher than that

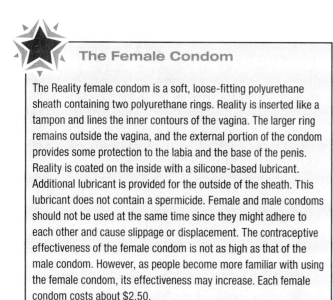

The Female Condom

The Reality female condom is a soft, loose-fitting polyurethane sheath containing two polyurethane rings. Reality is inserted like a tampon and lines the inner contours of the vagina. The larger ring remains outside the vagina, and the external portion of the condom provides some protection to the labia and the base of the penis. Reality is coated on the inside with a silicone-based lubricant. Additional lubricant is provided for the outside of the sheath. This lubricant does not contain a spermicide. Female and male condoms should not be used at the same time since they might adhere to each other and cause slippage or displacement. The contraceptive effectiveness of the female condom is not as high as that of the male condom. However, as people become more familiar with using the female condom, its effectiveness may increase. Each female condom costs about $2.50.

Prescription methods of contraception are those that include hormones, such as combined oral contraceptives and the contraceptive patch, and those that require expert fitting, such as the diaphragm and FemCap.

of other methods. Typically, it costs $15–$75 for a diaphragm and $4–$8 for the spermicidal cream or jelly. An examination may cost between $50 and $200, but it will be less at family planning clinics. Also, a high level of motivation to follow the instructions *exactly* is important.

Diaphragms and other vaginal barrier methods (caps and shields) do not provide reliable protection against STDs and HIV infection. Recent concerns about the spermicide nonoxynol-9 should prompt users to ask their physicians to recommend which spermicidal cream or jelly to use with diaphragms. If you are concerned about possible HIV infection, either avoid sexual activity or use a latex condom.

Lea's Shield and FemCap

The two newest barrier methods for women were approved by the FDA in 2002. Both methods are used with a spermicide. *Lea's Shield* is a reusable oval device made of silicone rubber that fits closely over the cervix. An attached loop helps in the removal from the vagina. The Lea's Shield works much like a diaphragm, but it has a central air valve that permits air to move out from beneath the shield and permit a closer fit. This device comes in only one size and must be prescribed by a physician. The first year, use effectiveness of this device (85 percent) is about the same as that for diaphragms (84 percent).[5]

The *FemCap* is a reusable hat-shaped silicone rubber cap that completely covers the cervix. Coated with spermicide, the FemCap's brim fits snugly against the deep vaginal walls. An attached strap helps in the removal of this device. The FemCap must be prescribed by a physician and comes in three sizes. Among women who have never been pregnant or given birth vaginally, the first year use effectiveness of this device is 86 percent. Costs for these new devices are similar to those for diaphragms.[5]

Intrauterine Device (IUD)

The **intrauterine device (IUD)** is the most popular reversible contraceptive method in the world, although the number of users in the United States is relatively small. It can be an excellent choice for women who desire a long-term, hassle-free, reversible, highly effective method of contraception. The IUD is especially advantageous to women who have already had at least one child, are in a stable, monogamous relationship, and perhaps are unable to take daily birth control pills.

Two types of IUDs are available in the United States: a T-shaped one containing the hormone progestin (Mirena) and a T-shaped one wrapped with copper wire (ParaGard). The Mirena IUD works by thickening cervical mucus, inhibiting sperm survival, and producing a thin endometrial lining that will not support a fertilized ovum. In some women, the Mirena inhibits ovulation.

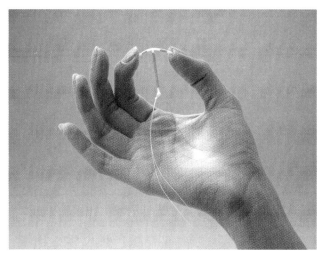

The T-shaped ParaGard IUD works by releasing copper ions that impair sperm function and prevent fertilization.

The ParaGard works by releasing copper ions that impair sperm function and prevent fertilization.[4] The Mirena IUD substantially reduces menstrual flow, but the Para-Gard may increase menstrual flow. About 20 percent of women who use the Mirena IUD stop having their periods altogether.[12]

The Mirena provides highly effective contraceptive protection for 5 years and the ParaGard for 12 years. Only a skilled physician can prescribe and insert an IUD. As with many other forms of contraception, IUDs do not offer protection against STDs, including the AIDS virus.[11]

For many years, the public has been concerned about two potentially serious side effects: *uterine perforation* (in which the IUD embeds itself into the uterine wall) and pelvic inflammatory disease (PID, a widespread infection of the abdominal cavity). Recent research, however, indicates that these events rarely happen, especially when the IUD is inserted by a skilled clinician. Between 2 and 10 percent of IUD users experience *expulsion* (muscular contractions which force the IUD out of the uterus) within the first year of use.[4]

As Table 16.1 indicates, IUDs are very effective birth control devices, surpassed in effectiveness only by abstinence, sterilization, and hormonal (pill, injection, implant, ring, patch) contraceptives. The cost for an IUD

> **Key Terms**
>
> **intrauterine device (IUD)** A small, plastic, medicated or unmedicated contraceptive device that prevents pregnancy when inserted in the uterus.

ranges from \$175–\$500, which includes an exam, insertion, and a follow-up visit.[5]

Oral Contraceptives

Developed in the late 1950s, the **oral contraceptive pill** provides the highest effectiveness rate of any single reversible contraceptive method used today. Worldwide, more than 100 million women are currently using oral contraceptives.[4]

Use of the pill requires a physician's examination and prescription. Because oral contraceptives are available in a wide range of formulas, follow-up examinations are important to ensure that a woman is receiving an effective dosage with as few side effects as possible. Matching the right prescription with the woman may require a few consultations.

Combined Pills All oral contraceptives contain synthetic (laboratory-made) hormones. The typical *combined pill* uses both synthetic estrogen and synthetic progesterone in each of 21 pills. With *triphasic pills,* the level of estrogen remains constant, but the level of progestin varies every 7 days.

The FDA has approved two *extended-cycle oral contraceptives* (Seasonale and Seasonique) that contain active hormones for 84 days (12 weeks) followed by 1 week of pills containing inactive ingredients.[3] Women using Seasonale or Seasonique have only four menstrual periods each year. In early 2007, the FDA approved the newest extended-cycle pill, called Lybrel. This contraceptive pill contains low-dose hormones that are taken each day for a full year. Despite having no menstrual periods for 365 days, most women in Wyeth Pharmaceuticals' clinical trials reported having some breakthrough bleeding or spotting during the early months of use.[13]

The contraceptive effect of the pill can be compromised in women who are also taking certain medicines or supplements. The antibiotic rifampin reduces the pill's effectiveness. Interestingly, other antibiotics do not make the pill less effective. But certain antifungal drugs taken orally for yeast infections, certain anti-HIV protease inhibitors, some anti-seizure medications, and the over-the-counter plant supplement St. John's Wort (sometimes used for mild depression) all have the ability to make the pill less effective. Thus it is very important for a woman to talk with her clinician about the medicines she is taking before she is given any prescription method of birth control.[5]

Oral contraceptives function in several ways. The estrogen in the pill tends to reduce ova development. The progesterone in the pill helps reduce the likelihood of ovulation (by lowering the release of luteinizing hormone). The progesterone in the pill also causes the uterine wall to develop inadequately and helps thicken cervical mucus, thus making it difficult for sperm to enter the uterus. As with many forms of contraception, *oral contraceptives do not protect against the transmission of STDs, including HIV infection.*

The physical changes produced by the oral contraceptive provide some beneficial side effects in women. Because the synthetic hormones are taken for 21 days and then are followed by **placebo pills** or no pills for 7 days, the menstrual cycle becomes regulated. Even women who have irregular cycles immediately become "regular." Because the uterine lining is not developed to the extent seen in a non-pill-taking woman, the uterus is not forced to contract with the same amount of vigor. Thus menstrual cramping is reduced, and the resultant menstrual flow is diminished. Research indicates that oral contraceptive use can provide protection against anemia, PID, noncancerous breast tumors, acne, recurrent ovarian cysts, ectopic pregnancy, endometrial cancer, endometriosis, and ovarian cancer.[4]

The negative side effects of the oral contraceptive pill can be divided into two general categories: (1) unpleasant and (2) potentially dangerous. The unpleasant side effects generally subside within two or three months for most women. A number of women report some or many of the following symptoms:

- Tenderness in breast tissue
- Nausea
- Mild headaches
- Slight, irregular spotting
- Weight gain
- Fluctuations in sex drive
- Mild depression
- More frequent vaginal infections

The potentially dangerous side effects of the oral contraceptive pill are most often seen in the cardiovascular system. Blood clots, strokes, hypertension, and heart attack seem to be associated with the estrogen component of the combined pill. However, when compared with nonusers, the risk of dying from cardiovascular complications is only slightly increased among healthy young oral contraceptive users. Additionally, over 50 scientific studies have determined that oral contraceptive use has little, if any, effect on the development of breast cancer, even among women with a family history of breast cancer.[4]

Most health professionals agree that the risks related to pregnancy and childbirth are much greater than those associated with oral contraceptive use. Certainly, a woman who is contemplating the use of the pill must discuss all of the risks and benefits with her physician.

There are some **contraindications** for the use of oral contraceptives. If you have a history of blood clots, migraine headaches, liver disease, a heart condition, high blood pressure, obesity, diabetes, hepatitis, cirrhosis,

Learning from Our Diversity

The Male Contraceptive Pill

Having males be responsible for the medical control of fertility would be a big shift in the sexuality responsibility roles for men and women. Forty-five years after the breakthrough of the female contraceptive pill, researchers are gaining confidence that a version of a male contraceptive pill will be commercially available in the not-too-distant future, perhaps between 5 and 10 years.*

For decades, difficulties have surrounded the development of a male contraceptive pill. Although many people believe that the primary reason for the slow development was the fact that the researchers were male, the most plausible explanations deal with male physiology. The typical male ejaculate contains 300–500 million sperm cells. A contraceptive method that is over 99 percent effective would still leave thousands and thousands of sperm cells available. In contrast, female contraceptives must block the viability of only one egg each cycle, arguably an easier task.

The drug being tested that blocks sperm development is actually a female hormone. While it is effective at blocking sperm production, it also reduces the amount of testosterone that the male produces. Without adequate levels of testosterone, the male sex drive diminishes considerably. For this reason, researchers are testing the effects of replacement androgen, often in the form of an injection or an implant. It is also possible that a slow-release patch, similar to the nicotine-replacement patch, could be used in the future.

Critics claim that a safe, effective, and inexpensive form of male contraception already exists in the form of a vasectomy. They argue, why not use an approach that already has shown its effectiveness for years? Besides, are women going to trust a man who claims he is using an oral contraceptive pill? Would the pill also have to make a man's eyeballs turn blue as proof that he was using an effective method? When would a woman know that a man is being truthful? Unfortunately, the track record for honesty among couples in sexual relationships isn't particularly good.

Within the next decade, the obstacles that prevent a safe and effective male contraceptive pill from being manufactured may be overcome. But questions will still remain, especially for women, since after all is said and done, they will always be the ones who must bear the brunt (as well as the joy) of pregnancy, labor, and childbirth.

*Health news: Will men use a contraceptive pill? Will women trust them? InteliHealth Online, August 29, 2000, www.intelihealth.com/enews?296075.

---

breast or uterine cancer, or if you are too young to have started consistent menstrual cycles, the pill probably should not be your contraceptive choice. Providing a physician with a complete and accurate health history is important before a woman starts to take the pill.

Two additional contraindications continue to draw considerable attention by the medical community. Cigarette smoking and advancing age are highly associated with an increased risk of potentially serious side effects. Increasing numbers of physicians are not prescribing oral contraceptives for their patients who smoke. The risk of cardiovascular-related deaths is greatly enhanced in women over age 35. The risk is even higher in female smokers over 35. The data are quite convincing.[4]

For the vast majority of women, however, the pill, when properly prescribed, is safe and effective. Careful scrutiny of one's health history and careful follow-up examinations when a problem is suspected are essential elements that can provide a good margin of safety. Monthly pill packs cost $15–$35 at drugstores and less at clinics. An exam may cost $35–$175.[5]

What about an oral contraceptive for men? See the box "The Male Contraceptive Pill" for information on the medical and social challenges of developing a pill for men.

Minipills   Some women prefer not to use the combined oral contraceptive pill. Thus to avoid some of the potentially serious side effects of the combined pill, some physicians are prescribing **minipills.** These oral contraceptives contain no estrogen—only low-dose progesterone in all pills in the 28-day pill pack. The minipill seems to work by thickening cervical mucus, preventing ovulation, and producing a thin endometrial lining.[4] The effectiveness of a minipill is slightly lower than that of the combined pill. *Breakthrough bleeding* and **ectopic pregnancy** are more common in minipill users than in

---

> ### Key Terms
>
> **oral contraceptive pill** A pill taken orally, composed of synthetic female hormones that prevent ovulation or implantation; "the pill."
>
> **placebo pills** (pla **see** bo) Pills that contain no active ingredients.
>
> **contraindications** Factors that make the use of a drug inappropriate or dangerous for a particular person.
>
> **minipills** Low-dose progesterone (progestin) oral contraceptives.
>
> **ectopic pregnancy** A pregnancy in which the fertilized ovum implants at a site other than the uterus, typically in the fallopian tubes.

combined-pill users. The cost of minipills is similar to that of combined pills.

 TALKING POINTS You've tried two different types of oral contraceptives and had unpleasant side effects with both. Your doctor says you should consider another birth control method, but you disagree. How could you talk with her about this in a matter-of-fact way?

Injectable Contraceptive

Depo-Provera is a highly effective (99 percent+) injectable progestin contraceptive that provides protection for 3 months. This hormone shot works primarily by preventing ovulation and thickening the cervical mucus to keep the sperm from joining the egg.

The most common side effects of Depo-Provera are irregular bleeding and spotting followed by *amenorrhea* (the absence of periods).[4] In particular, new users of Depo-Provera report occasional breakthrough bleeding as the most common unpleasant side effect.[4] When the woman's body adjusts to the presence of this drug, breakthrough bleeding diminishes, and the most common side effect is amenorrhea. This is understandable, because the drug inhibits ovulation. Many women consider amenorrhea to be a desirable effect of Depo-Provera use. Women who stop using Depo-Provera may experience infertility for a period of up to one year.[4] The cost of Depo-Provera ranges from $30 to $75 per injection.[5]

Contraceptive Implant

In July 2006, the FDA approved the use of a progestin-based contraceptive implant called Implanon. This thin, flexible plastic device is about the size of a matchstick and is inserted just under the skin of the upper arm. Implanon works by slowly releasing progestin for up to three years. The progestin inhibits ovulation and also thickens the cervical mucus to prevent the sperm from joining with an egg. Early studies indicate that this contraceptive implant will be up to 99.9 percent effective.

Many of the health concerns that apply to other hormone-based contraceptives (including drug interactions that can lower its effectiveness) apply to the implant as well. At the time of this writing, the implant is not yet widely available, in part because clinicians must be trained to correctly insert and remove the device. The costs of the device and its insertion have not yet been fully established.[5]

Contraceptive Ring

One of the newest contraceptives on the market is the vaginal **contraceptive ring** (NuvaRing). Available by prescription, NuvaRing is a thin polymer ring (2⅛ inches in diameter and ⅛ inch thick) that contains synthetic

The NuvaRing contraceptive ring is a flexible ring about 2⅛ inches in diameter. When inserted into the vagina, it delivers a low dose of hormones similar to those found in oral contraceptives.

estrogen and progestin. Users insert this device deep into the vagina where it remains for 3 weeks. At the end of the third week, the device is removed for a week and the woman has her period. The NuvaRing provides effective contraception (99 percent+ effective when used perfectly) for the entire 4-week time frame.

The ring functions in a manner similar to the oral contraceptive pill: it reduces the chances of ovulation and thickens cervical mucus. Women who use the ring cannot at the same time use shields, caps, or diaphragms as a backup method. The contraceptive ring does not protect against sexually transmitted diseases, including the virus that causes HIV/AIDS. As with all prescribed forms of contraception, women should discuss all the benefits, risks, and possible side effects with their health care provider. The costs of the contraceptive ring are about $30–$35 per month for the device and $35–$125 for the exam.[5]

Contraceptive Patch

In 2002 the Ortho Evra **contraceptive patch** became available to women. This patch contains continuous levels of estrogen and progestin delivered from a 1¾-inch square patch that is applied weekly to one of four areas on the woman's body: the buttocks, abdomen, upper chest (front and back, excluding the breasts), or upper outer arm.[14] The patch remains attached even while a woman bathes, swims, or exercises. After 3 weeks of patches, the woman uses no patch for the fourth week, during which time the woman has her period. The patch functions in a manner similar to the oral contraceptive pill. Like all hormonal measures of contraception, the patch does not protect against sexually transmitted diseases, including the virus that causes HIV/AIDS. The patch costs about $30–$40 per month. The exam may cost $35–$175.[12]

Many women have used the patch successfully, but some concerns have risen over possible increased cardiovascular risks (blood clots, strokes, heart attacks) due to the way the hormones are delivered to the user. On the home page of the Ortho Evra website, the manufacturer clearly states that patch users will be exposed to about 60 percent more estrogen than if they were taking a typical oral birth control pill that contains 35 μg of estrogen.[14] For this reason, it is especially important that potential users discuss with their health care provider whether this is a good contraceptive choice for them. This precaution is even more important for women who are smokers and women over the age of 35.

Emergency Contraception

Emergency contraception is designed to prevent pregnancy after unprotected vaginal intercourse such as when a condom breaks, when a couple uses no method of contraception, or when someone forces another to have intercourse. This method is also called postcoital or "morning after" contraception. (Emergency contraception is not the "abortion pill" or RU-486.) Emergency contraception is available in two forms: emergency hormonal contraception and the insertion of an IUD.

Currently, the FDA has approved one oral contraceptive (Plan B) for use specifically as emergency contraception, although physicians may prescribe other oral contraceptives for this purpose. Plan B is a progestin-only pill, the first dose of which should be taken as soon as possible (but not later than 120 hours or 5 days) after unprotected intercourse. Typically, a second dose follows 12 hours after the first pill. (The sooner the first dose is taken after intercourse, the better the contraceptive protection.) Plan B reportedly reduces the risk of pregnancy by 89 percent.[4]

Emergency contraception works by preventing ovulation or fertilization. If a woman is already pregnant, Plan B will not cause an abortion or affect the pregnancy. In 2006 the FDA decided to allow Plan B to be sold as an over-the-counter product, similar to the way nicotine-replacement medications are made available to the public. Thus, Plan B is available behind the pharmacy counter (not on aisle shelves) to women ages 18 and older. Some pharmacists may ask for identification to verify a young woman's age. Girls younger than 18 will need a prescription to get Plan B.[5]

The most commonly reported side effects of emergency hormonal contraception are nausea and vomiting. About 25 percent of users of progestin-only pills experience nausea, and 10 percent experience vomiting. The use of antinausea medication can help offset the nausea and vomiting. Some women also report fatigue, breast

Plan B emergency contraception consists of two doses of hormones taken about 12 hours apart. Nonprescription behind-the-counter access to Plan B was approved for women ages 18 and older in 2006.

tenderness, abdominal pain, headaches, and dizziness. These side effects subside within a day or two after treatment.[4] Costs for Plan B are estimated to be $8–$35.[5]

A copper IUD is a less commonly used, but highly effective, form of emergency contraception. To function as an emergency contraceptive, however, the ParaGard IUD must be inserted by a clinician within 5 days of unprotected intercourse.

Permanent Contraceptive Methods

All the contraceptive mechanisms or methods already discussed have one quality in common: they are reversible. Although microsurgical techniques are providing medical breakthroughs, **sterilization** should still be

> **Key Terms**
>
> **contraceptive ring** Thin, polymer contraceptive device containing estrogen and progestin; placed deep within the vagina for a 3-week period.
>
> **contraceptive patch** Contraceptive skin patch containing estrogen and progestin; replaced each week for a 3-week period.
>
> **emergency contraception** Contraceptive measures used to prevent pregnancy within 5 days after unprotected intercourse; also called post-coital or "morning after" contraception.
>
> **sterilization** Generally permanent birth control techniques that surgically disrupt the normal passage of ova or sperm.

Figure 16-4 The Most Frequently Used Forms of Male and Female Sterilization **A:** Vasectomy. **B:** Tubal ligation.

considered an irreversible procedure.[15] When you decide to use sterilization, you no longer control your own fertility because you will no longer be able to produce offspring. Attempts to reverse sterilization are quite difficult and very expensive.

Therefore, couples considering sterilization procedures usually must undergo extensive discussions with a physician or family planning counselor to identify their true feelings about this finality. People must be aware of the possible changes in self-concept they might have after sterilization. If you are a man who equates fertility with masculinity, you may have trouble accepting your new status as a sterile man. If you are a woman who equates motherhood with femininity, you might have adjustment problems after sterilization. Some people later regret not being able to have children. Sterilization does not protect one against STDs, including HIV infection.

Male Sterilization

The male sterilization procedure is called a *vasectomy.* Accomplished with a local anesthetic in a physician's office, this 20- to 30-minute procedure consists of the surgical removal of a section of each vas deferens. After a small incision is made through the scrotum, the vas deferens is located and a small section removed. The remaining ends are either tied or *cauterized* (Figure 16-4a).

Immediately after a vasectomy, sperm may still be present in the vas deferens. A backup contraceptive is recommended until a physician microscopically examines a semen specimen. This examination usually occurs about six weeks after the surgery. After a vasectomy,

men can still produce male sex hormones, get erections, have orgasms, and ejaculate. (Recall that sperm account for only a small portion of the semen.) Some men even report increased interest in sexual activity because their chances of impregnating a woman have been virtually eliminated.

What happens to the process of spermatogenesis within each testicle? Sperm cells are still being produced, but they are destroyed by specialized white blood cells called *phagocytic leukocytes.*

The future may hold a reversible form of vasectomy, as researchers experiment with injecting a plug-forming material into the vas deferens, with the intention that the plug could be removed at a later date if desired. The cost of a vasectomy ranges from $350–$1,000.[5]

Female Sterilization

The most common method of female sterilization is called *tubal ligation.* During this procedure, the fallopian tubes are cut and the ends tied back. Some physicians cauterize the tube ends to ensure complete sealing (Figure 16-4b). The fallopian tubes are usually reached through the abdominal wall. In a *minilaparotomy,* a small incision is made through the abdominal wall just below the navel. The resultant scar is small and is the basis for the term *band-aid surgery.*

Female sterilization requires about 20 to 30 minutes, with the patient under a local or general anesthetic. The use of a laparoscope has made female sterilization much simpler than in the past. The laparoscope is a small tube equipped with mirrors and lights. Inserted through a single incision, the laparoscope locates the fallopian tubes before they are cut, tied, or cauterized. When a laparoscope is used through an abdominal incision, the procedure is called a *laparoscopy.*

In 2002, a new method of female sterilization was approved by the FDA. This is a nonincision approach (the Essure coil), whereby a physician inserts a small, soft metallic coil into the vagina, through the cervix, and directly into each fallopian tube. This procedure is done under local anesthetic and takes about one half-hour. Once inserted, the coils encourage scar tissue growth that eventually blocks the fallopian tubes. If the tubes are obstructed, sperm are blocked from meeting the ovum. After 3 months, a woman returns to her physician for an x-ray test that determines whether the tubes are fully obstructed. During these first 3 months, couples must use another form of birth control. Cramping is the most common side effect. In rare cases, Essure coils can be expelled or perforate the fallopian tube.[3] Reports indicate that Essure has a 99.8 percent effectiveness rate.[5]

Women who are sterilized still produce female hormones, ovulate, and menstruate. However, the ovum cannot move down the fallopian tube. Within a day of its release, the ovum will start to disintegrate and be absorbed by the body. Freed of the possibility of becoming pregnant, many sterilized women report an increase in sex drive and activity.

Female sterilization is very effective, with failure rates of only 1 to 2 per 1,000 procedures. The complications tend to be few and minor, and there appear to be no serious long-term side effects. Tubal ligation costs $1,500–$6,000.[5]

Two other procedures produce sterilization in women. *Ovariectomy* (the surgical removal of the ovaries) and *hysterectomy* (the surgical removal of the uterus) accomplish sterilization. However, these procedures are used to remove diseased (cancerous, cystic, or hemorrhaging) organs and are not primarily considered sterilization techniques.

 TALKING POINTS You and your husband have children. And you'd like to stop taking the pill for health reasons. Your husband says you're pressuring him to have a vasectomy. How can you keep the dialogue going in a cooperative way?

Abortion

Regardless of the circumstances under which pregnancy occurs, women may now choose to terminate their pregnancies. No longer must women who do not want to be pregnant seek potentially dangerous, illegal abortions. On the basis of current technology and legality, women need never experience childbirth. The decision will be theirs to make.

Abortion is a highly controversial, personal decision—one that needs serious consideration by each woman. On the basis of the landmark 1973 U.S. Supreme Court case *Roe v. Wade,* the United States joined many of the world's most populated countries in legalizing abortion within the following guidelines:

1. For the first 3 months of pregnancy (first trimester), the decision to abort lies with the woman and her doctor. Most abortions are performed in the first trimester.
2. For the next 3 months of pregnancy (second trimester), state law may regulate the abortion procedure in ways that are reasonably related to maternal health.
3. For the last weeks of pregnancy (third trimester) when the fetus is judged capable of surviving if born, any state may regulate or even prohibit abortion except where abortion is necessary to preserve the life or health of the mother.

In 2002, 1.29 million women made the decision to terminate a pregnancy in the United States.[16] Thousands of additional women probably considered abortion but elected to continue their pregnancies.

First-Trimester Abortion Procedures

The first trimester consists of the first 13 weeks (91 days) of pregnancy. During the first 49 days after a woman's last menstrual period, a woman has two options for terminating a pregnancy: *vacuum aspiration* or *medication abortion.* Once 63 days have passed, only vacuum aspiration is an abortion option.

Vacuum Aspiration There are two common methods of performing vacuum aspiration abortions. Both procedures can be performed in a physician's office or in a hospital. Both procedures require **dilation** of the cervix. The method used depends on how long the woman has been pregnant. Together, these methods represent the most widely used abortion procedures in the United States. In 1999, 96 percent of all abortions in the United States were performed through aspiration procedures.[4]

The **manual vacuum aspiration (MVA)** procedure can be performed in the earliest part of the first trimester,

<table>
<tr><td>

Key Terms

abortion Induced premature termination of a pregnancy.

dilation Gradual expansion of an opening or passageway, such as the cervix.

manual vacuum aspiration (MVA) The abortion procedure performed in the earliest weeks after a pregnancy is established.

</td></tr>
</table>

from the time a woman knows she is pregnant up to 10 weeks after her last period. After a physician injects a local anesthetic into the cervix, dilators can be used to enlarge the cervical opening. The physician then inserts a small tube into the uterus and applies suction with a handheld instrument. By rotating and moving this small tube across the uterine wall, the physician can empty the uterus. A return visit to the physician is an important follow-up procedure.[4]

After the first month of pregnancy and throughout the first trimester, physicians typically select **dilation and suction curettage (D&C)** (frequently called *vacuum aspiration*) as the abortion procedure of choice. D&C is similar to MVA, but the clinician uses a vacuum machine rather than a manually operated suction instrument. The clinician tends to use more sedation for the woman, in addition to the local cervical anesthetic. The cervix is stretched open with dilators that gradually enlarge the opening to permit the insertion of a tube into the cervix. This tube is attached to a vacuum machine that empties the uterus with gentle suction. If the physician believes that additional endometrial tissue remains in the uterus, he or she can use a **curette** to scrape the wall of the uterus. A subsequent visit to the clinician is an important follow-up procedure. Costs range from $350–$700.[5]

Medication Abortion Mifepristone (RU-486) and methotrexate are drugs that can be used to induce a **medication abortion** during the first trimester of pregnancy. RU-486 was developed in France in the 1980s and has been widely used in Europe. Finally, after years of testing in the United States, the FDA gave approval to the so-called "abortion pill." The pill is being marketed under the name Mifeprex and is available only through physicians. The cost of using mifepristone is about the same as the cost of first-term surgical procedures, or about $350–$650.[5]

Under the FDA's regimen, women must use mifepristone within 49 days of their last menstrual period. Mifepristone blocks the action of progesterone and causes the lining of the uterus to break down. Women take three pills at the first doctor visit and then return 48 hours later to take a second drug, misoprostol, which causes menstruation to occur, usually within about 5 hours.

A third visit to a physician is necessary to ensure that the woman is recovering well from the procedure. Physicians will want to make certain that there is no infection or excessive bleeding and that the uterus is fully emptied. Over a decade of research studies have indicated that the use of mifepristone is around 95 percent effective, when used during the first 7 weeks of pregnancy.[17]

Methotrexate is a drug used since the 1950s for cancer treatment. Physicians have found that it is effective in inducing an early-term medication abortion. Typically, a woman receives an injection of methotrexate and, during an office visit 3 to 7 days later, receives misoprostol, usually through vaginal suppositories. The fetal contents are expelled, generally within 12 hours. A third visit to the physician is necessary to ensure that the woman is recovering well and that the abortion is complete. Costs of a medication abortion range from $350–$650.[5] If these and other new drugs continue to gain favor with women and their physicians, it is likely that more women will use physicians' offices, rather than abortion clinics, for abortion services.

Second-Trimester Abortion Procedures

When a woman's pregnancy continues beyond the thirteenth week of gestation, termination becomes a more difficult matter. The procedures at this stage become more complicated and take longer to be completed.

Dilation and Evacuation Between 13 and 16 weeks of pregnancy, the abortion method of choice is **dilation and evacuation (D&E).** Some physicians use this method up through 20 weeks or more of pregnancy.[4] The D&E is a more involved surgical procedure than is D&C and generally requires greater dilation of the cervix, larger medical instruments (including forceps), suction, and curettage (see Figure 16-5). Some women may be given a general anesthetic during D&E procedures. After D&E, a return visit to the clinician is an important follow-up procedure.

In the 1970s and the 1980s, it was not uncommon for women reaching the end of the second trimester of pregnancy to undergo an abortion using a **hypertonic saline procedure** or a *prostaglandin procedure.* In the saline procedure, a strong salt solution was injected directly into the amniotic sac. This caused the uterine contents to dehydrate and be expelled from the uterus within

---

Key Terms

dilation and suction curettage (D&C) (kyoo re taage) A surgical procedure in which the cervical canal is dilated to allow the uterine wall to be scraped; vacuum aspiration.

curette A metal scraping instrument that resembles a spoon, with a cup-shaped cutting surface on its end.

medication abortion An abortion caused by the use of prescribed drugs.

dilation and evacuation (D&E) Second-trimester abortion procedure that requires greater dilation, suction, and curettage than first-trimester vacuum aspiration procedures.

hypertonic saline procedure A salt solution with a concentration higher than that found in human fluids.

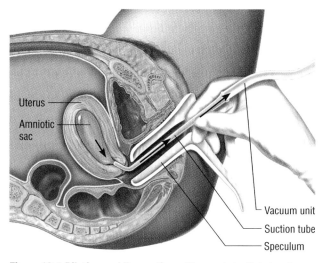

Uterus

Amniotic sac

Vacuum unit

Suction tube

Speculum

Figure 16-5 Dilation and Evacuation The cervix is dilated and the contents of the uterus are aspirated (removed by suction). This procedure is used to perform abortions during the second trimester.

24–36 hours. In the prostaglandin procedure, an injection or a vaginal suppository of prostaglandin was administered. The prostaglandin produced strong uterine contractions that expelled the fetal contents. Both of these procedures are rarely used today.[4] The D&E remains the abortion method of choice for the second trimester.

Partial-Birth Abortion

In the late 1990s the United States saw the beginning of many contentious legal issues concerning a rarely used, middle-to-late second-trimester abortion procedure called intact D&E (dilation and extraction), or more commonly, *partial-birth abortion.* Many legislators believed the procedure was too gruesome to be permitted, and many states banned this procedure. However, almost all of these state bans were blocked by various courts because the laws were either too vague or provided no exception for the health of the pregnant woman facing a medical emergency.

In 2003 the U.S. Congress passed the Federal Partial-Birth Abortion Ban and President George W. Bush signed this into law. However, this law was challenged and eventually overturned by federal appeals courts. The Justice Department appealed these rulings to the U.S. Supreme Court in early 2006. In April 2007, in a sharply divided 5–4 ruling, the Supreme Court upheld the original federal ban.[18] Concerned observers on both sides of the abortion debate now wonder whether this decision makes it more likely that this conservative Supreme Court will eventually revisit the 1973 *Roe v. Wade* ruling that guaranteed the constitutional right to abortion.

Clearly, this Supreme Court ruling has paved the way for states to approve new partial-birth abortion ban statutes. The first state to do this was Louisiana, which passed its new law within three months of the April 2007 high court decision. (For the current status of laws pertaining to partial-birth abortion, go to www.guttmacher.org.)

Third-Trimester Abortion Procedures

If an abortion is required in the latter weeks of the gestational period, a surgical procedure in which the fetus will be removed (*hysterotomy*) or a procedure in which the entire uterus is removed (*hysterectomy*) can be undertaken. As you can imagine, these procedures are more complicated and involve longer hospitalization, major abdominal surgery, and an extended period of recovery.

A Final Word

In the heat of passion, people often fail to think rationally about the potential outcomes of unprotected sex. Therefore, the time to prepare for the romantic moment is *before* you are in a position where you don't want to think about the possibility of an unintended result. If you choose to be sexually active, find a form of protection that works well for you and use it consistently. If you choose not to be sexually active, realize that this is a viable choice that can be 100 percent effective.

Taking Charge of Your Health

- Use the Personal Assessment at the end of this chapter to help you determine which birth control method is best for you.

- If you have a partner, discuss your personal preferences with him or her.

- Talk to your doctor about the health aspects of different types of birth control before making your decision.

- Find out as much as you can about the newest types of contraception (Seasonale, NuvaRing, Mirena, FemCap, Lea's Shield, Implanon, Essure, and Ortho Evra).

- Think about your likelihood of becoming pregnant or contracting an STD, and discuss with your partner how you might handle these possibilities if they should occur.

SUMMARY

- Each birth control method has both a theoretical-effectiveness rate and a use-effectiveness rate.
- Many factors should be considered when deciding which contraceptive is best for you.
- Sterilization is usually considered an irreversible procedure.
- The birth control pill is safe and effective for the vast majority of women, but it does not protect against sexually transmitted diseases.
- Among the newest hormonal contraceptives are the ring, the patch, the implant, and extended-cycle oral contraceptives.

- The contraceptive sponge has returned to the U.S. market.
- Two types of IUDs are available: a hormone-containing IUD and a copper IUD.
- Emergency contraception is safe and effective in preventing pregnancy when used within 5 days of unprotected intercourse.
- The FDA has approved the drug mifepristone (RU-486) to induce a medication abortion during the first trimester of pregnancy.
- Abortion procedures vary according to the stage of the pregnancy.

REVIEW QUESTIONS

1. Explain the difference between the terms *birth control* and *contraception*. Give examples of each.
2. Identify some of the factors that should be given careful consideration when selecting a contraceptive method. Explain each factor.
3. What is periodic abstinence? Identify and describe each of the five approaches to this birth control strategy.
4. What are the current concerns over the use of the spermicide nonoxynol-9?

5. How do minipills differ from the combined oral contraceptive pills?
6. What is emergency contraception? For what circumstances might this be used?
7. In what form is Depo-Provera delivered to a woman?
8. Describe the various sterilization procedures.
9. Identify and describe the different abortion procedures that are used during each trimester of pregnancy.
10. What is a medication abortion?

ANSWERS TO THE "WHAT DO YOU KNOW?" QUIZ

1. False   2. True   3. False   4. False   5. True   6. False   7. False

ENDNOTES

1. Bruckner H, Bearman P. After the promise: The STD consequences of adolescent virginity pledges. *Journal of Adolescent Health* (36): 271–278. 2005.
2. Hyde JS, DeLamater JD. *Understanding Human Sexuality* (9th ed.). New York: McGraw-Hill, 2006.
3. Crooks RL, Baur K. *Our Sexuality* (9th ed.). Belmont, CA: Wadsworth, 2005.
4. Hatcher RA, et al. *Contraceptive Technology* (18th ed.). New York: Ardent Media, 2004.
5. Planned Parenthood Federation of America. *Birth Control.* www.plannedparenthood.org/birthcontrol-pregnancy.
6. Carroll JL. *Sexuality Now: Embracing Diversity* (2nd ed.). Belmont, CA: Thomson Higher Learning, 2007.
7. Allgeier ER, Allgeier AR. *Sexual Interactions* (5th ed.). New York: Houghton Mifflin, 2000.
8. DeNoon D. Best Condoms Still Latex, WebMD Health. March 21, 2003. www.my.webmd.com.
9. Steiner MJ, et al. Contraceptive effectiveness of a polyurethane condom and a latex condom: A randomized controlled trial. *Obstetrics and Gynecology* 101 (3): 539–547. 2003.
10. Weise E. Contraceptive sponge is back, but why did it leave? *USA Today*, p. 7D. April 25, 2005.

11. Strong B, DeVault C, Sayad BW, Yarber WL. *Human Sexuality: Diversity in Contemporary America* (5th ed.). New York: McGraw-Hill, 2005.
12. Berlex Laboratories website. What Is Mirena?, www.mirena-us.com.
13. Wyeth Pharmaceuticals. Lybrel, First Low Dose Combination Oral Contraceptive with Unique 365-Day Dosing, Now Available in U.S. www.wyeth.com. July 30, 2007.
14. Ortho Evra website. New Important Labeling Information. www.orthoevra.com.
15. Kelly GF. *Sexuality Today: The Human Perspective* (8th ed.). New York: McGraw-Hill, 2006.
16. Finer LB, Henshaw SK. Estimates of U.S. Abortion Incidence in 2001–2003, www.guttmacher.org. August 3, 2006.
17. Creinin MD, et al. Mifepristone and misoprostol and methotrexate/misoprostol in clinical practice for abortion. *American Journal of Obstetrics and Gynecology* 188 (3): 664–669. 2003.
18. CNN.com. Justices uphold ban on abortion procedure. www.cnn.com/2007/LAW/04/18/scotus.abortion/index.html, April 18, 2007.

Personal Assessment

Which birth control method is best for you?

To assess which birth control method would be best for you, answer the following questions, and check the interpretation section.

	Yes	No
1. Need a contraceptive right away?	_____	_____
2. Want a contraceptive that can be used completely independent of sexual relations?	_____	_____
3. Need a contraceptive only once in a great while?	_____	_____
4. Want something with no harmful side effects?	_____	_____
5. Want to avoid going to the doctor?	_____	_____
6. Want something that will help protect against sexually transmitted diseases?	_____	_____
7. Have to be concerned about affordability?	_____	_____
8. Need to be virtually certain that pregnancy will not result?	_____	_____
9. Want to avoid pregnancy now but want to have a child sometime in the future?	_____	_____
10. Have any medical condition or lifestyle that may rule out some form of contraception?	_____	_____

Interpretation

If you have checked **Yes** to number:

1. Condoms, spermicides, and sponges may be easily purchased without prescription in any pharmacy.
2. Sterilization, oral contraceptives, hormone rings, patches, or injections, implants, and periodic abstinence techniques do not require that anything be done just before sexual relations.
3. Diaphragms, condoms, sponges, or spermicides can be used by people who have coitus only once in a while. Periodic abstinence techniques may also be appropriate but require a high degree of skill and motivation.
4. IUD use should be carefully discussed with your physician. For most women, IUDs are quite safe. Sometimes the use of oral contraceptives or hormone products results in some minor discomfort and, on rare occasions, may have harmful side effects.

5. Condoms, spermicides, and sponges do not require a prescription from a physician.
6. Condoms help protect against sexually transmitted diseases. Nonoxynol-9 may increase STD transmission in some users. No method (except abstinence) can guarantee complete protection.
7. Be a wise consumer: check prices, ask pharmacists and physicians. The cost of sterilization is high, but there is no additional expense for a lifetime.
8. Sterilization provides near certainty. Hormone-based contraceptives, IUDs, or a diaphragm-condom-spermicide combination also give a high measure of reliable contraceptive protection. Periodic abstinence, withdrawal, and douche methods should be avoided. Outercourse may be a good alternative.
9. Although it is sometimes possible to reverse sterilization, it requires surgery and is more complex than simply stopping use of any of the other methods.
10. Smokers and people with a history of blood clots should probably not use oral contraceptives or other hormone approaches. Some people have allergic reactions to a specific spermicide or latex material. Some women cannot be fitted with a diaphragm, shield, or cap. The woman and her health care provider will then need to select another suitable means of contraception.

TO CARRY THIS FURTHER . . .

There may be more than one method of birth control suitable for you. Always consider whether a method you select can also help you avoid an STD. Study the methods suggested here, and consult Table 16.1 to determine what method may be most appropriate.

Source: Adapted from K. Haas and A. Haas, *Understanding Sexuality*, 3rd ed. St. Louis, 1993, Mosby. Used with permission by Adelaide Haas.

Becoming a Parent

What Do You Know about Pregnancy and Parenting?

◉ If a fetus has a heartbeat above 140, then it's a boy. True or False?

◉ The acidic level in the vagina is destructive to sperm. True or False?

◉ In each human pregnancy, there are four trimesters. True or False?

◉ Typically, the longest stage of labor is the third stage. True or False?

◉ Amniocentesis helps to identify chromosomal abnormalities. True or False?

◉ Women's health issues are responsible for more cases of infertility than men's health issues. True or False?

◉ IVF-ET is the most frequently used assisted reproductive technology. True or False?

Check your answers at the end of the chapter.

Online Learning Center Resources
www.mhhe.com/payne10e

Visit the Online Learning Center for tools to improve your grade and get the most out of your course—chapter objectives, practice quizzes, key terms flashcards, chapter summaries for your digital audio player, Web activities, self-assessments, and many other study aids.

Although birth control is especially important for many young couples, most couples eventually want to have children and raise a family. In the past, couples had their children very soon after either high school or college. Now the trend seems to be to wait longer before having children. Most likely, educational, economic, contraceptive, and occupational factors have laid the groundwork for this trend. To the relief of many people, medical research indicates that women over the age of 30 or 35 are quite able to have healthy babies.

Parenting Issues for Couples

Before deciding to have children, couples should frankly discuss the effects that pregnancy and a newborn child will have on their lives (see the box "Parenthood Expands Personal Growth"). In addition, couples who are sexually active should consider these same issues, because very few contraceptive methods are

Parenthood Expands Personal Growth

Becoming a parent is almost always an exciting experience. Through nine months of pregnancy, anticipation of the baby increases on a daily basis. What sex will the baby be? How much hair will he or she have? How large will the baby be? Will the baby be a healthy child? Will the labor and delivery go smoothly? How will the household be changed as a result of the baby? How will the parents interact with each other after the baby enters the picture?

All these parental thoughts are centered on the baby and its presence. This is natural. Carrying a pregnancy to term and adjusting to the new baby are exciting, challenging, and exhausting experiences for the parents. There are times when new parents wonder how they ever got themselves into this situation. But there are many more times when parents are likely to be immensely thankful and proud to be parents of a newborn child.

Sometimes as we watch the growth and development of a newborn baby, we fail to think about the opportunities parenthood provides for the parents themselves to grow and develop. Parenthood presents an extra dimension to the lives of most parents. Although one can see this extra dimension in a number of ways, perhaps the most noticeable change is in the depth and quality of human relationships.

Perhaps most easily seen is the connection between mother and child. Living together, sharing nutrients (ideally only good ones), and protecting each other for nine months forges a spiritual bond between mother and child that remains for a lifetime. They experience labor and delivery in a way unique to themselves. Although fathers may be able to sense how strong this bond is, they never can fully understand or feel how close this mother-child connection is and how strong it tends to remain. *Parenthood is a life-altering experience for a woman.*

After becoming parents, fathers also tend to forge close, intimate bonds with their children, but these bonds are more likely related to the interactions they experience with the children as they grow and develop. Sometimes to their surprise, fathers find out that they have marvelous capabilities to adjust to the new demands a baby presents. Many fathers develop unexpected talents at nurturing their children. Perhaps because of this, more and more fathers are choosing to stay at home and raise their children, while their spouse works to support the family financially. This arrangement was virtually unheard of just three decades ago. *Indeed, parenthood is also a life-altering experience for a man.*

Parenthood encourages men and women to expand their focus from themselves (and their careers, their interests, their friends) to a broader spectrum of other people. This spectrum will certainly include the child, but also health care providers, teachers, school officials, their child's friends, the friends' parents and perhaps religious leaders, law enforcement personnel, and sports coaches. Parents will be required to expand their communication skills, their patience, and their insights as they try to raise their children the best way they can. Through this struggle comes added personal growth for the parents.

A final area in which parenthood offers a new dimension for the parents concerns the intimate bond between the parents themselves. Although it doesn't always happen (and the divorce statistics tell a compelling story), the process of conceiving a child, birthing a child, and raising a child to adulthood can make two people grow together in a way unmatched by any other experience. Older adult couples will often say that their most significant shared experience was raising their children. Many agree that it was through this experience that they gained a depth of understanding about each other that enriched their lives and established their most intimate connection. *In this sense, parenthood is a spiritual, life-altering experience for the parents.*

---

100 percent effective all the time, and pregnancy can result from nearly any act of intercourse. For students contemplating single parenthood, we ask that you consider these issues as they relate to your particular situation and to excuse our consistent use of plural pronouns.

Deciding to Become Parents

Here are some questions to consider before deciding to become parents:

- What effect will pregnancy have on us individually and collectively?
- Why do we want to have a child?
- What effect will a child have on the images we have constructed for ourselves as adults?
- Can we afford to have a child and provide for its needs?
- How will the responsibilities related to raising a child be divided?
- How will a child affect our professional careers?
- Are we ready now to accept the extended responsibilities that can come with a new child?
- How will we rear our child in terms of religious training, discipline, and participation in activities?
- Are we ready to part with much of the freedom associated with late adolescence and the early young adult years?
- How will we handle the possibility of being awakened at six o'clock or earlier each morning for the next few years?
- What plans have we made in the event that our baby (or fetus) has a serious birth defect?
- Are we capable of handling the additional responsibilities associated with having a disabled child?

For many young couples, the rewards of raising a family outweigh the stress that inevitably accompanies parenthood.

- Are we comfortable with the thought of bringing another child into an already overcrowded, violent, bigoted, and polluted world?

If these questions seem strikingly negative in tone, there is indeed a reason for this. We believe that all too frequently the "nuts and bolts" issues related to childbearing and parenting are ignored or at least are placed on the back burner. Of course, future parents will consider how cute and cuddly a new baby will be, how holidays will be enhanced with a new child, and how pleased the grandparents will be; however, we consider these issues to be secondary to the serious realities of having a child enter your lives. Complete the Personal Assessment at the end of this chapter to explore your feelings about parenting.

TALKING POINTS If you think you would like to have children someday, would you feel comfortable discussing these issues with your partner? How would you start the conversation?

Becoming a Parent through a Stepfamily

Some people will become parents through a marriage in which one or both adult partners bring children from a previous relationship.[1] This newly constituted household is called a stepfamily.

Although some people call this a *blended family,* the National Stepfamily Resource Center (NSRC) believes the preferred term is a *stepfamily.* Children in stepfamilies do not lose their individual identities and instantly "blend" into a new family while losing attachments to the parent who is not a part of the new marriage. Things are rarely that smooth. If both parents remarry, a child may become a member of two stepfamilies and, perhaps, face even more obstacles concerning family loyalty. It is natural for children to wonder where they fit in or where they belong. Calling a newly constituted family a blended family may set up too many unrealistic expectations for children and adults and make adjustments more difficult. For example, children may balk when told that they are to consider their new family to be the family that deserves all their attention and loyalty.[1]

It is beyond the scope of this chapter to outline the challenges (and joys) that come with becoming a parent through a stepfamily arrangement. The NSRC, a clearinghouse for research-based information about stepfamily relationships, indicates that for stepfamilies to be successful, parents should:

- Nurture and enrich the couple relationship.
- Reveal and understand emotions.
- Have realistic expectations.
- Develop new roles.
- Seek support and see the positive.

Throughout the merging of families into stepfamilies, clear communication, honest feelings, and a positive attitude about one's new role can help the process run more smoothly. It is quite possible that new family relationships can be wonderful experiences for all involved.

Parenting across Cultures

In their recent text *Transcultural Health Care,* Purnell and Paulanka describe the various ways ethnic groups in America tend to view babies and young children.[2] In the Amish culture, children are seen as gifts from God and are enthusiastically welcomed into families. Amish families have an average of seven children per family and, unlike in other ethnic groups in America, this fertility pattern has not changed for the past century. Large families prize children because they are not only gifts from God, but they are also valuable resources on low-tech, labor-intensive family farms.

Children are considered a blessing to Jewish families. Children are to be afforded an education that prepares them for progress in society as well as increased understanding of their Jewish heritage. To that end, many Jewish children attend public school but also attend Hebrew school a couple of afternoons each week during the school year. Jewish children play important roles in most of the holiday celebrations and religious services. Parents are expected to treat their children fairly and to be flexible, caring, and attentive to discipline.[2]

Although there is much change taking place as Chinese increase their assimilation into the United States,

Which Personal Media Should You Trust for Information on Pregnancy?

Some sources of communication and information are the "personal media" to which we are exposed on a daily basis. These media include our immediate family members, our relatives, our friends and peer groups, and people we respect in our communities. Frequently, these personal media have had a wealth of experiences that, at least to us, give them a measure of credibility. They have "walked the walk" and, in a strange way, we now feel obligated to hear them "talk the talk."

And perhaps that's all we should do with our personal media sources—just listen. Here are some of the "pearls of wisdom" we might hear:

- If the baby's heart rate is above 140, then it's a boy.
- Mixing a common cleaning solution with a mother's urine will show you the sex of her forthcoming child.
- If the Mom craves sweets, it will be a girl. If she craves salty foods, it will be a boy.
- Pregnant women should drink plenty of water, or the amniotic fluid will get dirty.
- Pregnant women should not take baths.
- Having sex on even days of the month will produce boy babies.
- If you sleep on your right side while pregnant, you will have a girl.
- If you hold your hands above your head while pregnant, you could strangle the fetus.
- Eating spicy food near the baby's due date will cause early contractions.

If you check the Internet, you will find many sources of pregnancy folklore through advertised books, websites, and publications. Some of these sources of folklore are indeed fascinating, especially ones coming from non-Western cultures far away from the United States.

Because pregnancy and childbirth are such beautiful, complex, and mysterious events, they lend themselves easily to folklore. And "gems of wisdom" coming from folklore are easily passed on to couples having their first child. These couples are so new to pregnancy that they don't know what to believe. They may believe the most ridiculous information because they trust their personal media sources—friends, family, and older relatives.

What would be good advice for a pregnant woman who feels a bit overwhelmed with traditional "pearls of wisdom" and folklore recommendations about how to handle her pregnancy? We would encourage her to simply listen, nod her head, and smile. Then, if she has a question or feels uncomfortable about a pregnancy question or topic, make certain she asks her physician, nurse, or health care provider during her next visit. Undoubtedly, they have heard all of the urban legends, latest medical breakthroughs, or bits of folklore before and are willing to set the record straight.

For instance, regarding those "pearls of wisdom" listed previously—they are all—*False*.

---

many Chinese American families still hold on to Chinese traditions. Children are highly valued, but the number of children in a family tends to be small, perhaps because of China's one-child rule. Independence is usually not fostered, and parents make many decisions for the children even into young adulthood. Teens are expected to work hard in school, score well on exams, and help with chores around the home.[2]

In discussing Arab Americans' views of children, Purnell and Paulanka write that high fertility rates tend to be favored because of the belief that "God decides family size" and because families follow Islamic dictates regarding birth control, treatment of infertility, and abortion. Procreation is considered the primary reason for a marriage, since it enhances family strength. As with a number of cultures around the world, pregnancy tends to occur early in the marriage, and the preference for boys over girls is a reality. The sex of a child can be a great concern for the pregnant woman, and observers will often note the way in which the mother "carries" her baby during the pregnancy (girls are thought to be carried high and boys to be carried low).[2] See the box "Which Personal Media Should You Trust for Information on Pregnancy?" for more on folklore related to pregnancy.

Pregnancy: An Extension of the Partnership

Pregnancy is a condition that requires a series of complex yet coordinated changes to occur in the female body. This chapter follows pregnancy from its beginning, at fertilization, to its conclusion, with labor and childbirth. Fathers-to-be share many of the joys and worries of pregnancy and childbirth.

Physiological Obstacles and Aids to Fertilization

Many sexually active young people believe that they will become pregnant (or impregnate someone) only when they want to, despite their haphazard contraceptive practices. Because of this mistaken belief, many young people do not consistently use contraceptives, Young adults must remember that, to ensure the survival of our species, our bodies were designed to promote pregnancy. It is estimated that about 85 percent of sexually active women of childbearing age will become pregnant within one year if they do not use some form of contraception.[3]

The surface of an ovum is penetrated by sperm at fertilization.

With regard to pregnancy, each act of intercourse can be considered a game of physiological odds. Obstacles exist that may reduce a couple's chance of pregnancy, including the following.

Obstacles to Fertilization

1. *The acidic level of the vagina is destructive to sperm.* The low pH of the vagina kills sperm that fail to enter the uterus quickly.
2. *The cervical mucus is thick during most of the menstrual cycle.* Sperm movement into the uterus is more difficult, except during the few days surrounding ovulation.
3. *The sperm must locate the cervical opening.* The cervical opening is small and may not be located by most sperm.
4. *Half of the sperm travel through the wrong fallopian tube.* Most commonly, only one ovum is released at ovulation. The two ovaries generally "take turns" each month. The sperm have no way of "knowing" which tube they should enter. Thus it is probable that half will travel through the wrong tube.
5. *The distance sperm must travel is relatively long compared with the tiny size of the sperm cells.* Microscopic sperm must travel about seven or eight inches after they are inside the female.
6. *The sperm's travel is relatively "upstream."* The anatomical positioning of the female reproductive structures necessitates an "uphill" movement by the sperm.
7. *The contoured folds of the tubal walls trap many sperm.* These folds make it difficult for sperm to locate the egg. Many sperm are trapped in this maze.

There are also a variety of aids that tend to help sperm and egg cells join. Some of these are listed next.

Aids to Fertilization

1. *An astounding number of sperm are deposited during ejaculation.* Each ejaculation contains about a teaspoon of semen.[4] Within this quantity are between 200 and 500 million sperm cells. Even with large numbers of sperm killed in the vagina, millions are able to move to the deeper structures.
2. *Sperm are deposited near the cervical opening.* Ejaculation into the vagina by the penis places the sperm near the cervical opening.
3. *The male accessory glands help make the semen nonacidic.* The seminal vesicles, prostate gland, and Cowper's glands secrete fluids that provide an alkaline environment for the sperm. This environment helps sperm be better protected in the vagina until they can move into the deeper, more alkaline uterus and fallopian tubes.[5]
4. *Uterine contractions aid sperm movement.* The rhythmic muscular contractions of the uterus tend to cause the sperm to move in the direction of the fallopian tubes.
5. *Sperm cells move rather quickly.* Despite their tiny size, sperm cells can move about one inch per hour. Powered by sugar solutions from the male accessory glands and the whiplike movements of their tails, sperm can reach the distant third of the fallopian tubes in less than 8 hours as they swim in the direction of the descending ovum.
6. *After they are inside the fallopian tubes, sperm can live for days.* Some sperm may be viable for up to a week after reaching the comfortable, nonacidic environment of the fallopian tubes. Most sperm, however, will survive an average of 48–72 hours. Thus they can "wait in the wings" for the moment an ovum is released from the ovary.
7. *The cervical mucus is thin and watery at the time of ovulation.* This mucus allows for better passage of sperm through the cervical opening when the ovum is most capable of being fertilized.

Signs of Pregnancy

Aside from pregnancy tests done in a professional laboratory, a woman can sometimes recognize early signs and symptoms. The signs of pregnancy have been divided into three categories.

Presumptive Signs of Pregnancy

Missed period after unprotected intercourse the previous month

Nausea on awakening (morning sickness)

Increase in size and tenderness of breasts

Darkening of the areolar tissue surrounding the nipples

Probable Signs of Pregnancy

Increase in the frequency of urination (the growing uterus presses against the bladder)

Increase in the size of the abdomen

Cervix becomes softer by the sixth week (detected by a pelvic examination by a clinician)

Positive pregnancy test (see the box "Home Pregnancy Tests")

Positive Signs of Pregnancy

Determination of a fetal heartbeat

Feeling of the fetus moving (*quickening*)

Observation of the fetus by ultrasound or optical viewers

Agents That Can Damage a Fetus

A large number of agents that come into contact with a pregnant woman can affect fetal development. Many of these (rubella and herpes viruses, tobacco smoke, alcohol, and virtually all other drugs) are discussed in other chapters of this text. The best advice for a pregnant woman is to maintain close contact with her obstetrician during pregnancy and to consider carefully the ingestion of any over-the-counter (OTC) drug (including aspirin, caffeine, and antacids) that could possibly harm the fetus.

Pregnant women should also avoid exposure to radiation. Such exposure, most commonly through excessive x-rays or radiation fallout from nuclear testing, can irreversibly damage fetal genetic structures. In addition, pregnant women should avoid Accutane, a drug prescribed for the treatment of cystic acne that can severely damage the fetus.[6]

Intrauterine Development

Intrauterine development takes place over the course of three **trimesters.** Most pregnancies last from 38–42 weeks. For purposes of illustration, we will consider each trimester to be 13 weeks. The growth and development during these trimesters occurs in a typical pattern for most pregnancies.

First Trimester The first 13-week trimester starts at conception, when the egg and sperm unite to form a structure called the **zygote** (Figure 17-1). The zygote, or fertilized egg, undergoes a series of cellular changes as it grows and makes its week-long journey down the fallopian tube to the uterus. About the tenth day after conception, the zygote, now called a **blastocyst,** imbeds itself into the endometrial lining of the uterus. From the end of 2 weeks after conception until the end of the eighth week, the growing structure is called an **embryo.** After 8 weeks and until the birth, it is called a **fetus.**

The first trimester is characterized by rapid cellular growth. By the end of the first trimester, the fetus weighs only about one ounce, yet most body organs are formed and the fetus can move.[7] It is currently thought that about half of all pregnancies end in **spontaneous abortion** during the early weeks of the first trimester, usually before the woman realizes she is pregnant. These miscarriages usually result from a genetic defect or a serious developmental problem.

Key Terms

trimester A 3-month period; human pregnancies encompass three trimesters.

zygote A fertilized ovum.

blastocyst Early stage of the developing life form that imbeds into the endometrial lining of the uterus.

embryo Developmental stage from the end of the second week after conception until the end of the eighth week.

fetus Developmental stage from the beginning of the ninth week after conception until birth.

spontaneous abortion Any cessation of pregnancy resulting from natural causes; also called a miscarriage.

Fallopian tube

FERTILIZATION

Sperm cells

Ovum

Graafian follicle

Follicle

Corpus luteum

Primary follicles

Ovary

Zygote dividing as it travels toward uterus

Uterine cavity

Endometrium

Cervix

Blastocyst is implanted in endometrium (at 8 days)

Embryo (at 4 weeks)

Figure 17-1 Fertilization and Implantation   After its release from the follicle, the ovum begins its week-long journey down the fallopian tube. Fertilization generally occurs in the outermost third of the tube. Now fertilized, the ovum progresses toward the uterus, where it embeds itself in the endometrium. A pregnancy is established.

Second Trimester   The second trimester is characterized by continued growth and maturation. During this time, the organs continue to grow and physicians can hear the fetal heartbeat with a stethoscope. The bone structures are fully evident during the second trimester. The fetus starts to look more and more like an infant.

Additionally, the mother's breast weight increases by about 30 percent because of the deposition of 2–4 pounds of fat. This fat serves as a reserve energy source for the mother should she decide to nurse her baby. For this reason, good maternal nutrition is essential during the second trimester.[7]

Third Trimester   The third trimester is another critical time for the developing fetus. At the beginning of this trimester, the fetus generally weighs 2–3 pounds. Over the final 13 weeks of gestation, the fetus will double in length and multiply its weight by up to five times.

This is also the time when the fetus absorbs considerable amounts of the minerals iron and calcium from the mother. For this reason, the mother must maintain sound eating patterns and avoid her body's depletion of mineral stores, perhaps by taking a vitamin and mineral supplement containing iron, which would reduce her risk of developing anemia during the final trimester.[7]

Maintaining a Healthy Pregnancy   Having a healthy pregnancy and delivering a healthy child actually should begin in the months before conception. During these pre-conception months, obstetricians advise women to stop smoking, stop drinking alcoholic beverages, eat well, get physical exercise, avoid or treat infections, avoid unnecessary exposure to toxic chemicals, and ask a physician before consuming any drug (prescription or over-the-counter).

Why the early start? Many women do not know that they are pregnant until after they miss a menstrual period. If they wait to alter their lifestyle until after they are

The fetus at 16 weeks' gestation within the amniotic sac.

Strategies for maintaining a healthy pregnancy include consuming a well-balanced diet, engaging in appropriate physical activity, and avoiding tobacco, alcohol, and other drugs.

certain of the pregnancy, they could inadvertently put the child's health at risk. Tremendous embryonic and fetal growth and development take place in the earliest weeks after conception. So it's best to plan ahead—before conception.

Once the pregnancy is established, it is important to follow additional guidelines:

- Arrange for prenatal care.
- Consume a well-balanced diet.
- Take a vitamin supplement that contains folic acid.
- Exercise according to your physician's recommendation.
- Avoid and treat infections.
- Avoid alcohol, tobacco, and other drugs.
- Limit your caffeine intake.
- Stay away from x-rays, hot tubs, and saunas.
- Stay away from toxic chemicals.

An expectant dad can also participate in this healthy approach by matching the woman's lifestyle changes. This provides sound emotional support for the pregnancy and, as an added bonus, improves the overall health of the dad.

Childbirth: The Labor of Delivery

Childbirth, or *parturition,* is one of the true peak life experiences for both men and women. Most of the time, childbirth is a wonderfully exciting venture into the unknown. For the parents, this intriguing experience can provide a stage for personal growth, maturity, and insight into a dynamic, complex world.

During the last few weeks of the third trimester, most fetuses move deeper into the pelvic cavity in a process called *lightening.* During this movement, the fetus' body rotates and the head begins to engage more deeply into the mother's pelvic girdle. Many women report that their babies have "dropped."

Another indication that parturition may be relatively near is the increased reporting of *Braxton Hicks contractions.*[8] These uterine contractions, which are of mild intensity and often occur at irregular intervals, may be felt throughout a pregnancy. During the last few weeks of pregnancy (*gestation*), these mild contractions can occur more frequently and cause a woman to feel as if she is going into labor **(false labor).**

Labor begins when uterine contractions become more intense and occur at regular intervals. The birth of a child can be divided into three stages: (1) effacement and dilation of the cervix, (2) delivery of the fetus, and (3) expulsion of the placenta (Figure 17-2). For a woman having her first child, the birth process lasts an average of 12–16 hours. The average length of labor for subsequent births is much shorter—from 4 to 10 hours on the average. Labor is very unpredictable: labors that last from 1 to 24 hours occur daily at most hospitals.

Stage One: Effacement and Dilation of the Cervix

In the first stage of labor the uterine contractions attempt to thin (*efface*) the normally thick cervical walls and to enlarge (*dilate*) the cervical opening.[4] These contractions are directed by the release of prostaglandins and the hormone oxytocin into the circulating bloodstream. In women delivering their first babies, effacement will occur before dilation. In subsequent deliveries, effacement and dilation usually occur at the same time.

The first stage of labor is often the longest. The cervical opening must thin and dilate to a diameter of 10 cm before the first stage of labor is considered complete.[5] Often this stage begins with the dislodging of

---

Key Terms

false labor Conditions that resemble the start of true labor; may include irregular uterine contractions, pressure, and discomfort in the lower abdomen.

(A) First stage: Effacement and dilation. Uterine contractions thin the cervix and enlarge the cervical opening.

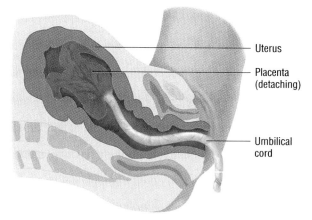

(B) Second stage: Delivery of the fetus. Uterine contractions are aided by mother's voluntary contractions of abdominal muscles. The fetus moves through dilated cervical opening and birth canal.

(C) Third stage: Delivery of the placenta. Placenta detaches from uterine wall and is delivered through the birth canal.

Figure 17-2 Labor and Delivery

the cervical mucus plug. The subsequent *bloody show* (a mucus plug and a small amount of blood) at the vaginal opening may indicate that effacement and dilation have begun. Another indication of labor's onset may be the bursting or tearing of the fetal amniotic sac. "Breaking

the bag of waters" refers to this phenomenon, which happens in various measures in expectant women.

The pain of the uterine contractions becomes more intense as the woman moves through this first stage of labor. As the cervical opening effaces and dilates 0–3 cm, many women report feeling happy, exhilarated, and confident. In the early phase of the first stage of labor, the contractions are relatively short (lasting 15–60 seconds) and the intervals between contractions range from 20 minutes to 5 minutes as labor progresses. However, these rest intervals will become shorter and the contractions more forceful when the woman's uterus contracts to dilate 4–7 cm.

In this second phase of the first stage of labor, the contractions usually last about 1 minute each, and the rest intervals drop from about 5 minutes to 1 minute over a period of 5–9 hours.

The third phase of the first stage of labor is called *transition*. During transition, the uterus contracts to dilate the cervical opening to the full 10 cm required for safe passage of the fetus out of the uterus and into the vagina (birth canal).[6] This period of labor is often the most painful part of the entire birth process. Fortunately, it is also the shortest phase of most labors. Lasting 15–30 minutes, transition contractions often last 60–90 seconds each. The rest intervals between contractions are short and vary from 30 to 60 seconds.

An examination of the cervix by a nurse, midwife, or physician will reveal whether full dilation of 10 cm has occurred (see the box "Midwifery on the Rise" for more on the role of midwives). Until the full 10 cm dilation, women are cautioned not to "push" the fetus during the contractions. Special breathing and concentration techniques help many women cope with the first stage of labor.

Stage Two: Delivery of the Fetus

When the mother's cervix is fully dilated, she enters the second stage of labor, the delivery of the fetus through the birth canal. Now the mother is encouraged to help push the baby out (with her abdominal muscles) during each contraction. In this second stage the uterine contractions are less forceful than during the transition phase of the first stage and may last 60 seconds each, with a 1- to 3-minute rest interval.

This second stage may last up to 2 hours in first births.[4] For subsequent births, this stage will usually be much shorter. When the baby's head is first seen at the vaginal opening, *crowning* is said to have taken place. Generally, the back of the baby's head appears first. (Infants whose feet or buttocks are presented first are said to be delivered in a *breech position*.) After the head is delivered, the baby's body rotates upward to let the shoulders come through. The rest of the body follows quite quickly. The second stage of labor ends when the fetus is fully

Midwifery on the Rise

For the past century, most of the women in the United States who went into labor followed a fairly standard procedure. This included a trip to the hospital and a lengthy wait in a labor room. The actual birth then took place in a delivery room, which was a surgical room equipped to handle most medical emergencies. Doctors and nurses were always close by to watch the expectant mother and to track the high-tech monitors.

This scenario is rapidly changing with the increased use of midwives, many of whom help deliver babies within hospital settings, at free-standing birthing centers, or in the homes of the pregnant women. Two types of nurse-midwives are certified by the American College of Nurse-Midwives (ACNM). A Certified Nurse-Midwife (CNM) is trained and certified in the two disciplines of nursing and midwifery, while the Certified Midwife (CM) has training and certification in midwifery. All Certified Nurse-Midwives have baccalaureate degrees and 72 percent also have master's or doctoral degrees.[*]

Both CNMs and CMs operate within a framework of a health care system that provides for consultation, collaborative management, or referral to additional medical care according to the health needs and condition of the pregnant woman. If the woman needs specialized help during the pregnancy or emergency care during labor, certified midwives do not hesitate to access the traditional medical system. Since 97 percent of midwife deliveries take place within hospitals, this care is usually easily attainable. Presently, less than 3 percent of midwife-assisted births occur at free-standing birthing centers or in private homes.

For many years, the traditional medical establishment discounted the use of midwives, believing that midwives were incapable of providing professional prenatal care and birthing assistance to women. However, this position has softened considerably. Indeed, most pregnancies and births follow a natural, standard pattern in which trained midwives can function in a very cost-effective, low-tech, patient-friendly manner.

Today, over 10 percent of all births in the United States are attended by midwives. In the year 2003, certified midwives attended more than 310,000 births. With certified midwifery training programs in place at some of the most prestigious universities in the country (for example, Vanderbilt University, Baylor College of Medicine, the University of Michigan, and Yale University), this trend will likely continue.

[*]American College of Nurse-Midwives. *About the Midwifery Profession*, www .midwife.org.

---

expelled from the vagina. In the past, deliveries were often performed with an *episiotomy,* a surgical incision of the **perineum** intended to prevent lacerations (tearing) during delivery.

Immediately after the birth, and again 5 minutes later, the newborn's physical health frequently is evaluated by obstetrical assistants using the Apgar score system. The baby will be judged (rated either 0, 1, or 2) on five criteria including appearance (color), pulse, response to foot stimulation, muscle tone, and respiration. After 5 minutes, 98 percent of infants score 7 or above. An Apgar score of less than 5 after 5 minutes indicates the possibility of a serious defect.

Newly delivered babies often look "unusual." Their heads are often cone-shaped as a result of the compression of cranial bones that occurs during the delivery through the birth canal. Within a few days after birth, the newborn's head assumes a much more normal shape. Most babies (of all races) appear bluish at first until they begin regular breathing. All babies are covered with a coating of *vernix,* a white, cheeselike substance that protects the skin.

Stage Three: Delivery of the Placenta

Usually within 30 minutes after the fetus is delivered, the uterus again initiates a series of contractions to expel the placenta (or *afterbirth*). The placenta is examined by the attending physician to ensure that it was completely expelled. Torn remnants of the placenta could lead to dangerous hemorrhaging by the mother. Often the physician manually examines the uterus after the placenta has been delivered.

After the placenta has been delivered, the uterus continues with mild contractions to help control bleeding and start the gradual reduction of the uterus to its normal, nonpregnant size. This final aspect of the birth process is called **postpartum.** External abdominal massage of the lower abdomen seems to help the uterus contract, as does an infant's nursing at the mother's breast (see the box "Benefits of Successful Breast-Feeding").

Cesarean Deliveries

A **cesarean delivery** (cesarean birth, C-section) is a procedure in which the fetus is surgically removed from the

---

> ### Key Terms
>
> **perineum** In the female, the region between the vulva and the anus.
>
> **postpartum** The period after the birth of a baby during which the uterus returns to its prepregnancy size.
>
> **cesarean delivery** (si **zare** ee an) Surgical removal of a fetus through the abdominal wall.

mother's uterus through the abdominal wall. This type of delivery, which is completed in up to an hour, can be performed with the mother having a regional or a general anesthetic.

In 2003, the percentage of deliveries by cesarean section reached an all-time high of 27.5 percent.[9] The increasing use of cesarean deliveries is questioned by some medical experts, although others point to the need for this kind of delivery when one or more of the following factors are present:

- The fetus is improperly positioned.
- The mother's pelvis is too small.
- The fetus is especially large.
- The fetus shows signs of distress.
- The umbilical cord is compressed.
- The placenta is being delivered before the fetus.
- The mother's health is at risk.

Key Terms

bonding Important initial recognition established between the newborn and those adults on whom the newborn will depend.

teratogenic agent Any substance that is capable of causing birth defects.

Although a cesarean delivery is considered major surgery, most mothers cope well with the delivery and postsurgical and postpartum discomfort. The hospital stay is usually a few days longer than for a vaginal delivery. The mother can still nurse her child and may still be able to have vaginal deliveries with later children. More and more hospitals are allowing the father to be in the operating room during cesarean deliveries. Fortunately, research indicates that early **bonding** between child, mother, and father can still occur with cesarean deliveries. Cesarean deliveries are much more expensive than vaginal deliveries.

Problems in Fetal Development and Pregnancy

Most women progress through their three trimesters of pregnancy without any major complications for either their own health or the health of the baby. Sometimes there are difficulties, but fortunately, many of these problems can be identified and successfully managed. Genetic and prenatal counseling can be especially helpful.

Genetic and Prenatal Counseling

Genetic and prenatal (before birth) counseling are two of the most beneficial advances in medical technology. Genetic counselors can provide timely, accurate, and complete information to patients, while maintaining the attitude that the patient's values should guide the decisions.

The March of Dimes is the nation's preeminent organization with the mission to "improve the health of babies by preventing birth defects, premature birth, and infant mortality."[10] The March of Dimes indicates that people who should be especially interested in genetic counseling include:

- Women who plan to be pregnant after age 35 (see the box "Pregnancy and Parenting after 40").
- Couples who already have a child with an inherited disorder, birth defect, or mental retardation.
- Women who have had three or more miscarriages or had babies who died in infancy.
- Men or women who think that their job, lifestyle, or medical history might pose a risk to a current or future pregnancy. Such concerns might be exposure to certain medications, chemicals, radiation, drugs, or infections. These substances are frequently called **teratogenic agents.**
- Couples who understand that certain genetic defects occur in their ethnic group. Examples are Tay-Sachs disease, a fatal nervous system disease that can occur in people of Eastern European Jewish ancestry, and sickle-cell disease, a blood disorder that can occur in African Americans.

Learning from Our Diversity

Pregnancy and Parenting after 40

Women who become pregnant in their 40s are not a new phenomenon. What is new is women becoming pregnant (or adopting or using surrogate mothers) at a time when many women begin menopause.* For example, Susan Sarandon delivered a child when she was in her mid-40s, and presidential hopeful John Edwards's wife, Elizabeth, delivered a child in her late 40s and another in her early 50s. Other examples are Sharon Stone (adopted a child in her late 40s), Diane Keaton (adopted two children in her 50s), and Cheryl Tiegs (had twins in her 50s using the services of a surrogate mother).

The reasons for births after age 40 are several. Some couples may have tried to conceive for years and only succeeded when in their 40s. Other women and couples delayed pregnancy in order to build their careers, travel, or become more financially secure. In addition, fertility technology, microsurgery, and the use of donor eggs or sperm have finally given many couples the baby they long wanted.

It is not unusual to see men becoming fathers in their later 50s or 60s. Well-known people like Rod Stewart, Larry King, Michael Douglas, and Paul McCartney became new fathers in later middle age. Indeed, there is plenty of evidence that sperm function in older men does not diminish much from that seen in younger men.†

However, women experience a decline in fertility as they age. Traditionally, women have been discouraged from becoming pregnant for the first time in their 40s because of the health risks to the mother and the risk of birth defects for the baby. The risk of having a child with a birth defect also increases as the mother's age increases. For example, about 1 out of 1,400 babies born to women in their 20s has Down syndrome, while 1 out of 100 babies is born with Down syndrome to women in their 40s.††

Older women suffer more complications than younger women during pregnancy and childbirth. The risk of miscarriage is 12–15 percent for women in their 20s but rises to 25 percent in women at age 40. Older women are more likely than younger women to develop gestational diabetes or high blood pressure during a pregnancy. Older moms also are more likely to have low-birth-weight babies (under 5.5 pounds) or stillbirths (births of a baby who has died). The incidence of cesarean births is slightly higher for older moms as well.††

If this sounds discouraging, remember that women who want to have a baby in their 40s should use this information to *prevent problems* rather than let it discourage them from having a baby. Revisit the recommendations in the section "Maintaining a Healthy Pregnancy." These guidelines are important for all pregnant women to follow. Women in their 40s who want to start their families should consider the following additional points:

- To identify all of your options, consult with your obstetrician/gynecologist before trying to become pregnant.
- Make sure you have early prenatal (before birth) care. The first 8 weeks of development are especially important for the baby.
- Don't skip any doctor appointments. Your health must be carefully monitored.
- Get appropriate prenatal screening tests, including ones that test for genetic disorders. Your doctor will advise you on these tests.

Following these strategies will help a woman minimize the chances of having complications for herself and her baby. The odds for success are still in her favor.

* Hesse, M. Famous Older Moms. AARP Online. www.aarpmagazine.org/lifestyle/famous_older.html.
† Crooks RL, Baur K. *Our Sexuality* (9th ed.). Belmont, CA: Wadsworth, 2005.
†† WebMD. Preganncy: Having a Baby after Age 35. www.webmd.com/content/Article/51/40823.htm.

- Couples who are first cousins or other close blood relatives.
- Pregnant women who have had screening tests that indicate that their pregnancy may be at increased risks for complications or birth defects.[11]

The genetic counselor might use a variety of methods to gather information about the couple, including DNA testing, other medical tests, medical records, family histories, and autopsy reports. When a couple receives genetic counseling before conception and learn that they have a high risk of conceiving a child with a birth defect, then they have a variety of options still open to them, such as artificial insemination by a donor, ovum donation, and adoption.

If you have already become pregnant, you should still work with your physician to identify risk factors in your first prenatal visit. This allows time for tests to be conducted and medical records to be reviewed. (These tests are explained in the next section of this chapter.) In general, couples may want to consider receiving genetic counseling and testing while they still have the legal option to terminate the pregnancy.

TALKING POINTS You have a concern that makes you want to get genetic testing and prenatal counseling, but your partner balks at this suggestion. How can you get a dialogue going so you can change his or her mind about this?

Testing for Fetal Abnormalities

Many women undergo tests during pregnancy to check for birth defects, genetic disorders, and other problems.[12] A few of the most common tests are ultrasound scans, the quad marker screen, amniocentesis, and chorionic

Ultrasound scans are used to check the growing fetus for possible abnormalities, as well as size, development, position, and many other factors.

villus sampling (CVS). Each of these tests can be helpful in diagnosing problems, but the tests are not necessary for every pregnancy. Women should check with their doctor about which, if any, are appropriate.

Ultrasound Ultrasound technology uses high-frequency sound waves to form pictures of the fetus on a computer screen. The test can verify a due date; determine causes of bleeding; check the overall health, development, sex, and position of the baby; measure the amniotic fluid; and check the position of the placenta. There are no known risks from the tests, and many women have one or two ultrasounds in routine pregnancies. However, there is no known evidence that normal pregnancies benefit from ultrasound tests.[12]

Quad Marker Screen The quad marker screen is a simple blood test that predicts the likelihood of a certain problem occurring with the pregnancy or the fetus. The quad marker screen does not diagnose the problem, however.[13] The test is only used during the fifteenth and twentieth weeks of pregnancy. It analyzes the mother's blood sample for levels of four substances (two proteins produced by the baby's liver and two hormones produced by the placenta). The quad marker screen results can indicate a variety of possible problems, including brain and spinal cord defects and genetic disorders like Down syndrome. The results provide additional information about the possibility of twins and the age of the fetus.

In over 98 percent of pregnancies, normal test results predict healthy babies and uncomplicated births. Abnormal results from a quad marker screen do not necessarily mean that a problem exists. A small percentage of women with elevated, abnormal results will be carrying a fetus with a birth defect. Follow-up tests, such as amniocentesis, may be used to make a more definitive diagnosis.

Amniocentesis This test examines skin cells shed by the fetus into the surrounding amniotic fluid. Performed about 16 weeks into pregnancy, the test involves inserting a long, thin needle through the mother's abdomen to extract less than an ounce of fluid from the womb. A local anesthetic reduces any discomfort. The cells must be cultured in a laboratory, and it may take 2 or 3 weeks for test results to be ready. The test is a reliable indicator of chromosomal abnormalities such as Down syndrome or genetic disorders such as Tay-Sachs disease, Hunter's syndrome, and sickle-cell disease. Amniocentesis can also identify neural tube defects. The accuracy of test results is 99.4 percent.[14]

While usually quite safe, amniocentesis can trigger cramping, leakage of amniotic fluid, and vaginal bleeding, and it may increase the risk of miscarriage by about 0.5 to 1 percent. The test is done only on women at increased risk of having babies with genetic disorders or to assess the maturity of the baby's lungs in the last trimester.

Chorionic Villus Sampling Performed between 10 and 12 weeks of pregnancy, CVS can detect the same genetic abnormalities as amniocentesis, with the exception of neural tube defects. CVS is undertaken earlier in a pregnancy than amniocentesis. The results are usually available within 10 days. The test involves inserting a needle or catheter into the womb and extracting some of the chorionic villi (cells from the placenta that originate from the fertilized egg). These villi have the same genes as the fetus.

The test is quite safe, but CVS has a slightly greater risk of causing miscarriage than amniocentesis, since it takes place earlier in the pregnancy. Rare cases of babies born with finger and toe defects after CVS have been reported, but these seem to have been in tests undertaken before the ninth week. The accuracy of CVS results is 98 percent.[15]

Complications in Pregnancy and Childbirth

Most women progress through pregnancy and delivery without complications, but once in a great while something goes wrong. Complications are usually the result of genetics, an environmental factor (such as the use of drugs or alcohol by the mother), or some combination of these. Pregnant women should remember that the following complications are unusual if they are consuming a healthy diet, avoiding agents that can damage a fetus, such as alcohol and drugs, and following their doctor's recommendations.

- *Ectopic pregnancy.* This is a pregnancy in which the embryo implants outside the uterus, most often in a fallopian tube. It can be serious and even life threatening, especially if not discovered early, but treatment can remove most of the risk for the mother while preserving future fertility.

- *Miscarriage.* Early miscarriage is very common, occurring in as many as half of all conceptions, often passing unnoticed by the woman. It is usually related to a chromosomal abnormality or other problem in the fetus. Late miscarriage, on the other hand, is usually related to the mother's condition, her exposure to drugs or other toxins, or problems of the placenta.

- *Gestational diabetes.* This is a temporary condition in which the mother's body does not produce enough insulin to handle the increased blood sugar of pregnancy. Symptoms include unusual thirst, frequent urination, and fatigue. If treated, it is not a threat to the mother or baby.

- *Hyperemesis gravidarum.* This term literally means "excessive vomiting during pregnancy." This is a very unusual condition that is more serious than typical morning sickness. If untreated, it can result in malnutrition, dehydration, or damage to the fetus. It can be treated, however, with measures ranging from rest and antacids to hospitalization if necessary.

- *Preeclampsia (pregnancy-induced hypertension; toxemia).* This is a condition in which the woman's blood pressure becomes elevated during pregnancy; it occurs in one of every 10–20 pregnancies, and if untreated, preeclampsia can be serious and even life threatening. Fortunately, physicians almost invariably identify the disease if the mother is receiving regular prenatal care, and a poor outcome is rare. Treatment depends on the severity of the disease and can include an immediate induction of labor or hospitalization of the mother until the fetus is sufficiently developed to survive outside the uterus.

- *Eclampsia.* The final stage of preeclampsia, this disease is very unusual when the mother is receiving regular prenatal care. Symptoms include convulsions and coma. Treatment includes preventing convulsions and inducing labor or performing a cesarean delivery as soon as possible.

- *Intrauterine growth retardation (IUGR).* This term is used to describe insufficient growth of the fetus, which can occur because of genetic factors, maternal disease, or fetal malnutrition. With regular prenatal care, this condition can be identified and reversed.

- *Premature rupture of the membranes (PROM).* Rupture of the chorionic membranes, often called "breaking of the water," can occur prematurely. Infection is a risk because the protective membrane has been broken. Doctors typically try to delay delivery as long as possible up to about 37 weeks.

- *Premature labor.* Labor that begins after the fetus is considered viable and before term, at about 37 weeks, is called *premature labor.* It carries a variety of risks, but in many cases premature labor can be halted, and the mother can carry the baby to term. Quick medical attention is paramount.

- *Fetal distress.* This term describes a category of fetal problems, in particular a lack of oxygen caused by any of a variety of factors. The treatment usually is immediate delivery, by cesarean if necessary.

 TALKING POINTS Are there people in your life who you can comfortably ask, "What was it like to go through labor and delivery?" Will you feel open enough to express any personal concerns you might have about your own fears of this process?

Infertility

Most traditional age college students are interested in preventing pregnancy. However, other people are trying to do just the opposite: they are trying to become pregnant. It is estimated that about 10 percent of the U.S. population has a problem with *infertility.* These couples wish to become pregnant but are unsuccessful.

Causes of Infertility

What causes infertility? About 40 percent of infertility problems are attributed to male factors and about 40 percent are explained by female factors. Approximately 10 percent of the problems stem from a combination of female and male factors, while the remaining 10 percent come from unknown origins.[16]

Problems of infertility that may come from males include low sperm count, inability of the sperm to move properly, or structural abnormalities of the sperm. Female factors related to infertility center on lack of ovulation and obstructions in the fallopian tubes.

Preventing Infertility

Can you do anything to prevent infertility? There are many ways you can increase your chances of remaining fertile. Avoiding sexually transmitted diseases is one crucial factor. (See the guidelines for safe sex in Chapter 12.) The risk from multiple partners should encourage responsible sexual activity. Men and women should avoid working around hazardous chemicals or using psychoactive drugs. Being overweight or underweight, smoking, and heavy alcohol consumption are risk factors that reduce one's fertility.[17] Maintaining overall good health and having regular medical (and, for women, gynecological) checkups are excellent ideas. Because infertility is directly linked with advancing age, couples may not want to indefinitely delay having children.

Consumer and Safety Issues

Part Six includes chapters on consumer health and safety. The decisions you make in each of these areas can have a profound effect on your well-being in each dimension of your health.

1. Physical Dimension

The physical dimension of health is directly influenced by consumer decisions, such as the physician you choose. And, of course, it is crucial to learn how to protect yourself from physical harm caused by intentional or unintentional injury.

2. Emotional Dimension

The effect of an overcrowded, highly industrialized society on your emotional health is often evident. Yet an even more powerful influence is the potential for violence or unintentional injury. Many people who are rape survivors or victims of other crimes feel fearful or angry for years afterward. Those who have behaved violently themselves may find that the knowledge of their actions erodes their emotional health.

3. Social Dimension

Good health care consumers are made, not born. The decisions you make about your health are shaped by many people. Your doctor, for example, may give you information about behavior change, or your insurance agent may offer you several managed care options from which to choose. Effective interaction with these professionals and many other people can help you meet your health care needs.

4. Intellectual Dimension

Understanding violence-related issues and consumer options requires critical thinking skills. Isolating causes of safety-related problems and devising workable solutions are complex tasks. In addition, you must be able to analyze a number of variables to make difficult decisions about your health.

5. Spiritual Dimension

Nurturing our spirituality and caring for the well-being of others are inextricably intertwined. As we search for solutions to complex social and health-related issues, we must often make difficult decisions: For example, will we someday deny health insurance coverage to persons based on the existence of high-risk health behaviors such as tobacco use and a sedentary lifestyle? Or, might we someday legally define smoking by parents as a form of child abuse? To build a better world for future generations may be the most serious challenge to our spiritual commitment to serve others.

6. Occupational Dimension

Your occupational health can be enhanced by making sound decisions about your health care and personal safety. For example, choosing a health care provider who emphasizes prevention and positive behavior change will promote your overall well-being and minimize the number of days you are unable to work because of illness. In addition, avoiding intentional and unintentional injuries will allow you to perform at your peak.

part six

chapter 18

Becoming an Informed Health Care Consumer

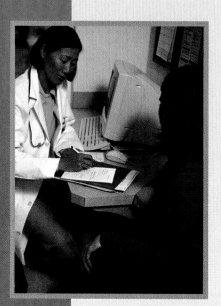

Online Learning Center Resources
www.mhhe.com/payne10e

Visit the Online Learning Center for tools to improve your grade and get the most out of your course—chapter objectives, practice quizzes, key terms flashcards, chapter summaries for your digital audio player, Web activities, self-assessments, and many other study aids.

What Do You Know about Health Care?

◉ In terms of assessing the honesty of health-related advertising, testimonials represent the highest level of trustworthiness. True or False?

◉ On the basis of current educational standards and state licensing examinations, a doctoral degree in allopathic medicine (MD) and a doctoral degree in osteopathic medicine (DO) are essentially interchangeable. True or False?

◉ Nurse practitioners are primary care providers who are permitted to diagnose and treat patients, doing so under the supervision of physicians. True or False?

◉ To be permitted to practice in the United States, practitioners in all fields of complementary and alternative medicine (CAM) must pass licensing examinations supervised by the U.S. Department of Health and Human Services. True or False?

◉ The sale of a generic version of a prescription medication is permitted upon the expiration of the patent protection period of the brand name medication. True or False?

◉ You must have a prescription to purchase over-the-counter (OTC) medications in any state other than the state where you obtained your driver's license. True or False?

◉ The safety and effectiveness of dietary supplements is established and carefully monitored by the Food and Drug Administration (FDA). True or False?

Check your answers at the end of the chapter.

Health care providers often evaluate you by criteria from their areas of expertise. The nutritionist knows you by the food you eat. The physical fitness professional knows you by your body type and activity level. In the eyes of the expert in health consumerism, you are the product of the health information you believe, the health-influencing services you use, and the products you consume. When you make your decisions about health information, services, and products after careful study and consideration, your health will probably be improved. However, when your decisions lack insight, your health, as well as your pocketbook, may suffer.

Health Information

The Informed Consumer

The Pew Charitable Trust's ongoing study of Internet use (Internet & American Life Project)[1] provides current information on health-related Internet use. The breadth of this interest is informative. Of the 95 million Americans who in 2004 conducted health-related searches, 66 percent of the searchers sought information pertaining to specific conditions and problems, 51 percent to treatment and management of conditions, 51 percent to nutrition and diet, 42 percent to exercise and fitness, 40 percent to prescription medications and over-the-counter (OTC) products, and 30 percent to alternative treatments. Further, 31 percent sought information regarding health insurance, 18 percent investigated environmental health issues, and 11 percent pursued sexual health information. Among the 16 areas searched, only 8 percent sought information pertaining to drug and alcohol use, whereas 7 percent investigated information pertaining to smoking cessation, the area least visited.

In light of the breadth of these interest areas and the complexity associated with each, it is very likely that most people turn to a variety of sources for the information and access that they seek. Some sources are easily accessed, while others are more difficult to find but perhaps contain more appropriate information. In the section that follows you will be introduced to several sources of health-related information. Complete the Personal Assessment at the end of this chapter to rate your own skills as a consumer of health-related information, products, and services.

Sources of Information

Your sources of information on health topics are as diverse as the number of people you know, the number of publications you read, and the number of experts you see or hear. No single agency or profession regulates the quantity or quality of the health-related information you receive. Readers will quickly recognize that all are familiar sources and that some provide more accurate and honest information than others.

Family and Friends   The accuracy of information you get from a friend or family member may be questionable. Too often the information your family and friends offer is based on "common knowledge" that is wrong. In addition, family members or friends may provide information they believe is in your best interest rather than facts that may have a more negative effect on you.

Advertisements and Commercials   Many people spend much of every day watching television, listening to the radio, and reading newspapers or magazines. Because many advertisements are health oriented, these are significant sources of information. The primary purpose of advertising, however, is to sell products or services. One newer example of this intertwining of health information with marketing is the "infomercial," in which a compensated studio audience watches a skillfully produced program that trumpets the benefits of a particular product or service. In spite of the convincing nature of these infomercials, however, the validity of their information is often questionable.

In contrast to advertisements and commercials, the mass media routinely offer public service messages, as mandated by the FCC, that give valuable health-related information. For example, the FCC ordered antismoking public-service announcements on television following the release of the first Surgeon General's Report on Smoking and Health (1964). These ads were powerful players in fostering a significant drop in smoking during the late 1960s and the 1970s.

Labels and Directions   Federal law requires that many consumer product labels, including all medications and many kinds of food (see Chapter 5), contain specific information. For example, when a pharmacist dispenses a prescription medication, he or she must give a detailed information sheet describing the medication.

Many health care providers and agencies give consumers helpful information about their health problems or printed directions for preparing for screening procedures. Generally, information from these sources is accurate and current and is given with the health of the consumer foremost in mind.

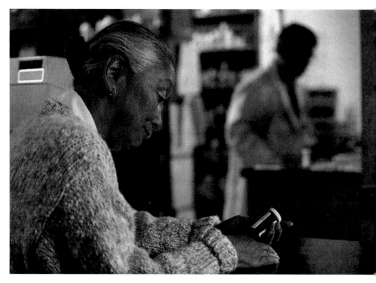

Labels and directions that accompany prescription medications are a good source of information for consumers.

Folklore   Because it is passed down from generation to generation, folklore about health is the primary source of health-related information for some people.

The accuracy of health-related information obtained from family members, neighbors, and coworkers is difficult to evaluate. As a general rule, however, one should exercise caution relying on its scientific soundness. A blanket dismissal is not warranted, however, because folk wisdom is occasionally supported by scientific evidence. In addition, the emotional support provided by the suppliers of this information could be the best medicine some people could receive. In fact, for some ethnic groups, indigenous health care is central to overall health care. For example, within the Chinese American community, practitioners of traditional healing arts represent primary health care. Even though many Americans would consider this form of care "folk medicine," it is highly valued and trusted by those who find it familiar.

Testimonials   People eagerly want to share information that has benefited them. Others may base their decisions on such testimonials. However, the exaggerated testimonials that accompany the sales pitches of the medical quack or the "satisfied" customers appearing in advertisements and on commercials and infomercials should never be interpreted as valid endorsements.

Mass Media   Health programming on cable television stations, stories in lifestyle sections of newspapers, health care correspondents appearing on national network news shows, and the growing number of health-oriented magazines are sources of health information in the mass media.

In terms of the public's priority for specific media sources of health information, a gradual evolution is occurring. As recently as 1999, television, followed by magazines and newspapers, were the three principal sources of health-related news for American adults. Now, with more than 200 million Americans having cable or phone access,[2] these traditional sources of information are gradually losing popularity to the Internet. Most likely this trend will continue until a new information-sharing technology moves into the mainstream of American life.

Health-related information in the mass media is generally accurate, but it is sometimes presented so quickly or superficially that its usefulness is limited. The consumer who wants more complete coverage of a health topic might acquire it by subscribing to a cable channel devoted partly or entirely to health-related programming, such as the Discovery Health Channel or The Learning Channel.

Practitioners   The health care consumer also receives much information from individual health practitioners and their professional associations. In fact, today's health care practitioner so clearly emphasizes patient education that finding one who does not offer some information to a patient would be difficult. Education improves patient **compliance** with health care directives, which is important to the practitioner and the consumer.

Another important development in the trend toward health-related education is the evolution of the hospital as an educational institution. Moving beyond traditional educational activities, such as physician/staff in-house education and patient education, hospitals are extending their educational activities into the communities in a variety of ways, including newspapers, online websites, and public speaking bureaus. Wellness centers and larger multispecialty group practices are also engaged in informational outreach.

Online Computer Services   We have already discussed the rapidly growing utilization of the Internet as a primary source of health-related information. We have even, in a sense, concluded that you are or would be one of those users. This assumption may not, however, be as predictable as we believe.

In spite of the fact that today's health care system depends on computer technology to diagnose and treat illness and injury, medical professionals are perhaps the professionals least likely to use the Internet to correspond with their clients. In a study of medical practitioners across a wide range of medical specialties, only 16 percent had ever used e-mail to correspond with patients, and less than 3 percent had done so with any frequency.[3] It is not clear why physicians seem reluctant to correspond in this manner, but the medical establishment states concerns over privacy and issues of liability.

 TALKING POINTS A family member considers herself good at diagnosing health problems. Since she hasn't been wrong in years, she no longer relies on physicians. What questions could you ask her to point out the dangers associated with her approach?

Health Reference Publications   A substantial portion of all households own or subscribe to a health reference publication, such as the *Encyclopedia of Complementary Health Practices,* the *Physicians' Desk Reference (PDR),* or a newsletter such as *The Harvard Medical School Health Letter* or *The Johns Hopkins Medical Letter: Health after 50.* Some consumers also use personal computer programs and DVDs or CDs featuring health-related information.

┌─ **Key Terms** ─────────────────────────────

compliance Willingness to follow the directions provided by another person.

Table 18.1 Consumer Protection Agencies and Organizations

These agencies and organizations can be found in a variety of forms. Many are located within the organizational makeup of various federal agencies, while others, taking the form of free-standing organizations, are sustained in part by the validity of products, services, and corporate "good citizenship" of companies engaged in retail sales. Yet a third arena of operation for consumer protective services is within the confines of a highly creditable professional organization, such as the American Medical Association. Several consumer protective agencies and organizations are listed below.

Federal Agencies

Office of Consumer Affairs, Food and Drug Administration
(301) 827-5006
www.fda.gov/oca/aboutoca.htm

Federal Trade Commission
www.ftc.gov

Fraud Division, U.S. Postal Inspection Service
(202) 268-4299
www.usps.gov

Consumer Information Center
(719) 948-3334
www.pueblo.gsa.gov

U.S. Consumer Product Safety Commission Hotline
(800) 638-CPSC

Consumer Organizations

Consumers Union of the U.S., Inc.
(914) 378-2000
www.consumerreports.org

Professional Organizations

American Medical Association
(312) 464-5000
www.ama-assn.org

American Hospital Association
(312) 422-3000
www.aha.org

American Pharmaceutical Association
(202) 628-4410
www.aphanet.org

Reference Libraries Public and university libraries continue to be popular sources of health-related information. One can consult with reference librarians and check out audiovisual collections and printed materials. More and more of these holdings can be accessed through the home computer.

Consumer Advocacy Groups A variety of nonprofit consumer advocacy groups patrol the health care marketplace (Table 18.1). These groups produce and distribute information designed to help the consumer recognize questionable services and products. Large, well-organized groups, such as The National Consumers' League and Consumers Union, and smaller groups at the state and local levels champion the right of the consumer to receive valid and reliable information about health care products and services.

Voluntary Health Agencies Volunteerism and the traditional approach to health care and health promotion are virtually inseparable. Few countries besides the United States can boast so many national voluntary organizations, with state and local affiliates, dedicated to improving health through research, service, and public education. The American Cancer Society, the American Red Cross, the National Multiple Sclerosis Society, and the American Heart Association all are voluntary (not-for-profit) health agencies. Consumers can, in fact, expect to find a voluntary health agency for virtually every health problem. College students should also note that volunteerism on their part, perhaps with a health agency like the Red Cross or the AHA, is both a personally satisfying experience and an activity viewed favorably by potential employers.

Government Agencies Government agencies are also effective sources of information to the public. Through meetings and the release of information to the media, agencies such as the Food and Drug Administration, Department of Agriculture, Federal Trade Commission, U.S. Postal Service, and Environmental Protection Agency publicize health issues. Government agencies also control the quality of information sent out to the buying public, particularly through labeling, advertising, and the distribution of information through the mail. The various divisions of the National Institutes of Health regularly release research findings and recommendations to clinical practices, which in turn reach the consumer through clinical practitioners.

Despite their best intentions, federal health agencies are often less effective than the public deserves. A variety of factors, including inadequate staff, poor administration, lobbying by special interest groups, and political pressures prevent these federal agencies from enforcing consumer-protection legislation. As a result, the public is left with a sense of false confidence in the consumer protection provided by the federal government.

State governments also distribute health-related information to the public. State agencies are primary sources of information, particularly in the areas of public health and environmental protection. (For an example of health care activism at work, see the box "Americans with Disabilities Act—New Places to Go.")

Qualified Health Educators Health educators work in a variety of settings and offer their services to diverse groups. Community health educators work with virtually all of the agencies mentioned in this section; patient

Trager bodywork, and a host of other practices that include pressing on muscles, bones, joints, soft tissue, and underlying blood and lymphatic vessels.[7] So varied are the techniques, including location of pressure, depth of pressure, and interval between applications of pressure, that it is difficult to compare one with another. That said, all techniques are based on the common agreement that the body is self-regulating and can heal itself, and that its parts are interdependent. Beyond that, the professional organizations, education and licensing of practitioners, and conduct of clinically based research are too variable to allow meaningful comparisons. Some have suggested, however, that all of these modalities do have in common the structuring of their practices to fit the expectations of their patients.

Although chiropractic, osteopathic, and physical therapy programs do sponsor research that appears in the medical literature (as identified by National Library of Medicine searches), the majority of the other techniques mentioned here have produced relatively little research, or research limited largely to patient observations and self-reporting. The research that does exist includes little or no use of imaging technology; little documentation of anatomical, physiological, or biomechanical changes occurring with treatment; and no evaluation of biochemical alterations occurring at the cellular or subcellular levels.[7] As a result, these practices remain "highly alternative" and are not covered by health insurance. On the positive side, relatively little risk is reported, particularly when practitioners are experienced.

Homeopathy   Widely accepted in Europe, **homeopathy** is the leading alternative therapy in France. Homeopathy uses infinitesimal doses of herbs, minerals, or even poisons to stimulate the body's curative powers. The theory on which homeopathy is based, the *law of similars,* contends that if large doses of a substance can cause a problem, tiny doses can trigger healing. A few small studies showed homeopathy to be at least somewhat effective in treating hay fever, diarrhea, and flu symptoms, but members of the scientific community call the studies flawed or preliminary and suggest that the placebo effect was occurring. Much more informative, however, are reports from three meta-analysis studies, funded by the National Center for Complementary and Alternative Medicine, involving the reassessment of 240 individual studies, in which it was concluded that major methodology weaknesses existed in most studies of homeopathy conducted to date. It was further concluded that on the basis of these studies there was no strong evidence in favor of homeopathy over conventional treatment methods. The Center recommended that larger, more carefully controlled studies be conducted.[8] Since the report on homeopathic medication was released by the National Center for Complementary and Alternative Medicine, recent studies continue to experience methodological

difficulties, principally related to the small sample sizes used by researchers.[9]

An interesting dimension to the marketing of homeopathy as an effective alternative to conventional medical care relates to the contention of some homeopathy physicians that the "molecular essence" of their homeopathic medicines can be sent via the Internet, thus allowing treatment to occur through cyberspace.

Naturopathy   The core of naturopathic medicine is what Hippocrates called *medicatrix naturae,* or the healing power of nature. Proponents of **naturopathy** believe that when the mind and the body are in balance and receiving proper care, with a healthy diet, adequate rest, and minimal stress, the body's own vital forces are sufficient to fight off disease. Getting rid of an ailment is only the first step toward correcting the underlying imbalance that allowed the ailment to take hold, naturists believe. Correcting the imbalance might be as simple as rectifying a shortage of a particular nutrient, or as complex as reducing overlong work hours, strengthening a weakened immune system, and identifying an inability to digest certain foods.

Naturopathy was popular in the nineteenth century and began a comeback in the 1970s in the Pacific Northwest, spurred by the back-to-nature themes of the counterculture. In some states, naturopaths are licensed, and health insurance plans must cover treatment they provide.

Herbalism   **Herbalism,** also known as herbology, phytotherapy, and herbal medicine, is without a doubt the most ancient form of medical treatment. As long ago as the Neandertal period (60,000 years ago), evidence indicates the use of plants for both food and medicine. Today herbalism is the principal form of medical treatment in developing areas of the world and is strongly supported in many developed areas as well. In the United States, botanicals provide the molecular models for many prescription medications and are principal players in the field of dietary supplementation. If prayer is excluded, herbal medicine is the most popular form of complementary and alternative medicine used in America.

Because plants contain active biochemical systems, they are known to produce a wide array of chemical compounds and bioactive metabolites. An experienced herbalist will know how to prepare such plants for human use. However, as with any bioactive material, there is a risk of toxic reaction rather than therapeutic response.[10] Herbalists can be formally trained (undergraduate degrees in herbology can be earned in England, Australia, and Germany) or traditionally trained; both forms of training should make the practitioner knowledgeable about formulating herb-based medications in an appropriate (safe and effective) manner.

Herbal medications and supplements can be dispensed in a variety of forms, including teas, coffees, tinctures, fluid and solid extracts, poultices (plasters), ointments, oils, pills, capsules, and powders. Even though many prescription medications are botanically based, the FDA classifies herbal preparations as dietary supplements because their safety and effectiveness have not been subjected to rigorous testing. Consumers use these preparations knowing relatively little about their safety and effectiveness, processing, formulation, and packaging/labeling. These risks must be taken seriously, particularly by anyone who uses herbal supplements in large quantities or in combination with prescription medications.

Today mainstream American and European pharmaceutical companies are gradually moving into the herbal supplement market. This may improve herbal safety and effectiveness, but the more sophisticated research/testing, manufacturing, marketing, and distribution could raise prices.

Therapeutic Touch (Biofield Therapy) The *biofield* (or energy field) is believed by therapeutic touch practitioners to dwell within and immediately surround the body. For thousands of years, practitioners of biofield therapy, as exemplified by therapeutic touch, have attempted to identify irregularities or contractions in this electrical field and through appropriate touching (or near-touching of the body) restore its appropriate configuration. Once the biofield is aligned appropriately, the negative forces that have been disruptive to the physical and emotional balance required for healthful living are released. A second perception of biofield therapies is that through manipulation of the biofield a pathway or entry point is established that allows other health modalities, such as medications, to influence the restoration of the holistic balance needed for good health.

Practitioners of biofield therapies, including healing touch, therapeutic touch, and SHEN (Specific Human Emotional Nexus) therapy, describe their practice as noninvasive, deeply relaxing, gentle, and both safe and effective. Treatment sessions are usually conducted in a quiet and relaxed location, with the patient fully clothed and lying on a softly padded table or in bed. Sessions generally last from several minutes to an hour, often including a period of dialogue between the patient and the practitioner, and may be delivered for several days or for only a day or two.

Sessions may be delivered within a hospital (before or following surgery) or in the home following discharge from the hospital. Therapeutic touch is generally an adjunct therapy to more conventional therapies, given in conjunction with cancer treatment or during postsurgical recovery or as part of the treatment to alleviate the anxiety associated with traumatic injury recovery. Nurses are the most likely practitioners of therapeutic touch and related therapies in the hospital setting. In fact, it is in

nursing journals that the most literature related to the practice is found. When therapeutic touch is used in a wellness-oriented manner, it is most often delivered by a certified practitioner. This is often a nurse practicing in a fee-for-service manner, a chiropractor, a naturopathic physician, or a psychologist.

The scientific literature regarding the effectiveness of therapeutic touch is very difficult to interpret. This is largely because of the difficulty of establishing double-blind experiments to study a therapeutic approach (that is, experiments in which neither practitioner nor patient knows whether the actual therapy versus a sham therapy is being delivered). A second difficulty is the problem of quantifying the outcome of the therapy. At this point it appears that therapeutic touch is somewhat effective in reducing anxiety, enhancing mood, improving sleep, and producing a higher level of relaxation among patients experiencing various emotionally traumatic medical treatments, such as breast cancer surgery. Its efficacy in enhancing holistic health and a sense of wellness is based largely on self-reported improvement and various inventories designed to assess feeling states.

If you would like to consult a practitioner in one of the alternative disciplines but you don't know where to start, see the box "Researching and Evaluating CAM Practitioners" for advice.

National Center for Complementary and Alternative Medicine At the urging of many people in both the medical and complementary health care fields, the National Institutes of Health requested federal funding to establish a scientific center for the study of alternative medical care. Today the National Center for Complementary and Alternative Medicine assembles information about alternative approaches to medical care and provides a framework for well-controlled research into the effectiveness of each approach. Double-blind studies, so called because neither the participants nor the researchers know which treatment each participant is receiving, are being conducted. The first substantial recommendation regarding an alternative form of care, acupuncture, was released in 1998.

Key Terms

homeopathy (hoe mee **op** ah thee) The use of minute doses of herbs, minerals, or other substances to stimulate healing.

naturopathy (na chur **op** ah thee) A system of treatment that avoids drugs and surgery and emphasizes the use of natural agents, such as sunshine, to correct underlying imbalances.

herbalism An ancient form of healing in which herbal preparations are used to treat illness and disease.

It will be interesting to note whether all the branches of complementary medical care will want their theories of treatment and prevention tested under the rigorous criteria used by the National Center for Complementary and Alternative Medicine and to see how they respond if the results are not favorable.

Restricted-Practice Health Care Providers

We receive much of our health care from medical physicians. However, most of us also use the services of various health care specialists who also have advanced graduate-level training. Among these professionals are dentists, psychologists, podiatrists, and optometrists.

Dentists (Doctor of Dental Surgery, DDS) deal with a wide range of diseases and impairments of the teeth and oral cavity. Dentists undergo undergraduate predental programs that emphasize the sciences, followed by four additional years of study in dental school and, with increasing frequency, an internship program. State licensure examinations are required. As with physicians, dentists can also specialize by completing a postdoctoral master's degree in fields such as oral surgery, **ortho-dontics,** and **prosthodontics.** Dentists are also permitted to prescribe therapy programs (such as the treatment of temporo-mandibular joint [TMJ] dysfunction) and drugs that pertain to their practices (primarily analgesics and antibiotics).

As discussed in Chapter 2, *psychologists* provide services to help patients understand behavior patterns or perceptions. More than 40 states have certification or licensing laws that prohibit unqualified people from using the term *psychologist.* The consumer should examine a psychologist's credentials. Legitimate psychologists have received advanced graduate training (often leading to a PhD or EdD degree) in clinical, counseling, industrial, or educational psychology. Furthermore, these practitioners will have passed state certification examinations and, in many states, will have met further requirements that allow them to offer health services to the public. Psychologists may have special interests and credentials from professional societies in individual, group, family, or marriage counseling. Some are certified as sex therapists.

Unlike psychiatrists, who are medical physicians, psychologists cannot prescribe or dispense drugs. They may refer to or work collaboratively with medical physicians about clients who might benefit from drug therapy.

Podiatrists are highly trained clinicians who practice podiatric medicine, or care of the feet (and ankles). Although not MDs or DOs, doctors of podiatric medicine (DPM) treat a wide variety of conditions related to the feet, including corns, bunions, warts, bone spurs, hammertoes, fractures, diabetes-related conditions, athletic injuries, and structural abnormalities. Podiatrists perform surgery, prescribe medications, and apply orthotics (supports or braces), splints, and corrective shoes for structural abnormalities of the feet.

Doctors of podiatric medicine follow an educational path similar to that taken by MDs and DOs, consisting of a four-year undergraduate preprofessional curriculum, four additional years of study in a podiatric medical school, and an optional residency of one or two years. Board-certified areas of specialization include surgery, orthopedics, and podiatric sports medicine. Hospital affiliation generally requires board certification in a specialized area.

Optometrists are eye specialists who primarily treat vision problems associated with **refractory errors.** They examine the eyes and prescribe glasses or contact lenses to correct visual disorders. Additionally, optometrists prescribe prescription medications, such as antibiotic drops for application in the eye. Optometrists sometimes attempt to correct certain ocular muscle imbalances with specific exercise regimens. Optometrists must complete undergraduate training and additional years of course-work at 1 of 16 accredited colleges of optometry in the United States or 3 Canadian colleges before taking a state licensing examination.[11] Residency programs in areas of specialization are also available, and are one to two years in length.

Opticians are technicians who manufacture and fit eyeglasses or contact lenses. Although they are rarely licensed by a state agency, they perform the important function of grinding lenses to the precise prescription designated by an optometrist or ophthalmologist (physicians who have specialized in vision care). To save money and time, many consumers take an optometrist's or ophthalmologist's prescription for glasses or contact lenses to optician-staffed retail stores that deal exclusively with eyewear products.

Nurse Professionals Nurses constitute a large group of health professionals who practice in a variety of settings. Their responsibilities usually depend on their academic preparation. Registered nurses (RNs) are academically prepared at two levels: (1) the technical nurse and (2) the professional nurse. The technical nurse is educated in a two-year associate degree program. The professional nurse receives four years of education and earns a bachelor's degree. Both technical and professional nurses must successfully complete state licensing examinations before they can practice as RNs.

In light of the important role that nurse professionals play in today's health care system, it is worrisome that a significant shortage of nurses exists. On the basis of enrollment data for nursing programs in this country, and the number of nurses who have apparently left the workforce for various reasons, the current shortage of registered nurses is estimated to be 110,000. Projecting through 2012, it is estimated that 1.1 million new and replacement openings for nurses will exist in the United States,[12] a need that will most likely not be met.

Compounding the shortage of nurses is an equally acute shortage of nursing faculty to staff the nursing education programs that currently exist. As can be imagined, the demand for nurses has increased salaries, generated competition between health care institutions to recruit nurses, and increased the nurse-to-patient ratio to dangerously high levels in many areas of the country. In this final regard, it should not be surprising that patient ratios exceeding 1 to 3 or 1 to 4, depending on area

---

Key Terms

orthodontics A dental specialty that focuses on the proper alignment of the teeth.

prosthodontics A dental specialty that focuses on the construction and fitting of artificial appliances to replace missing teeth.

refractory errors Abnormal patterns of light wave transmission through the structures of the eye.

of care, has been shown to result in higher levels of job dissatisfaction, increased job burnout, and, of course, adverse patient outcomes (for surgical patients), including increased rates of *failure-to-rescue* (from adverse events) and increased mortality within the 30-day period following discharge.[13]

Many professional nurses continue their education and earn master's and doctoral degrees in nursing or other health-related fields. Some professional nurses specialize in a clinical area (such as pediatrics, gerontology, public health, or school health) and become certified as *advanced practice nurses* (APNs). Currently four APN fields, including nurse midwives, nurse anesthetists, nurse practitioners, and nurse case managers, can be found in larger communities. Working in close association with physicians, APNs perform an array of diagnositic, treatment, and administrative activities once limited to physicians. The ability of these highly trained nurses to function at this level gives communities additional primary care providers and frees physicians to deal with more complex cases. With the expansion of managed care, the role of APNs is growing. This increases access to medical care and allows physicians to use their time more cost-effectively.

Licensed practical nurses (LPNs) are trained in hospital-based programs that last 12 to 18 months. Because of their brief training, LPNs' scope of practice is limited. Most LPN training programs are gradually being phased out. Additionally, some hospitals are financially assisting LPNs to transition into associate degree programs leading to the RN degree, or to be redefined as a nursing care technologist, at a lower rate of pay, if they do not receive the RN degree.

Allied Health Care Professionals   Our primary health care providers are supported by a large group of allied health care professionals, who are often responsible for highly technical services and procedures. These professionals include respiratory and inhalation therapists, radiographic technologists, nuclear medicine technologists, pathology technicians, general medical technologists, operating room technicians, emergency medical technicians, physical therapists, occupational therapists, cardiac rehabilitation therapists, dental technicians, physician assistants, and dental hygienists. Depending on the particular field, the training for these specialty support areas can take from one to five years of postsecondary school study. Programs include hospital-based training leading to a diploma through associate, bachelor's, and master's degrees. Most allied health care professionals must also pass state or national licensing examinations.

Self-Care/Home Care

The emergence of the **self-care movement** suggests that many people are becoming more responsible for

Self-care is appropriate in the management of certain chronic conditions, including diabetes. People with diabetes can monitor their blood sugar at home and make appropriate adjustments to their diet and medication schedule.

maintaining their health. They are developing the expertise to prevent or manage many types of illness, injuries, and conditions. They are learning to assess their health status and treat, monitor, and rehabilitate themselves in a manner that was once thought possible only through a physician or some other health care specialist.

The benefits of this movement are that self-care can (1) reduce health care costs, (2) provide effective care for particular conditions, (3) free physicians and other health care specialists to spend time with other patients, and (4) increase interest in health-related activities.

Appropriate Self Care   Self-care is an appropriate alternative to professional care in three areas. First, self-care may be appropriate for certain acute conditions that have familiar symptoms and are limited in their duration and seriousness. Common colds and flu, many home injuries, sore throats, and nonallergic insect bites are often easily managed with self-care. That said, there are some symptoms that might seem somewhat familiar that should not be responded to through self-care, but rather by seeing a physician promptly. These include a feeling of pressure or squeezing in the chest, a sudden severe headache, markedly blurred vision, difficulty talking or walking, dizziness and confusion, blood in urine or stool, unrelieved depression, and a cough with a yellow-green discharge. Self-care might be useful at some point, but not until the symptoms have been evaluated by a physician.

A second area in which self-care might be appropriate is therapy. For example, many people administer injections for diabetes mellitus, allergies, and migraine headaches and continue physical therapy programs in their homes. Asthma and hypertension are also conditions that can be managed or monitored with self-care.

A third area in which self-care has appropriate application is health promotion. Weight loss programs,

Table 18.2 Patients' Institutional Rights

Regardless of the type of institution in which you are a patient, you have a
financial loss. The hospital too can expect your cooperation as a patient.

As a patient, you can expect all of the following from the institution:

- To be treated with respect and dignity
- To be afforded privacy and confidentiality consistent with federal and st&
- To be provided services on request, as long as they are reasonable and
- To be fully informed of the identity of the physicians and staff providing
- To be kept fully updated about your condition, including its management
- To be informed of any experimental or other research/educational projec
- To have the opportunity to specify advance directives (a living will, a life
  order to facilitate health care decisions
- To receive an explanation of your bill for services regardless of the sourc
- To present a complaint and receive a response about any aspect of your
- To be involved in ethical considerations that arise during the course of y

The institution can expect you, as a patient:

- To keep all appointments
- To provide all background information pertinent to your condition
- To treat hospital personnel with respect
- To ask questions and seek clarification about matters that affect you
- To follow the treatment prescribed by your physician
- To be considerate and respectful of other patients and to ensure that you
- To satisfy your financial obligation to health care providers through the p

As a patient, you may at any time:

- Refuse treatment
- Seek a second opinion
- Discharge yourself from the institution

Beyond the "universal" patient/institutional rights listed above, a wide arra
based needs, sensory perception deficiencies (including access to commu
hospitalized patients. Information pertaining to these needs can be found i
ment of Health and Human Services, March 7, 2007, www.hhs.gov/ocr/hos

---

---

year for which statistics are available) nearly 45.8 million Americans were without health insurance for the entire year.[16] Some believe that adding those people who lacked coverage for a portion of the year to the preceding figure would result in a total number of 75 million people with less than full health care. No age group is more likely to be uncovered than are young adults between 18 and 24 years of age. Demographic differences in the pool of uninsured reflect the unevenness of the problem. Again using the most recent figures available, approximately 19 percent of persons under the age of 18 were uninsured. When race and ethnicity were viewed, 33 percent of Hispanics, 30 percent of Native Americans and Native Alaskans, 20 percent of African Americans, and 15 percent of whites lacked health insurance coverage. Household income also reflects the same unevenness of health insurance coverage, as nearly a quarter of households with incomes below $25,000 lack coverage, in comparison to only 8.5 percent of households earning over $75,000.[17] Employed persons, regardless of age or race, who work in the service sector and lack benefits, such as food workers, and the self-employed often find access to individual

physical conditioning activities, smoking cessation, and stress-reduction programs are particularly well suited to self-care (see the box "Good Health—What's It Worth, Now and Later?").

A potential fourth area in home care, self-diagnosis, is emerging, and not without some concern. Perhaps beginning with the thermometer, progressing to the home pregnancy test and the mail-in HIV diagnostic kit, today in-home genetic testing is available. These genetic screening tests are readily available and consist of a swab that is used to obtain a scraping of cells from the inner cheek and a mail-in envelope. Upon processing cells for their DNA, persons can obtain a genetic profile as it relates to specific disease predispositions. Principal concerns associated with the use of these tests are the shortcutting of primary care physicians (although some brands require physician consent) and the absence of genetic counselors to work with clients after they receive the results of their tests. Currently, in-home genetic screening tests cost $200–$400 and are readily available over the Internet.

Over a thousand diseases can now be tested for using genetic screening. However, test results based on self-collected samples of genetic material are not necessarily reliable. For example, laboratories processing such materials do not consistently demonstrate analytical validity (getting the right technological outcome from the tissue sample submitted) and clinical validity (verifying that the DNA results are related to a medically recognized condition). When samples submitted to online genetic testing services (by the U.S. Genetics and Public Policies Center) were retested, it was found that many of the initial test results did not meet acceptable criteria for validity. Furthermore, companies that were marketing dietary and exercise prescriptions based on genetic findings

(nutrigenomic testing) were often returning advice inconsistent with genetic findings.[14] Today there is little governmental supervision over this growing form of self-care.

Home Health Care   As the U.S. population ages, it is becoming increasingly common for family members to provide home care to older relatives. As the number of frail older people increases, home care can significantly reduce the need for institutional care. Home care also can be delivered by home health care specialists. In fact, this form of care is proving so cost-effective that some insurance programs, including *Medicare* and *Medicaid,* cover portions of the cost of home health care for older adults. (See the sections on Medicare and Medicaid on pages 523–524.)

With the rapid development of the home health care industry during the 1980s and 1990s, concerns mounted about the lack of regulation over aspects of the industry, particularly the background and training of personnel, and existence of fraud in the billing of services to Medicare and Medicaid. Although personnel issues remain to some degree, the financial aspects of professional home care have been addressed at the federal level. In 1999 the Healthcare Integrity and Protection Data Bank was established to better supervise the billing by home

> **Key Terms**
>
> **self-care movement**   The trend toward individuals' taking increased responsibility for prevention or management of certain health conditions.

health care providers for services covered under Medicare and Medicaid.

A decision to provide family-based home care, particularly for older adults, is often made for admirable and understandable reasons, including love for the relative who needs care and the high cost of professional home care and institutional care. For the millions of families who have made this decision, providing home health care can be highly rewarding. It also can be very demanding, however, because of the needs and limitations of the person who requires care and the compromises the caregivers must make.[15] Particularly when a spouse or family decides to provide care without the assistance of professional caregivers, they can jeopardize their own health long before the recovery or death of the person for whom they are caring. Even when their physical stamina seems unaffected, factors such as fatigue, emotional strain, postponement of personal and family goals, loss of social contact, and even physical abuse of caregivers by those receiving care can be substantial.

Health Care Facilities

Most of us have a general idea of what a hospital is. However, all hospitals are not alike. They usually fall into one of three categories—private, publicly owned, or voluntary. *Private hospitals* (or proprietary hospitals) function as profit-making hospitals. They are not supported by tax monies and usually accept only clients who can pay all their expenses. Although there are some exceptions, these hospitals are generally smaller than tax-supported public hospitals. Commonly owned by a group of business investors, a large hospital corporation, or a group of physicians, these hospitals sometimes limit their services to a few specific types of illnesses.

Publicly owned hospitals are supported primarily by tax dollars. They can be operated by government agencies at the state level (such as state mental hospitals) or at the federal level (such as the Veterans Administration Hospitals and various military service hospitals such as Walter Reed Army Medical Center in Washington, D.C., about which so much has been written in regard to conditions surrounding the care of wounded soldiers from Iraq and Afghanistan). Large county or city hospitals are frequently public hospitals. These hospitals routinely serve indigent segments of the population. They also function as *teaching hospitals.*

The most commonly recognized type of hospital is the *voluntary hospital.* Voluntary hospitals are maintained as nonprofit public institutions. Often supported by religious orders, fraternal groups, or charitable organizations, these hospitals usually offer a wider range of comprehensive services than do private hospitals or clinics. Voluntary hospitals are supported by patient fees (covered by health insurance), Medicare reimbursement,

In its current configuration Medicare is divided into two portions. Part A helps pay for care while in hospitals, as well as for care in skilled nursing facilities and hospice care, and for some home health care. Persons become eligible for Part A coverage on turning 65, on the condition of having paid Medicare taxes while working. Medicare Part A does require an annual deductible of $992 (historically deemed to be the equivalent of the first three days of hospital care). Additionally, beginning in 2007, Part A–related deductions from Social Security monthly payments will be increased progressively for individuals with a total retirement income above $80,000 and for couples with a combined income above $160,000.[23] This Medicare Modernization Act legislation is intended to more equitably share the burden of the "universal" Part A portion of Medicare.

Part B is an optional portion of Medicare that can be chosen at the time of becoming eligible for Part A, or at selected times following initial eligibility. Unlike Part A, there is a monthly charge for Part B coverage. Currently, that charge is $93.50 per month but is subject to annual adjustment. Part B helps pay for doctor's services, outpatient hospital care, and some other medical services not covered under Part A, including physical and occupational therapy, medical devices, and some home health care. Routine dental and vision care are not included. Like Part A, Medicare Part B also has a deductible, currently $131.

Because of the universal nature of Medicare Part A and the affordable monthly charge for Part B, group health insurance plans to which many retirees belong require that Medicare be the "first payer" for services, thus allowing the group plan to be responsible for only that portion of health-related charges not covered by Medicare.

The Medicare Prescription Drug Improvement and Modernization Act of 2003 (now referred to as Part D) provides new prescription coverage options for Medicare recipients. Beginning in 2006, it provides prescription coverage through third-party providers for a premium of about $35 per month. In 2007, after meeting an annual deductible of $265 Medicare covers 75 percent of the costs of prescription drugs, up to $2,250 per year; there is then a gap (the "donut hole") in coverage until out-of-pocket expenses reach $3,600 in a single year, at which point Medicare kicks in again and covers 95 percent of further costs for the remainder of the year. The Medicare prescription drug program is expected to cost the Medicare system $724 billion during the first decade of its existence.

After its initial implementation in 2006, Medicare Part D remains confusing for many older persons, largely due to the large number of Part D coverage plans available in the marketplace, "windows" during which coverage can be changed, in combination with the array of medications that are frequently added or subtracted from the lists of medications covered, thus making some plans a "better fit" than other plans. That said, at this point

acceptance of Part D has been strong, and first-year costs were slightly lower than initially anticipated. Further refinements in Medicare-based drug coverage will likely occur with time.

Medicaid

Unlike Medicare, a program that is almost exclusively for persons 65 or older, *Medicaid* is a program designed to assist in meeting the health care needs of qualified persons regardless of age. Also unlike Medicare, which is a federal program entirely funded through Medicare tax withholdings (Part A), user-paid elected enrollment fees (Part B), and the new Part D, Medicaid is a federal- and state-funded program administered by each of the individual states.

Qualification for receiving Medicaid assistance can be perplexing. Federal Medicaid law sets mandatory eligibility standards, while optional eligibility standards allow each state to tailor many aspects of the program to fit its unique needs. Central to the majority of the federally mandated eligibility standards is the current Federal Poverty Level (FPL), as well as the standards related to the Aid to Families with Dependent Children (AFDC) program and the Temporary Assistance to Needy Families (TANF) program. Optional eligibility standards allow states to define some aspects of eligibility for pregnant women, disabled children, certain working disabled persons, and those designated as medically needy.

Federally mandated Medicaid services are wide ranging and include hospital services, physician services, laboratory/x-ray procedures, immunizations, family planning services, home health care services, transportation for medical care services, and nursing home services. This final service is of critical importance to older adults in that it pays for the majority of nursing home care required by this age group. Optional services, which are under state control, include prescription drugs, rehabilitation and physical therapy services, prosthetic devices, vision services, hearing services, and dental services, to include a few.

Health Maintenance Organizations

Health maintenance organizations (HMOs) are health care delivery plans under which health care providers agree to meet the covered medical needs of subscribers for a prepaid amount of money. For a fixed monthly fee, enrollees are given comprehensive health care with an emphasis on preventive health care. Enrollees receive their care from physicians, specialists, allied health professionals, and educators who are hired (group model) or contractually retained (network model) by the HMO.

Managed care, and HMOs in particular, was a reaction to the sharply climbing costs of health care that began in the 1980s. Businesses, which paid a large portion of health care costs through employee-benefit plans, complained that no one in the health care loop had an incentive to control costs. Employers complained that consumers paid only a deductible and a small copayment, giving them little cause to question prices; doctors faced little financial oversight; and insurance companies merely rubber-stamped the bills.

When HMOs presented an alternative, employers began offering their workers incentives to select HMOs over traditional fee-for-service coverage and thus attempted to rein in the runaway costs of health care. HMOs now cover nearly 74 million Americans. Membership is rising again following a gradual decline during mid-2005 when HMOs discontinued serving Medicare recipients (as a Medicare carve-out program) due to the cost of their prescription medication needs. However, in spite of growing enrollment, HMO premiums continue to rise at rates commensurate with other forms of health care coverage.[24]

HMOs are usually the least expensive but most restrictive type of managed care. The premiums are 8–10 percent lower than those for traditional plans, they charge no deductibles or coinsurance payments, and copayments are $15–$20 per visit. However, you are limited to using the doctors and hospitals in the HMO's network, and you must get approval for treatments and referrals.

In theory, HMOs were to be the ideal blend of medical care and health promotion. Today, however, many observers are concerned that too many HMOs are being too tightly controlled by a profit motive in which physicians are being paid large bonuses to *not* refer patients to specialists or are prevented by "gag rules" from discussing certain treatment options with patients because of their costs to the HMOs.

Concerns, in addition to the "gag rules" mentioned above, have also arisen over the years. Among these have been concerns related to the right of members to sue their HMOs for medical negligence, the provision of better ob-gyn coverage, and the development of a more efficient mechanism to appeal denial of services. However, in the last regard, in 2004 the Supreme Court ruled that HMO patients could not use more permissive state laws to sue HMOs for damages resulting from their refusal to approve particular medical services.

In spite of the problems just mentioned, HMOs remain, in theory, more cost-efficient than the traditional fee-for-service health care model. Cost containment is achieved, in part, because most of the medical services within a group model HMO are centralized, and there is little duplication of facilities, equipment, or support staff.

Other new approaches to reducing health costs are independent practice associations (IPAs) and preferred provider organizations (PPOs). An IPA is a modified form of an HMO that uses a group of doctors who offer prepaid services out of their own offices and not in a central HMO facility. IPAs are viewed as "HMOs without walls." A PPO is a group of private practitioners who sell their services at reduced rates to insurance companies. When a policyholder chooses a physician who is in that company's PPO network, the insurance company pays the entire physician's fee less the deductible and copay amounts. When a policyholder selects a non-PPO physician, the insurance company pays a smaller portion of that physician's fee. Today, more than 80 percent of Americans with health benefits are enrolled in a managed care plan (HMO, IPA, or PPO).

Extended or Long-Term Care Insurance

With the aging of the population and the greater likelihood that nursing home care will be required (at nearly $64,240 per year in 2005 for a semiprivate room), insurers have developed extended care policies.[25] When purchased at an early age (by one's mid-50s), these policies are much more affordable than if purchased when a spouse or family member will soon require institutional care. However, not all older adults will need extensive nursing home care, so an extended or long-term care policy could be an unnecessary expenditure.

Access to Health Care

With nearly 46 million (or perhaps more) Americans lacking any health insurance and with nearly a quarter of those with insurance being underinsured, Americans are finding it increasingly difficult to access their country's highly sophisticated health care system. The unemployed poor, working poor, and minorities have the most difficulty accessing health care. African Americans, Hispanic Americans, and Native Americans have the worst health status of all Americans, yet they receive the fewest health care services. Even for older Americans with Medicare, gaping holes exist in the types of care covered (for example, glasses and hearing aids are not covered) and the prices of prescription medications far exceed the coverage provided. Currently, the United States and South Africa are the only two major industrialized nations lacking a comprehensive and unified approach to meeting the health care needs of their populations.

There is today, however, renewed interest at the federal level in finding a solution to our health care crisis, and at the state level, California and Massachusetts have formulated statewide plans to provide more effective health care coverage for their residents. Whether these efforts will stimulate more comprehensive federal planning remains to be seen.

Health-Related Products

As you might imagine, prescription and over-the-counter (OTC) drugs constitute an important part of any discussion of health-related products.

Prescription Drugs

Caution: Federal law prohibits dispensing without prescription. This FDA warning appears on the labels of approximately three-fourths of all medications. Prescription drugs must be ordered for patients by a licensed practitioner. Because these compounds are legally controlled and may require special skills in their administration, the public's access to these drugs is limited.

Although the *Physicians' Desk Reference* lists more than 2,500 compounds that can be prescribed by a physician, only 200 drugs made up the bulk of the nearly 3,383 million new prescriptions and refills dispensed by online, mail-order, supermarket, mass-market, corporate, and independent pharmacies in 2005.[25] Total retail prescription sales of $253.7 billion for 2005 represent a 5.8 percent increase over the previous year's sales and are projected to be in the 6–9 percent range through 2010. This modest upward trend reflects in large part the greater variety of prescription medications being prescribed each year by physicians. It is projected that by the year 2015 approximately $446 billion will be spent on prescription medications.[26]

Research and Development of New Drugs

As consumers of prescription drugs, you may be curious about the process by which drugs gain FDA approval. The rigor of this process may be the reason that only about 17 new drugs were approved in 2006, the lowest number approved in several years.[27]

The nation's pharmaceutical companies constantly explore the molecular structure of various chemical compounds in an attempt to discover important new compounds with desired types and levels of biological activity. Once these new compounds are identified, companies begin extensive in-house research with computer simulations and animal testing to determine whether clinical trials with humans are warranted. Of the 125,000 or more compounds under study each year, only a few thousand receive such extensive preclinical evaluation. Even fewer of these are then taken to the FDA to begin the evaluation process necessary to gain approval for further research with humans. When the FDA approves a drug for clinical trials, a pharmaceutical company can obtain a patent, which prevents the drug from being manufactured by other companies for the next 17 years.

If the 7 years of work needed to bring a new drug into the marketplace go well, a pharmaceutical company enjoys the remaining 10 years of legally protected retail sales. Today new "fast-track" approval procedures at the FDA are progressively reducing the development period, particularly for desperately needed breakthrough drugs such as those used to treat AIDS. Concern was expressed in 2000 that this "rush to approval" forced the FDA to utilize the services of independent evaluators, many of whom had ties to the pharmaceutical industry that could have influenced their assessments of a drug's readiness for marketing.

Figure 18-2 maps the long, arduous, and expensive process whereby a scant few of the tens of thousands of compounds, often derived from botanical sources, are, after nearly 7 years of testing and review, approved for market as the newest prescription medications. During these carefully monitored stages, pharmaceutical companies take biologically active molecules through computer modeling, synthesizing, testing in vitro, testing in animals, and human trials, and eventually some are approved for marketing. Note that in this example, of the 5,000 compounds initially introduced into the process, only 1 successfully completes the approval process to become a marketable prescription medication. For more information on the drug approval process, visit the website for the FDA Center for Drug Evaluation and Research (www.fda.gov/cder/handbook).

For decades the process of testing and reviewing new prescription medications involved human testing only on adult males (such as medical students, prisoners, patients). In the latter decades of the twentieth century, concerns were raised about the absence of women, and then children and older adults, in the testing process, and most recently testing using pregnant women. Today, when deemed appropriate for the best use of a new medication, these groups are included in the human testing protocol. Now when a new medication comes onto the market, it is no longer necessary to extrapolate from adult male dosages in order to determine safe and effective use with women, children, or older adults.[28]

An additional area of concern related to the research and development of prescription medications includes the extent to which the pharmaceutical industry will continue to voluntarily use children (and pregnant women) in reassessment of drug dosages initially determined for adult men and nonpregnant women.

Generic Drugs

When a new drug comes into the marketplace, it carries three names: its **chemical name,** its **generic name,** and its **brand name.** While the 17-year patent is in effect, no other drug with the same chemical formulation can be sold. When the patent expires, other companies can manufacture a drug of equivalent chemical composition and market it under the brand name drug's original generic name. Because extensive research and development are unnecessary at this point, producing generic drugs is far less costly than is developing the original brand name drug. Nearly all states allow pharmacists to substitute generic drugs for brand name drugs, as long as the prescribing physician approves. For those interested in viewing all of the current approved

Figure 18-2 New Drug Development and Approval Only about 5 of 5,000 investigated compounds make it to human testing (clinical trials), and only about 1 in 5 drugs tested in people are eventually approved. The FDA is involved in two stages of drug development: A company files an Investigational New Drug Application (IND) to request approval to test a new drug in humans. If clinical trials indicate that the drug is safe and effective, the drug developer will then file a New Drug Application (NDA) seeking FDA approval to make the drug available for physicians to prescribe to patients. Additional testing and surveillance may be required after drug approval in order to evaluate long-term effects.

Source: Used with permission by Pharmaceutical Research and Manufacturers of America.

	Preclinical Testing		Clinical Trials				FDA		Phase IV
			Phase I	Phase II	Phase III				
Years	3.5		1	2	3		2.5	12 Total	
Test Population	Laboratory and animal studies	File IND at FDA	20 to 80 healthy volunteers	100 to 300 patient volunteers	1,000 to 3,000 patient volunteers	File NDA at FDA	Review process/ approval		Additional post-marketing testing required by FDA
Purpose	Assess safety and biological activity		Determine safety and dosage	Evaluate effectiveness, look for side effects	Verify effectiveness, monitor adverse reactions from long–term use				
Success Rate	5,000 compounds evaluated		5 enter trials				1 approved		

generics, the FDA updates each month its Generic Drug Approvals list.[29]

 TALKING POINTS Your mother insists on using the brand-name drug that she has used for years to control her arthritis pain, even though her doctor has prescribed a generic version that has recently become available. What might you say to help her consider the less expensive option?

In recent years the pharmaceutical industry has actively attempted to extend the patent protection on several of the most profitable drugs on the market because their period of protected sales is expiring. In some cases the manufacturers have appealed directly to Congress for waivers to the current patent law, contending that they need the additional time to recoup research and development costs. This reason seems highly questionable to some people in light of the $4.35 billion spent by the drug industry in 2004 for advertising, most of which was directed to consumers through skillfully crafted televisions commercials (such as those for erectile dysfunction drugs). In addition to direct appeals to Congress, other manufacturers have quietly "layered" additional patents onto their products to prevent manufacturers of generic versions from using the same shape or color used in brand name versions, even though the chemical formulations are no longer protected. In another approach, manufacturers of highly profitable brand name drugs have offered to pay manufacturers of generic drugs to not make generic versions of their products once the patent protection has expired.

Today a variety of reference books are available to inform consumers about the availability of generic drugs and the prescription drugs that they can legally be substituted for. *Mosby's Drug Consult* series is a widely used reference focusing on both brand name drugs and generic equivalents. Updated annually, this publication is currently available in the 2007 edition.[30]

Over-the-Counter Drugs

When people are asked when they last took some form of medication, for many the answer might be, "I took aspirin (or a cold pill, or a laxative) this morning." In making this decision, people engaged in self-diagnosis, determined a course for their own treatment, self-administered their treatment, and freed a physician to serve people whose illnesses are more serious than theirs. None of this would have been possible without readily available, inexpensive, and effective OTC drugs.

Although 2,500 prescription drugs are available in this country, there are easily as many as 100,000 different OTC products,[31] now classified as belonging to one or more of 80 different categories[32]—such as acne medications, laxatives, skin-bleaching agents, cold and cough suppressants, diaper rash ointments, and wart removal compounds. Incorporated into these thousands of products are 1 or more of the 800 FDA-approved (as safe and effective) active ingredients. Like prescription drugs, nonprescription drugs are regulated by the FDA. However, for OTC drugs, the marketplace is a more powerful determinant of success.

The regulation of OTC drugs is based on a provision in a 1972 amendment to the 1938 Food, Drug, and Cosmetic Act. As a result of that action, OTC drugs were

---

Key Terms

chemical name A name used to describe the molecular structure of a drug.

generic name A common or nonproprietary name of a drug.

brand name A specific patented (proprietary) name assigned to a drug by its manufacturer.

Drug Facts

Active Ingredient (in each tablet)   **Purpose**
Chlorpheniramine maleate 2 mg   Antihistamine

Uses temporarily relieves these symptoms due to hay fever or other upper respiratory allergies:

- sneezing ■ runny nose ■ itchy, watery eyes ■ itchy throat

Warnings

Ask a doctor before use if you have
- glaucoma ■ a breathing problem such as emphysema or chronic bronchitis
- trouble urinating due to an enlarged prostate gland

Ask a doctor or pharmacist before use if you are taking tranquilizers or sedatives

When using this product
- you may get drowsy ■ avoid alcoholic drinks
- alcohol, sedatives, and tranquilizers may increase drowsiness
- be careful when driving a motor vehicle or operating machinery
- excitability may occur, especially in children

If pregnant or breast-feeding, ask a health professional before use.
Keep out of reach of children. In case of overdose, get medical help or contact a Poison Control Center right away.

Directions

adults and children 12 years and over	take 2 tablets every 4 to 6 hours; not more than 12 tablets in 24 hours
children 6 years to under 12 years	take 1 tablet every 4 to 6 hours; not more than 6 tablets in 24 hours
children under 6 years	ask a doctor

Other information
- store at 20-25°C (68-77°F) ■ protect from excessive moisture

Inactive ingredients D&C yellow no. 10, lactose, magnesium stearate, microcrystalline cellulose, pregelatinized starch

Figure 18-3 Over-the-Counter Drug Label   The FDA now requires over-the-counter drugs to carry standardized labels, such as the one at the left.

placed in three categories (I, II, and III) based on the safety and effectiveness of their active ingredient(s). Today, only category I OTC drugs that are safe, effective, and truthfully labeled are to be sold without prescription. The FDA's drug-classification process also allows some OTC drugs to be made stronger and some prescription drugs to become nonprescription drugs by reducing their strength through reformulation. Whether the reformulation of a prescription drug into an OTC formulation is always to the consumer's advantage is questionable. For example, in 2003 Prilosec, a drug for reducing esophageal reflux disease, became available over the counter. Although Prilosec as an OTC drug is less expensive than it was as a prescription product, it is now no longer covered by health insurance. The loss of insurance coverage (usually 80 percent of the price once deductibles are met) makes the medication as expensive, if not more expensive, than it was initially, at least for patients who have prescription coverage. Of course, by being an OTC drug a doctor appointment and resultant prescription are not required, but even this savings will soon be offset by the lack of insurance coverage if the medication is used over a long period of time.

Like the label shown in Figure 18-3, current labels for OTC products reflect FDA requirements. The labels must clearly state the type and quantity of active ingredients, alcohol content, side effects, instructions for appropriate use, warning against inappropriate use, and risks of using the product with other drugs (polydrug use). Unsubstantiated claims must be carefully avoided in advertisements of these products. In addition, under new labeling laws, the use of Black Boxes will be required when it is known that OTC medications hold risks, particularly when used in combination with other medications. When used on a routine basis, OTC medications should be carefully discussed with a physician or a pharmacist.

As described in Chapter 5, dietary supplements are not regulated in the same way as OTC drugs; see the box "Dietary Supplements and the Self-Care Movement" for more information.

Currently, more than 50 percent of American adults are using an array of vitamins, minerals, herbal products, hormones, amino acids, and glandular extracts in their quest for improved health. People turn to dietary supplements rather than the dietary recommendations discussed in Chapter 5 for many reasons, including concern over their own morbidity and mortality, dissatisfaction with today's impersonal health care system, distrust in the safety of the food supply, and people's increasing inability to control other aspects of life. As a result, we are now spending an estimated $20 billion annually on dietary supplements—many of which appear unnecessary and some of which may be unsafe and ineffective. Recall that dietary supplement makers are not required to submit evidence of safety or effectiveness to the Food and Drug Administration, as is the case with prescription medications and, to a lesser degree, the OTC products.

In spite of the lack of available data on safety and effectiveness, the traditional medical community is showing increasing interest in the potential benefits of dietary supplements. A growing number of teaching hospitals are establishing departments of complementary medicine, and medical students are learning about the documented role (to the extent that it is known) that these

supplements can play in promoting health. Additionally, major international pharmaceutical companies are beginning to market dietary supplements. The reputation and resources of these companies are likely to generate more carefully controlled research into the safety and efficacy of these products. However, the extent to which the National Center for Complementary and Alternative Medicine (within the National Institutes of Health) will undertake carefully controlled studies of dietary supplements remains uncertain.

In the 1994 Dietary Supplement Health and Education Act, some degree of "clarity" was brought to the largely self-regulated dietary supplement industry. For the FDA little was gained in terms of having increased supervision over the safety and effectiveness of supplements or their production and packaging, as they remained "foods" by definition. The regulation of advertising of dietary supplements was retained by the Federal Trade Commission (FTC). Critics of this division of labor have contended that the FTC's regulation of dietary supplement advertising is less focused than it needs to be. The FTC has issued some guidelines regarding questionable claims in this advertising and urges concerned consumers to contact the FTC. The following are examples of advertising claims that would be the basis of such reporting:[*]

- A claim that the product is an effective cure-all for a wide variety of diseases, or can function as a diagnostic tool for identifying a health problem
- A claim that the product can treat or cure a specific disease or condition
- Phrasing such as "scientific breakthrough," "miraculous cure," or "ancient remedy"
- Technologically unfamiliar words such as *thermogenesis*, *hypothalamic appetite center*, or *metabolic substrates*
- Undocumented personal testimonials from patients or practitioners claiming spectacular results
- A claim that availability is limited or that a "holding deposit" is needed
- A promise of a no-risk guarantee

If you find such claims or wording in advertisements for a particular dietary supplement in a pamphlet, an infomercial, or other media, contact the FTC at www.ftc.gov. Similar claims or wording on a supplement's packaging should be reported to the FDA.

[*] *"Miracle" Health Claims: Add a Dose of Skepticism.* Federal Trade Commission. Sept. 2001. www.ftc.gov/bcp/conline/pubs/health/frdheal.htm.

Health Care Consumer Fraud

A person who earns money by marketing inaccurate health information, unreliable health care, or ineffective health products is called a fraud, a **quack,** or a charlatan. **Consumer fraud** flourished with the old-fashioned medicine shows of the late 1880s. Unfortunately, consumer fraud still flourishes. You need look no further than large city newspapers to see questionable advertisements for disease cures and weight loss products. Quacks have found in health and illness the perfect avenues to indulge in **quackery**—to make maximum gain with minimum effort. Fraud can even occur after death, see the box "Modern 'Grave Robbing.'"

When people are in poor health, they may be afraid of becoming disabled or dying. So powerful are their desires to live and avoid suffering that people are vulnerable to promises of health improvement or a cure. Even though many people have great faith in their physicians, they also want access to experimental treatments or

products touted as being superior to currently available therapies. When tempted by the promise of help, people sometimes abandon traditional medical care. Of course, quacks recognize this vulnerability and present a variety

Key Terms

quack A person who earns money by purposely marketing inaccurate health information, unreliable health care, or ineffective health products.

consumer fraud Marketing of unreliable and ineffective services, products, or information under the guise of curing disease or improving health; quackery.

quackery The practice of disseminating or supplying inaccurate health information, unreliable health care, or ineffective health products for the purposes of defrauding another person.

Perhaps one of the most distressing examples of health-related consumer fraud reached headline status in 2006 when it was discovered that a body-parts procurement business was working in conjunction with a mortuary (or individual mortuary employees) to harvest marketable human body parts for sale to medical schools for medical research or to hospitals for transplantation into living recipients. Modern "grave robbing" is, of course, illegal. All organ donations must have been legally authorized by the donor, or by the immediate family of the deceased. In addition to stealing and selling body parts, the mortuary deceived the survivors of the deceased into believing that the body had been handled properly in preparation for viewing before burial or cremation. This scandal reached public attention when investigators released x-rays showing that the mortuary had inserted PVC pipes and other "filler" to normalize the appearance of the body in areas where parts had been illegally removed.

In light of the high demand for, and limited supply of, human body parts for use in modern medical education, medical research, and medical practice, a cadaver is worth thousands of dollars, as virtually every type of tissue, individual body part, anatomical region (pelvis, intact leg, head, and so on), and, of course, the intact body, can be used. This said, how can a family be assured that no illegal harvesting has occurred? The answer, beyond only using the services of a "trusted" mortuary in the local community, is to request viewing of the prepared body before dressing and placement in the casket or in the retort prior to cremation—something many a grieving family member would be uncomfortable doing.

of "reasons" to seek their help (see the box "Recognizing Quackery"). Gullibility, blind faith, impatience, superstition, ignorance, or hostility toward professional expertise eventually carry the day. In spite of the best efforts of agencies at all levels, no branch of government can protect consumers from their own errors of judgment that so easily play into the hands of quacks and charlatans.

Regardless of the motivation that leads people into consumer fraud, the outcome is frequently the same. First, the consumer loses money. The services or products are grossly overpriced, and the consumers have little recourse to help them recover their money. Second, the consumers often feel disappointed, guilty, and angered by their own carelessness as consumers. Far too frequently, consumer fraud may lead to unnecessary suffering.

Becoming a Skilled Health Care Consumer

After reading this discussion of health information, services, and products, you should be a wiser, more prepared consumer. However, information alone is not enough. Consider these six suggestions to help you become a more skilled, assertive consumer:

1. *Prepare yourself for consumerism.* In addition to offering this personal health course, your university may offer a course on consumerism. Libraries and bookstores offer trade books on a variety of consumer topics. Consumer protection agencies can guide you in some subjects. Government agencies also may help you in your choices. Unfortunately,

most Americans have, at best, an intermediate level of health literacy, and many, particularly those for whom English is a second language, have even less. This is true in spite of attempts to add "plain language" to communications between health professionals and the general public.[33] Consumers must insist on receiving understandable explanations of information related to health issues.

2. *Comparison shop.* In our free-enterprise system, virtually every service or product can be duplicated on the open market. Very few items or services are one-of-a-kind. Take the time to study your choices before you purchase a product or service.

3. *Insist on formal contracts and dated receipts.* Under the consumer laws in most states, you have a limited time in which to void a contract. Formal documentation of your actions as a consumer will give you the maximum protection available.

4. *Obtain written instructions and warranties.* Be certain of the appropriate use of any product you purchase. If you use a product inappropriately, you might void its warranty. Be familiar with what you can reasonably anticipate from the products and services you buy. In addition, be aware that a written warranty supersedes any verbal assurances a salesperson might make.

5. *Put your complaints in writing.* A carefully constructed record of your complaints is vital. Accurate records of the names and addresses of all companies and people with whom you have done business will enable you to document your actions as a consumer.

6. *Press for resolution of your complaints.* As a consumer, you are entitled to effective products and services. If your consumer complaints are not resolved, you have legal recourse through the courts. You should not hesitate to assert your rights, not only for your own sake, but for consumers who might later become victims.

Consumerism is an active relationship between you and a provider. If the provider is competent and honest and you are an informed and active consumer, both of you will profit from the relationship. However, if the provider is not competent or honest, you can protect yourself by employing the preceding six suggestions.

Taking Charge of Your Health

- Keep yourself well informed about current health issues and new developments in health care.

- Analyze the credibility of the health information you receive before putting it into practice.

- Select your health care providers by using a balanced set of criteria (see pages 509 and 510).

- Explore alternative forms of health care, and consider using them as a complement to traditional health care.

- In selecting a health insurance policy, compare various plans on the basis of several key factors, not simply cost (see page 523).

- Assemble a complete personal/family health history as soon as possible. Be sure to include information from older family members.

- Comply with all directions regarding the appropriate use of prescription and OTC medications.

SUMMARY

- Physicians can be either Doctors of Medicine (MDs) or Doctors of Osteopathy (DOs). They receive similar training and engage in similar forms of practice.
- Although alternative health care providers, including chiropractors, naturopaths, herbalists, and acupuncturists, meet the health care needs of many people, systematic study of these forms of health care is only now under way.
- Nursing at all levels is a critical health care profession. Advanced practice nurses represent the highest level of training within nursing.
- Self-care is often a viable approach to preventing illness and reducing the use of health care providers.
- Our growing inability to afford health care services has reached crisis proportions in the United States.

- Health insurance is critical to our ability to afford modern health care services.
- Medicare and Medicaid are governmental plans for paying for health care services.
- The development of prescription medication is a long and expensive process for pharmaceutical manufacturers. The cost of prescription medication is the most rapidly increasing aspect of health care affordability.
- OTC products have a role to play in the treatment of illness, but their safe use is based on following label directions.
- Critical health consumerism, including avoiding health quackery, requires careful selection of health-related information, products, and services.

Personal Assessment

Are you a skilled health care consumer?

Circle the selection that best describes your practice. Then total your points for an interpretation of your health consumer skills.

1 Never
2 Occasionally
3 Most of the time
4 All of the time

1. I read all warranties and then file them for safekeeping.   1   2   3   4
2. I read labels for information pertaining to the nutritional quality of food.   1   2   3   4
3. I practice comparative shopping and use unit pricing, when available.   1   2   3   4
4. I read health-related advertisements in a critical and careful manner.   1   2   3   4
5. I challenge all claims pertaining to secret cures or revolutionary new health devices.   1   2   3   4
6. I engage in appropriate medical self-care screening procedures.   1   2   3   4
7. I maintain a patient-provider relationship with a variety of health care providers.   1   2   3   4
8. I inquire about the fees charged before using a health care provider's services.   1   2   3   4
9. I maintain adequate health insurance coverage.   1   2   3   4
10. I consult reputable medical self-care books before seeing a physician.   1   2   3   4
11. I ask pertinent questions of health care providers when I am uncertain about the information I have received.   1   2   3   4
12. I seek second opinions when the diagnosis of a condition or the recommended treatment seems questionable.   1   2   3   4
13. I follow directions pertaining to the use of prescription drugs, including continuing their use for the entire period prescribed.   1   2   3   4
14. I buy generic drugs when they are available.   1   2   3   4
15. I follow directions pertaining to the use of OTC drugs.   1   2   3   4
16. I maintain a well-supplied medicine cabinet.   1   2   3   4

TOTAL POINTS _____

Interpretation

16–24 points   A very poorly skilled health consumer
25–40 points   An inadequately skilled health consumer
41–56 points   An adequately skilled health consumer
57–64 points   A highly skilled health consumer

TO CARRY THIS FURTHER . . .

Could you ever have been the victim of consumer fraud? What will you need to do to be a skilled consumer?

Protecting Your Safety

What Do You Know about Safety?

- Unintentional injuries harm more people than intentional injuries. True or False?

- Suicides (self-directed violence) take more lives than homicides (interpersonal violence). True or False?

- The rate of criminal victimization in the United States is at an all-time high. True or False?

- The incidence of family violence, including intimate partner violence, maltreatment of children, and maltreatment of elders, has declined in recent years. True or False?

- Children are safer from interpersonal violence after school than while in school. True or False?

- More injuries occur at home than at any other location. True or False?

- Motor vehicle crashes take more lives than any other type of injury. True or False?

Check your answers at the end of the chapter.

Online Learning Center Resources
www.mhhe.com/payne10e

Visit the Online Learning Center for tools to improve your grade and get the most out of your course—chapter objectives, practice quizzes, key terms flashcards, chapter summaries for your digital audio player, Web activities, self-assessments, and many other study aids.

It is nearly impossible to read a newspaper or watch the television news without seeing evidence of violence in our world. In addition to international terrorist incidents, which seem to be occurring with increasing regularity, there are reports of robberies, assaults, sexual offenses, and homicides. The newsroom adage "If it bleeds, it leads" seems to determine which items will receive top billing on the evening news. Is there that much violence in our communities, or are the news media just providing us with the kind of news we demand? After all, programs such as *Cops, Law and Order,* and *CSI: Miami* are among the most popular on television.

We can all think of examples of interpersonal violence in our communities, such as family violence, including intimate partner violence and child and elder maltreatment or school violence. There is violence on college campuses, where the binge-drinking rate is 40 percent, and there is violence in our streets as well, where youth gangs compete for territory. Needless to say, everyone is at some risk for becoming a victim of violence. For tips on ways to reduce your risk for becoming a victim of interpersonal violence, see the box "Don't Be a Victim of Violent Crime."

While it is true that interpersonal violence and the resulting injuries are a serious problem in our society, it is important to keep the threat of interpersonal violence in perspective. The fact is, unintentional injuries injure and kill many more people than interpersonal violence. For example, you are more than twice as likely to die from a motor-vehicle-related injury as from an intentional injury. Each year thousands of people die from motor vehicle crashes, unintentional poisonings, falls, fires, drowning, and firearms accidents, and millions more are injured. Even though the most serious unintentional injuries and injury deaths are reported in the media, they do not seem to carry the same "shock value" as intentional violence. Perhaps we assume that these were chance occurrences—"accidents." However, many of these unintentional injuries and injury deaths could have been prevented with proper precautions.

In the first part of this chapter we discuss intentional injuries, injuries that result from interpersonal violence, and ways you can keep yourself safe. In the second part of this chapter, we examine unintentional injuries and suggest ways to prevent and control them. Our goal is to help you, the student, protect your health, by reducing your risk of becoming an injury victim. Complete the Personal Assessment at the end of this chapter to see whether you are adequately protecting your own safety.

Intentional and Unintentional Injuries

In 2005 in the United States there were 33.2 million injuries and poisonings for which individuals sought or received medical care.[1] Injuries are the fifth leading cause of death in this country, and they cause significant pain and suffering to people and families while placing a heavy financial burden on individuals and on the economy.[2]

Intentional and unintentional injuries are part of living in an imperfect world, and we cannot expect to eliminate these injuries completely. But we can take steps together, and as individuals, to reduce the number and seriousness of injuries. Many federal, state, and local agencies are involved in the prevention and control of injuries.

These agencies include the National Center for Injury Prevention and Control, the National Center for Occupational Safety and Health, the National Highway Traffic Safety Administration, the Federal Trade Commission, the U.S. Coast Guard, numerous law enforcement agencies, and a large number of nongovernmental agencies.

You, too, can take steps to prevent and control injuries. In this chapter you will learn about types of injuries, their prevalence, and ways you can lower your risk of becoming the victim of an intentional or unintentional injury.

Intentional Injuries

Intentional injuries are injuries purposely inflicted either by the victim or by another person. Each year in the United States intentional acts of violence, including suicides, result in approximately 50,000 deaths and another 2 million nonfatal injuries.[3] Included in these 50,000 fatal intentional injuries are approximately 30,000 suicides, the leading cause of intentional injury deaths, and 20,000 fatalities resulting from *interpersonal violence*. (See Chapter 2 for more information about suicide and suicide prevention.) In this chapter we discuss only those intentional injuries that result from interpersonal violence.

Interpersonal Violence

Interpersonal violence occurs in our homes and communities, including our schools, places of work, and college campuses. Interpersonal violence can be perpetrated by family members, friends, colleagues, acquaintances, strangers, or gang members. Motivations for these acts include material gain, power, anger, jealousy, and religious, racial, or ethnic hatred.

In 2005 an estimated 5.2 million violent crimes were committed against U.S. residents 12 years of age and older. This is equivalent to 21 violent crime victims for every 1,000 people living in the United States. While these figures may seem high, they represent a continuing downward trend in criminal victimization that began in 1994; the 2005 rate is less than half the 1994 rate.[4] An estimated 1.8 million persons were treated for non-fatal physical-assault-related injuries in emergency departments in 2004.[5] Although the physical assault rate is higher for males, the rate of assault-related visits to emergency departments is higher for females. The highest intentional injury rates for both genders were for the 20- to 24-year-old age group.[4]

Homicide The spectrum of interpersonal violence includes homicide, robbery, rape and other sexual assault, and simple and aggravated assault (assaults with a weapon). Homicide, or murder, is the intentional taking

of one person's life by another person. Sadly, the United States leads the industrialized world in homicide rates. The homicide rate for 2004 was 5.5 per 100,000.[6] Homicide ranked as the thirteenth leading cause of death in the United States in 2003, accounting for 17,732 deaths.[7] Among 15- to 24-year-olds, of whom 5,085 were murdered, homicide was the second leading cause of death in 2004.[3] Three-fourths of all homicide victims are male.[4]

While the U.S. homicide rate is higher than that of any European country, it has steadily declined since 1991, when it was 9.8 per 100,000 population.[6] The higher homicide rates in the early 1990s have been attributed to illegal drug trafficking in large cities.[8] The lower homicide rates of more recent years have been attributed to better community policing, tougher state laws regulating hand guns, and mandatory prison sentences. No other country has such a large proportion of its population in prison. It is estimated that 1 in every 15 people (6.6 percent) of the entire U.S. population will spend time in a state or federal prison. The chances of going to prison are higher for men (9.1 percent) than for women (1.8 percent).[9]

Other Types of Interpersonal Violence Homicide is just one type of interpersonal violence. There are also robberies, rapes and other sexual assaults, and aggravated and simple assaults. Since 1993 the rate of violent victimization has fallen from 50 to 21 violent victimizations per 1,000 persons. Victims of violent crimes tend to be male, black, under 25 years of age, and in the lower income brackets.[4] Except for rape and other sexual assault, every violent crime victimization rate is higher for males than for females. In 2005 the overall victimization rate for males was 49 percent higher than for females. Females were more likely to be victimized by someone they knew (64 percent), while males were more often victimized by a stranger (54 percent). The rate of violent victimization for blacks was 34 percent higher than that for whites, and the victimization rate for 16- to 24-year-olds was more than twice that for the overall population. While violent crimes against females (55 percent) were more likely to be reported than those against males (42 percent), it is estimated that only 38 percent of rapes and other sexual assaults were reported. Less than half of all violent crimes committed in 2005 were reported to police.[4]

> ### Key Terms
>
> **intentional injuries** Injuries that are purposely inflicted either by the victim or by another person.
>
> **homicide** The intentional taking of one person's life by another person.

Your neighbor, an elderly adult, stays locked in her house all day, afraid to open the door to anyone. Too many hours of watching local TV news, you think. But it's not just older people who are living in fear. Parents, women, gays, and minorities are all looking over their shoulders.

Some parents who walked to school when they were children wouldn't think of letting their kids do that. What about child molesters and kidnappers? A young woman at a party guards her drink all night—afraid that someone might put a drug in it. She's afraid of being raped. The gay person who goes to his old neighborhood to visit his grandmother feels uneasy. Is it his imagination, or are people looking at him in a threatening way? An African American man walking down the street hears a racial slur. Should he ignore it, or stop and say something?

All of these situations call for caution. If you're a parent, you need to be careful about your child's safety. But your child can walk to school—accompanied by you, another parent, or an older child. If you're a woman, you can keep an eye on your drink at a party without making that the focus of your attention. If you're a gay man who feels uncomfortable in an unfamiliar part of town, stay focused on where you're going. Walk quickly and confidently, without being intimidated. If you're a minority member who's being taunted, keep your dignity and remain calm.

Putting fear in perspective takes practice. First, stay reasonable. Recognize that acts of violence represent the extreme elements of society. There's a good reason you probably haven't met many (or any) murderers, robbers, or rapists. They make up a small segment of society. The people you usually encounter, who are basically good, represent the large majority. Second, be aware. Pay attention to what's going on around you. See things in a neutral way. If you do, you'll realize when an argument is about to turn into a fistfight or worse. Third, use common sense. Don't put yourself at risk, but don't stop living. You can't build your life around avoiding a potential act of violence. Fourth, trust your senses. If someone is walking too close to you and you feel uncomfortable, cross the street and go into a store. Last, practice what-if situations. For example, what would you do if you were in your car at a stoplight and someone held a gun up to your window? Considering your possible actions ahead of time, without dwelling on them, is one way of preparing yourself for real-life threats.

Living in fear is something that happens gradually—as fear takes control of a person's life. But that doesn't need to happen to you. You can take control of fear in a healthy, positive way—to build a life of rich experiences balanced by caution and good sense.

Stalking In recent years the crime of **stalking** has received considerable attention. Stalking is "behavior directed at a specific individual involving repeated visual or physical proximity; nonconsensual communication; explicit or implied threats; or a combination thereof that would cause fear in a reasonable person."[10] Most stalkers are male. (One notable exception was the convicted female stalker of talk show host David Letterman.) Many of these stalkers are excessively possessive or jealous and pursue people with whom they formerly had a relationship. Some stalkers pursue people with whom they have had only an imaginary relationship.

Some stalkers have served time in prison and have waited for years to "get back" at their victims. In some cases, stalkers go to great lengths to locate their intended victims and frequently know their daily whereabouts. Although not all stalkers plan to batter or kill their victims, their presence and potential for violence are enough to create an extremely frightening environment for the intended victim and family (see the box "Putting Fear in Perspective").

Fortunately, since 1990 virtually all states have enacted or tightened their laws related to stalking and have created stiff penalties for stalkers. In many areas the criminal justice system is proactive in letting possible victims of stalking know, for example, when a particular prison inmate is going to be released. In other areas,

citizens are banding together to provide support and protection for people who may be victims of stalkers.

A recent report indicates that about 13 percent of college women are stalked in a given year.[11] If you think you are or someone you know is being stalked, contact the police (or a local crisis intervention hot line number) to report your case.

 TALKING POINTS You suspect that someone is stalking you, but your friends think you're being dramatic. How would you get objective advice on what to do?

Rape and Other Sexual Assault As violence in our society increases, the incidence of *rape* and other *sexual assault* correspondingly rises. The victims of these crimes fall into no single category. Survivors of rape and other sexual assault include young and old, male and female. They can be people with mental retardation, prisoners, hospital patients, college students. We are all potential victims, and self-protection is critical. Table 19.1 deals with the myths surrounding rape.

Sometimes a personal assault begins as a physical assault that may turn into a rape (see the box "Rape Awareness Guidelines"). Rape is generally considered a crime of sexual aggression in which the victim is forced to have sexual intercourse. Current thought concerning rape

Table 19.1 Rape: Myth versus Fact

Myth	Fact
Only women are raped.	Nearly 10 percent of rape victims (19,670) in 2003 were males.
Most rapists are strangers.	Seventy-four percent of male victims and 70 percent of female victims describe the offender as a nonstranger (intimate, other relative, or friend/acquaintance).
Most rapes occur in streets, alleys, and deserted places.	Ninety percent of rapes occur in living quarters—60 percent in the victim's residence.
Rapists are easily identified by their demeanor or psychological profile.	Most experts indicate that rapists do not differ significantly from nonrapists.
Rape is an overreported crime.	Only one in five rapes is reported.
Rape happens only to people in low socioeconomic classes.	Rape occurs in all socioeconomic classes. Each person, male or female, young or old, is a potential victim.
There is a standard way to avoid rape.	Each rape situation is different. No single method to avoid rape can work in every potential rape situation. Because of this we encourage personal health classes to invite speakers from a local rape prevention services bureau to discuss approaches to rape prevention.

characterizes this behavior as a violent act that happens to be carried out through sexual contact.

Psychiatrists and psychologists have long contended that the psychodynamic underlying the act of rape is that of a deviant urge to control and dominate others that is in no way related to the fulfillment of sexual desire. They support this contention by pointing out that rapists often experience impotence during the rape, that rapists are emotionally aroused by images of violent behavior directed toward people, and that rapists choose as victims those people whom they perceive to be most vulnerable. These traits are viewed by mental health professionals as being largely unrelated to sexually based needs.

In stark contrast to this approach, two evolutionary biologists have proposed myt rape is an extreme expression of the evolutionary urge to reproduce common to all males.[12] According to the authors, their controversial theory in no way excuses rape, nor does it speak against the incarceration of rapists, but rather it suggests an alternative interpretation of rape's underlying causation that might eventually lead society to determine more effective ways to prevent the crime from occurring. Although thought provoking, this interpretation is unlikely to change many minds about the heinous nature of the act.

Acquaintance rape refers to forced sexual intercourse between individuals who know each other. *Date rape* is a form of acquaintance rape that involves forced sexual intercourse by a dating partner. Studies on a number of campuses suggest that about 20 percent of college women report having experienced date rape; a recent report from the Bureau of Justice Statistics puts the figure at about 3 percent per year. This figure includes completed and attempted rapes.[11] A higher percentage of women report being kissed and touched against their will. Alcohol is frequently a significant contributing factor in these rape situations. (See Chapter 8 concerning alcohol's role in campus crime.) Some men have reported being psychologically coerced into intercourse by their female dating partners. In many cases the aggressive partner will display certain behaviors that can serve as warning signs (see the box "Avoiding Date Rape").

In addition to alcohol as an adjunct to acquaintance rape or date rape, the use of additional drugs such as Rohypnol (roofies), ketamine hydrochloride (Special K), and gamma-hydroxybutyrate (GHB) (see Chapter 7) are playing a greater role in date rapes reported on or near college campuses. Because of the inconspicuous nature of these drugs, they are easily incorporated into drinks without intended victims knowing it. The effects of these drugs are disinhibition, increasing confusion (including the inability to give sexual consent), relaxation of voluntary muscles, and eventual unconsciousness.[13] The amnesic effect of these drugs reduces the ability of victims to supply information important in the apprehension of date rapists.

Psychologists believe that aside from the physical harm of date rape, a greater amount of emotional damage may occur. Such damage stems from the concept of broken trust. Date rape survivors feel particularly violated because the perpetrator was not a stranger; it

> **Key Terms**
>
> **stalking** Repeated visual or physical proximity, nonconsensual communication, or threats that would cause fear in a reasonable person.

was someone they initially trusted, at least to some degree. Once that trust has been broken, developing new relationships with other people becomes much more difficult for the date rape survivor.

Nearly all survivors of date rape seem to suffer from *posttraumatic stress disorder.* They can have anxiety, sleeplessness, eating disorders, and nightmares. Guilt concerning their own behavior, self-esteem, and judgment of other people can be overwhelming, and the individual may require professional counseling. Indeed, all students should be aware of the risk of date rape.

Sexual Harassment   Sexual harassment consists of unwanted attention of a sexual nature that creates embarrassment or stress. Examples of sexual harassment include unwanted physical contact, excessive pressure for dates, sexually explicit humor, sexual innuendos or remarks, offers of job advancement based on sexual favors, and overt sexual assault. Unlike more overt forms of sexual victimization, sexual harassment may be applied in a subtle manner and can, in some cases, go unnoticed by coworkers and fellow students. Nevertheless, sexual harassment produces stress that cannot be resolved until the harasser is identified and forced to stop. Both men and women can be victims of sexual harassment.

Sexual harassment can occur in many settings, including employment and academic settings. On the college campus, harassment may be primarily in terms of the offer of sex for grades. If this happens to you, think carefully about the situation and document the specific times, events, and places where the harassment took place. Consult your college's policy concerning harassment. Next, you should report these events to the appropriate administrative officer (perhaps the affirmative action officer, dean of academic affairs, or dean of students). You may also want to discuss the situation with a staff member of the university counseling center.

If harassment occurs in the work environment, the victim should document the occurrences and report them to the appropriate management or personnel official. Reporting procedures will vary from setting to setting. Sexual harassment is a form of illegal sex discrimination and violates Title VII of the Civil Rights Act of 1964.

In 1986 the U.S. Supreme Court ruled that the creation of a "hostile environment" in a work setting was sufficient evidence to support the claim of sexual harassment. This action served as an impetus for thousands of women to step forward with sexual harassment allegations. Additionally, some men are also filing sexual harassment lawsuits against female supervisors.

Bias and Hate Crimes   One sad aspect of any society is how some segments of the majority treat certain people in the minority. Nowhere is this more violently pronounced than in **bias and hate crimes.** These crimes, which account for just 3 percent of all violent crimes, are defined as crimes that occur "when offenders choose a victim because of some characteristic—for example, race, ethnicity, or religion—and provide evidence that the hate prompted them to commit the crime." [14] During the period from July 2000 through December 2003, about 191,000 hate crimes occurred annually. More than half (55.4 percent) of these incidents were motivated by race, another 30.7 percent were motivated by the victims' association with persons with certain characteristics such as multiracial marriage, 28.7 percent by ethnicity, 18.0 percent

Avoiding Date Rape

What can I do to prevent date rape?

First, consider your partner's attitudes and behaviors. Sexual stereotypes play a role in date rape. Society may encourage men to be aggressive and competitive and encourage women to avoid confrontation. Some people still believe that women say "no" to sex when they really mean "yes"—an idea that may lead to misunderstanding and miscommunication. Signs that a man may adhere to social norms that support male sexual entitlement include difficulty managing frustration and anger, disregard for what others are saying, use of threats or violence to solve problems, extreme competitiveness, and inability to take no for an answer, even in nonsexual situations. Below are some specific ways both men and women can avoid a date rape situation.

Men

- Think about your own sexual stereotypes and how they may affect your attitudes and actions toward women. For example, what do you assume about the sexual desires of your dates? How do you interpret a woman's dress and behavior? Have you ever tried to get a clearly reluctant partner to agree to sex?
- If you aren't clear about what sexual activities someone wants to engage in, ask in a direct but non-threatening way.
- If a woman says "no," believe and accept that she means "no." Don't try to bully her, make her feel guilty, or accuse her of being uptight. She isn't responsible for your assumptions and reactions.
- Don't use alcohol or other drugs in sexual situations; intoxication will impair your judgment and understanding. Being drunk or high is not an excuse for raping someone.

- Realize that forcing a woman to have sex against her will is rape—a criminal act. If your date is drunk, high, or impaired in any way, she cannot legally consent to sex.

Women

- Talk openly about sex and make your feelings and limits clear.
- Don't use alcohol or other drugs in sexual situations; intoxication will impair your ability to make sensible decisions and assert yourself.
- Be aware of your dress and manner. There's nothing wrong with dressing in a sexy manner and flirting, but your appearance and actions send a message that could be misinterpreted.
- Go to parties with a group of friends. Keep an eye on each other, and leave together. Do not leave a party, club, or bar with someone you just met or don't know well.
- Get your own drink and keep it with you, even when you go to the bathroom. Date rape drugs are odorless and tasteless and can easily be added to any type of beverage without your knowledge.
- Trust your instincts. If a situation doesn't feel right, leave.
- If someone is forcing you to do something you don't want to do, loudly and directly say "stop" or "no." Stand up for yourself, even if you feel you are being rude—a polite or passive response may be misunderstood or ignored. If the person continues to ignore your objections, it is okay to respond physically, to push the person away, and to scream.

---

by sexual orientation, 12.9 percent by religion, and 11.2 percent by disability (see the box "Violence against the Disabled").[14] Victims of hate crimes are often verbally abused, their property is damaged or destroyed, and too frequently they are physically attacked. Two recent hate-motivated killings shocked the nation. One case involved the beating death of Matthew Shepard, a gay college student who was taken from a Wyoming bar, driven to a rural area, tied to a fence post, and savagely beaten to death. Aaron McKinney, one of the two men accused in the killings, based his defense on "gay panic," contending that he was traumatized by a homosexual advance as a young child. A second case that shocked the nation was that of James Byrd, Jr., a 49-year-old African American man who was accosted by two white men as he walked along a rural roadway in Texas. After being beaten, spray-painted black, and chained to the rear of a pickup, Byrd was then dragged behind the truck for an extended distance. The trauma Byrd experienced was so severe that he was decapitated and his torso dismembered.

Typically, the offenders in bias or hate crimes are fringe elements of a larger society who believe that the mere presence of someone with a racial, ethnic, sexual orientation, or religious difference is inherently bad for the community, state, or country. Examples of groups commonly known to commit bias and hate crimes in the United States are skinheads, the Ku Klux Klan, and other white supremacist groups. Increasingly, state and federal laws have been enacted to make bias and hate crimes serious offenses.

With a small but growing presence of neo-Nazi groups in Europe and clear evidence that ethnic cleansing took place in Kosovo, Bosnia, Serbia, Croatia, Rwanda, Iraq, Darfur, and the former Soviet Union, bias and hate crimes are a worldwide problem. The recent push on college campuses to promote multicultural education and the celebration of diversity may help today's generation

---

Key Terms

bias and hate crimes Criminal acts directed at a person or group solely because of a specific characteristic, such as race, religion, sexual orientation, ethnic background, or other difference.

Hate crimes are directed at a person or group solely because of a characteristic such as race, religion, or sexual orientation. Celebrating tolerance and diversity and promoting inclusion can help combat the bigotry that contributes to hate crimes.

of college graduates understand the importance of tolerance and inclusion and avoid bigotry and exclusion.

Family Violence

Unfortunately, some victims of interpersonal violence are family members. During much of America's relatively brief history, many families were multigenerational, with mothers, fathers, children, and grandparents living together as a family. By the 1950s this arrangement became unusual; the more common family arrangement was mothers and fathers living together with their children. Today, families are more varied and, in some cases, more complex. Many married couples do not have children, and there are also many "blended families" with children from previous and current marriages all living together. In 2005 there were an estimated 10.4 million single-mother families and 2.5 million single-father families in the United States.[15] For our discussion, we'll use the U.S. Census Bureau's definition of a family "a group of two or more people who reside together and who are related by birth, marriage, or adoption."

Another way contemporary families differ from families in the past is that today many more women work outside of the home. Since 1950, the labor force participation rate of women has nearly doubled, so that today more than half of all women work. In 2005, women made up 46 percent of the American workforce.[16] Although it is stressful for working spouses to juggle work and domestic responsibilities, and many children are left to take care of themselves after school, the increased income does reduce financial stress at home. Furthermore, female spouses bringing home paychecks may not feel as powerless as those who stay at home all day. Thus, the higher percentage of women in the workforce may be one reason the level of family violence has been declining.

Family violence is the use of physical force by one family member against another, with the intent to hurt, injure, or cause harm. The spectrum of family violence includes intimate partner violence, maltreatment of children, sibling violence, and violence directed at elder family members. One in every six homicides is the result of family violence.

Intimate Partner Violence **Intimate partner violence** is rape, physical assault, or stalking perpetrated by current and former dates, spouses, and cohabiting partners (cohabiting meaning living together at least some of the time as a couple).[10] Most of the victims are women, and a significant percentage of these women are spouses or former spouses of the assailant. Intimate partner violence can include murder, rape, other sexual assault, robbery, aggravated assault, and simple assault. Violent acts that constitute abuse range from a slap on the face to murder.

According to the Bureau of Justice Statistics, injuries from intimate partner violence have declined in recent years. The number of fatal injuries among intimate partners has declined from 2,944 in 1976 to 1,544 in 2004. Interestingly, almost all of this decline has been in the numbers of male victims. Nonfatal injuries among intimate partners have also declined, from 5.8 per 1,000 in 1993 to 2.6 per 1,000 in 2004.[17] The reasons for the decline in intimate partner violence include the high incarceration rates of violent offenders, better social services for families at risk, and lower levels of unemployment.

The most vulnerable female victims are African American and Hispanic, live in large cities, are young and unmarried, and are from lower socioeconomic groups. However, these trends do not mean that only women from these classifications are vulnerable to violent behavior. Men and women across all economic, racial, and age categories are potential victims.

One of the real difficulties related to intimate violence is the vast underreporting of this crime to law enforcement authorities. The U.S. Department of Justice estimates that about half of the victims of intimate violence do not report the crime to police. Too many victims view their violent situations as private or personal matters and not actual crimes. Despite painful injuries, many victims view the offenses against them as minor. Even psychological abuse, the least frequently reported form of intimate violence, can lead not only to feelings of loss of control and emotional dysfunction, but also to a wide array of physical health problems. Victims of psychological abuse are twice as likely as others to report chronic pain, spastic colon, irritable bowel syndrome, infections, and migraine headaches.[18]

Of course, it is easy to criticize the victims of intimate violence for not reporting the crimes committed against them, but this may be unfair. Why do women stay in these relationships? Many women who are injured

Learning from Our Diversity

Violence against the Disabled

No one is totally free from the risk of senseless violence—children, adults, or college students. No single group, however, is a more tragic target of violence than the disabled. Despite the protective efforts of laws such as the Fair Housing Amendments Act, the Americans with Disabilities Act, and the Rehabilitation Act, the disabled remain an easily victimized segment of the population.

Because of the high level of vulnerability that disabled persons face, national advocacy groups, such as All Walks of Life, are working to assist the disabled, their caregivers, and the general population in reducing the risk of violence to this group. However, much can also be accomplished on an individual basis. If you are an able-bodied college student, you can probably implement the following suggestions on your campus:

- Encourage your disabled peers to remain vigilant by staying tuned in to their environment. Remind them that simply because they appear disabled does not guarantee that they will be protected from harm.
- Support your disabled friends in the challenges imposed by their limitations, particularly when they are in unfamiliar environments or experiencing unusual situations.
- Suggest that your peers with disabilities carry or wear a personal alarm device. Such devices, also frequently carried by ablebodied

students, can be purchased in bookstores or sporting goods stores.
- Remind your disabled friends to inform others about their schedule plans, for example, when they will be away from school and when they are likely to return.
- Encourage people with disabilities to seek the assistance of an escort (security personnel) when leaving a campus building or a shopping mall to enter a large parking area.
- Be an advocate for your disabled friends. For example, if residence hall room doors do not have peepholes at wheelchair height, find out if the doors can be modified.

One additional approach remains controversial. That is the teaching of self-defense techniques to people with disabilities. Groups that advocate instruction to the disabled in the martial arts, such as judo, remind us that "doing nothing will produce nothing." Others contend that a limited ability to use a martial art leads to a false sense of confidence that encourages a disregard for other forms of protection. They further argue that if disabled persons try to counter aggression with ineffectively delivered martial arts techniques, they may anger their attacker and actually increase the aggression against themselves.

---

may fear being killed if they report the crime. Women may also fear for the safety of their children. Women who receive economic support may fear being left with no financial resources.

However, help is available for victims of intimate abuse. Most communities have family support or intimate violence hot lines that abused people can call for help. Communities are establishing shelters where abused women and their children can seek safety while their cases are being handled by the police or court officials. If you are being abused or know of someone who is the victim of intimate violence, do not hesitate to use the services of these local hot lines or shelters. Also, check the resources listed in the Health Reference Guide at the back of this text.

 TALKING POINTS A close friend confides that her boyfriend sometimes "gets rough" with her. She's afraid to talk to him about it because she thinks that will make things worse. What immediate steps would you tell her to take?

Maltreatment of Children Like many cases of intimate partner violence, **child maltreatment** tends to be a silent crime. It is estimated that nearly 1 million children are victims of child abuse and neglect each year.[19] Some children are victims of repeated crimes, and since many

victims do not report these crimes, the actual incidence of child abuse is difficult to determine.

Child maltreatment includes child abuse and child neglect. Children are abused in various ways. Physical abuse reflects physical injury, such as bruises, burns, abrasions, cuts, and fractures of the bones and skull. Sexual abuse includes acts that lead to sexual gratification of the abuser. Examples include fondling, touching, and various acts involved in rape, sodomy, and incest. Psychological abuse is another form of child abuse. Certainly, children are scarred by family members and

> **Key Terms**
>
> **family violence** The use of physical force by one family member against another, with the intent to injure or otherwise cause harm.
>
> **intimate partner violence** Violence committed against a person by a current or former spouse, date, or cohabiting partner.
>
> **child maltreatment** The act or failure to act by a parent or caretaker that results in abuse or neglect of a child or that places the child in imminent risk of serious harm.

others who routinely damage their psychological development. However, this form of abuse is especially difficult to identify and measure.

Child neglect is failure to provide a child with adequate clothing, food, shelter, and medical attention. The incidence of child neglect is approximately three times the incidence of physical abuse and about seven times the incidence of child sexual abuse. Child maltreatment deaths are more often associated with child neglect than with any type of abuse.[19] Educational neglect, such as failure to see that a child attends school regularly, is one of the most common types of child neglect. Each form of abuse can have devastating short- and long-term consequences for the child.

Research studies in the various areas of child maltreatment reveal some interesting trends. Abused children are much more likely than are nonabused children to grow up to be child abusers. Abused children are more likely to suffer from poor educational performance, increased health problems, and low levels of overall achievement. Abused children are significantly more likely than are nonabused children to become involved in adult crime and violent criminal behavior. Finally, neglected children's rates of arrest for violence were almost as high as those of physically abused children.[20]

It is beyond the scope of this book to discuss in detail how to reduce child abuse. However, the violence directed against children can likely be lessened through a combination of early identification measures and violence prevention programs. Teachers, friends, relatives, social workers, counselors, psychologists, police, and the court system must not hesitate to intervene early in cases of suspected child abuse. In fact, every adult is responsible for reporting suspected child abuse and neglect. To do so, persons should call their local police department or Child Protective Services (within the Department of Public Welfare) and request assistance in filing a report. So long as the report is filed in good conscience (without malice) there will be no negative ramifications for the person filing. The later the intervention, the more likely that the abuse will have worsened. When an individual has abused once, he or she is likely to do it again.

Violence prevention programs can help parents and caregivers learn how to resolve conflicts, improve communication, cope with anger, improve parenting skills, and challenge the view of violence presented in movies and television. These programs may help to stop violence before it begins to damage the lives of young children. The box "Twelve Alternatives to Lashing Out at Your Child" provides helpful guidelines for parents.

Maltreatment of Elders Among the 37 million adults 65 years of age and older, between 1 and 2 million have been injured, exploited, or otherwise mistreated.[21, 22] Particularly vulnerable are women over the age of 75 years. Ninety percent of all known abusers are family members; two-thirds are the victims' adult children or their spouses.[23]

Many older adults are hit, kicked, attacked with knives, or denied food and medical care; others are robbed of their Social Security checks and automobiles. These crimes probably reflect a combination of factors, particularly the stress of caring for failing older people by middle-aged children who also face the additional demands of dependent children and careers. In many cases, the middle-aged children were themselves abused, or there may be a chemical dependence problem. The alternative, institutionalization, is so expensive that it is often not an option for either the abused or the abuser.

Although protective services are available, abuse of older adults is frequently unseen and unreported. In many cases, the older adults themselves are afraid to report their children's behavior because of the fear of embarrassment that they were not good parents to their children. Regardless of the cause, however, abuse of older adults must be reported to the appropriate protective service so that intervention can occur.

Violence in Our Communities

When family members go to school, attend college, or engage in other community activities, we do not expect them to be injured by the intentional acts of another.

School Violence Usually, students are safe at school, but occasional, highly publicized fatal school shootings, like the ones at Columbine High School and Red Lake Indian Reservation, cause parents to ask how safe their children are at school. The National Center for Educational Statistics collects data to determine the frequency, seriousness, and incidence of violence in elementary and high schools. During the 2003–2004 school year, 81 percent of U.S. public schools reported at least one crime incident. During that year, 77 percent of schools reported instances of physical attacks or fights without a weapon, 53 percent reported threats of physical attacks without a weapon, 51 percent reported vandalism, 46 percent reported theft or larceny, and 15 percent reported possession of a knife or other sharp object. Six percent of public schools reported a student in possession of a firearm or explosive device, and 5 percent reported an attack or fight with a weapon. Only 3 percent reported sexual battery other than rape, and only 1 percent reported rape or attempted rape.[24] According to the Youth Risk Behavior Surveillance surveys, the rate of carrying a weapon to school declined from 11.8 percent in 1993 to 5.4 percent in 2005.[25] Nonetheless, the fact that 1 in 20 high school children carried a weapon to school within the past 30 days is frightening.

Weapon carrying is related to another form of interpersonal violence at school—bullying. Bullying includes making fun of another person; spreading rumors about a person; threatening to harm another person; pushing, shoving, tripping, or spitting on a person; pressuring someone to do something he or she does not want to do; excluding someone; or destroying someone's property. In 2005, 28 percent of 12- to 18-year-olds reported that they were bullied at school within the past six months.[24] One natural response to being bullied might be to carry a weapon to school.

In spite of these statistics, the odds of a student suffering a school-associated violent death are less than one in a million. Only 19 of the more than 1,437 children nationwide who were murdered, and only 3 of the 1,285 children who committed suicide, during the 2003–2004 school year were at school, on school property, at a school-sponsored event, or on their way to school or a school-sponsored event at the time of their death. So while violence at schools has captured the headlines, schools are really a relatively safe place for children to be. Most of the violent crimes committed by juveniles on school days occur after school.[26]

Violence at College A recent report has summarized violent victimization of college students. Perhaps the

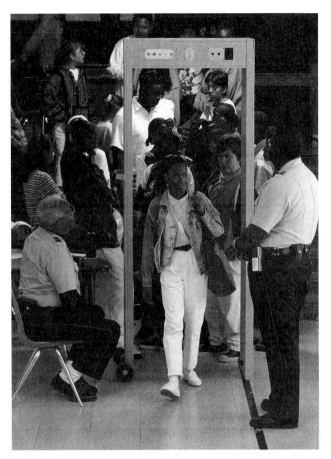

Although young people are safer at school than outside of school, some types of school violence—including fights, threats, vandalism, and weapons carrying—are relatively common. Some schools have instituted strategies such as video surveillance and metal detectors to help reduce the risk of school violence.

most important finding was that college campuses are a relatively safe place to be. College students (ages 18–24 years) experience less violence than do nonstudents in the same age group. Violence rates have declined for both groups since 1995, when rates were 88 per 1,000 for college students and 102 per 1,000 for nonstudents. The 2002 rates are 41 and 56, respectively.[27]

During the period 1995–2002, simple assault (assault without a weapon) accounted for 63 percent of the violent victimizations, whereas rape/sexual assault accounted for 6 percent. Males were about twice as likely to be victims of violence as women were. About 93 percent of the crimes occurred off campus and 72 percent occurred at night.[27]

One factor that increases the risk of interpersonal violence on American college campuses is the consumption of alcohol and other drugs. More than 40 percent of victims of violent crimes in college settings perceived their offenders to be using drugs or alcohol. The percentage was even higher for aggravated and simple assault.[27] It should be noted that this is higher than the level of drug use perceived by victims in all settings.[27, 28] To reduce your risk of becoming a victim of interpersonal violence, consider reducing your alcohol intake, pay attention to the alcohol consumption of those around you, and stay away from places where others are drinking heavily.

Campus Safety   Although many of the topics in this chapter are quite unsettling, students and faculty must continue to lead normal lives in the campus environment despite potential threats to our health. The first step in being able to function adequately is knowing about these potential threats. You have read about these threats in this section on intentional injuries; now you must think about how this information applies to your campus situation.

The campus environment is not immune to many of the social ills that plague our society. At one time the university campus was thought to be a safe haven from the real world. Now there is plenty of evidence to indicate that significant intentional and unintentional injuries can happen to anyone at any time on the college campus.

For this reason, you must make it a habit to think constructively about protecting your safety. In addition to the personal safety tips presented earlier in this section, remember to use the safety assistance resources available on your campus. One of these might be your use of university-approved escort services, especially in the evenings as you move from one campus location to another. Another resource is the campus security department (campus police). Typically, campus police have a 24-hour emergency phone number. If you think you need help, do not hesitate to call this number. Campus security departments frequently offer short seminars on safety topics to student organizations or residence hall groups. Your counseling center on campus might also offer programs on rape prevention and personal protection.

If you are motivated to make your campus environment safer, you might wish to contact an organization that specifically focuses on campus crime. Safe Campuses Now is a nonprofit student group that tracks legislation, provides educational seminars, and monitors community incidents involving students. (For information about Safe Campuses Now, including how to start a chapter on your campus, call 706-354-1115. Visit the Web page for Safe Campuses Now, www.safecampusesnow.org. Another useful website is www.securityoncampus.org. The mission of this organization is to promote on-campus safety for students. We encourage you to become active in making your campus a safer place to live.)

Youth and Gang Violence   In the last 30 years, gangs and gang activities have been increasingly responsible for escalating violence and criminal activity. Before that time, gangs used fists, tire irons, and occasionally, cheap handguns ("Saturday night specials") as tools of enforcement. Now, gang members do not hesitate to use more lethal semiautomatic weapons.

The gang problem is most persistent in cities of greater than 50,000 population, where 82 percent of law enforcement agents report experiencing youth gang activity.[29] These are areas where many socially alienated, economically disadvantaged young people live. Convinced that society has no significant role for them, gang members can receive support from an association of peers that has well-defined lines of authority. Rituals and membership initiation rites are important in gang socialization. Gangs often control territories within a city. Frequently, gangs are involved in criminal activities, the most common of which are illicit drug trafficking and robberies. In the late 1990s, gang-related murders and drive-by shootings contributed to the high death rate among young people and especially inner-city youth. In 1999 the rate of gang-related murders of young persons reached, on average, 24 deaths every two days—the equivalent of a classroom of dead young persons (below the age of 20) every other day. Perhaps no single example of youth violence, with a measure of gang affiliation included, is more vivid than the April 20, 1999, shootings that occured at Columbine High School in Littleton, Colorado. On that day Eric Harris and Dylan Klebold, dressed in their gang-affiliated black trench coats, entered their high school and began a planned and systematic gun and bomb rampage that resulted in the deaths of 14 students and 1 teacher. To this day, no one is certain why Harris and Klebold, and their closest friends, felt such anger toward and sense of disenfranchisement from their classmates and community.

It is not only older male teenagers and young adults who are members of today's gangs. Law enforcement officials see younger people (ages 12, 13, and 14) joining gangs. Some gangs have recently included young women as members, and some cities report a growing number of all-female gangs. Some female gangs are reported to be every bit as ruthless as the male gangs. Only about 6 percent of gang members were female in 2000.[29]

Attempting to control gang and youth violence is particularly expensive for communities. When you consider that for every gang-related homicide, there are about 100 nonfatal gang-related intentional injuries, it becomes obvious that gang violence is an expensive health care proposition. Furthermore, gang and youth violence takes an enormous financial and human toll on law enforcement, the judicial system, and corrections departments.

Fortunately, the recent decline in murders and other serious crimes also applies to gang-related crimes. Once again, some observers credit more aggressive police tactics for the decline. Some of the tactics being used to meet this problem are the aggressive "quality of life" policing in some cities and President Clinton's COPS program (Community Oriented Policing Services) to hire new police officers and put them on foot patrols, so they become acquainted with residents. Others believe that the drop in crime should be attributed to factors such as a stronger economy and the fading of the crack market. In Boston, a campaign aimed at youth gangs offered summer jobs to gang members, combined with threats of federal prison sentences for gun violence. This program has significantly reduced firearm-related fatalities among Boston youth.

Regardless, reducing gang and youth violence will be a continuing challenge for the nation in the twenty-first century.

Factors That Contribute to Intentional Injuries

The use and abuse of alcohol and other psychoactive drugs, as discussed in Chapters 7 and 8, are contributing factors to interpersonal violence and the toll of intentional injuries in our society. In 2004, 4 percent of homicides, 10 percent of other violent crimes, and 26 percent of property crimes were drug related.[30] A psychological manifestation of alcohol intoxication is the lowering of inhibitions, and for some this results in a loss of behavior control resulting in acts of interpersonal violence. A drunk or drugged person is more likely than a sober person to become either a victim or a perpetrator of violence. In 2004, 49 percent of state and federal inmates imprisoned for violent crimes reported having used drugs in the month before their offense, and roughly 25 percent reported use at the time of their crime.[31]

Another factor that contributes to the prevalence and deadliness of interpersonal violence is the availability of firearms. Firearms are present in more than half of American homes. In 2002, firearms were the second leading cause of death, after automobiles, accounting for 18.8 percent of all injury deaths. That year, guns were involved in two-thirds of all homicides in the United States.[32] The ratio of fatalities to nonfatalities for firearm injuries compared to that ratio for all injuries, reveals the lethality of gun violence. For each injury death there are 9 hospitalizations and 189 more people treated and released. But for firearm injuries, for each injury death, only 1.2 people are hospitalized and only 1 person is treated and released.[33] Firearm deaths are a leading cause of deaths of teenage and young adult men, ages 15 to 24 years. In 2004 there were 3,796 deaths attributed to homicide and legal intervention in this population, a death rate of 17.71 deaths per 100,000.[3] Evidence of the availability of guns is clear from the Youth Risk Behavior Survey conducted by the Centers for Disease Control and Prevention. In 2005, nearly 10 percent of male high school students had carried a gun to school on 1 or more of the past 30 days.[34] Colleges and universities are not immune to gun violence. A recent study found that 4.3 percent of college students had a working firearm at college. Of these students, nearly half stated that they had the gun for protection.[35]

See the box "Violence in the Media: Does It Affect Behavior in the Real World?" for more information on factors contributing to intentional injuries.

The proliferation of firearm use has prompted serious discussions about the enactment of gun control laws. For years, gun control activists have been in direct battle with the National Rifle Association (NRA) and its congressional supporters. Gun control activists want fewer guns manufactured and greater controls over the sale and possession of handguns. Gun supporters believe that such controls are not necessary and that people (the criminals) are responsible for gun deaths, not simply the guns. This debate will certainly continue.

Identity Theft

In today's cashless, wired society, we make several transactions each day in which personal information is transferred: we write checks, pay bills online, use credit and debit cards at restaurants and for purchases, and withdraw cash from ATMs; we might be asked to provide a Social Security number when we write a check, or give our phone number or address when we shop at a particular store. Each of these transactions provides an opportunity for thieves to obtain your personal information and use it fraudulently.

Identity theft has been on the rise since the early 1990s. Here are some of the common ways ID theft occurs. Identity thieves (1) rummage through trash looking for bills and other papers bearing your personal information ("dumpster diving"), (2) steal credit or debit card numbers using a special storage device when processing your card ("skimming"), (3) pretend to be a financial institution or other business and try to get you to reveal personal information ("phishing"), (4) divert your mail by submitting a change of address form for you, or (5) simply steal your wallet, purse, or mail, such as pre-approved credit offers, new checks, or other papers. They might also steal your information from your employer by bribing a dishonest employee who has access to it.[36]

Thieves use falsely obtained names, addresses, and Social Security numbers to open credit card accounts and bank accounts, purchase cell phone services, and secure loans to buy automobiles and other big ticket items. They might even avoid paying taxes by working under false Social Security numbers, or use your identity for other purposes—if they are arrested, for example. Identity thefts can drain a person's bank account and ruin

> ### Key Terms
>
> **identity theft** A crime involving the fraudulent use of a person's name, Social Security number, credit line, or other personal financial or identifying information.

Violence in the Media: Does It Affect Behavior in the Real World?

Does watching violent movies and television make a person more likely to be violent in real life? Does playing violent video games lead to aggressive behavior? There are clearly many other social, economic, and interpersonal factors that influence behavior, and evidence conflicts on whether exposure to violent media content causes aggression or desensitizes people to violence.

But some studies have found links between media violence and increased rates of aggression and violent behavior. In one recent study, college students were found to have a lower emotional and physical response to video images of real-life violence after exposure to violent games, suggesting they had become desensitized. A study of adolescents found that playing violent video games stirs up the brain's emotional response center while reducing activity in regions of the brain involved in inhibition, concentration, and self-control—a clear effect on brain activity, at least in the short term. Another study of teens found an association between watching professional wrestling and engaging in dating violence.

Some researchers are particularly concerned about the effects of media violence on children, who may not be able to clearly distinguish between the fantasy world offered in various forms of media and the real world. The more television children watch—whether or not the programs contain violent content—the more likely they are to behave aggressively and have other social problems. And the more violent television a child watches, the less time she or he spends with friends.

What can concerned parents do? It makes sense for parents to monitor their children's viewing, choose programs that are appropriate for a child's age and level of maturity, watch programs with children whenever possible, and set a good example by limiting their own television and Internet time. If violent content does appear on programs or in games, parents can discuss it with their children, talking about appropriate behavior, the consequences of violence, and other, better ways to solve problems and resolve conflicts. Praise positive examples of interpersonal behavior, such as friendship and cooperation.

Sources: Carnagey NL, Anderson CA, Bushman BJ, 2006, The effect of video game violence on physiological desensitization to real-life violence, *Journal of Experimental Social Psychology* 43(3): 489–496; DuRant RH, Champion H, Wolfson, M, 2006, The relationships between watching professional wrestling on television and engaging in date fighting among high school students, *Pediatrics* 118: e265–e272; Do violent video games change teen brains? *Research at Indiana University*, www.research.indiana.edu/news/stories/0096games.html, November 2006; Violence in the Media, *JAMA* Patient Page, May 24/31, 2000, vol. 283, no. 20. p. 2748.

her credit rating before she knows she's become a victim. Often the crime is not discovered until a person wants to make a major purchase—such as a house or a car that requires a credit check.

The Federal Trade Commission suggests a three-prong attack against identity theft, which it labels "Deter-Detect-Defend." See the box "Reducing Your Risk for Identity Theft" for specific guidelines.

Terrorism

Although definitions vary, the United Nations defines **terrorism** as any act "intended to cause death or serious bodily harm to civilians or noncombatants with the purpose of intimidating a population or compelling a government or an international organization to do or abstain from doing any act."[37] Over the past 30 years the world has witnessed dozens of acts of terrorism in countries such as Germany, Spain, Indonesia, Kenya, London, Northern Ireland, Japan, and Russia. The United States has not been immune from terrorist acts. To list a few: the World Trade Center bombing in 1993, the Oklahoma City bombing in 1995, the Olympic Park bombing in Atlanta in 1996, and the attacks on the World Trade Center and Pentagon in 2001.

By their very nature, terrorist acts are difficult to prevent. However, it is less likely that your health will be affected by a terrorist act than by your everyday health behavior. As an educated person, you should become knowledgeable about world events and support federal, state, and local security efforts. If you travel abroad, keep in mind that American-style restaurants and night clubs might be more attractive targets for anti-American terrorist acts than locally owned or natively owned establishments.

Key Terms

terrorism Any actions intended to harm or kill civilians in order to intimidate a populace or force a government to take some action.

unintentional injuries Injuries that have occurred without anyone's intending that harm be done.

Unintentional Injuries

The vast majority of injuries that occur each year are **unintentional injuries,** injuries that occur without anyone intending harm. Nearly half of all these injuries occur in or around the home.[1] Nearly twice as many injuries occurred in the home as occurred outside, and falls are the leading cause of medically consulted injuries in the home. The next most common locations for injuries were recreation areas, and streets and highways.[1] Even though we spend a lot of time at schools and places of work, these venues are relatively safe.

Unintentional injuries account for about two-thirds of all injury deaths annually in the United States. More fatal injuries occur on streets and highways than anywhere else. Of the 112,012 unintentional injury deaths reported in 2004, 40 percent were caused by motor vehicle crashes, 18 percent by unintentional poisonings, 17 percent by falls, and 7.9 percent by unintentional suffocation. Other causes were drowning, exposure to smoke, fire, and flames, and the accidental discharge of firearms.[38] In 2004, injuries cost an estimated $575 billion, including $298 billion in lost wages and productivity, $99 billion in medical expenses, $112 billion in insurance administration costs, and $65 billion in motor vehicle damage and other costs.[39]

Motor Vehicle Injuries and Safety

Motor vehicle crashes are the leading cause of injury deaths in the United States and, for the 16- to 24-year age group (a majority of those reading this textbook), motor vehicle crashes are the leading cause *all* deaths. In 2005, 43,433 people were killed and an estimated 1.9 million more were injured in motor vehicle crashes on U.S.

streets and highways. The rates of involvement in fatal crashes are highest for drivers in the 16- to 20-year and the 21- to 24-year age groups; the rates of involvement for male drivers are twice as high as for female drivers (Figure 19-1). Weekends and nights are more dangerous driving times. The most dangerous hours are from midnight to 3 a.m. on Saturdays and Sundays.[40]

As with intentional injuries, alcohol intoxication is often a contributing factor to the number and seriousness of unintentional injuries. This is especially true for motor vehicle crashes. Alcohol involvement increases the likelihood that a crash will occur and that it will result in a fatality. In some age groups the percentage of alcohol involvement for fatal crashes is five times as high as it is for nonfatal injury crashes (Figure 19-2).

Motor vehicle crashes also cause disabling injuries. With nearly 2 million such injuries each year, all college students should be concerned about avoiding motor vehicle crashes. With this thought in mind, we offer some important safety tips for motor vehicle operators:

- Make certain that you are familiar with the traffic laws in your state.
- Do not operate an automobile or motorcycle unless it is in good mechanical order. Regularly inspect your brakes, lights, and exhaust system.

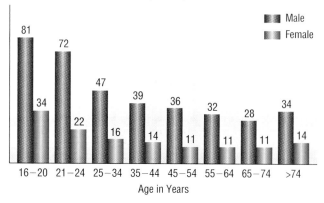

Driver Involvement Rate per 100,000 Licensed Drivers

Figure 19-1 Fatal Motor Vehicle Crashes by Gender and Age
Males are more likely than females to be involved in fatal motor vehicle crashes; rates are highest among young drivers. What could be done to reduce the number of driving fatalities involving young males?
Source: National Highway Traffic Safety Administration. *Traffic Safety Facts 2005.* Washington, DC: U.S. Department of Transportation.

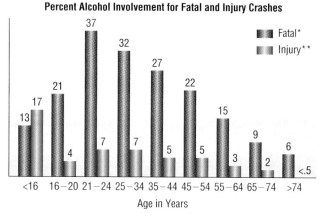

Percent Alcohol Involvement for Fatal and Injury Crashes

* For fatal crashes, alcohol involvement is a blood alcohol concentration (BAC) of 0.01 grams per deciliter (g/dl) or greater.

** For injury crashes, alcohol involvement is police-reported alcohol involvement.

Figure 19-2 Alcohol and Fatal Motor Vehicle Crashes Alcohol is more often involved in fatal motor-vehicle crashes than in nonfatal crashes.
Source: National Highway Traffic Safety Administration. *Traffic Safety Facts 2005.* Washington, DC: U.S. Department of Transportation.

- Do not exceed the speed limit. Observe all traffic signs.
- Always wear safety belts, even on short trips. Require your passengers to buckle up. Always keep small children in child restraints.
- Do not drive if you have been drinking alcohol. Give your car keys to a sober, trusted friend.
- Avoid horseplay and other distractions inside a car (see the box "Distractions and Safe Driving").
- Be certain that you can hear the traffic outside your car. Keep the car's music system at a reasonable

Distractions and Safe Driving

Max Jones was a very popular youth soccer coach who was tragically killed when his car left the road while he was driving to an early morning practice. His family and his players and their parents were all devastated when they heard the news. It was only later, after the funeral, when several of Max's close friends were chatting, that someone mentioned how Max would drive with a cup of coffee between his legs. Then another friend noted that Max had a habit of picking up fast food on his way to soccer practice. He would sometimes eat a breakfast sandwich and drink coffee while driving. His friends began to wonder whether these distractions could have contributed to Max's crash.

A recent research study found that drivers are distracted an average of 16 percent of the time with activities that take their attention away from the road and their driving environment. Activities such as manipulating vehicle controls (air-conditioning or windows), music/audio controls, or talking to a child or baby in the car distracted drivers. Approximately three-fourths of those observed ate or drank something. Searching or reaching for an object while driving was also observed in a majority of the drivers who were observed. Forty percent were observed reading, writing, or grooming while the vehicle was moving.

To lower your risk of injuring yourself or others, avoid distractions while driving. Do not eat or drink while driving. If you are driving alone, make sure you have all of the vehicle's controls set appropriately before you embark on your trip. Use highway rest stops wisely to eat, read maps, arrange music, and reorganize the inside of your car so that you won't be distracted while at the wheel.

Source: Stutts J, Feaganes J, Rodgman E, Hamlett C, Meadows T, Reinfurt D, Gish K, Mercadante M, Staplin L. *Distractions in Everyday Driving.* Washington, DC: AAA Foundation for Traffic Safety, 2003.

decibel level. (See the box "Cell Phone Safety while Driving" for more information.)

- Give pedestrians the right of way.
- Drive defensively at all times. Do not challenge other drivers. Refrain from drag racing.
- Look carefully before changing lanes.
- Be especially careful at intersections and railroad crossings.
- Carry a well-maintained first aid kit that includes flares or other signal devices.
- Drive even more carefully during bad weather.
- Do not drive when you have not had enough sleep.
- Do not ride with a driver who has been drinking.

In spite of the best efforts that people make to prevent motor vehicle crashes, when they occur there is, of course, not only damage to property but also the very real possibility of injury and even death. Remember, poor decisions also affect family members and friends, who pay an emotional price when they experience the

Anything that distracts a driver—talking on a phone, reading a map or notes, eating and drinking, or adjusting vehicle controls—can decrease concentration and slow reaction time. Driver distraction is a key contributing factor in many crashes.

loss of companionship when people for whom they care a great deal have been in serious motor vehicle crashes. The effects of motor vehicle–related injuries and injury deaths are also felt in the workplace where they result in economic losses of employers and employees alike.

 TALKING POINTS You're in a car with a friend when another driver starts tailgating you very closely. Your friend, who is driving, slows down to annoy the tailgater. How would you convince your friend that his action is dangerous?

Motorcycle Safety Some emergency-room physicians call motorcycles "murder-cycles" because of their experience with motorcycle crash victims. The statistics support this grim view. With the death rate for motorcycles at 43 per 100 million vehicle miles of travel compared to a death rate for cars of 1.55, motorcycles are nearly 28 times more deadly.[40] Therefore, our first recommendation is to not operate or ride on the back of a motorcycle.

If you choose to ride a motorcycle, you can reduce your risk of injury or death by following these suggestions:

- Most important of all, wear a helmet. A variety of studies have supported the effectiveness of helmets in preventing head injuries. Warriors and athletes have worn helmets for centuries to protect themselves from head injuries. Modern examples include construction workers, football players, race car drivers, and military aircraft pilots.

- Wear boots, gloves, and heavy clothing to protect your skin from serious injury when you slide on pavement in a crash.

- Get proper training, such as the Motorcycle Safety Foundation course offered in some states.

- Your risk increases in wet weather. Consider whether a ride in the rain is necessary.

- Do not ride after taking medication that can affect your alertness or performance.

- Never ride after drinking alcohol or taking drugs. About half of motorcyclists killed in accidents had alcohol in their blood.

- Ride defensively. Remember that many drivers do not see you or may not give you the right-of-way you deserve.

For all the reasons discussed in conjunction with automobile accidents, motorcycle accidents can influence the well-being of a wide array of people. However, because of the very high probability of serious injury and death associated with these accidents, the distress suffered by family, friends, witnesses, and coworkers may be even more extensive.

Residential Injuries and Safety

Although more injury deaths occur on our highways and streets, more injuries of all types occur at home. Approximately 1 person in 10 is injured each year at home. It is not that our homes (residence halls, apartments, houses) are particularly dangerous; it is simply that we spend more time at home than anywhere else. Injuries that occur where we live include poisonings, falls, burns, and suffocations.

Poisonings The leading cause of unintentional injury deaths in homes is poisonings.[41] A few of these are attributable to alcohol, pesticides, or carbon monoxide; but most, by far, are caused by prescription drugs or illegal drugs, particularly prescription narcotics and cocaine. The rate of unintentional poisoning deaths increased 62 percent from 1999 to 2004. The largest increases were among 15- to 24-year-olds (113.3 percent), females (103 percent), and whites (75.8 percent). Unlike some earlier epidemics of drug abuse, the greatest increase in unintentional poisoning rates have occurred not in East Coast or West Coast cities, but in the Midwest (85.5 percent) and the South (113.3 percent).[41]

Prevention of poisoning by prescription drugs requires an understanding of the potency of these agents, particularly the opioid analgesics such as oxycodone. These, and similar drugs, depress respiration to the point where there is insufficient oxygen in the body to sustain a heartbeat. To reduce your risk of a drug overdose, adhere to the following precautions:

- Always read all information provided with your prescription.

ANSWERS TO THE "WHAT DO YOU KNOW?" QUIZ

1. True 2. True 3. False 4. True 5. False 6. True 7. True

ENDNOTES

1. Adams PF, Dey AN, Vickerie JL. Summary Health Statistics for the U.S. Population: National Health Interview Survey, 2005. *Vital and Health Statistics* 10 (233). Hyattsville, MD: National Center for Health Statistics, Centers for Disease Control and Prevention, U.S Department of Health and Human Services. January, 2007.

2. Miniño AM, Heron M, Murphy SL, Kochanek KD. *Deaths: Final Data for 2004*. National Center for Health Statistics, www.cdc.gov/nchs/products/pubs/pubd/hestats/finaldeaths04/finaldeaths04.htm.

3. Centers for Disease Control and Prevention, National Center for Injury Prevention and Control, WISQARS (Web-based Injury Surveillance Query and Reporting System), www.cdc.gov/ncipc/wisqars/.

4. Catalano SM. National Crime Victimization Survey: Criminal Victimization, 2005. U.S. Department of Justice, Office of Justice Programs, *Bureau of Justice Statistics: Bulletin.* NCJ 214644, September 2006.

5. McCaig L, Nawar EW. National Ambulatory Medical Care Survey: 2004 Emergency Department Summary. *Advance data from vital and health statistics.* No. 372. Hyattsville, MD: National Center for Health Statistics, 2006.

6. Fox, JA. *Homicide Trends in the U.S.* Department of Justice, Office of Justice Programs, Bureau of Justice Statistics, 2006, www.ojp.usdoj.gov/bjs/homicide/tables/totalstab.htm.

7. Hoyert EL, Heron MP, Murphy SL, Kung H. Deaths: Final Data for 2003. *National Vital Statistics Reports.* 54 (13): 1–120, 2006.

8. Blumstein A, Rivara FP, Rosenfeld R. The rise and decline of homicide—and why. *Annu. Rev. Public Health* 21:505–541, 2000.

9. Bonczar, TP. "Prevalence of Imprisonment in the U.S. Population, 1974–2001." U.S. Department of Justice, Office of Justice Programs, Bureau of Justice Statistics, *Bureau of Justice Statistics: Special Report*, NCJ 197976, 2003, www.ojp.usdoj.gov/bjs/pub/pdf/llgsfp.pdf.

10. Tjaden P, Thoennes N. *Extent, Nature, and Consequences of Intimate Partner Violence: Findings from the National Violence Against Women Survey.* NCJ 181867, Washington D.C.: National Institute of Justice, 2000.

11. Fisher BS, Cullen FT, Turner MG. *The Sexual Victimization of College Women.* U.S. Department of Justice, Bureau of Justice Statistics, NCJ 182369. Washington, D.C., 2001.

12. Thornhill R, Palmer CT, Wilson M. *A Natural History of Rape.* Cambridge: MIT Press, 2000.

13. Schwartz RH, Milteer R, LeBeau MA. Drug-facilitated sexual assault ("date rape"). *South Med 2000.* 93 (6):558–561.

14. Harlow, CW. Hate crimes reported by victims and police. *Bureau of Justice Special Report, National Criminal Victimization Survey and Uniform Crime Reporting.* U.S. Department of Justice, Office of Justice Programs, NCJ 209911, 2005.

15. U.S. Census Bureau. *Families and Living Arrangements, March 2005.* Washington, D.C.: U.S. Census Bureau, www.census.gov/population/www/socdemo/hh-fam/cps2005.html.

16. U.S. Department of Labor, Bureau of Labor Statistics (2006). Employment and fatality profiles by gender of worker, 2005. In *Census of Fatal Occupational Injuries Charts, 1992–2005*, www.bls.gov/iif/oshcfoi1.htm#charts.

17. Catalano S. Intimate Partner Violence in the United States. Bureau of Justice Statistics, U.S. Department of Justice, www.ojp.usdoj.gov/bjs/intimate/ipv.htm.

18. Coker AI et al. Physical health consequences of physical and psychological intimate partner violence. *Arch Fam Med 2000*; 9 (5):451–457.

19. U.S. Department of Health and Human Services, Administration on Children, Youth and Families. *Child Maltreatment 2004*, www.acf.hhs.gov/programs/cb/pubs/cm04/cm04.pdf.

20. National Institute of Justice, *The cycle of violence revisited.* Washington D.C.: U.S. Department of Justice, Office of Justice Programs, NIJ, Research in Progress Seminar Series, February, 1996.

21. U.S. Census Bureau, *Population Estimates*, www.census.gov/popest/estimates.php.

22. National Research Council, *Elder Mistreatment: Abuse, Neglect, and Exploitation in an Aging America.* Washington D.C.: National Academies Press, 2003.

23. National Center on Elder Abuse (1998). "The National Elder Abuse Incidence Study: Final Report," www.elderabusecenter.org/default.cfm?p=nis.cfm.

24. U.S. Department of Education, National Center for Education Statistics (2007). "Indicators of School Crime and Safety: 2006." NCES 2007-003, nces.ed.gov/programs/crimeindicators/.

25. Centers for Disease Control and Prevention. "Youth Risk Behavior Surveillance—United States, 1993." *Morbidity and Mortality Weekly Report,* CDC Surveillance Summaries 44 (SS-1): 1–55. 1995.

26. Bilchik S. Violence after School. *1999 National Report Series, Juvenile Justice Bulletin,* Washington, D.C.: U.S. Department of Justice, Office of Justice Programs, Office of Juvenile Justice and Delinquency, Prevention. NCJ 178992, November 1999.

27. Baum K, Klaus P. Violent victimization of college students, 1995–2002. U.S. Department of Justice, Office of Justice Programs, *Bureau of Justice Statistics: Special Report National Crime Victimization Survey* NCJ 206836, January, 2005, www.ojp.usdoj.gov/bjs/pub/pdf/vvcs02.pdf.

28. Bureau of Justice Statistics (2006). *Criminal Victimization in the United States, 2005, Statistical Tables, Table 32,* www.ojp.usdoj.gov/bjs/abstract/cvusst.htm#one.

29. Egley Jr. A, Ritz CE. Highlights of the 2004 National Youth Gang Survey. *OJJDP Fact Sheet.* April 2006 #01. U. S. Department of Justice, Office of Justice Programs, Office of Juvenile Justice and Delinquency Prevention, www.iir.com/nygc/publications/fs200601.pdf.

30. Dorsey TL, Zawitz MW, Middleton P. *Drugs and Crime Facts.* U.S. Department of Justice, Office of Justice Program, Bureau of Justice Statistics, NCJ 165148, www.ojp.usdog.gov/bjs/pub/pdf/dcf.pdf.

31. Mumola CJ, Karberg JC. Drug Use and Dependence, State and Federal Prisoners, 2004. U.S. Department of Justice, Office of Justice Programs, *Bureau of Justice Statistics: Special Report,* NCH 213530, 2006, www.ojp.usdoj.gov/bjs/pub/pdf/dudsfp04.pdf.

32. Miniño AM , Anderson RN. Deaths: Injuries, 2002. *National Vital Statistics Reports.* 54 (10): 1–128, 2006.

33. Centers for Disease Control and Prevention. Surveillance of fatal and nonfatal firearm-related injuries—United States, 1993–1998. *Morbidity and Mortality Weekly Report* 50 (SS-2): 1–34.

34. Centers for Disease Control and Prevention. Youth Risk Behavior Surveillance—United States, 2005. *Morbidity and Mortality Weekly Report* 55 (SS-5): 1–110.

35. Miller M, Hemenway D, Wechsler H. Guns and Gun Threats at College. *J. Am. Coll. Hlth* 51 (2): 57–65, 2002.

36. Federal Trade Commission. Deter•Detect•Defend Avoid ID Theft: Fighting back against identity theft, www.ftc.gov/idtheft.

37. Annan, K. [In the second part of the report titled] *Larger Freedom.* A commentary issued by the United Nations at the Security Council Meeting. March 17, 2005, www.un.org/unifeed/script.asp?scriptId=73.

38. Miniño AM, Heron MP, Smith BL. Deaths: Preliminary Data for 2004. *National Vital Statistics Reports* 54 (19): 1–52. 2006.

39. National Safety Council. *Injury Facts, 2005–2006.* Itasca, IL. 2006.

40. U. S. Department of Transportation, National Highway Traffic Safety Administration. (2007). *Traffic Safety Facts 2005: A compilation of motor vehicle crash data from the fatality analysis reporting system and the general estimates system.* Washington, D.C.: US DOT, DOT HS 810 631, www-nrd.nhtsa.dot.gov/Pubs/TSF2005.pdf.

41. Centers for Disease Control and Prevention. Unintentional Poisoning Deaths—United States, 1999–2004. *Morbidity and Mortality Weekly Report* 56 (5): 93–96. 2007.

42. National Safety Council. *Injury Facts, 2004.* Itasca, IL: Author, 2004.

43. U.S. Coast Guard. *Boating Safety*, www.uscgboating.org/statistics/accidentstats.htm.

Personal Assessment

How well do you protect your safety?

This quiz will help you measure how well you manage your personal safety. For each item, circle the number that reflects the frequency with which you do the safety activity. Then, add up your individual scores and check the interpretation at the end.

3 I regularly do this
2 I sometimes do this
1 I rarely do this

1. I am aware of my surroundings and do not get lost.
   3   2   1
2. I avoid locations in which my personal safety would be compromised.
   3   2   1
3. I intentionally vary my daily routine (such as walking patterns to and from class, parking places, and jogging or biking routes) so that my whereabouts are not always predictable.
   3   2   1
4. I walk across campus at night with other people.
   3   2   1
5. I am careful about disclosing personal information (address, phone number, Social Security number, my daily schedule, etc.) to people I do not know.
   3   2   1
6. I carefully monitor my alcohol intake at parties.
   3   2   1
7. I watch carefully for dangerous weather conditions and know how to respond if necessary.
   3   2   1
8. I do not keep a loaded gun in my home.
   3   2   1
9. I know how I would handle myself if I were to be assaulted.
   3   2   1
10. I maintain adequate insurance for my health and my property.
    3   2   1
11. I keep emergency information numbers near my phone.
    3   2   1
12. I keep my first aid skills up to date.
    3   2   1
13. I use deadbolt locks on the doors of my home.
    3   2   1
14. I use the safety locks on the windows at home.
    3   2   1
15. I check the batteries used in my home smoke detector.
    3   2   1
16. I have installed a carbon monoxide detector in my home.
    3   2   1

17. I use adequate lighting in areas around my home and garage.
    3   2   1
18. I have the electrical, heating, and cooling equipment in my home inspected regularly for safety and efficiency.
    3   2   1
19. I use my car seat belt.
    3   2   1
20. I drive my car safely and defensively.
    3   2   1
21. I keep my car in good mechanical order.
    3   2   1
22. I keep my car doors locked.
    3   2   1
23. I have a plan of action if my car should break down while I am driving it.
    3   2   1
24. I use appropriate safety equipment, such as flotation devices, helmets, and elbow pads, in my recreational activities.
    3   2   1
25. I can swim well enough to save myself in most situations.
    3   2   1
26. I use suggestions for personal safety each day.
    3   2   1

TOTAL POINTS _____

Interpretation

Your total may mean that:

72–78 points	You appear to carefully protect your personal safety.
65–71 points	You adequately protect many aspects of your personal safety.
58–64 points	You should consider improving some of your safety-related behaviors.
Below 58 points	You must consider improving some of your safety-related behaviors.

TO CARRY THIS FURTHER . . .

Although no one can be completely safe from personal injury or possible random violence, there are ways to minimize the risks to your safety. Scoring high on this assessment will not guarantee your safety, but your likelihood for injury should remain relatively low. Scoring low on this assessment should encourage you to consider ways to make your life safer. Refer to the text and this assessment to provide you with useful suggestions to enhance your personal safety. Which safety tips will you use today?

The Environment and Your Health

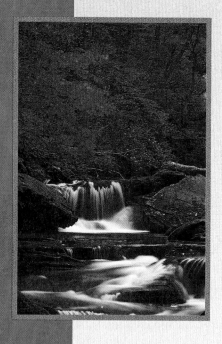

What Do You Know about Environmental Health?

◉ The vast majority of your exposure to potentially harmful pollutants occurs in the home and workplace. True or False?

◉ Electromagnetic radiation from electrical power lines, microwave ovens, and cell phones has been shown to cause cancer. True or False?

◉ If you live in an old house, you and your family are at greater risk for lead poisoning, which can reduce intelligence and increase behavior problems in young children. True or False?

◉ The government has tested all chemicals used in household and personal hygiene products to ensure that they do not cause adverse health effects in people. True or False?

◉ If you suffer from asthma or other lung diseases, it would be good for your health to move to Los Angeles. True or False?

◉ Tap water from a municipal water supplier can contain measurable amounts of potentially harmful pollutants. True or False?

◉ Warming of Earth's climate associated with increasing carbon dioxide in the atmosphere from burning fossil fuels can have negative impacts on your health. True or False?

Check your answers at the end of the chapter.

Environmental issues are important concerns for many college-age students as they perceive disturbing trends that may affect their future health and well-being. News programs regularly present the latest bad news about environmental problems such as overpopulation, pollution, global warming, damage to the ozone layer, loss of wilderness to economic exploitation, and endangered species. Movies such as *Water World, Blade Runner, Batman, The Matrix*, and *The Day After Tomorrow* depict fictional futures that are dismal environmental disasters. Some college students join environmental organizations that work to clean up litter, encourage recycling, regulate pollution emissions, control human population growth, and protect endangered species and natural areas. Others feel there is nothing they can do, lose hope for the future and may become depressed and apathetic. The impact of environmental quality on your health is influenced by both the nature of your environment and your intellectual, emotional, social, and spiritual responses (see the box "Religious Perspectives on Our Relationship with the Environment").

Reducing Risk of Waterborr

If water comes out of a tap, it'

If you travel to other countries, e
Asia, Africa, or South America, b
of these countries may be conta
One report estimated that 30 pe
of traveler's diarrhea during a ty
minimize your risk, consider the

1. Drink only bottled water or s
   (read the label). Do not drink
2. If you cannot find bottled dri
   with purification tablets any
   ing when you brush your tee
3. Avoid using ice, which is oft
4. Eat only well-cooked foods,
   meat, and raw fruits or vege
   wash. You are more likely to
   than from water.
5. As much as possible, keep
   ers are not uncommon in m
   lay their eggs in the sewers

phones for over 10 years
likely to have cancer in t
or eye (tissues close to w
when in use) than people
However, a smaller 2006 s
905 people with malignar
domly chosen people with
cer patients were more lik
cell phones (analog or di
over long periods.[12] Cell p
nology, and the authors
cancers that may be cause
to develop. Hence, there
to study effects of long-te
use cell phones more, be
some suggest that it may
to RFR from these devic
using a headset, so that t
will be farther away fro
RFR from cell phones d
small distances. Advanc
also reducing the amour
phones.

Another common s
in the human environme
wires and electronic devi
lines. A few studies have

Discovering Your Spirituality

Religious Perspectives on Our Relationship with the Environment

Can the root of modern environmental problems be found in Judeo-Christian-Islamic scriptures? All three religious traditions revere the Old Testament of the Bible, including the Genesis story. Passages in this part of the Bible imply that the purpose of all of creation is to serve humankind and include exhortations to "go forth and multiply" and "subdue the Earth." These passages established a dualism (human versus not-human) that did not exist in earlier Earth-based religions that perceived divinity in all of creation. This humans-versus-nature dualism encourages population growth and exploitation, resulting in the many environmental problems facing us today.

Earth-based religions of many indigenous cultures of the world (pre-Christian Europe, Native American, African religions) believed that many or all aspects of the natural world were manifestations of one or more gods. Humans performed religious rituals to gain favors or atone for sins against nature. While many of these cultures appear to have lived in ecological balance with their environment, it is unknown if this is due to their religious beliefs, small populations, limited technologies, or a combination of these factors. Modern Earth-based religions, including paganism, Wicca, Druidism, and Goddess religions, also worship the natural world as a manifestation of the energy of God or Creation. Many people who follow these religious traditions are dedicated to protecting the environment.[*]

Teachings of the major Eastern religious traditions are also more environmentally sensitive. Traditional Hinduism teaches that humans, gods, and nature are all parts of a single organic whole; any abuse of nature is considered a sacrilegious act.[†] Buddhism teaches followers to understand change in the natural world and condemns pollution and global alteration as evidence of the sins of greed, hatred, and delusion. Confucian scholars teach that humans are not lords of nature, but rather, filial sons and daughters of the universe who should care for the world around them.[‡]

While traditional Earth-based and Eastern religious traditions encouraged followers to live in ecological balance with their environment, many of these cultures now face a modern dualism: economic development versus environmental protection. Some people working for economic development in India and on Native American reservations sacrifice traditional beliefs, resulting in environmental degradation. In many cases these environmentally destructive decisions occur in the context of grinding poverty and a breakdown in traditional social systems associated with globalization of economies and cultures.

Some people read the Judeo-Christian-Islamic scriptures and find messages that encourage protection of the natural world. The Bible states that at the end of each day of creation God saw that each of his creations was "good," suggesting that the Creator valued all aspects of creation, not just humankind. Passages in the Bible and Qur'an (Koran) exhort believers to be "good stewards" over the other parts of Creation. Muslims are encouraged to be moderate in consumption, including the use of natural resources. Taken together, passages from the Qur'an encourage Muslims to protect and manage their environment for the common good.[§]

The National Religious Partnership for the Environment is an umbrella organization for Christians and Jews who believe that protecting the environment is a mandate well-founded in their scriptural traditions.[**] This association encourages its members to support environmental protection. For people who are committed to protecting the environment and dedicated to their Judeo-Christian religion, this organization offers a community of like-minded people working toward similar goals.

[*]Pagan and Earth-based Religions, www.beliefnet.com/index/index_10015.html.
[†]Narayanan V. Water, Wood and Wisdom: Ecological Perspectives from the Hindu Traditions. *DÆDALUS: Journal of the American Academy of Arts and Sciences*, www.amacad.org/publications/fall2001/narayanan.aspx. 2001.
[‡]Rohrman D. Religion, law, and the environment. *Frontiers in Ecology and the Environment*. 5 (1): 51. 2007.
[§]Alhilaly TH. 1993. Islam and Ecology. www.ummah.com/islam/taqwapalace/fitness/microcosmpage2.html.
[**]National Religious Partnership for the Environment. www.nrpe.org.

Your **environment** includes a range of conditions that can influence your health, such as the availability of resources (oxygen, water, food) and environmental characteristics, such as temperature, humidity, toxins, allergens, pathogens, noise, and radiation. Conditions in your environment operate across a wide range of spatial scales, from the air immediately surrounding your body to the global earth, air, and ocean system. Your physical health is influenced primarily by your *personal environment,* comprised of conditions immediately around your body, in the home, neighborhood, and workplace. However, this personal environment is influenced by conditions in the larger *community* and *regional environment,* including such conditions as air pollution and water pollution. These local and regional conditions are influenced by conditions of the *global environment,* such as climate and solar radiation.

Your health can be influenced by changes in environmental conditions at the home/workplace, community/region, or global levels. Excessive noise in the workplace

Key Terms

environment The physical conditions (temperature, humidity, light, presence of substances) and other living organisms that exist around your body.

ment. Disease-causing vir
cold, flu, measles) are put in
ple or animals sneeze or cou
handling systems can be bre
dew, and bacteria and can tl
nants throughout the home
cause disease, allergic react
have allergic reactions (itc
ing, coughing, stuffy chest
ache, and/or dizziness) to s
on moist surfaces inside bu
cates that exposure to indoo
your risk of developing adu
plants around the home or
reactions (hay fever) in m
rats, mice, and cockroache
feces, and skin dander that
lergic reactions.[8]

You can minimize yo
door air pollutants by ma
ity in your home within th
will minimize the growth
can cause health problem:
ity by installing exhaust fa
(major sources of water
water vapor accumulates
spaces), and using air-cor
You should also eliminate
been damaged by leaks or
surfaces.[8]

To minimize allergic
air pollutants, you should
your home. While this wil
mites, pollen, and animal
tially reduce the amounts
verity of allergy symptom
leave the house while it is
may temporarily increase
gens and other biological
try to keep your house fr
as these pests are sources

Radon   **Radon** is an er
seeps into buildings fro
foundation. It is invisible,
be detected only by using

Key Terms

radon A naturally occurr
ted during the decay of u

nonionizing radiation
tion that cannot break c
electrons or heat biolog

Approximately 23 million people in the United States obtain their drinking water from groundwater (that is, from private wells), streams, or cisterns that collect rainwater.[17] These households are responsible for ensuring the safety of their own drinking water. Private drinking water supplies that rely on surface waters, or wells that tap shallow groundwater layers, are at risk of contamination by pathogens from home septic systems, contaminants from leaking underground fuel storage tanks, improper disposal of various household chemicals (cleaners, automotive fluids, and pesticides), and agricultural chemicals applied to surrounding farm fields.

Drinking Water Contaminants and Their Health Effects   *Nitrate* from agricultural fertilizer that leaches into shallow groundwater supplies poses a widespread health risk in rural areas. The U.S. Geological Survey estimates that 10–20 percent of groundwater sources of drinking water may have levels of nitrate contamination that pose risks to human health. Excessive consumption of nitrate in contaminated drinking water can cause serious illness and death. Nitrate interferes with the oxygen-transport function of the blood (methemoglobinemia). This effect is most pronounced in children, resulting in "blue-baby" syndrome.[18] Nitrate can also cause reproductive problems and is linked to development of several types of cancer.

Pathogenic bacteria, protozoans, and viruses may be found in drinking water from shallow wells that are located near home septic systems. These organisms cause diarrhea and sometimes more life-threatening dehydration and kidney failure.

Rural wells contaminated by nitrate may also have high levels of other agricultural chemicals. See the section "Endocrine Disrupters" below for more information on the health effects of pesticides and herbicides. Leaching of substances from pipes in the plumbing of older homes is another potential source of contamination to drinking water in the home.[19] Metallic pipes can re-

Key Terms

fecal coliform bacteria   A category of bacteria that live within the intestines of warm-blooded animals; the presence of these bacteria is used as an indicator that water has been contaminated by feces.

endocrine disrupting chemicals   Substances that interact with the glands, hormones, and tissues that regulate many physiological processes in humans, including growth, development from fetus to adult, metabolism, reproduction, and development of the brain and nervous system.

---

lease toxic metals such as lead and copper into the water. Polyvinyl chloride (PVC) pipes manufactured before 1977 may release toxic vinyl chloride into the water. Vinyl chloride is a known human carcinogen.

Taking Action to Keep Your Drinking Water Safe Leaching of toxic substances from pipes into the drinking water supply is most problematic in small–diameter pipes (less than a two-inch diameter), with high water temperatures, and when the water is stagnant in the pipes for long periods (more than 24 hours).[19] A relatively easy way to reduce contaminants from household plumbing in your drinking water is to regularly flush fresh water through the plumbing. Let the water run from the tap for a couple of minutes before taking water to drink, especially first thing in the morning and if you have been away from home for long time periods. In some cases it may be advisable to replace the old plumbing, but this can be very expensive.

Private water supplies should be tested annually for nitrate and **fecal coliform bacteria.** If you suspect there may be a problem with radon or pesticide contamination, you may need to test your water even more frequently. Testing generally requires that you send samples of your water to a laboratory that tests water quality. You can get a listing of local certified laboratories from your local or state public health department. Some local health departments test private water for free. A private laboratory will charge $10–$20 to perform a nitrate and bacteria test. Testing for pesticides or organic chemicals may cost from several hundred to several thousand dollars. Most laboratories mail back the sample results within a few days, or several weeks if the analyses are more complex. The results indicate the concentrations of contaminants and indicate whether each contaminant exceeds a drinking water quality standard.

If your drinking water contains contaminants that exceed safety standards, you should retest the water supply immediately and contact your public health department for assistance. High bacteria concentrations can sometimes be easily controlled by disinfecting a well. Water filters may also remove some contaminants. However, other problems may require a new source of water, such as a deeper well. Alternatively, you may need to rely on bottled water until a new water source can be obtained.[17] You can obtain technical assistance with residential drinking water supply problems from the organization Farm˙A˙Syst/Home˙A˙Syst (see the websites www.uwex .edu/farmasyst and www.uwex.edu/homeasyst). See the box "Reducing Your Contribution to Water Pollution" for steps you can take to help keep drinking water safe.

Endocrine Disrupters

Endocrine-disrupting chemicals include a number of infamously dangerous pollutants (dioxin, PCBs, DDT), a large number of pesticides, herbicides, and antiseptics, and chemicals used in the manufacture of plastics (phthalates, bisphenol A) and Teflon (perfluorooctanoic acid, PFOA). These chemicals enter the home and work environment as contaminants of air, food, and water, in household plastics, nonstick cookware, and popcorn popping bags, and in a range of personal products such as cosmetics, hair spray, perfumes, soap, shampoo, and insect repellant. Many of these substances are not readily eliminated from the body and tend to accumulate; large proportions of the human population in the United States have measurable amounts of these substances in their body.[20]

Agricultural pesticides and herbicides that act as endocrine disrupters include some of the most widely used chemicals in our food production system (for example, the herbicide Atrazine). Your exposure to these chemicals can occur via pesticide residues on fruit and vegetables or contamination of well water (in areas with large areas of farmland). These chemicals have been linked to testicular and breast cancer, reduced sperm production in men, and nervous disorders in children.[21]

Phthalates are a class of endocrine disrupters that has recently become a source of concern after analyses of urine from a random sample of people in the United States indicated that virtually the entire population has measurable quantities of one or more of these chemicals in their bodies.[20] This is likely due to the almost ubiquitous use of phthalates in soft plastics, including food packaging, plastic storage containers, children's soft plastic toys, and medical tubing, and in many personal hygiene products. Phthalates are released from plastics to air, water, and food and are readily absorbed across the skin and via the lungs and digestive tract. Phthalates have been shown to disrupt the action of estrogen and testosterone, affecting both reproductive development of fetuses and children and reproductive function of adults.[22] Disruption of hormonal balance at critical stages in the development of a fetus or child can have long-lasting effects.[23] Some have suggested that increases in the occurrence of breast and testicular cancer, and decreases in human sperm quality, in recent decades may be linked to exposure to endocrine-disrupting chemicals like phthalates.[24]

Given their widespread use in agriculture and home products, it is difficult to see how you can eliminate your exposure to endocrine disrupters. However, you might reduce exposure by eating organic foods that are not contaminated with pesticides and herbicides, reducing your use of personal hygiene products that contain any ingredient with the word *phthalate*, avoiding the use of nonstick cookware, and minimizing the use of soft plastic containers for food and drinks, choosing glass or metal containers when possible. This might be especially important for women who are pregnant and families with young children. Soft plastic toys and pacifiers that

usually end up in the mouths of small children contain phthalates, and might be avoided.

Noise

Noise can be defined as any undesirable sound. What constitutes "undesirable sound" will vary from one person to the next, but it often involves loud sounds that occur at irregular intervals and cannot be controlled by the listener.[25] In the personal environment of the home, neighborhood, and workplace, noise may include overly loud music, barking dogs, motorcycles and cars with broken, missing, or volume-enhanced muffler systems, loud machinery, appliances and power tools, airplanes flying overhead, and train whistles.

Health Effects of Noise The health effects of environmental noise depend on the intensity, frequency, and nature of the noise. Excessively loud noise can cause physical damage to sensory tissues in your ears, resulting in partial or total hearing loss that can be temporary or permanent. This physical damage will depend on both the intensity (as measured in decibels) and the duration of exposure to the loud noise. A common source of long-term exposure to loud sound that causes hearing loss in many young people is amplified music. Occasional loud rock music at 110 to 120 db may cause only temporary damage. However, daily exposure to such sound levels will cause permanent hearing loss. Jacking up the volume of your iPod or car stereo may be fun today, but is it worth a lifetime of incessant ringing in your ears and diminished hearing later in life? Ironically, damage caused by excessively loud sounds robs you of one of your most important senses, the ability to hear the unamplified human voice.

Even noise at lower levels can cause adverse health effects. The American Speech-Language-Hearing Association reports that low-level noise can elevate blood pressure, reduce sleep, cause fatigue, and disturb digestion. These physical effects of low-level noise can diminish emotional, intellectual, social, and occupational health. Effects reported by the World Health Organization include increased frustration and anxiety, impaired

ability to concentrate, reduced productivity and ability to learn, and increased absenteeism and accidents. These effects of noise can increase your feeling of stress and cause you to exhibit anger and aggression that are out of proportion to the immediate source of your irritation.[25] This antisocial behavior may have negative consequences in your personal relationships and occupational health (see the box "Reducing Health Risks of Noise Pollution").

The Community and Regional Environment

The community and regional environment is made up of the outdoor air you breathe, local rivers and lakes that provide water and recreation opportunities, surrounding lands (urban, industrial, suburban, rural, agricultural, natural communities), and all the people and other species that live in these areas. A wide range of human activities can degrade this community environment in ways that affect personal health. Air, water, and land pollution include many substances that have significant negative effects on physical health. Loss of natural areas and other recreational and aesthetic "green space" to roads, cities, and industrial development can adversely affect your perceived quality of life, with negative effects on emotional and spiritual health. Degraded environmental conditions in many communities discourage new economic development and may limit occupational health.

While you can exert some influence on the environmental conditions in your community, the influence of any one individual is usually small. Your control over how the community environment affects your personal health is often limited to controlling your exposure to known health risks, such as contaminated water and land or outdoor air pollution. You can also choose to reduce your own contributions to community/regional air, water, and land pollution through conservation of energy and water and recycling solid waste.

Because one person cannot have a significant impact on community environmental problems, many people join organizations that work to improve the environment and quality of life in their community. By working with others of like mind in the political process and in environmental organizations, you become "part of the solution" to major environmental problems that can affect your health and that of your family. For many people, getting involved in solving local environmental problems can provide significant benefits to emotional and spiritual health.

In this section you will learn about aspects of the community and regional environment that can affect your health, and what you can do to exert some level of personal control over these environmental influences.

Learning from Our Diversity

Race, Economic Status, and Exposure to Pollution

When it is impossible to prevent all pollution, it is important to know if the risk of adverse health effects due to exposure is fairly distributed across the population. The "environmental justice" movement studies whether people of color and people who are economically or politically disadvantaged are disproportionately exposed to environmental hazards and more likely to suffer associated injury or disease than the general population. This movement gained prominence after a report found that new hazardous waste dumps were being disproportionately located in communities with high proportions of racial minorities and low-income families.[*] In the years since, researchers have studied this issue in various regions of the United States. Many, but not all, studies have found evidence that environmental hazards are more likely to be in or near areas with a high percentage of minority and low-income population.

Two hypotheses have been proposed for this association between race, class, and pollution: (1) *Industrial siting decisions:* pollution producers prefer to locate their facilities in areas that have cheap real estate and/or where the community is less able to resist (poor and uneducated); and (2) *move-in decisions:* hazardous pollution sources reduce the value of surrounding housing and land, attracting low-income renters and homeowners who tend to be disproportionately of racial and ethnic minorities.[†] While there is evidence for both phenomena, siting decisions appear to be the primary factor.

Issues of environmental justice are not restricted to industrial pollution and hazardous waste dumps. In recent years, the siting of large confined-animal feeding operations (CAFOs) has stirred much controversy in rural areas of the United States. These mainly corporate-affiliated facilities generate millions of gallons of animal waste that is stored in sewage lagoons. Sewage lagoons can emit large amounts of hydrogen sulfide (rotten egg smell) and ammonia into the atmosphere. These very unpleasant-smelling air pollutants result in adverse physical health effects, diminished quality of life, and reduced land value in the area around the CAFO.[‡] Studies in the southeastern United States have provided evidence that new hog CAFOs were being preferentially sited in areas with high proportions of African American and low-income families.[§]

Studies of the impact of increased exposure to air pollutants in low-income and minority-dominated communities have documented increased risk of cancer and respiratory distress and decreased academic performance of students in schools located in these communities.[**] This latter effect acts to strengthen the cycle of poverty, as lowered academic performance by children in poor neighborhoods contributes to reduced future opportunities for economic advancement.

These and other studies have motivated a social and political environmental justice movement that helps disadvantaged communities resist attempts to build new pollutant sources near their neighborhoods. Governmental recognition of the environmental justice issue has resulted in new laws and regulations for land-use planning and permits that require builders of new pollutant sources to specifically address issues of disproportionate pollution exposure of minority and low-income populations. If we all benefit from the products made by industries that produce pollutants, fairness requires that we also share equally the health costs of associated pollutants. If we all share equally the costs and benefits of industry, perhaps there will be greater motivation to develop less-polluting technologies.

[*] United Church of Christ. *A National Report on the Racial and Socio-Economic Characteristics of Communities with Hazardous Waste Sites.* 1987. UCC Committee for Racial Justice, New York.
[†] Pastor M, et al. Which came first? Toxic facilities, minority move-in, and environmental justice. *Journal of Urban Affairs* 23 (1): 1–21. 2001.
[‡] Donham K, et al. Community health and socioeconomic issues surrounding concentrated animal feeding operations. *Environmental Health Perspectives* 115: 317–320. 2006.
[§] Wing S, et al. Environmental justice in North Carolina's hog industry. *Environmental Health Perspectives* 108: 225–231. 2000.
[**] Pastor M, et al. Reading, writing, and toxics: Children's health, academic performance, and environmental justice in Los Angeles. *Environment and Planning C: Government and Policy* 22: 271–290. 2004.

Air Pollution

Air pollution includes substances that naturally occur in the air (pollen, microbes, dust, sea salt, volcanic ash) and substances produced by human activities (engine exhaust, ozone, various volatile organic compounds, and acid rain). In this section on community and regional environmental influences on health, we focus on those components of air pollution that are produced within a specific region and that have substantial health effects within that community or region.

Sources of Air Pollutants The primary sources of human-caused air pollutants are various kinds of internal combustion engines associated with electric power plants, industry, and transportation (trucks, automobiles, and farm/construction equipment). Oil refineries and chemical production factories also contribute to air pollution in some communities. Electric power stations, industrial facilities, and chemical factories are classified as *point sources* that produce large amounts of pollution from a single location (see the box "Race, Economic Status, and Exposure to Pollution"). Automobiles, trucks, heavy construction/farm equipment, gas stations, lawn mowers,

---

Key Terms

air pollution Substances in the atmosphere that can have adverse effects on human health, crop productivity, and natural communities.

Tropospheric ozone is a key component of smog, which is especially common in certain parts of the United States.

and charcoal grills are *nonpoint sources* of air pollutants. Individually, nonpoint sources produce relatively small amounts of pollution, but when added together account for a large proportion of community air pollution.

Health Effects of Air Pollutants   Air pollutants that are directly produced by internal combustion engines include *carbon monoxide, nitrogen dioxide, sulfur dioxide, polycyclic aromatic hydrocarbons,* and *particulate matter.* Carbon monoxide is a toxic gas that impairs respiration, as described under indoor air quality in the previous section. Nitrogen and sulfur oxides interact with water vapor in the air to form small particulates (diameter <2.5 μm) that are inhaled into the deepest parts of the lungs. These substances can damage lung tissues, reduce lung capacity, cause coughing and chronic bronchitis, and make worse such ailments as hypersensitivity to allergens, asthma, emphysema, and heart disease. The U.S. Environmental Protection Agency estimates that over 70 million people in the United States live in counties where levels of small particulate air pollutants exceed human health standards for at least some part of the year.[26] It has been estimated that small-particulate air pollution

---

causes as many as 50,000 to 100,000 premature deaths in the United States per year.[27]

Polycyclic aromatic hydrocarbons (PAHs)   have been shown to be carcinogenic to both test animals and humans. Several new studies indicate that PAHs can cross the placenta and cause adverse health effects on a developing human fetus.[28, 29] Increased maternal exposure to PAHs was associated with lower birth weight, smaller head circumference, and reduced birth length of newborn children.[28] A study of mothers and newborns living in large cities in the United States, Poland, and China documented a significant association between maternal exposure to PAHs and PAH-linked DNA damage in newborns that is associated with increased risk of cancer.[29] This type of DNA damage was detected in 42 percent and 61 percent of two groups of newborns in New York City (where PAH exposure was lowest), 71 percent of newborns in Krakow, Poland, and 80 percent of newborns in Tongliang, China (where PAH exposure was highest).

Tropospheric ozone is produced when hydrocarbons, nitrogen oxides, and other small particle matter chemically interact in the presence of sunlight. The result is a brownish haze over affected cities, often called *smog.*

Ozone levels are particularly high in locations with warm, sunny climates (southern California) and where natural vegetation produces volatile organic compounds that contribute to the photochemical process that produces ozone (eastern United States). The U.S. Environmental Protection Agency estimates that over 110 million people in the United States live in counties where ozone levels exceed human health standards for at least some part of the year.[26] Most of these people live in southern California and near the East Coast between Virginia and southern Maine (see Figure 20-2).

Inhalation of ozone can cause lung damage that reduces lung capacity. This is a particular health risk to individuals who suffer from asthma, emphysema, or heart disease. On days when ozone concentrations are highest, local hospital emergency room visits associated with respiratory distress increase from 10–20 percent.[30] If you suffer from asthma or a chronic cardiovascular disease, you may want to think carefully before living in any of the noncompliance areas shown in Figure 20-2. There is also some evidence that childhood exposure to ozone can actually cause children to become asthmatic.[30, 31]

Air toxics are a diverse collection of hazardous air pollutants produced mainly by electric power plants and industrial sources that constitute a widespread environmental health risk in the United States. When lifetime cancer risks for all carcinogenic air toxics are combined, 200 million people in the United States live in counties where that risk exceeds 10 in 1 million, and 20 million people live in areas where the risk exceeds 100 in 1 million.[32] However, these risk estimates are based on a lifetime of exposure to toxic air pollutant levels as they were last

---

> **Key Terms**
>
> **polycyclic aromatic hydrocarbons (PAHs)** Air pollutants from fossil fuel combustion.
>
> **tropospheric ozone** Ozone comprises three oxygen atoms that are bound into a single molecule; tropospheric ozone refers to this substance as it occurs in the lower layer of the atmosphere, close to the ground.
>
> **air toxics** A class of 188 toxic air pollutants identified by the U.S. Environmental Protection Agency as known or suspected causes of cancer or other serious health effects, such as reduced fertility, birth defects, or adverse environmental effects.

Figure 20-2 Exposure to Unhealthy Air This map shows counties classified by the EPA as in "nonattainment" of ozone standards in the year 2007, meaning levels of ozone in the county exceeded the limit set by the EPA.

Source: U.S. Environmental Protection Agency.

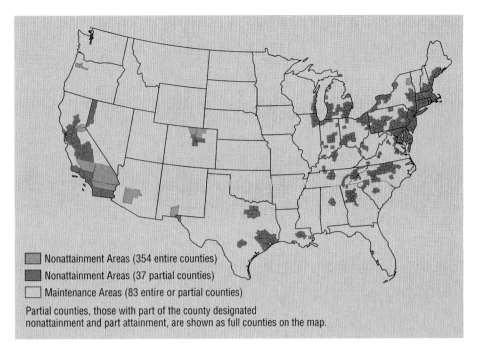

Nonattainment Areas (354 entire counties)
Nonattainment Areas (37 partial counties)
Maintenance Areas (83 entire or partial counties)

Partial counties, those with part of the county designated nonattainment and part attainment, are shown as full counties on the map.

inventoried in 1996. With continued progress on reducing toxic air pollution, risks associated with air toxics might be expected to decrease in the future. Since Congress passed the Clean Air Act in 1970, substantial progress has been made in reducing most human-caused air pollution in the United States. However, further reduction of air pollution poses serious technological and/or economic challenges, and efforts to strengthen regulations often face tough political opposition. For more information about air toxics, go to the U.S. EPA website at www.epa.gov/ttn/atw.

Taking Action on Air Pollution Unfortunately, the degree to which you can control your own exposure to regional air pollution and the associated health risks is limited. In many larger urban areas, where air pollution levels are highest, weather reports in newspapers and on television often include information about air pollution. This information is often conveyed in color-coded alerts. A "yellow" air pollution alert means people who suffer from respiratory or cardiac diseases, or hypersensitivity to allergens, should stay indoors. An "orange" air pollution alert indicates that everyone should limit their outdoor activities to the minimum possible.

You can also help to lower air pollution levels by limiting contributions from your own automobile, lawn mower exhaust, and charcoal grill. You can carpool, use mass transit, or telecommute (work at home via a computer network) to reduce air pollution associated with automobile exhaust. You can fill your car gas tank, mow your lawn, and use your grill during the cooler evening hours to reduce your contribution to tropospheric ozone. You can conserve electricity to reduce emissions of air

toxics, sulfur and nitrogen oxides, and particulates from electric power plants. In areas of the United States where air pollution is especially problematic, local laws may require that you do some of these things on days when conditions result in a "pollution emergency."

Water Pollution

We humans have had a very "schizophrenic" relationship with our rivers and lakes. Water is an essential resource for all living things on our planet, including humans and the plants and animals we use for food. We also value our rivers and lakes for the recreational opportunities and aesthetic benefits they provide. Yet for decades we used these water bodies as convenient dumps for our sewage and industrial wastes.

The problem of water pollution came to national attention on a day in 1968 when children playing with matches set on fire chemical pollutants that covered the Cuyahoga River in Ohio. The subsequent public outcry resulted in major national legislation, including the Clean Water Act of 1972 and the Safe Drinking Water Act of 1974. Since then, substantial progress has been made in reducing water pollution and ensuring safe drinking water supplies. However, the job of cleaning up rivers and lakes in the United States is not complete, and people who come into close contact with contaminated waters or fish from these areas are still at risk for a variety of health problems.

Sources of Water Pollution Water pollutants in surface waters come from obvious point sources (sewer overflows, confined livestock feedlot operations, sometimes

Agricultural runoff and the flow of untreated sewage into rivers during urban flooding are key sources of biological water pollutants.

called "factory farms") and from nonpoint sources such as water runoff from urban streets and agricultural areas that carries various chemicals and animal waste into local rivers. In some areas, water drainage from mines carries toxic metals into nearby streams. Some of the most troublesome water pollutants in the United States today are described below.

Biological water pollutants from untreated sewage and drainage from leaking home septic systems include various species of disease-causing viruses, bacteria, and protozoa found in rivers and lakes. The largest sources of biological water pollutants in United States surface waters today are overflows from urban combined septic and storm sewers during heavy rainfall and animal wastes that are carried by runoff of rainfall from agricultural areas. Although much has already been done to eliminate biological contamination from municipal sewer systems, billions of dollars are still required to dig up old combined sewer systems and replace them with separate systems for sewage and storm water run-off. As large animal "factory farms" have become more common in rural America, government agencies have established regulations for the proper handling of the huge amounts of animal sewage they generate. Even so, violations of regulations and occasional accidents result in contamination of local surface waters with animal waste.

A wide variety of **toxic pollutants** can be found in surface and groundwater sources of drinking water. These substances include naturally occurring toxic elements (such as arsenic and mercury) produced by breakdown of minerals in certain kinds of rock. Various industrial and agricultural human activities produce a wide range of toxic chemicals that find their way into U.S. surface waters, including metals, solvents, plastics, and PCBs (polychlorinated biphenols). Some toxic substances, including arsenic and mercury, have both natural and human-caused sources. While the dumping of toxic substances into surface waters is now illegal, some of these toxins are very stable and can be found in large quantities in the sediments of rivers and lakes that were polluted before 1972. Cleaning up these toxic sediments can be very costly. A recent decision to dredge and dispose of PCB-contaminated sediments in the Hudson River near Albany, New York, will cost hundreds of millions of dollars.

Agricultural pesticides can be significant toxic water pollutants in parts of the United States where large areas of land are used for crop production. These chemicals include insecticides, fungicides, and herbicides to kill organisms that consume or compete with crop plants. Rainfall can carry these chemicals from crop lands into local streams and rivers.

Health Effects of Water Pollution The organisms present in biological pollution cause diseases that are at best uncomfortable (diarrhea) and at worst potentially lethal (dysentery, hepatitis, typhoid fever, and cholera). In the late 1800s, diseases associated with drinking water contaminated by biological pollution were the third leading cause of death in the United States.[33] When surface water polluted with these organisms is used for crop irrigation of fruit and vegetables, these foods can become contaminated and cause disease or death (as seen in recent foodborne *E. coli* outbreaks).

Health effects of agricultural chemicals and other toxic substances depend on the specific chemical.[33] Taken as a group, these substances have been linked to adverse effects on the blood, liver, spleen, kidney, adrenal gland, thyroid gland, reproductive system (fertility), and cardiovascular system. Some are known or suspected human *carcinogens* (substances that cause cancer), *mutagens* (substances that cause cell mutations), or *teratogens* (substances that cause birth defects). Obvious health effects that occur immediately after exposure to high concentrations of these substances include nausea, fatigue, headache, skin and eye irritation, or tremors. The risks for these adverse immediate health effects are greatest for workers who come in direct contact with the concentrated chemicals. More insidious are health effects such as cancer and birth defects that develop slowly,

---

Key Terms

biological water pollutants Disease-causing organisms that are found in water.

toxic pollutants Substances known to cause cancer or other serious health effects.

solid waste Pollutants that are in solid form, including nonhazardous household trash, industrial wastes, mining wastes, and sewage sludge from wastewater treatment plants.

imperceptibly, after long-term exposure to low concentrations of these chemicals in the environment.

Taking Action on Water Pollution At present, your personal risk of exposure to biological water pollution in the United States is relatively small. Public health departments monitor local surface waters for the presence of fecal coliform bacteria in every U.S. county. While they may or may not cause illness or disease, the presence of fecal coliform organisms is an indicator that water has been contaminated by sewage. All municipal drinking water systems and many private households in the United States treat their water to kill pathogenic organisms. By the end of the twentieth century, deaths due to water pathogens in the drinking water supply were very rare in the United States.[33] It is also important to wash fresh vegetables before eating them, just in case they have been contaminated by polluted irrigation water.

The best way for you to minimize physical health risks posed by waterborne biological or toxic contaminants is to be well informed. Read the annual water quality report from your municipal water supplier that lists the amounts of biological contaminants, agricultural pesticides, and toxic substances detected in their water. If your supplier does not provide a report, you can access the supplier's annual report to the U.S. Environmental Protection Agency at www.epa.gov/safewater/dwinfo .htm. These reports list mean and range (minimum and maximum) concentrations for all regulated contaminants for all samples analyzed in a year. Look at the maximum value to determine if your water system occasionally fails to adequately remove any regulated contaminants. If your water supplier fails to meet health standards, consider drinking bottled, boiled, or filtered water until the supplier fixes the problems. Reverse osmosis water filters can be installed under a household sink and will remove most contaminants from drinking water at a cost of pennies per gallon.

You can also be exposed to toxic water pollutants by eating contaminated fish. Some toxic substances, such as mercury and PCBs, accumulate in high levels in the bodies of shellfish and fish that live in contaminated water. This problem can occur even in remote, apparently pristine areas if there are natural sources of toxic substances such as mercury. People who regularly consume fish from contaminated waters may be at high risk of adverse health effects. To reduce health risks associated with consuming fish, you should be aware of health advisories issued by the public health department or state agencies responsible for fish and game. These advisories are often stated in terms of limits on how much fish may be safely consumed in a specified time period. Pregnant women should be especially careful about consuming shellfish or fish; mercury and PCBs can cause birth defects in the fetus they carry. See Chapter 5 for more information.

You can also be exposed to waterborne pollutants as a result of recreational activities, such swimming, boating, and backpacking. You can limit your personal risk of exposure to health risks from contaminated water by being aware of "Don't swim" warnings for your local rivers and lakes, usually issued by the public health department. If you are backpacking in an apparently pristine wilderness area, never assume that crystal-clear water in the mountain stream is safe to drink. Backpackers should always filter, boil, or chemically treat drinking water to kill pathogens that may be present even in such remote water sources.

TALKING POINTS How can you approach your political representatives about environmental policy? What are some effective ways of keeping health-related environmental issues on the national agenda?

Land Pollution

We do not physically consume land or soil the way we do air and water, but pollution of land can still result in serious adverse health effects. Disposal of toxic wastes often involves burying them in the ground. When done with proper safeguards, this disposal method can isolate these dangerous materials so they can do no harm to humans or natural systems. If done improperly, these toxic pollutants leach into groundwater or are carried into surface waters by the runoff of rain, where they cause serious ecological problems and pose significant human health risks.

Sources and Components of Solid Waste Most land pollution today is associated with the disposal of **solid waste.** *Municipal solid waste* consists of everyday items such as product packaging, grass clippings, furniture, clothing, bottles, food scraps, newspapers, appliances, paint, and batteries. Other solid waste produced by business and industry includes waste tires, concrete, asphalt, bricks, lumber, and shingles from demolished buildings, and *sewage sludge* (solids remaining after wastewater treatment). In 1999 the U.S. population produced 230 million tons of solid waste, or about 4.6 pounds of waste per person per day (or 1,680 pounds per person per year).[34]

Disposal of Solid Waste Municipal sanitation departments and private disposal companies are very efficient at removing these wastes from our homes and businesses and putting them someplace where we don't see them. These waste disposal locations include sanitary landfills (wastes are compacted and buried under soil), ocean dumping in garbage barges (with trash sometimes escaping to wash up on beaches), and incinerators (where solid wastes are burned).

As we run out of places to dump our solid waste, some have proposed that we burn it in large incinerators. However, many concerns have been raised about

Recycling can reduce land pollution and consumption of natural resources.

incinerators because they can release toxic substances into the atmosphere. Furthermore, the ash from these incinerators contains concentrated toxic chemicals in forms that can easily leach into ground and surface waters.

Taking Action on Land Pollution Most of the potential health effects of land pollution have already been described in this chapter under the topics of air and water pollution. Most human exposure to pollutants that are deposited on land occurs when those toxic substances end up in the air or water. You can limit your risk of these health effects by being aware of where solid wastes are disposed, both at the present time and in the past. You should be particularly aware of proximity to a local landfill or waste disposal site if your water source is a private well that draws from groundwater that might be contaminated.

You can reduce your personal contribution to the solid waste problem of your community by following the Three R's: Reduce, Reuse, Recycle. You can reduce the amount of solid waste you produce by consuming less and accepting less packaging materials on the products you buy. You can compost your yard waste for use as a mulch and fertilizer in flower beds, or use a lawn mower with a mulching blade to eliminate grass clippings and leaves in the autumn. Reusing items such as bottles, zipper-closure storage bags, cloth shopping bags, and cloth diapers reduces the amount of solid waste you throw away each week. Many items in typical household trash

(newspapers and magazines, aluminum and steel cans, glass bottles, and many plastic containers) can be recycled and the materials used to make new products. Diverting these solid wastes away from the landfill toward reuse can greatly reduce the solid waste problem of your community. However, recycling will work only if you also buy products that are made from recycled materials, such as recycled paper and plastic "wood" products. Electronic equipment poses special waste and recycling challenges; see the box "The High-Tech Revolution and E-Waste."

Loss of Green Space

Loss of **green space** represents another kind of land pollution that can affect your quality of life and health. In many parts of the United States, green space is being converted to housing developments, shopping malls, industrial sites, and highways. Hundreds of large, brightly lit signs along the highways pollute the visual environment. Wildlife species disappear from your community and surroundings as their habitats are destroyed.

While development of green space for human uses may provide job opportunities and be beneficial for your occupational health, the "urban sprawl" nature of much of this development can adversely impact your physical, emotional, and spiritual health. Recent studies have shown that urban development that increases commute times to work or school is associated with decreased physical activity and increased prevalence of obesity and high blood pressure.[35] Increased time spent in a car commuting to work often comes at the expense of time spent in physical activities. Schoolchildren who lived within walking distance of parks had significantly more physical activity per week than those who did not have ready access to parks.[36] Likewise, children who lived close to their schools had more physical activity than children who lived far from school and had long bus rides every day.[37] The replacement of green space with urban sprawl can also adversely affect your emotional health and quality of life when you no longer see wild animals in your backyard or you feel that your community is becoming ugly.

Some communities have created land-use (zoning) plans that allow for economic development while protecting recreational and aesthetic values in their communities. These zoning plans can be controversial, as they try to balance the rights of private property owners with the welfare of the entire community. You can contribute toward protecting environmental quality in your community by supporting land-use planning and enforceable zoning laws that protect green space while allowing for responsible economic development.

Ionizing Radiation

Sources and Effects of Radiation *Radiation* is a general term that refers to various forms of energy that are

★ The High-Tech Revolution and E-Waste

The high-tech revolution has a hidden dark side—mountains of accumulating obsolete electronic equipment that contains large amounts of toxic substances. Hundreds of millions of old computers, containing millions of pounds of lead, cadmium, chromium, and mercury, need to go somewhere. These toxic metals cause a wide range of severe health effects if they end up in the air, drinking water, or food supply.[*†]

Computers contain more than a thousand different substances, making recycling a complex, labor-intensive process. Only 6 percent of obsolete computers disposed of after 1998 were recycled. The remainder were deposited in landfills across the country. It is estimated that 70 percent of heavy metals such as lead and mercury going into U.S. landfills today comes from electronic waste. To protect groundwater, several states, including California and Massachusetts, have banned disposal of computer monitors in landfills.[*]

While recycling of computers is seen as the ideal solution to the problem of waste disposal, it is estimated that 50–80 percent of computers "recycled" before the year 2002 were actually shipped to poor Asian countries. Workers in these countries disassemble computers to recover useful materials; they earn very low wages and have minimal or no protection from the toxic materials to which they are exposed. Materials that cannot be recycled are dumped into rivers or burned in open-air pits, exposing the workers and surrounding local populations to toxic substances. The practice of shipping toxic computer waste to underdeveloped countries is now banned by international treaty. The United States is the only developed nation that has not ratified this treaty. The "free market" justification for the practice of shipping toxic computer waste to underdeveloped countries is that this provides jobs and helps poor people. The question is, is it moral to give poor people the choice between poverty and poisons?[*]

Given that the use of computers and electronics will only increase in the future, many argue that we must develop environmentally responsible computer-recycling systems. Some computer manufacturers are already initiating computer take-back programs. In 2002, Rep. Mike Thompson introduced the Computer Hazardous-Waste Infrastructure Program (CHIP) Act, which would require the Environmental Protection Agency to help set up computer recycling across the United States. The program would be funded by a fee of up to $10 on all retail sales of desktop and laptop PCs and computer monitors. As of 2006, this legislation is still pending in Congress. Similar legislation is also appearing in many state legislatures.

The other, and perhaps most important, approach to the computer waste problem is to develop electronic equipment that is less toxic and more easily recycled. This will require development of, and investment in, new technologies. In our free-market system, this will happen only when the electronics manufacturers must share the cost of dealing with computer waste.

[*]Puckett, J, et al. *Exporting Harm: The High-Tech Trashing of Asia*. www.ban.org/E-waste/techno trashfinalcomp.pdf. 2002.
[†]U.S. Environmental Protection Agency. *WasteWise Update: Electronics Reuse and Recycling*. 2003. www.epa.gov/wastewise/pubs/wwupda14.pdf.

---

emitted by atoms and molecules when they undergo change, including radio waves, infrared waves, visible light, ultraviolet waves, x-rays, and gamma rays. Each kind of radiation has different effects on biological materials and health. **Ionizing radiation** causes damage to biological structures such as DNA that can result in serious adverse health effects. Ionizing radiation is produced by nuclear reactions, and sources include medical x-rays, naturally occurring radioactive minerals such as uranium and radon, various radioactive materials used by industry, nuclear reactors and their waste products, and nuclear bomb explosions.

The health effects of exposure to x-rays and gamma radiation depend on many factors, including the duration, type, and dose of radiation and your individual sensitivity. Heavy exposure to these forms of radiation can occur if you are near a nuclear bomb blast or downwind of a major nuclear reactor accident. In such cases, exposure can cause *radiation sickness,* including intense fatigue, nausea, weight loss, hair loss, fever, bleeding from the mouth, and compromised immune system, usually resulting in death.

Exposure to lower levels of nuclear radiation can cause damage to eyes, skin, and reproductive organs and may result in birth defects in children. Since September 11, 2001, government officials have warned about the possibility of terrorists using "*dirty bombs,*" whereby conventional explosives are combined with radioactive materials. The resulting dispersion of radioactive matter by the conventional bomb blast and wind would contaminate land well beyond the area affected by the blast.

The Challenge of Nuclear Waste Disposal In the coming years, huge amounts of radioactive waste must be permanently stored where it cannot escape into our environment. Nuclear reactors that generate 20 percent of the U.S. electricity supply have been accumulating highly

> ### Key Terms
>
> **green space** Areas of land that are dominated by domesticated or natural vegetation, including rural farmland, city lawns and parks, and nature preserves.
>
> **ionizing radiation** Electromagnetic radiation that is capable of breaking chemical bonds, such as x-rays and gamma rays.

Chapter Twenty The Environment and Your Health

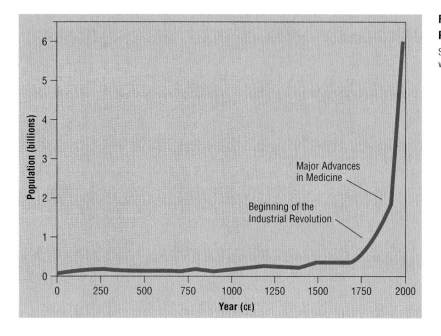

Figure 20-3 Growth of the Earth's Human Population
Source: U.S. Census Bureau, www.census.gov/ipc/www/worldhus.html.

radioactive wastes on-site. The U.S. government plans to store these wastes permanently in underground salt caves below Yucca Mountain, Nevada. A major health concern raised about the U.S. nuclear waste disposal program is the need to transport large quantities of highly radioactive waste by truck or train across the United States. However, the current situation is not safe either. Hundreds of tons of high-level radioactive waste are dispersed across the country in shallow, water-filled temporary holding tanks adjacent to nuclear power plants.

The Global Environment

The global environment is made up of the atmosphere, oceans, continental land masses, and all the living organisms that exist on Earth. Interactions among these components of the global environment influence the characteristics of solar radiation at the ground level, climate (temperature, precipitation, seasonal variation), production of food plants and animals, availability of freshwater, energy requirements for heating and cooling of human habitations, the geographic distribution of diseases, the composition of natural communities (deserts, tundra, rain forest), and the survival and extinction of species.

Some of the characteristics of the global environment have obvious and direct effects on human physical health, such as the presence of disease-causing organisms or solar UV radiation that can increase the risk of skin cancer. Other effects of the global environment on personal health are less well documented, such as the adverse effects on emotional or spiritual health associated with the extinction of species or destruction of beautiful natural communities. Many scientists warn that the

global environment is being degraded by the combined forces of ever more powerful technology being used by a rapidly increasing global human population. In this section we briefly describe major concerns regarding the global environment and how these might affect personal health. We end this section and the chapter with some thoughts about how you can take some degree of personal control over these global environmental problems and their influence on your health.

Human Population Explosion

Many scientists warn that the human population is increasing at a rate that cannot be sustained by the resources of the Earth (see Figure 20-3). There are currently over 6 billion people in the global human population, and this is projected to increase to over 10 billion in the next 50 years. Every year the world's population grows by about 78 million people, with 97 percent born into the poorest countries.[38]

Effects of Human Population Growth   The effects of the human population explosion on personal health depend on who you are and where you live. Many of the poorer nations of Asia, Africa, and South America will not be able to feed their people; starvation and associated diseases will be major health problems for these populations. Growing populations in dry regions are exceeding their freshwater supply, and hundreds of millions of people must drink from contaminated water sources. Every year, 5 million children die from waterborne diarrhea diseases associated with unsanitary drinking water.[38] By 2025, 2.5 billion people may live in regions where available freshwater is insufficient to meet their needs.

In many extremely poor countries, hungry people will destroy most or all of the remaining natural communities (tropical rain forests, African savanna) in vain efforts to grow food on lands that are not suited for agriculture. Overcultivation of farmlands to meet the demand for food has already degraded the fertility of a land area equivalent to that of the United States and Canada combined.[38] Hungry people who live on oceanic islands often destroy their coral reefs trying to make a living by using dynamite or cyanide to catch fish. In Africa hungry people hunt wild game for food, putting more and more species at risk of extinction.

Competition among nations for limited supplies of water and oil is often a root cause of political tensions, terrorism, and war. Political upheaval in the Middle East, recent terrorist attacks on U.S. targets, and the war in Iraq can be partially explained by competition for scarce resources (water, land, and oil). The genocide that killed hundreds of thousands in Rwanda in 1994–1995 has been traced to inequitable distribution of land and associated hunger in some parts of that country.[39] Many fear that such social instability and strife will be the inevitable result of competition for scarce resources, associated with excessive human population growth and overconsumption of limited resources.

Reducing Human Population Growth   The solutions to the human population growth problem are simple in theory, but often complex in their implementation. Basic population ecology theory states that the rate of population growth can be reduced if: (1) women have fewer children over their lifetime and (2) if they delay the start of their reproduction. A somewhat counterintuitive pattern is that population growth rate slows when infant survival rate is increased by better health care. It has been documented in many countries that women choose to have fewer children if they are confident that their children will survive.

Simply providing education opportunities to girls can have major and long-lasting effects that act to reduce population growth. Girls who become educated delay having their first child; educated women have half the pregnancies of their uneducated sisters.[38] Educated women are more likely to be employed outside the home. This has two effects: working women are too busy to care for large numbers of children, and women with an independent income have greater status and influence in deciding how many children they will have. Of course, universal access to birth control information and affordable contraception are also needed to allow women to have only as many children as they desire.

While this combination of commonsense actions can drastically reduce future human population growth, these proactive initiatives are often held hostage to political and cultural controversies. The sad result is that human populations may ultimately be controlled by

increased death rates associated with starvation, disease, and war rather than reduced birth rates. For more information on issues related to population growth, visit the websites listed in the box "Organizations Related to Environmental and Population Control Concerns."

Global Climate Change

Greenhouse Gases   A wide range of human activities add **greenhouse gases** to the atmosphere that trap heat and cause a net gain of energy and increase in temperature in the Earth system. This increase in global temperature is called the "greenhouse effect" or "global warming." Greenhouse gases include water vapor, carbon dioxide, methane, chlorofluorocarbons, ozone, and nitrous oxides. Human-caused sources of greenhouse gases include carbon dioxide from both industrial and agricultural activities, including the burning of coal, oil, and natural gas, conversion of natural communities (grasslands, forests, and wetlands) to human uses, methane emissions from leaking natural gas pipelines, flatulence from large herds of cattle, flooded rice fields, tropospheric ozone (described earlier in this chapter), chlorofluorocarbons from air-conditioner fluids, and nitrous oxide from agricultural fertilizer use. The average concentration of carbon dioxide in the atmosphere has increased 35 percent since the 1700s and currently exceeds the range of natural variation over the past 650,000 years. This increase is mostly due to burning of fossil fuels, and the rate of fossil fuel burning continues to increase. Atmospheric concentrations of the other greenhouse gases (methane and nitrous oxides) have also increased substantially during this period.[40]

There is growing evidence that increases in atmospheric greenhouse gases are associated with changes in global climate. Chemical analyses of gas bubbles in glacial ice core samples from the polar ice caps indicate that atmospheric carbon dioxide and methane concentrations have been closely related to changes in global temperature through several cycles of ice ages and warm periods during the past 420,000 years; when carbon dioxide and methane concentrations increased, so did atmospheric temperature.[41] The current increase in greenhouse gases is also associated with increasing global

---

Key Terms

greenhouse gases   A category of gases in the atmosphere that allow solar radiation to pass through the atmosphere to the Earth but then trap the heat that is radiated from the Earth back toward space; greenhouse gases include water vapor, carbon dioxide, methane, nitrous oxide, and tropospheric ozone.

temperature. According to the websites for the National Oceanic and Atmospheric Administration (NOAA) and the World Meteorological Association, the year 2006 was the warmest ever recorded in the United States and the sixth warmest year for the entire Earth; the nine years from 1998 to 2006 were among the 25 warmest years in the United States since 1895. The rate of increase in temperature has been accelerating since the mid-1970s.

Most scientists around the world believe that the changes in global climate described previously are the first evidence of global climate change related to human activities. However, a vocal minority of scientists still question the relative contributions of humans versus natural processes, and whether or not this warming trend is a short-term phenomenon or the beginning of a long-term trend (see the box "Hype versus Useful Information").

Effects of Climate Change   Because climate is such a fundamental characteristic of the environment, global warming is expected to have diverse and widespread effects, including melting of the polar ice caps that raises sea level and floods coastal areas (including major coastal cities) and increased frequency and severity of hurricanes and other destructive weather events. Effects of climate change on human health include increased heat stress, loss of life in storms and floods, expansion of the ranges of disease-carrying insects (such as mosquitoes) from subtropical regions into temperate regions (such as the United States), increased abundance of waterborne pathogens, decreased air and water quality, and decreased food availability associated with severe weather and water shortages. In 2003 a highly unusual heat wave in western Europe killed 35,000 people. While it is unknown if this event was linked to global warming, it proved the potential for severe climate events to have major impacts, even in economically developed countries. In less developed countries, millions of people have died from drought-related famine and severe storms (hurricanes and typhoons).

Taking Action on Climate Change   Your ability as an individual to take personal responsibility for addressing the global warming problem is limited, but all good things must start with individuals willing to do the right thing. You can reduce your personal contribution to global warming by conserving electricity at home, driving the most fuel-efficient automobile that meets your needs, using mass transit where available, recycling/reusing, and purchasing appliances that are rated as highly efficient. Compact fluorescent lights consume only

Hype versus Useful Information

An obscure scientist predicts a major shift in global climate. His warnings are brushed off by the powers that be. Within a month there are massive polar hurricanes encircling Earth's Northern Hemisphere. Within another month, the northern half of the United States is buried under ice and uninhabitable, millions of Americans are dead, and the survivors have permanently moved to Mexico. In the span of two hours, the movie *The Day After Tomorrow* brought the complex process of global climate change to a tidy storyline conclusion. Television pundits predicted that the movie would raise public awareness of this looming environmental problem. A few weeks later, the issue had fallen off the public radar. Two years later, another movie, the documentary *An Inconvenient Truth,* has been a surprising box office success. This "slide show" presentation by Al Gore again raises public awareness about the problem of global climate change. Gore's science-based presentation has been widely acclaimed for effectively communicating the intricacies of this complex issue in a manner that was accepted by a wide audience.

The media are among the most powerful forces in American society, and their influence extends to most of the Earth's human population. However, large multinational corporations have come to control many media producers, and information and news are increasingly being filtered for entertainment value. That which is deemed sufficiently entertaining is often hyped, with the most titillating aspects repeated over and over. Information that is deemed uninteresting is simply ignored.

The "entertainment filter" of many media producers often does not interact well with issues of environmental health. Many environmental problems are complex and affect human health in subtle ways over long time periods. For example, the U.S. population is being exposed to hundreds, if not thousands, of chemicals that have not been tested for human toxicity. They are found in our air, water, and food supply. They are found in our body fluids and hair. Some have been shown to cause cancer and birth defects in experimental animals. The EPA estimates that air pollution in major U.S. cities contributes to thousands of deaths due to respiratory and cardiovascular disease each year. In the last 20 to 30 years, cancer rates in the U.S. population have increased substantially, while fertility of men as measured by sperm counts has been declining by 1–3 percent per year. When was the last time you heard about these issues on the evening news or read about them in a newspaper or magazine? While Al Gore demonstrated in *An Inconvenient Truth* that it is possible to communicate environmental health issues in an entertaining manner, most media producers lack the motivation to do this with other complex issues.

Even when the news media do cover an environmental health story, their efforts to make it entertaining can present false or misleading information. Sometimes the story is presented as a debate to make it more interesting. Ideally, speakers from both sides of an issue present their perspectives and challenge incorrect or unsubstantiated claims from their opponents. All too often, these debates become shouting matches with more catchy sound bites, mischaracterizations, and name calling than useful information. The motivation of the speakers is to "win" rather than to communicate useful information. The media's efforts to objectively present both sides can also give the misperception that an environmental health issue is unresolved, leading to inaction. For example, the vast majority of the world's scientists believe that global warming is real and that the consequences are potentially very harmful.* However, there is a small vocal minority of scientists, many of whom receive funding from the fossil fuel industry, who dispute the existence and potential consequences of global warming.* News programs that present one representative from each side of this issue may claim to be "fair and balanced," but they give a mistaken impression that the current state of scientific judgment regarding global warming is not yet sufficiently resolved to warrant preventive action.

On the positive side, it has never been easier to obtain information about environmental health issues. Just type a few words into the Google search line and you will have more information than you can handle. Detailed reports from the EPA and the Centers for Disease Control and Prevention can be copied from their websites to your computer in seconds. You can read articles in scientific journals and browse websites that present a diversity of information and opinion.

However, when you "Google" an environmental health issue, you will need to exercise some judgment about what you read. Environmental advocacy groups, industrial groups, and liberal and conservative think tanks all have their Web presence, where they promote their perspectives. The mainstream news media have self-correcting mechanisms; when someone makes inaccurate statements in public, someone else exposes the mistake. Similar mechanisms have not yet been fully developed for the Internet. When an industry group or environmental group criticizes some change in environmental regulations, you need to be aware of their motivations before you can assess whether or not you will believe their claims. In general, information from professional scientific journals and U.S. government websites will be more reliable, because these sources have review processes to minimize errors and eliminate statements that are not well supported by research data. Before you accept statements from other sources, you should sample many websites that present a diversity of opinions. This will help you identify important issues and questions and will give you a better basis upon which to make informed decisions.

Unfortunately, as our lives become progressively more complex and busy, we rely more heavily on the news media to help us identify issues of importance. If the mainstream news media are not talking about environmental health issues, how will you know what to type on the Google search line? We tend to seek information about topics that concern us. Without adequate news coverage, we remain ignorant, blissfully or otherwise. By the time an environmental health issue becomes sufficiently "entertaining" to be covered on the evening news, the damage is often already done. No wonder the environment is not perceived as a high-priority issue when we elect our leaders.

*Union of Concerned Scientists, 2007, "Smoke, mirrors, and hot air: How ExxonMobile uses Big Tobacco's tactics to manufacture uncertainty on climate science," www.ucsusa.org/assets/documents/global_warming/exxonreport.pdf.

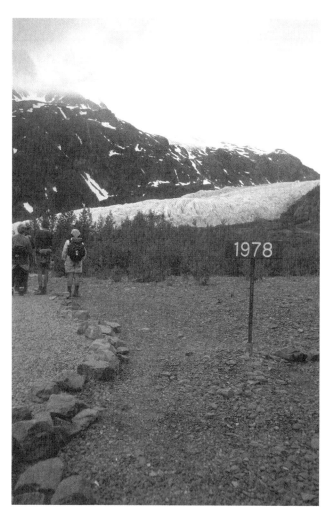

Global warming is expected to melt polar ice caps, raise sea level, and flood coastal areas. One result of recent warming is melting glaciers. The sign in this photo shows how far this Alaskan glacier has retreated since 1978.

Stratospheric Ozone Depletion

The *stratospheric ozone layer* is a concentration of ozone molecules located about 10 to 25 miles above the Earth's surface. This "ozone layer" contains about 90 percent of the planet's ozone. Stratospheric ozone is a naturally occurring gas formed by the interaction of atmospheric oxygen and components of solar radiation. Unlike tropospheric (low-elevation) ozone, which has many adverse health and ecological effects, the stratospheric ozone layer has beneficial health effects by protecting living organisms on the Earth's surface from harmful solar ultraviolet (UV) radiation.

Causes of Ozone Depletion It has been well documented that chemical reactions between stratospheric ozone and certain human-made air pollutants can significantly reduce the ozone layer, causing increased UV radiation at the Earth's surface. The chemicals that cause ozone depletion include chlorofluorocarbons (CFCs, used as coolants in many air-conditioning and refrigeration systems, in insulating foams, and as solvents), halons (used in fire suppression systems), and methyl bromide (used in pesticides). When these substances are released to the atmosphere and rise to the stratosphere, they release either chlorine or bromine molecules. One chlorine molecule can destroy 100,000 ozone molecules, and these substances can remain in the atmosphere for years.[42]

The vast majority of depletion of the ozone layer occurs in the atmosphere above the north and south poles; the colder temperatures and ice crystals in the atmosphere over the poles increases the breakdown of ozone. In 2006 the Antarctic "ozone hole" reached a record size of 10.6 million square miles. Thankfully, the Arctic ozone hole, which is much closer to major human population centers in Europe and North America, was not nearly so large. The decrease in the stratospheric ozone layer has been associated with as much as a 50 percent increase in UV radiation at the ground level in Antarctica.[42] The ozone layer above the United States has decreased by only 5–10 percent.

Effects of Ozone Layer Depletion and Increased UV Radiation For people, overexposure to UV rays can lead to skin cancer, cataracts (clouding of the lens of the eye), and weakened immune systems. Increased UV can also lead to reduced crop yield and reduced plant production in natural communities. The latter can result in less food for all the other species in the communities and disruption of the ocean's food chain.

Taking Action on Ozone Depletion In response to the well-documented links between certain air pollutants

10 percent of the electricity used by incandescent or halogen lights. As technologies improve, you may someday be able to contribute to the electricity needs of your home using photovoltaic roof coverings and solar or geothermal energy for heating and cooling. Government action will be required to support widespread technological and economic shifts toward energy conservation and reduction of greenhouse emissions. You could join and be active in environmental organizations that work to address global warming. When politicians see that their constituents want to protect our common global environment, they may find the political will to do the right thing.

TALKING POINTS How can you encourage your children to develop sound habits regarding their environment and their personal health? What changes can you make in your own habits to serve as a better example for them?

and depletion of the ozone layer, and links between UV radiation and adverse health and ecological effects, the world community has worked to eliminate the use of ozone-depleting chemicals. For example, a complete ban on the production of halons and CFCs went into effect in the mid-1990s. As the amounts of ozone-depleting chemicals in the atmosphere decrease, the ozone layer is projected to recover to natural levels by the year 2050.[42] However, there remain thousands of tons of CFCs in older refrigeration and air-conditioning systems, including those in older automobiles. You can contribute to reducing ozone-depleting chemicals in the atmosphere by always having your refrigerator and air-conditioning systems serviced by licensed technicians who have the equipment to capture and properly dispose of old CFC chemicals.

To limit your risk of skin cancer and other UV-related health problems that can be exacerbated by ozone layer depletion, you should limit your exposure to direct sunlight, and when you are outside you should wear sunscreen on exposed skin. You should also wear sunglasses that are rated as eliminating over 95 percent of UV radiation. When traveling to parts of North America, Europe, South Africa, South America, and Australia that are close to the polar ozone holes, you should be aware of UV index information presented by the popular media. During months when the polar ozone holes are larger, you may want to further restrict your exposure to direct sunlight.

TALKING POINTS Your sister is a sun worshipper who loves the look of a deep, dark tan. How might you persuade her to protect her skin from the rays of the sun?

Loss of Natural Habitats and Species Extinctions

Causes of Habitat Destruction and Species Extinctions On every continent, an exploding human population armed with ever more powerful technology is altering or completely taking over the habitats of other species that share our planet. Over 20 percent of the total land surface of Earth has been converted entirely for human uses, and as much as 40–50 percent has been degraded by human activities.[43] Humans currently use 50 percent of the Earth's fresh-water runoff, mostly for agricultural irrigation. Dams for electric power generation have impacted 94 percent of the rivers in the world.[44]

Human impact on the biosphere is not limited to the land. Humans consume 25–35 percent of the energy flow in coastal ocean waters.[43] As of 2003, 29 percent of all ocean fish populations exploited for human consumption had collapsed due to overharvesting. If current trends continue, all populations of ocean fish currently

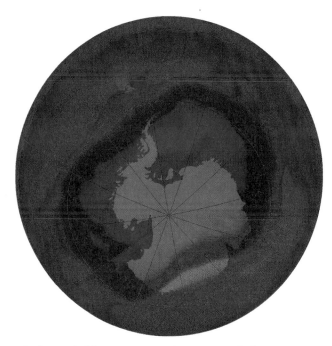

The "ozone hole" over Antartica in 2006 was the largest to date. The depleted ozone layer in the atmosphere is expected to recover, but the process is slow and will likely take until about 2050.

used for human food production will collapse by the year 2050.[45] Worldwide, 30 percent of all coral reefs have been destroyed by human activities. Coastal water pollution has been linked to increased frequency of fish kills and massive "dead zones" where nothing else can live.[44]

The cumulative effects of all these human-caused changes to the Earth's land and oceans have increased the species extinction rate by 100 to 1,000 times over rates estimated for the period before human domination. The primary causes of these extinctions are habitat loss due to human activities and overharvesting of species by humans.[44]

Personal Health Effects of Habitat Destruction and Species Extinctions The effects on personal health associated with worldwide loss of natural communities and species extinctions are highly variable from person to person. Pharmaceutical companies have found many substances produced by species in various natural communities to be useful sources of drugs to treat human illnesses. As the richness of species on Earth is depleted by extinction, we lose a wealth of genetic material that could be of great importance to human health. The degradation and loss of natural ecosystems also undermines the systems that function to make Earth a livable planet, contributing to such problems as global climate change, fresh water shortages, and increased frequency of destructive flooding.

Is Organic Food Good for the Environment?

Certified "organic" food in the United States is produced under guidelines set out by the Organic Foods Production Act. The guidelines in this law stipulate materials and practices that enhance the balance of natural systems and that integrate parts of the farming system into an ecological whole.

The primary goal of organic agriculture is to optimize the health and productivity of interdependent communities of soil life, plants, animals, and people. Organic farmers that produce grain, fruits, and vegetables may not use synthetic pesticides or fertilizers. Meat producers must feed their livestock only organically produced feedstuffs. In addition, many organic meat producers forgo the use of growth hormones and antibiotics that stimulate livestock growth rates. While organic foods have not been shown to be any more nutritious than non-organic food, organic foods have fewer chemical residues that may adversely impact human health.*

A recent study documented that when elementary school children were switched from a conventional diet to an organic food diet, pesticide residues in their urine dropped to nondetectable levels. As soon as the children were returned to a conventional diet, the concentration of pesticide residues in their urine increased again.[†]

The description of organic food above suggests that organic farming practices are good for the environment. Organic farming puts far less pollution into local water and air, and fewer chemicals into the food supply. Local farmers can often make greater profits through direct sales of organic produce to local cooperatives or other consumer-supported agriculture organizations. This may help to preserve local green space against encroachment by suburban developers. Hence, organic farming can certainly be good for the local community environment.

Whether or not organic farming is good for the global environment is an open question. While organic farms produce less pollution, they also produce less food per acre. Lower production per acre, higher labor costs, and the small number of organic farmers often make organic foods an expensive luxury for the well-to-do. Many environmentalists call for a widespread shift from chemical-dependent agriculture to more ecologically sustainable organic farming. However, it is doubtful that organic farming on existing agricultural lands could feed the current human population of 6 billion people. A worldwide shift to organic farming would likely require an expansion of agricultural lands into national parks, nature preserves, and wilderness areas. This loss of natural habitats would result in massive species extinctions.[‡] On the other hand, there is some uncertainty as to whether or not intensive, chemical-dependent agricultural systems will provide a sustainable food supply. Chemical fertilizers can replace lost nutrients but can't repair compacted soil nor replace eroded topsoil. Pesticides and herbicides can control pests and weeds now, but these species are already displaying signs of increased resistance that may prevent control in the future.

At the moment, your personal choices to buy organically grown, locally produced foods are probably most beneficial to your local environment and may benefit your personal health. It is much less clear whether or not a widespread shift to organic farming would be beneficial to the larger global environment.

*Cable News Network Interactive. *In-Depth: Organic Food.* 1998. www.cnn.com/HEALTH/indepth.food/organic/index.html.
[†]Lu C, et al., "Organic Diets Significantly Lower Children's Dietary Exposure to Organo-Phosphorous Pesticides," *Environmental Health Perspectives* 114 (2): 260–263. 2006.
[‡]Center for Global Food Issues. *Growing More Food per Acre Leaves More Land for Nature.* 2002. www.highyieldconservation.org.

Some have proposed that human evolution predisposes us to be most happy when we are surrounded by natural beauty; this is called the *Biophilia hypothesis.*[46] Many have written about the human psychological benefits from natural communities. John Muir, a famous early U.S. environmentalist wrote:

Climb the mountains and get their good tidings.
Nature's peace will flow into you as sunshine flows into
    trees.
The winds will blow their own freshness into you,
    and the storms their energy, while cares drop
    off like autumn leaves.

Wallace Stegner wrote a passage that appears in the Wilderness Act passed by the U.S. Congress in 1964 to protect areas of intact U.S. ecosystems for the enjoyment of future generations:

We simply need that wild country available to us, even if we never do more than drive to its edge and look in. For it can
be a means of reassuring ourselves of our sanity as creatures, a part of the geography of hope.

Both Muir and Stegner refer to the psychological benefits that humans derive simply from the knowledge that natural communities and wildlife species still exist somewhere on our planet. Try to imagine how you would feel about a world completely dominated and degraded by a massive human population; no great herds of caribou, zebra, and wildebeest moving like a tide across the landscape; no wolves, lions, tigers, or elephants to excite the imagination; no monarch butterflies sipping nectar in your backyard on their migration from Maine to Mexico; no dolphins and orcas playing in the ocean waves; no humpback whales singing in the depths; no coral reef wonderlands; no great, ancient trees stretching out of sight toward a clear blue sky; no expansive grasslands rippling in the breeze as far as the eye can see; the sky and waters tainted with pollution; the climate itself hostile to human civilization. The effects of such a dark and dismal world on the human psyche seem unimaginable. The thought of forever losing the natural wonders of our planet could have profoundly adverse effects on our emotional, psychological, and spiritual well-being. For many, the thought of such a dark future can cause anger, frustration, depression, hopelessness, and despair.[47]

Taking Action on Habitat Destruction and Species Extinction   How can you or any one person exert any degree of personal control over such a great and complex threat to your physical, emotional, and spiritual health? Start with the little things. Conserve energy, recycle and reuse, limit your consumption of resources to what you need, and join together with others to support organizations that are working to solve these big problems (see the listing in the box "Organizations Related to Environmental and Population Control Concerns"). If you want to make a bigger personal commitment to solving global environmental problems, you could limit your own family size to at most two children. For a list of many more ways to reduce your personal impact on the Earth, go to the website www.earthshare.org/get_involved/earth_saving_tips.html.

Another way you can reduce the negative environmental effects of your personal consumption of natural resources is to "buy green" when you can. In recent years, environmental organizations have begun certification programs so that the consumer can identify which products are produced by "Earth-friendly" means (for more information, see www.newdream.org/buy). Examples of such products include sustainably harvested timber, shade-grown coffee, and organic food and cotton (see the box "Is Organic Food Good for the Environment?"). These products are often more expensive, because they are produced by methods that lack the efficiency of environmentally destructive production systems. When you "buy green," you support Earth-friendly producers and reduce economic pressure to destroy natural communities. Many "buy-green" organizations also work to improve economic conditions in villages where their producers live. These efforts improve educational opportunities and health care, resulting in reduced birth rates, slowing the human population growth that is the root cause for many environmental problems.

The combined actions of 6 billion people making personal choices will determine the future of the Earth's environment and thus the future of humankind. The solutions to the great environmental problems looming in the future begin with you, today. Your positive actions and faith in fellow humans to do the right thing will not only benefit the future, but also enhance your emotional well-being in the present.

Taking Charge of Your Health

- All environmental problems and their associated health risks begin with personal choices regarding resource consumption, waste disposal, and electing leaders who set policies and regulations. When you make your choices, consider the environmental consequences and act in ways that promote a healthy environment for all people and other living things on Earth.

- Be aware of environmental hazards in the air, water, and materials in your personal environment and work to minimize or eliminate these hazards.

- Reduce your own consumption of natural resources, and dispose of wastes responsibly.

- Be aware of government policies regarding natural resource exploitation, pollution, and habitat destruction.

- Vote for leaders who are more concerned with the quality of the environment of all people and other species than they are for economic special interests.

- When that small voice inside you says, "Forget it, there is nothing I can do," don't listen! That voice is leading you toward a life of cynicism and despair. For your own psychological, emotional, and spiritual well-being, have faith that the actions of individuals can accumulate to bring about world change.*

*Ellison K. A question of faith. *Frontiers in Ecology and the Environment* 1(1): 56, 2003.

SUMMARY

- Environmental influences on personal health operate over a wide range of spatial scales, from the personal spaces of your home and workplace, to the common spaces of your community and region, to the global environment that supports all life on Earth.
- You can exert the greatest degree of control over your exposure to pollutants within the personal environment of your home and workplace. You can identify environmental health risks in your personal environment, and then eliminate or reduce these risks by changing your buying habits and eliminating pollutant sources.
- Air pollution in major urban areas can cause significant adverse health effects, especially for people who suffer from respiratory or cardiac disease.

- Much progress has been made in reducing community water pollution, but water and fish in many rivers and lakes still contains chemicals and pathogens that can adversely affect your health.
- Loss of green space in your community and regional environment, associated with urban sprawl and unregulated land development, can diminish your perceived quality of life, and reduce opportunities for exercise, which is important for maintaining good physical health.
- While you have limited personal control over the environment of your community and region, you can still work to enhance your environment by joining others of like mind in groups that advocate environmental protection through the democratic political process.
- At the current rate of human population growth, most scientists of the world warn of increased starvation and disease, decreased standards of living, and increased conflict over progressively decreasing supplies of natural resources.
- Pollutants produced by humans are responsible for changes in the atmosphere that are altering climate patterns and allowing harmful solar radiation to reach the surface of the Earth.
- Changes in the global environment have potential to increase risks to human health and to significantly harm many other species and natural communities.
- While individuals can do little to address global environmental problems, the solutions all start with individual choices about family size, resource consumption, and political candidates. The best path to a livable future for humankind is to do your part and have faith that others will do theirs.

REVIEW QUESTIONS

1. Identify the sources and the potential health effects of the following common indoor air pollutants: carbon monoxide, volatile organic compounds, and biological pollutants such as mold, mildew, pollen, and pet dander. Describe actions you could take to minimize health risks from these pollutants.
2. What health risks are associated with lead and asbestos? What actions can you take to minimize these risks?
3. Tropospheric ozone and small particulate matter are community and regional air pollutants that have been linked to serious health risks. For each of these substances, describe the main human sources, the effect(s) on human physical health, and what actions you could take to minimize your own risk of adverse health effects from these air pollutants.
4. What are "air toxics" and where do you think you are most likely to be exposed to these substances? What do you think you could do to minimize your personal health risk from air toxics?
5. What are some pollutants that might be in drinking water from a tap in your home? What are the main sources of these pollutants? What can you do to minimize the risk to your personal health from water pollutants?
6. What is "green space," and why is it important to your personal health? What personal actions could you take to protect green space in your community or region?
7. What policies should the U.S. foreign aid agencies implement in poor underdeveloped countries to help them reduce their population growth rate? Explain how these policies would work toward this goal.
8. Global warming and stratospheric ozone depletion are large-scale changes in the global environment with uncertain, but potentially significant, health consequences. For each of these global changes, describe the cause(s) of environmental change, the potential health effects, and what might be done to minimize these effects.
9. Loss of natural habitats and species extinctions are major ecological problems, but do these phenomena represent any risk to *your* personal health? Your answer should reflect your own perceptions and should provide some explanation for your assessment.
10. A well-known environmentalist slogan is "Think globally, but act locally." Based on what you've learned in this chapter, describe how you think this slogan applies to your personal actions in response to environmental health risks.

ANSWERS TO THE "WHAT DO YOU KNOW?" QUIZ

1. True   2. False   3. True   4. False   5. False   6. True   7. True

ENDNOTES

1. U.S. Environmental Protection Agency. *Health Buildings, Healthy People: A Vision for the 21st Century*. 2003. www.epa.gov/iaq/hbhp/index.html.
2. Consumer Product Safety Commission. *Carbon Monoxide Questions and Answers*. CPSC Document #466. 2003. www.cpsc.gov/cpscpub/pubs/466.html.
3. U.S. Environmental Protection Agency. *The Inside Story: A Guide to Indoor Air Quality*. 1995. www.epa.gov/iaq/pubs/insidest.html.
4. Thorn J, et al. Adult-onset asthma linked to mold and tobacco smoke exposure. *Allergy* 56: 287–292. 2001.
5. U.S. Environmental Protection Agency. *Sources of Indoors Air Pollution: Asbestos*. 2003. www.epa.gov/iaq/asbestos.html.
6. U.S. Environmental Protection Agency. 2003. *Sources of Indoor Air Pollution: Lead* (Pb). www.epa.gov/iaq/lead.html.
7. U.S. Department of Health and Human Services, Public Health Service, Agency for Toxic Substances and Disease Registry. *Case Studies in Environmental Medicine: Lead Toxicity*. 1995. www.atsdr.cdc.gov/HEC/CSEM/lead/.
8. U.S. Environmental Protection Agency. *Sources of Indoors Air Pollution: Biological Pollutants*. 2003. www.epa.gov/iaq/biologic.html.

9. National Safety Council. *Radon.* 2002. www.nsc.org/ehc/radon.htm.

10. National Academy of Science. *The Biological Effects of Ionizing Radiation (BEIR) VI Report: The Health Effects of Exposure to Indoor Radon.*1998. National Academy Press. books.nap.edu/books/0309056454/html/.

11. Schüz J, et al. Cellular telephone use and cancer: Update of a nationwide Danish cohort. *Journal of the National Cancer Institute* 98 (23): 1707–1713. 2006.

12. Hardell L, et al. Pooled analysis of two case-control studies on use of cellular and cordless telephones and the risk for malignant brain tumors diagnosed in 1997–2003. *International Archives of Occupational and Environmental Health* 79 (8): 630–639. 2006.

13. Ahlbom A, et al. Epidemiology of health effects of radiofrequency exposure. *Environmental Health Perspectives* 112 (17). 2004.

14. UK Childhood Cancer Study Investigators. Childhood cancer and residential proximity to power lines. *Brit J Cancer* 83: 1573–1580. 2000.

15. Savitz DA, Loomis DP. Magnetic field exposure in relation to leukemia and brain cancer mortality among electric utility workers. *American Journal of Epidemiology* 141 (2): 123–128. 1995.

16. Greenland S, et al. A pooled analysis of magnetic fields, wirecodes, and childhood leukemia. *Epidemiology* 11: 624–634. 2000.

17. U.S. Environmental Protection Agency. *Water on Tap: What You Need to Know.* 2003. www.epa.gov/safewater/wot/pdfs /book_waterontap_full.pdf.

18. U.S. Environmental Protection Agency. *Factsheet on: Nitrate/Nitrite.* 2002. www.epa.gov/safewater/dwh/t-ioc/nitrates.html.

19. U.S. Environmental Protection Agency. 2002. *Permeation and Leaching.* www.epa.gov/ogwdw/disinfection/tcr/pdfs/whitepaper_tcr_permation-leaching.pdf.

20. U.S. Centers for Disease Control and Prevention. *Second National Report on Human Exposure to Environmental Chemicals.* 2003. NCEH Pub No. 02-0716, National Center for Environmental Health, Atlanta.

21. Gray LE, Ostby J. Effects of pesticides and toxic substances on behavioral and morphological reproductive development: Endocrine versus non-endocrine mechanisms. *Toxicology and Industrial Health* 14: 159–184. 1998.

22. U.S. Environmental Protection Agency. *Endocrine Disrupting Chemicals Risk Management Research.* www.epa.gov/ord/NRMRL/EDC.

23. Adibi J, et al. Pre-natal exposures to phthalates among women in New York City and Krakow, Poland. *Environmental Health Perspectives* 111 (14): 1719–1722. 2003.

24. Landrigan P, Garg A, Droller D. Assessing the effects of endocrine disruptors in the National Children's Study. *Environmental Health Perspectives* 111 (13): 1678–1682. 2003.

25. Bell P. Noise, pollution, and psychopathology. In Ghadirian A, Lehmann H (eds.), *Environment and Psychopathology.* New York: Springer, 1993.

26. U.S. Environmental Protection Agency. *Draft Report on the Environment: Outdoor Air Quality.* 2003. www.epa.gov/indicators/roe/html/roeAirOut.htm.

27. Dockery D, Pope C III. Acute respiratory effects of particulate air pollution. *Annual Review Public Health* 15: 107–132. 1994.

28. Perera F, et al. Effects of transplacental exposure to environmental pollutants on birth outcomes in a multiethnic population. *Environmental Health Perspectives* 111 (2): 201–205. 2003

29. Perera F, et al. DNA damage from polycyclic aromatic hydrocarbons measured by Benzo[a] pyrene-DNA adducts in mothers and newborns from northern Manhattan, the World Trade Center area, Poland, and China. *Cancer, Epidemiology Biomarkers & Prevention* 14: 709–714. 2005.

30. National Institute of Environmental Health Sciences. *Children's Environmental Health: Asthma and Other Respiratory Diseases.* 2003. www.niehs.nih.gov/oc/factsheets/ceh/asthma.htm#ozone.

31. McConnell R, et al. Asthma in exercising children exposed to ozone. *Lancet* 359: 386–391. 2002.

32. U.S. Environmental Protection Agency. *The National Air Toxics Assessment.* 2002. www.epa.gov/ttn/atw/nata.

33. U.S. Environmental Protection Agency. 2003. *Drinking Water and Your Health, What You Need to Know, List of Drinking Water Contaminants & MCL's.* www.epa.gov/safewater/mcl.html#1.

34. U.S. Environmental Protection Agency. *Municipal Solid Waste: Basic Facts.* 2003. www.epa.gov/epaoswer/non-hw/muncpl/facts.htm.

35. Ewing R, et al. Relationship between urban sprawl and physical activity, obesity and morbidity. *American Journal of Health Promotion* 18 (1): 47–57. 2003.

36. Cohen D, et al. Public parks and physical activity among adolescent girls. *Pediatrics* 118 (5): 1381–1389. 2006.

37. Cohen D, et al. Proximity to school and physical activity among middle-school girls: The trial of activity for adolescent girls study. *Journal of Physical Activity and Health* 3 (suppl. 1): S129–S138. 2006.

38. The Population Institute. www.populationinstitute.org/.

39. Gasana J. Remember Rwanda? *World Watch* 15 (5): 24–33. 2002.

40. Intergovernmental Panel on Climate Change. *Climate Change 2007: The Physical Science Basis: Summary for Policy Makers.* 2007. www.ipcc.ch/SPM2feb07.pdf.

41. Petit JR, et al. Climate and atmospheric history of the past 420,000 years from the Vostok ice core, Antarctica. *Nature* 399: 429–436. 1999.

42. U.S. Environmental Protection Agency. The Science of Ozone Depletion. 2003. www.epa.gov/docs/ozone/science/index.html.

43. Vitousek P, et al. Human domination of Earth's ecosystems. *Science* 277: 494–499. 1997.

44. World Resources Institute. 2003. www.wri.org.

45. Worm B, et al. Impacts of biodiversity loss on ocean ecosystem services. *Science* 314: 787–790. 2006.

46. Wilson E. *Biophilia: The Human Bond with Other Species.* Cambridge, MA: Harvard University Press, 1984.

47. Gardner GT, Stern PC. *Environmental Problems and Human Behavior.* Needham Heights, MA: Allyn & Bacon, 1996.

Completing Life's Journey

This last part comprises a single chapter on a topic that inevitably affects each of us: dying and death. Traditional-age students may think that death will not touch their lives until they grow older. Yet many young people must face the reality of death much sooner, when a loved one is lost to an accident, a disease, suicide, or some other tragedy.

1. **Physical Dimension**

   Unless we die suddenly at a young age, most of us will enjoy years of good physical health before we begin a period of gradual decline. Eventually, we may experience an extended period of failing health before dying of a chronic condition, such as heart disease. However, many people today experience their highest level of physical health late in life. An adequate activity level, weight management, smoking cessation, and moderation of alcohol use can increase the likelihood that an older adult will be able to enjoy good physical health well into his or her later years.

2. **Psychological Dimension**

   The process of dying and death can be emotionally draining for both the dying person and his or her loved ones. The death of a spouse, close friend, or child, especially when it is unexpected, can be emotionally taxing. The grieving person may feel anger, sadness, regret, and a range of other complex emotions. Indeed, coping with death can be a great challenge to the emotional stability of even the healthiest person.

3. **Social Dimension**

   The dying process and the event of a loved one's death offer opportunities for reaching out to others. In fact, many people who have had these experiences report that having a social support system was essential to maintaining their emotional balance during the ordeal. The families of people who are dying must also deal effectively with health care professionals, funeral directors, and estate executors.

4. **Intellectual Dimension**

   As in any other crisis, a strong intellect is a valuable resource during the dying and death process. Complex decisions about treatment options must be made. Loved ones may be left to sort out the finances of a family member who has died. These difficult situations require an ability to analyze many variables in order to make sound choices.

5. **Spiritual Dimension**

   Confronting the reality of death requires drawing on spiritual resources. Those who have a strong religious faith may find comfort in their beliefs, while others may find that their faith is shaken by the experience. Those who are not religious may look for other ways to find meaning in the event.

6. **Occupational Dimension**

   The dying process often unfolds slowly. A person who is terminally ill may have to continue working for months or even years before he or she becomes so ill that work is no longer possible. Clearly, such an illness can make work difficult. However, some people find that their job provides a welcome diversion as well as a social support network.

part seven

Accepting Dying and Death

What Do You Know about Dying and Death?

◉ Signing a donor card or the organ-donor option on your driver's license ensures that your organs will be donated when you die. True or False?

◉ Death is defined as a state when one's heartbeat can no longer be detected and breathing has ceased. True or False?

◉ There is only one state in the United States where physician-assisted suicide is legal. True or False?

◉ It is advisable to bring children to funerals to help them better understand and accept death. True or False?

◉ Hospice care is provided primarily in the patient's home. True or False?

◉ The average cost for a funeral service is around $6,500. True or False?

◉ Only 25 percent of people choose cremation for disposal of their bodies. True or False?

Check your answers at the end of the chapter.

Online Learning Center Resources
www.mhhe.com/payne10e

Visit the Online Learning Center for tools to improve your grade and get the most out of your course—chapter objectives, practice quizzes, key terms flashcards, chapter summaries for your digital audio player, Web activities, self-assessments, and many other study aids.

The Experience of Dying

The primary goal of this chapter is to help people realize that accepting the reality of death can motivate us to live a more enjoyable, healthy, productive, and contributive life. Each day in our lives becomes even more meaningful when we have fully accepted the reality that someday we will die. We can then live each day to its fullest.

Our personal awareness of death can give us a framework from which to appreciate and conduct our lives. It helps us to prioritize our activities so that we can accomplish our goals (in our work, our relationships with others, and our recreation) before we die. Quite simply, death can help us to appreciate living.

Dying in Today's Society

Since the 1920s, the way people experience death in this society has changed. Formerly, most people died in their own homes, surrounded by family and friends. Young children frequently lived in the same home with their aging grandparents and saw them grow older and eventually die. Death was seen as a natural extension of life. Children grew up with a keen sense of what death meant, both to the dying person and to the grieving survivors.

Times have indeed changed. Today about 80 percent of people die in hospitals, nursing homes, and assisted living facilities, rather than in their own homes. The extended family is seldom at the bedside of the dying person.[1] Sometimes, frantic efforts are made to keep a dying person alive. Although medical technology has improved our lives, some people believe that it has reduced our ability to die with dignity. Some are convinced that our way of dying has become more artificial and less natural than it used to be. The trend toward hospice care may be a positive response to this high-tech manner of dying.

Many families are forced to deal with death unexpectedly when a loved one dies in an accident or by violence. The emotions they feel are somewhat different from the ones normally evoked when a friend or relative dies of a disease or failing health in old age.

As the baby boomers age over the next 30 years, the number of people age 85 and older will more than double, to 9 million. This means that the topic of death and dying will become increasingly common and relevant for us all as we cope with the loss of our parents, grandparents, friends, and other family members.

Definitions of Death

Death was once easy to define. People were considered dead when a heartbeat could no longer be detected and when breathing ceased. Now, with the technological advances in medicine, especially emergency medicine, some patients who give every indication of being dead can be resuscitated. Critically ill people, even those in comas, can now be kept alive for years with many of their bodily functions maintained by medical devices, including feeding tubes and respirators.

Thus death can be a very challenging concept to define.[2] Many professional associations and ad hoc interdisciplinary committees have struggled with this problem and have developed criteria by which to establish death. The Uniform Determination of Death Act of 1981 is adhered to by most states in defining death. It states, "An individual who has sustained either (1) irreversible cessation of circulatory and respiratory functions, or (2) irreversible cessation of all functions of the entire brain, including the brain stem, is dead."[3]

Clinical determinants of death measure bodily functions. Often judged by a physician, who can then sign a legal document called a *medical death certificate,* these clinical criteria include the following:

1. Lack of heartbeat and breathing.
2. Lack of central nervous system function, including all reflex activity and environmental responsiveness. This can often be confirmed by an *electroencephalograph* reading. If no brain wave activity is recorded after an initial measurement and a second measurement after 24 hours, the person is said to have undergone *brain death.*
3. The presence of *rigor mortis,* indicating that body tissues and organs are no longer functioning at the cellular level. This is sometimes called *cellular death.*

The legal determinants used by government officials are established by state law. A person is not legally dead until a physician, *coroner,* or health department officer has signed a death certificate. However, some argue that death should be defined as occurring when there is an irreparable lack of consciousness or loss of the structures that support thinking even if the brain stem is still functioning. This would allow faster harvesting of donor organs, such as hearts for transplant patients.

Psychological States of Dying

People who have a terminal illness undergo a process of self-adjustment (see the box "Challenging Death"). The stages in this process have helped form the basis for the modern movement of death education. Knowing these stages may help you understand how people adjust to other important losses in their lives.

Perhaps the most widely recognized name in the area of death education is Dr. Elisabeth Kübler-Ross. As a psychiatrist working closely with terminally ill patients at the University of Chicago's Billings Hospital, Kübler-Ross could observe the emotional reactions of dying people. In her classic book *On Death and Dying,* Kübler-Ross summarized the psychological stages that dying people often experience.[4]

- *Denial.* This is the stage of disbelief. Patients refuse to believe that they actually will die. Denial can serve as a temporary defense mechanism and can allow patients the time to accept their prognosis on their own terms.

- *Anger.* A common emotional reaction after denial is anger. Patients can feel as if they have been cheated. By expressing anger, patients can vent some of their fears, jealousies, anxieties, and frustrations. Patients often direct their anger at relatives, physicians and nurses, religious symbols, figures, and healthy people.

- *Bargaining.* Terminally ill people follow the anger stage with a bargaining stage. In an effort to avoid their inevitable death, they attempt to strike

Challenging Death: Unconventional Measures

People who learn that they have a terminal illness sometimes take unconventional measures in an attempt to avoid death. For example, they may travel to a foreign country to undergo a treatment regimen that is not approved in the United States, participate in a research study that is testing experimental drugs or treatment protocols, use alternative or complementary therapies, or use unproven, potentially dangerous, unorthodox treatments.

People who are confronted with a "death sentence" diagnosis might take an entirely new look at unconventional approaches. For terminally ill cancer patients, the *possibility* that shark cartilage capsules might cure their cancer gives them hope. The belief that driving to Mexico to obtain laetrile (found in the pits of apricots and peaches and touted to cure cancer) *gives some people hope,* despite the fact that in the early 1980s the National Cancer Institute reported that laetrile treatments were ineffective.

Some terminally ill patients turn to hands-on approaches to healing because they are put off by the hands-off, hurry-up approach of traditional biomedicine. They would rather deal with a practitioner who touches them with therapies (such as acupressure, acupuncture, therapeutic massage, or chiropractic) and patiently takes the time to listen to their concerns.

Other patients facing a terminal illness may choose to enroll in a research study involving the testing of experimental drugs or treatments. They are often referred to these studies by their primary care physicians. The research studies usually take place at major medical centers, universities, or training hospitals in metropolitan areas. Patients typically are cared for by a team of physicians, and their drugs and their hospital care are provided free of charge. However, candidates first must be deemed "suitable" for the treatment protocols. Determining factors may include how long they have had the condition, their age, what drugs or therapies they have already used, and their general health status. There is great joy—for the ill person, his or her family, and the team of researchers and physicians—when a person responds well to the treatment, and such good news offers encouragement to others who are facing death from a similar illness.

Perhaps the most unusual approach to confronting death is the use of cryonics. This is the unproven technology of freezing dead bodies (or parts of bodies, typically the head) in liquid nitrogen in the hope that a cure for the disease will be found in the future. This pseudoscience is so fraught with technical problems that most scientists believe it will never work successfully. Yet, several hundred people have consented to have their bodies frozen in an attempt to "cheat death."

How do you think you would react to receiving the diagnosis of a terminal illness? Would you consider any of the approaches described here?

---

bargains—often with God or a church leader. Some people undergo religious conversions. The goal is to buy time by promising to repent for past sins, to restructure and rededicate their lives, or to make a large financial contribution to a religious cause.

- *Depression.* When patients realize that, at best, bargaining can only postpone their fate, they may begin an unpredictable period of depression. In a sense, terminally ill people are grieving for their own anticipated death. They may become quite withdrawn and refuse to visit with close relatives and friends. Prolonged periods of silence or crying are normal components of this stage and should not be discouraged.

- *Acceptance.* During the acceptance stage, patients fully realize that they will die. Acceptance ensures a relative sense of peace for most dying people. Anger, resentment, and depression are usually gone. Kübler-Ross describes this stage as one without much feeling. Patients feel neither happy nor sad. Many are calm and introspective and prefer to be left either alone or with a few close relatives or friends.

The psychological stages of dying include two more important points. Just as each person's life is totally unique, so is each person's death. Unfolding deaths vary as much as do unfolding lives. Some people move through Kübler-Ross's stages of dying very predictably, but others do not. It is not uncommon for some dying people to avoid one or more of these stages entirely or to revisit a stage more than once.

The second important point about Kübler-Ross's stages of dying is that the family members or friends of dying people often pass through similar stages as they observe their loved ones dying. When informed that a close friend or relative is dying, many people also experience varying degrees of denial, anger, bargaining, depression, and acceptance. Because of this, as caring people we need to recognize that the emotional needs of the living must be fulfilled in ways that do not differ appreciably from those of the dying.[5]

Near-Death Experiences

Death ends our physical existence. Perhaps this is the ultimate connection between death and our physical dimension of health. Many people believe that, in a positive sense, death brings a sense of relief and comfort—two qualities one may need most when one is dying. The classic work of Raymond Moody,[6] who examined reports of people who had near-death experiences, suggests that we may have less to fear about dying than we have generally thought.

In a comprehensive study of more than 100 people who had near-death experiences, Kenneth Ring[7] reported that these people shared a core experience. This experience was composed of some or all of the following stages:

1. Acknowledgement of the person's death
2. An out-of-body experience in which the dying person floats above his or her body and witnesses the activities that are occurring
3. A movement into extreme blackness or darkness
4. Encountering loved ones who have died
5. A shaft of intense light that generally leads upward or lies in the distance
6. A sense of well-being and peace
7. A decision whether to enter into the light
8. Return to the body

Central to this experience is the need to decide whether to move toward death or to return to the body that has been temporarily vacated.

Experts do not agree whether near-death experiences are truly associated with death or more closely associated with the depersonalization that some people experience during particularly frightening situations. In a scientific sense, near-death experiences are impossible to prove. Science can neither verify nor deny the existence of out-of-body experiences.[1]

Regardless, for those who have had near-death experiences, simply knowing that death might not be such an unpleasant experience appears to be comforting. Most seem to have formed a more positive orientation toward living.[1]

Interacting with Dying People

Facing the impending death of a friend, relative, or loved one is a difficult experience. If you have yet to go through this situation, be assured that, as you grow older, your opportunities will increase. This is part of the reality of living.

Most counselors, physicians, nurses, and ministers who spend time with terminally ill people suggest that you display one quality when interacting with dying people: honesty. Just the thought of talking with a dying person may make you feel uncomfortable, especially if you have not had this experience before. Sometimes, to make ourselves feel less anxious or depressed, we may tend to deny that the person we are with is dying. Our words and nonverbal behavior reveal that we prefer not to face the truth. Our words become stilted as we gloss over the facts and merely attempt to cheer up both our dying friend and ourselves. This behavior is rarely beneficial or supportive—for either party.

As much as possible, we should attempt to be genuine and honest. We should not try to avoid crying if we feel the need to cry. At the same time, we can give dying people emotional support by allowing them to express

Talking honestly, answering questions, and providing support can help a child cope with loss.

their feelings openly. We should resist the temptation to try to pull someone out of the denial, anger, or depression. We should not feel obliged to talk constantly and to fill long pauses with idle talk. Sometimes nonverbal communication, including touching, may be much more appreciated than mere talk. Because our interactions with dying people help fulfill our needs, we too should express our emotions and concerns as openly as possible.

Talking with Children about Death

Because most children are curious about everything, we should not be surprised that they are also fascinated about death. From very young ages, children are exposed to death through mass media, adult conversations ("Aunt Emily died today," "Uncle George is very ill"), and their discoveries (a dead bird, a crushed bug, the death of a pet). The way children learn about death greatly affects their ability to recognize and accept their own mortality and to cope with the deaths of others.

Psychologists encourage parents and older friends to avoid shielding children from or misleading children about the reality of death. Young children need to realize that death is not temporary and is not like sleeping. Parents should make certain they understand children's questions about death before they give an answer. Most children want simple, direct answers to their questions, not long, detailed dissertations, which often confuse the issues. For example, when a 4-year-old asks her father, "Why is Tommy's dog dead?" an appropriate answer might be, "Because he got very, very sick and his heart stopped beating." Getting involved in a long discussion about "doggy heaven" or the causes of specific canine diseases may not be necessary or appropriate.

When a child suffers the loss of a near relative, inform-ing the child is a painful task. Adults are usually present when a near relative dies, but children in Western societies are unlikely to be present at the time of death. In the death of a parent, the surviving parent usually must tell the child. The surviving parent sometimes tells the child the news much later, and often in a misleading form.

Two crucial pieces of information that help children to cope with death are knowing that the person will never come back and that the body has been buried or burned to ashes.[8] It is for these reasons that it is recommended that children be brought to funerals, so that they can better understand and accept death. Children's fantasies about death and burial can be more frightening to them than reality, especially if they are not told the truth about death. For example, a common tendency is to tell young children that the deceased has "gone to sleep." Since children tend to take things literally, they may develop a fear of going to sleep themselves, since they now associate sleeping with dying. Seeing the dead body at the funeral can dispel these myths.

People often hide their feelings of loss in an effort to be strong and protect children from emotional pain. However, it is good role modeling for children to see how adults mourn and grieve the loss of a loved one and that mourning assists with normalizing this part of the life cycle.

By telling children about the death of a loved one, using language that is age-appropriate, straightforward, and honest, you can help them to begin to learn that death is not something to be feared but something to be accepted. Sharing feelings, answering questions truthfully without too much detail, and giving him or her sympathy and support to cope with losses is the best gift you can give to a grieving child.

End-of-Life Options and Decisions

Many decisions related to dying and death can be anticipated and discussed with family members. Areas to consider include the type of care you'd like at the end of your life and whether you plan to donate organs.

Hospice Care for the Terminally Ill

The thought of dying in a hospital ward, with institutional furniture, medical equipment, and strict visiting hours, leaves many people with a cold feeling. Perhaps this thought alone has helped encourage the concept of **hospice care.** Hospice care is an alternative approach to dying for terminally ill patients and their families. The goal of hospice care is to maximize the quality of life of dying people and their family members. Popularized in England during the 1960s, yet derived from a concept developed during the Middle Ages (where hospitable lodges took care of weary travelers), the hospice helps people die comfortably and with dignity by using one or more of the following strategies:

- *Pain control.* Dying people usually are not treated for their terminal disease; they are given appropriate drugs to keep them free from pain, alert, and in control of their faculties. Drug dependence is of little concern, and patients can receive pain medication when they feel they need it.

- *Family involvement.* Family members and friends are trained and encouraged to interact with the dying person and with each other. Family members often care for the dying person at home. If the hospice arrangement includes a hospice ward in a hospital or a separate building (also called a hospice), the family members have no restrictions on visitation.

- *Multidisciplinary approach.* The hospice concept promotes a team approach.[9] Specially trained physicians, nurses, social workers, counselors, and volunteers work with the patient and family to fulfill important needs. The needs of the family receive nearly the same priority as those of the patient.

- *Patient decisions.* Contrary to most hospital approaches, hospice programs encourage patients to make their own decisions. The patient decides when to eat, sleep, go for a walk, and just be alone. By maintaining a personal schedule, the patient is more apt to feel in control of his or her life, even as that life is slipping away.

Another way the hospice differs from the hospital approach is in the care given to the survivors. Even after the death of the patient, the family receives a significant amount of follow-up counseling. Helping families with their grief is an important role of the hospice team.

The number of hospices in the United States has climbed quickly to more than 4,100. According to the National Hospice and Palliative Care Organization, hospices served at least 1.2 million patients in 2005.[10] People seem to be convinced that the hospice system does work effectively. Part of this approval may be the cost factor. The cost of caring for a dying person in a hospice is usually less than the cost of full (inpatient) services provided by a hospital. Although insurance companies are delighted to see the lower cost of hospice care, many are still uncertain how to define hospice care. Thus not all insurance companies are fully reimbursing patients for their hospice care. Before you discuss the possibility of hospice care for members of your family, you may want to consider the extent of hospice coverage in your health insurance policy.

Euthanasia and Physician-Assisted Suicide

There are two types of euthanasia: **indirect (passive) euthanasia** and **direct (active) euthanasia.**

Indirect Euthanasia Indirect euthanasia is when people are allowed to die without being subjected to life-sustaining efforts such as being placed on life support. Examples of indirect euthanasia include physicians' orders of "do not resuscitate" (DNR) and "comfort measures only" (CMO).

Indirect euthanasia is increasingly occurring in a number of hospitals, nursing homes, and medical centers. Physicians who withhold lifesaving techniques or drug therapy treatments or who disconnect life-support systems from terminally ill patients are practicing indirect euthanasia. Although some people still consider this form of euthanasia a type of murder, indirect euthanasia seems to be gaining legal and public acceptance for people with certain terminal illnesses—near-death cancer patients, brain-dead accident victims, and hopelessly ill newborn babies.

Direct Euthanasia Direct euthanasia is when people are intentionally put to death. It is usually performed through the administration of large amounts of depressant drugs, which eventually causes all central nervous system functioning to stop. Although direct euthanasia is commonly practiced on house pets and laboratory animals, it is illegal for humans in the United States, Canada, and other developed countries. There have been accusations that medical personnel performed euthanasia on hospital patients who could not be given adequate treatment during Hurricane Katrina. There are documented cases of patients receiving seemingly lethal doses of morphine—some argue it was a palliative measure to alleviate pain, while others cry "murder." There is an ongoing investigation into the cause of patient deaths during this time to determine if these were indeed mercy killings. However, in 1992, the Netherlands became the first country to enact legislation that permits euthanasia under strict guidelines. Belgium and Switzerland have enacted similar laws.

Physician-Assisted Suicide In recent years, physician-assisted suicide has been the focus of some important news stories. In July 1997, the U.S. Supreme Court unanimously ruled that dying people have no fundamental constitutional right to physician-assisted suicide. In effect, this ruling left the decision to individual states to permit or prohibit physician-assisted suicide.

More than 30 states have enacted laws prohibiting assisted suicide, and many other states have essentially prohibited it through common law. Only the state of Oregon has passed a law, in 1994, that legalized assisted suicide, referred to as the Death with Dignity Act. This act allows doctors to prescribe fatal doses of barbiturates and other drugs to adults of sound mind who have less than 6 months to live. It requires the patient to be at least 18 years of age and of sound mind, make two oral and one written request for the medication with 15 days between the first request and the final one, consult with two physicians, and notify pharmacists and state health authorities before proceeding with physician-assisted suicide. A fatal drug is prescribed, and the patient may ingest it orally at his or her discretion, with or without the doctor present. It remains illegal for physicians to administer lethal injections. To date, there have been over 200 legal physician-assisted suicides in Oregon.

Even though physician-assisted suicide is legal in the state of Oregon, many physicians are unwilling to prescribe the lethal medication. Being confined to their bed or home, living a long way from a large urban area, experiencing difficulty finding a willing physician, dying before completing the requirements of the law, and encountering opposition from family and friends are some of the reasons why greater numbers of terminally ill patients are not obtaining medication to end their lives.

A second news story concerned the April 1999 Michigan conviction of Dr. Jack Kevorkian, a retired pathologist who has aided in the suicides of over 100 people. Kevorkian was convicted of second-degree murder and delivery of a controlled substance in the assisted suicide of Thomas Youk, a 52-year-old patient with Lou Gehrig's disease. This suicide had been televised on the CBS show *60 Minutes.* Kevorkian was sentenced to 10–25 years in prison and was paroled in 2007, contingent on his promise that he would not assist in any more suicides.[11]

Advance Health Care Directives

Because some physicians and families have difficulty supporting indirect euthanasia, many people are starting to use legal documents called *advance health care directives.*[12] One of these health care directives is the **living will** (Figure 21-1). This is a document that confirms a dying person's desire to be allowed to die

---

> **Key Terms**
>
> **hospice care** (**hos** pis) An approach to caring for terminally ill patients that maximizes the quality of life and allows death with dignity.
>
> **indirect (passive) euthanasia** Allowing people to die without the use of life-sustaining procedures.
>
> **direct (active) euthanasia** Intentionally causing death.
>
> **living will** A legal document that requires physicians or family members to carry out a person's wishes to die naturally, without receiving life-sustaining treatments.

Figure 21-1 Sample Living Will   Living wills and other advance directives must conform to specific state laws. To obtain a copy of the living will for your state, visit the website for the National Hospice and Palliative Care Organization (www.caringinfo.org).

Source: Copyright © 2007 National and Palliative Care Organization. All rights reserved. Reproduction and distribution by an organization or organized group without the written permission of the National Hospice and Palliative Care Organization is expressly forbidden.

peacefully and with a measure of dignity if a time should arise when little hope exists for recovery from a terminal illness or severe injury. All 50 states and the District of Columbia have living will statutes. The living will requires that physicians or family members carry out a person's wishes to die naturally, without receiving life-sustaining treatments.[12] About one-third of U.S. citizens have signed living wills. The Terri Schiavo case has drawn increased attention to health care advance directives, because she neither had a living will nor did she designate a health care agent; see the box "The Controversy Surrounding the Death of Terri Schiavo" for more information.

A second important document that can assist terminally ill or incapacitated patients is the **durable power of attorney for health care.** This legal document authorizes another person (sometimes called a *health care agent* or *proxy*) to make specific health care decisions about treatment and care under specified circumstances, such as when patients are in vegetative states and cannot communicate their medical wishes. This document helps tell hospitals and physicians which person will help make the critical medical decisions. You can complete both a living will and a durable power of attorney for health care document.

Organ Donation

For some, the decision to donate body tissue and organs is rewarding and comforting. Organ donors understand that their sacrifice can help give life or improve the qual-

---

Key Terms

durable power of attorney for health care A legal document that designates who will make health care decisions for people unable to do so.

Terri Schiavo's death became a legal battle, media event, religious debate, and was even brought into the political spotlight. She was 26 years old when she had heart failure because of a chemical imbalance that may have been caused by an eating disorder. This left her severely brain damaged for 15 years. While she was in hospice care in a vegetative state, her husband and her parents were in a legal battle over whether to remove the feeding tube that was keeping her alive. If she had had a living will, this would have helped to make her wishes more clear, but it may not have precluded the legal debate. Advance directives such as living wills and durable powers of attorney for health care are legal documents that communicate the person's wishes about being kept alive with life support should they become incapacitated.

Both Terri Schiavo's husband and her parents claimed to know her end-of-life wishes, but none of them was named as her health care agent or proxy, giving a specific person the legal right to make this determination. Michael, her husband, stated that she had made casual comments about not wanting to be on life support if she were ever incapacitated. She had further stated to him that she didn't ever want to be a burden to him or her family. Her parents countered by saying that she was a devout Roman Catholic who believed in the sanctity of life.

The tug of war that ensued between her family members, as well as the publicity surrounding her dying wishes, spurred thousands of people to consider completing living wills. In fact, the Aging with Dignity organization estimated that requests for advance directives increased 10-fold because of the Schiavo case. They further reported that they have distributed over 1 million copies of living wills since this case, and orders for more living wills continue to flood in at a rate of 200 an hour.

Bitter legal battles continued for 12 years between these families. The case was brought to the U.S. Supreme court six times and refused each time. The judges stated that any action on their part would be improper. There was a great deal of public outcry, with some referring to her death as "judicial homicide."

Terri Schiavo remained in hospice care for 5 years before she died. Because she didn't preplan her funeral, there was continued acrimony and disagreement concerning the disposition of her body. Her husband stated that Terri had expressed her wish to be cremated, but her parents asserted that because of her Roman Catholic faith, she would not have wanted cremation and would have wanted to be buried. Michael Schiavo had her cremated and her ashes buried at an undisclosed location so that her parents, her brother, and the media wouldn't create a disturbance.

This young woman's death brought to the forefront many important issues that we all must face regarding death and dying. Should your family keep you alive with life support, and if so, for how long? Who should make these decisions? Do we have a legal right to die? Should the courts decide our fate? Having a living will, health care agent, hospice care, and preplanned funeral arrangements could clarify your wishes and possibly preclude a court battle.

Sources: Life and death tug of war: The whole Terri Schiavo story. *World Net Daily*, March 24, 2005; Terri Schiavo dies in Florida hospice. *Fox News*, March 31, 2005; Terri Schiavo has died. *CNN.com*, March 31, 2005; Terri Schiavo dies, but battle continues. *U.S. News*, March 31, 2005.

---

ity of life for another person. In this sense, their death can mean life for others.

Certain states permit people to state on their driver's license that they wish to donate their organs. However, family consent (by next of kin) is also required at the time of death for organ or tissue donation to proceed. Recently, hospitals have been required by federal law to inform the family of a deceased person about organ donation at the time of death. Thus, those who wish to donate organs at the time of death should discuss these wishes with their family as soon as possible so that family members will support the donation after the individual has died.

The issue of major organ donation today is the shortage of donors—the need for organs is much greater than our current supply.[13] Other critical issues, including interagency cooperation and screening procedures for donated organs, have largely been resolved (see the box "Organ Donation: Fact or Fiction?"). The scarcity of suitable organs is a life-threatening issue for over 100,000 persons on waiting lists for transplant organs (Table 21.1). Demand for organs has risen considerably since 1990, but the number of donors has remained fairly stable. Currently, 77 people receive organ transplants each day; another 110 people join a waiting list every day—one person every 13 minutes. In 2006 nearly 7,000 people—19 per day—died waiting for an organ transplant.[14]

The death in 1999 of NFL Hall of Fame football star Walter Payton highlighted the need for organ donation in the United States. Payton died while on the waiting list for a liver transplant. Although he was a celebrity, Payton did not ask for special treatment, such as being put at the top of the waiting list. He faced his death with dignity and poise, and served as a beacon to help call for increased organ donation. You can fulfill Payton's dream and the dream of others by planning for your own organ donation and encouraging your friends and family to follow your example. See the box "Planning an Organ Donation" for information on completing an organ donor card.

Grief and Coping

The emotional feelings that people experience after the death of a friend or relative are collectively called *grief*. *Mourning* is the process of experiencing these emotional feelings in a culturally defined manner. (See the box "The Grieving Process" on page 602 for more information.)

Organ Donation: Fact or Fiction?

From people not really being dead when their organs are harvested, to medical personnel not doing all that they can to save people's lives in order to obtain more organ donors, there are many myths surrounding organ donation. Perhaps this is one of the biggest reasons the need for donated organs far surpasses the number of available organs. Here are some common myths and facts about organ donation.

If I donate my organs, then . . .

Myth #1 The medical staff will remove my organs as soon as possible to save somebody else, instead of working hard to save my life.

Reality When you go to the hospital for treatment, the doctor in charge of your care has nothing to do with organ donations, as this procedure is performed by a physician specializing in transplants. You will be treated by a physician whose sole focus is saving your life.

Myth #2 The medical staff might take my organs before I am actually dead, and I might have survived had they not done so.

Reality People who have agreed to organ donation are actually given more tests to determine that they are truly dead than are those who haven't agreed to organ donation, to ensure that organs are not taken from a living person.

Myth #3 My family will be charged thousands of dollars for the medical expenses related to my organ donation.

Reality The cost of organ removal is the responsibility of the transplant recipient. The organ donor's family is never charged for donating. Charges incurred for lifesaving efforts are sometimes misinterpreted as costs related to organ donation. Funeral expenses are not covered by the transplant recipient.

Myth #4 I wouldn't be able to have an open-casket funeral.

Reality Organ donation doesn't interfere with having an open-casket funeral. If organs are taken, the body is stitched up as if the person were alive and had undergone surgery. The body is clothed for burial, and the stitches aren't visible. Great care is taken to ensure that the body is treated with respect and dignity in preparation for funeral services. For example, with skin donation, a very thin layer of skin

is taken from the donor's back; because the donor is clothed and lying on his or her back in the casket, no one can see any difference. For eye donation, an artificial eye is inserted and the eyelids are closed. For bone donation, a rod is inserted where bone is removed. The body is stitched up and clothed.

Myth #5 No one would want my organs because I am not in the best of health—my organs would be thrown away.

Reality The decision to use an organ is based on strict medical criteria. Some organs may not be suitable for transplant, but other organs may be fine. Organs are never thrown away.

Myth #6 I would be violating my religious beliefs.

Reality Typically, organ donation is consistent with the beliefs of Catholicism, Protestantism, and most branches of Judaism. You might want to talk to a leader of your religious organization to get a better understanding of your religion's position on organ donation.

Myth #7 My family cannot stop me from donating my organs as long as I have signed a donor card or my driver's license indicating these are my wishes.

Reality Signing a donor card or indicating your wish to donate on your driver's license doesn't guarantee that your organs will be donated. Your family or medical personnel can prevent an organ donation from occurring. To ensure that your wishes are carried out, you need to inform your family and doctor of your intent and perhaps even assign a durable power of attorney to someone who will abide by your wishes.

It is hoped that knowing the real facts will ease people's minds about the process and enable them to make well-informed choices about organ donation and perhaps save another person's life.

Source: Adapted from MayoClinic.com. Organ Donation: Don't let myths stand in your way. April 3, 2006.

Grief and the Resolution of Grief

The expression of grief is seen as a valuable process that gradually permits people to accept the loss of the deceased. Expressing grief, then, is a sign of good health. Although people experience grief in remarkably different ways, most people have some of the following sensations and emotions:

- *Physical discomfort.* Shortly after the death of a loved one, grieving people display a similar pattern of physical discomfort. This discomfort is characterized by "sensations of somatic distress occurring in waves lasting from 20 minutes to an hour at a time, a feeling of tightness in the throat, choking with shortness of breath, need for sighing, and an empty feeling in the abdomen, lack of muscular power, and an intense subjective distress described as a tension or mental pain. The person soon learns that these waves of discomfort can be precipitated by visits, by mentioning the deceased, and by receiving sympathy."[4]

- *Sense of numbness.* Grieving people may feel as if they are numb or in a state of shock. They may deny the death of their loved one.

- *Feelings of detachment from others.* Grieving people see other people as being distant from them, perhaps because the others cannot feel the loss. A person in grief can feel very lonely. This is a common response.

Type of Transplant	Patients Waiting for Transplant
Kidney transplant	74,066
Liver transplant	17,471
Pancreas transplant	1,767
Intestine transplant	235
Heart transplant	2,844
Heart-lung transplant	133
Lung transplant	2,841
Total	*Total Patients: 101,794

*Some patients are waiting for more than one organ, therefore the total number of patients is less than the sum of patients waiting for each organ.

Note: UNOS policies allow patients to be listed with more than one transplant center (multiple-listing), thus the number of registrations is greater than the actual number of patients. Waiting lists are updated weekly at www.unos.org/data.

- *Preoccupation with the image of the deceased.* The grieving person may not be able to complete daily tasks without constantly thinking about the deceased.

- *Guilt.* The survivor may be overwhelmed with guilt. Thoughts may center on how the deceased was neglected or ignored. Sensitive survivors feel guilt merely because they are still alive. Indeed, guilt is a common emotion.

- *Hostility.* Survivors may express feelings of loss and remorse through hostility, which they direct at other family members, physicians, lawyers, and others. Sometimes survivors may feel anger at the deceased person, perhaps at the suddenness of the death, at leaving the survivor to deal with problems, or at abandoning the survivor. Such a feeling may cause the survivor to feel guilty and ashamed. Survivors should know that such hostility can be a normal part of grieving.

- *Disruption in daily schedule.* Grieving people often find it difficult to complete daily routines. They can suffer from an anxious type of depression. Seemingly easy tasks take a great deal of effort. Starting new activities and relationships can be difficult. Social interaction skills can be temporarily lost.

- *Delayed grief.* In some people, the typical pattern of grief can be delayed for weeks, months, and even years.

The grief process continues until the bereaved person can establish new relationships, feel comfortable with others, and look back on the life of the deceased person with positive feelings (see the box "Helping the Bereaved" on page 603). Although the duration of the

Changing for the Better

Planning an Organ Donation

I've thought about organ donation for a long time, and now I am ready. What steps do I need to take to do this?

Donating organs is one of the most compassionate, responsible acts a person can perform. Only a few simple steps are required:

1. You must complete a donor card. You can request a free national donor card online from ask.hrsa.gov/detail or obtain a card from a physician, hospital, or regional transplant or organ bank.

Organ/Tissue Donor Card

I wish to donate my organs and tissues. I wish to give:
- [ ] any needed organs and tissues
- [ ] only the following organs and tissues:

Donor
Signature _____ Date _____
Witness _____
Witness _____

2. Print or type your name on the card.
3. Indicate which organs you wish to donate. You may also indicate your desire to donate all organs and tissues.
4. Sign your name in the presence of two witnesses, preferably your next of kin.
5. Fill in any additional information (such as date of birth, city and state in which the card is completed, and date the card is signed).
6. Tell others about your decision to donate. Some donor cards have detachable portions to give to your family.
7. Always carry your card with you.
8. If you have any questions, you can call the United Network for Organ Sharing (UNOS) at 1-888-TXINF01, or visit this organization's website at www.unos.org.

grief resolution process varies with the emotional attachments one has to a deceased person, grief usually lasts for 18 months. One should seek professional help when grieving is characterized by unresolved guilt, extreme hostility, physical illness, significant depression, and a lack of other meaningful relationships. Trained counselors, physicians, and hospice workers can all play significant roles in helping people through grief.

Coping with Death from Specific Causes

Coping with Death from a Terminal Illness Watching a family member or friend slowly die can bring mixed emotions, from being glad to have that person with you as long as possible to wishing that the person

The grieving process consists of four phases, each of which varies in length and form in each individual. These phases are composed of the following:

1. *Internalization of the deceased person's image.* By forming an idealized mental picture of the dead person, the grieving person is freed from dealing too quickly with the reality of the death.

2. *Intellectualization of the death.* Mental processing of the death and the events leading up to its occurrence move the

grieving person to a clear understanding that death has occurred.

3. *Emotional reconciliation.* During this third and often delayed phase, the grieving person allows conflicting feelings and thoughts to be expressed and eventually reconciled with the reality of the death.

4. *Behavioral reconciliation.* Finally, the grieving person can comfortably return to a life in which the death has been fully reconciled. The survivor reestablishes old routines and adopts new

patterns of living where necessary. The grieving person has largely recovered.

The friends of a grieving person sometimes make the mistake of encouraging a return to normal behavior too quickly. When friends urge the grieving person to return to work right away, make new friends, or become involved in time-consuming projects, they may be preventing necessary grieving. It is not easy or desirable to forget about the fact that a spouse, friend, or child has recently died.

---

would not have to suffer. It can be painful to see the person you know gradually slip away. In addition, he or she may become someone who seems more like a stranger to you and may not even recognize you or acknowledge your presence. Some people say that they are thankful for the time they have with this person and to be able to say good-bye. However, others may feel a false sense of hopefulness that the person is beating the illness only to feel shocked and devastated when the illness begins to progress at a faster rate. The research does suggest that we cope better with loss when we are expecting it, when we have time to prepare and take whatever action we feel necessary in response to it. In this way, a protracted illness can facilitate the ability to cope that people who experience loss through accidental death, natural disaster, suicide, or murder do not have.

Coping with Death from Accident, Natural Disaster, Terrorism, or War Deaths that occur from natural disasters or accidental deaths bring some unique challenges. Accidental death is the number-one cause of death for 15- to 34-year-olds, and so college students may encounter this more often than terminal illnesses. Though any type of trauma or crisis is more difficult to deal with when it is unexpected, accidental death seems particularly devastating in that you are unprepared and shocked by the news. Often people have more trouble accepting this type of death because it is so unexpected that it seems unreal.

Death from natural disasters are typically uncommon and unlikely and so are even more difficult to comprehend and accept. We tend to cope better with events we can understand and explain. Yet this may be impossible to do with accidental deaths such as from a car accident or from incidents without a clear cause of death. Part of finding an explanation can also involve blaming someone: "I should have known he was too tired to drive." People can feel more vulnerable and fearful af-

ter accidents and disasters and become more hesitant in their day-to-day living. Things that you may not have questioned begin to seem potentially dangerous, such as going swimming after a friend has drowned or driving after a car accident.

Death associated with terrorism is something that Americans have not had to face, as other countries have, until 9/11. Since that time, Americans have felt less safe on their own soil and traveling abroad. People have changed their lifestyles in terms of the trips they take, having a survival kit at home, stockpiling food and water, and encountering stringent security. Organizations, hospitals, and government agencies are developing responses to bioterrorism and other types of terrorist attacks.

Those who say good-bye to a soldier going off to combat may dread that the soldier will die in the war. Even though we know this is a possibility, such a death is very difficult to accept, especially when the solider is young, as many are. Those who have lost a loved one to war might have mixed emotions—pride at the person's courage, heroics, and sacrifice, and anger at the enemy or the government. When a soldier goes missing in action, loved ones lack closure and may remain hopeful that he or she will be found alive and well. When people die in a war thousands of miles away, their deaths can seem unreal because of the distance and the different worlds people and their loved ones have been living in.

Coping with Death by Suicide People react similarly to suicides as they do to accidental death, because both means of death are sudden and unexpected. Making sense of these types of death is difficult, and coping with a completed suicide brings the added burden of understanding the reason and motivation behind the death. If you hold religious beliefs that tell you committing suicide is a sin, this can lead to additional misunderstanding and anger. As with death by murder, this type of death is a crime, and so there are legal as well as religious

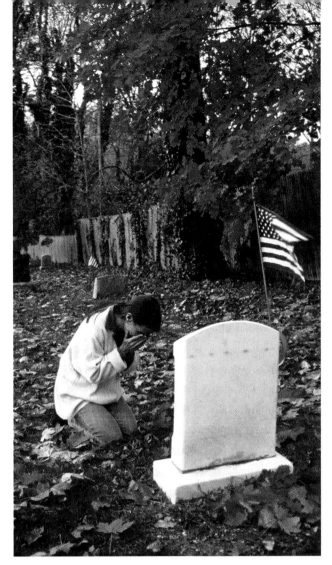

The cause and manner of death can affect the experience of grief. The death of a young soldier in war can be difficult to accept and can lead to a mix of emotions—pride, anger, and profound loss.

and moral implications in accepting a person's decision to take his or her own life.

Family members frequently say they feel ashamed and embarrassed by the suicide because of these connotations. They worry that others will see them and their family as crazy. All these concerns usually mean that coping with death by suicide can be a longer process than coping with other types of death. It is helpful for people to understand the events that led up to and contributed to a person's choosing to take his or her life.

Chapter 2 discussed the warning signs and factors that contribute to suicide. Often people blame themselves for not seeing the warning signs or not acting on those they did see. There can also be a sense of feeling unimportant or unloved by this person because you tell yourself "If she really cared about me, she would have fought to stay with me and not left me." Survivors of suicide often feel abandoned and rejected. If your relationship with this person was distant, if you hadn't talked to him or her for a while or you had recently had an argument, you may feel guilty and blame yourself, saying "If only I had been nicer or called her more often, this might not have happened."

Coping with Death by Murder   Shock, anger, guilt, confusion, and vulnerability are some of the emotions people commonly experience when they cope with a murder. Obviously, you don't expect murder to happen—certainly not to someone you know. It can be difficult to comprehend the taking of someone's life, which makes it even more difficult to accept such a loss. You may blame yourself for not protecting the victim in some way or not doing something to prevent it from happening. If the suspect hasn't been identified or apprehended, you may feel angry at the police for not doing more or feel frightened that you live in a world that seems suddenly very unsafe and frightening. If the murderer has been apprehended, it can take years before the trial is over, making it hard to have a sense of closure.

Coping with the Death of a Child

Adults face not only the death of their parents and friends but perhaps also the death of a child. Whether because of sudden infant death syndrome (SIDS), chronic illness, accident, or suicide, adults are sometimes forced to grieve the loss of someone who was "too young to die."

Parents and children are bound by physical and emotional ties like no other relationship. When the tragic death of a young child severs that bond, the pain and anguish the parents feel can be too much to bear. Getting through such a traumatic experience can be one of life's toughest challenges.

Miscarriage Most pregnancies progress to full term and result in the birth of a healthy child. However, researchers now believe that about one-third of pregnancies end in miscarriage. Since accurate home-pregnancy tests were developed, many women began learning early in the first trimester that they are pregnant. Thus, rather than mistaking the miscarriage for a late heavy menstrual period, more women now know that their pregnancy has ended. Most then go through a grieving process.

In addition, other couples may learn of complications that lead them to choose an elective abortion, or the baby may die during birth or during infancy. Though most people know that such things can happen, many believe that such tragedies happen only to others. When they face the death or potential loss of a child, parents often find their beliefs shaken and their faith tested.

Miscarriage can be especially difficult for the mother. She may think that something she did (or did not do) caused the miscarriage. The exact cause of a miscarriage may never be determined, and the woman needs to be reassured that she did not cause any abnormalities in the fetus.

A miscarriage can be painful and stressful for the woman. Physical symptoms may not occur when the baby dies but may be delayed for some time. Mild or moderate depression, sleeping difficulties, recurring images of the miscarriage, loss of appetite, and abdominal discomfort and cramping may occur weeks or months after a miscarriage. Not surprisingly, fathers can also experience similar symptoms of loss and depression after a miscarriage.

Supportive comments acknowledging how painful their loss is can be helpful to the parents. If an unhealthy fetus is miscarried or aborted, sometimes people try to rationalize the loss for the parents by saying it was "nature's way" of preventing the birth of an imperfect child. Such comments are not only insensitive, but they also imply that the parents should be grateful that they lost the baby. Even seemingly innocent comments can cause pain in the wrong context.

Losing an Infant or Young Child Even after a baby is delivered, there are health risks. Sometimes newborn babies die. The support of family and friends is especially important when a couple is trying to recover from the death of a child. Friends and coworkers can help by acknowledging the death of the child and offering support.

Often people will not mention the baby because they think that the parents will become upset, but not talking about the baby can cause greater pain for the parents. Calling to offer support or showing up in person can also help.

Parents often want to hold on to the memory of the child. Such feelings are normal and do not mean that the parents are clinging to their grief in an unhealthy way. Remembering the child can give a sense of meaning to parents' lives. Parents often do something constructive to help them remember their baby and accept this loss. Putting together a scrapbook, donating the baby's clothes and toys to charity, writing memoirs, or setting up a place for remembrance can help the family keep memories of the baby.

Eventually, the grief will lose its intensity. It may flare up again around "anniversaries" (the baby's due date or birthday, the date of the baby's death), but gradually things will become bearable. The family will be forever changed by the experience. The death of a child can change the parents' value system, and their spiritual beliefs may be challenged as well.

Sometimes parents become more protective and focused on their remaining children, creating a new set of problems. It is also not uncommon for parents to take their anger over their loss out on each other, sometimes resulting in so much distance, resentment, and bitterness that they eventually divorce.[9] So, how people come to terms with the loss of their child is important to the continued health and healing of the family unit.

Grieving for a Dead Child Coping with the death of a child is particularly difficult because it seems so unnatural and wrong for a child to precede his or her parents in death. Experts agree that grieving adults, particularly the parents, should express their grief fully and proceed cautiously to return to normal routines. They can avoid many pitfalls. Adults who are grieving for dead children should do the following:

- Avoid trying to cope with grief by using alcohol or drugs.
- Make no important life changes. Moving to a different home, relocating, or changing jobs usually doesn't help parents deal any better with the grief they are experiencing.
- Share their feelings with others. Grieving adults should share their feelings, particularly with other adults who have experienced a similar loss. Group support is available in many communities.
- Avoid trying to erase the death. Giving away clothing and possessions that belonged to the child cannot erase the adult's memories of the child.
- Give themselves the time and space to grieve. On the anniversary of the child's death or on the child's

birthday, family members should give themselves special time just for grieving.

- Don't attempt to replace the child. Do not quickly have another child or use the deceased child's name for another child.

For most adults, grief over the death of a child will require an extended time. Eventually, however, life can return to normal.

Coping with the Death of a Parent, Spouse, or Sibling

In some ways, coping with the death of a parent, spouse, or sibling is similar to coping with the death of a child. In each case, survivors must live with the significant loss of a family member. Each death produces some degree of emotional trauma for each survivor, followed by a period of grief. Gradually, the force of the grieving process lessens as the survivors put the death into a perspective that they can live with. Despite the similarities, there are some differences involving the death of a parent, spouse, or sibling.

Death of a Parent The death of a parent can be especially difficult because parents have formed a foundation in most people's lives. In a sense, parents have always "been there." There is a sense of a loss of security that a parent provided for his or her children. A "safety net" for the children disappears. Perhaps for the first time, adult children genuinely see themselves as getting older. When a parent dies, the children realize they have become the new matriarchs and patriarchs, the leaders of their families.

When a parent dies, adult children are reminded of their own mortality.[3] It is not unusual for this realization to push adult children into serious reflection about their own lives. They may, for the first time, evaluate their lives to determine whether the dreams they had as young adults have materialized. This evaluation can be a positive experience for midlife adults, if it encourages them to refocus on the real priorities in their lives.

Some may consider the death of a mother to be more traumatic than the death of a father.[3] Perhaps this is because the mother traditionally has had the role of the primary nurturing caregiver in a family. From the mother's nine months of pregnancy through a child's adult life, the maternal role produces a special bond between a mother and her child. Perhaps another reason why a mother's death is especially traumatic is the fact that men tend to die at younger ages than women do. Thus, a mother's death typically follows a father's death and leaves the adult child with the emptiness of "feeling orphaned."

Death of a Spouse There is great variability in the way a person adapts to the death of a spouse depending on the length of the marriage (or relationship), the age of the person at death, the children from that marriage, financial resources, the vitality of the relationship, the manner in which the spouse died, and the health status of the widow or widower.

For many couples, the death of a spouse is the most traumatic of all deaths.[3] Some couples become so interconnected that the death of one leaves the survivor feeling utterly alone and not whole. A spouse's death might also create a single-parent family, thereby making day-to-day activities quite challenging for the survivor. Some couples may need to assume roles and responsibilities that are unfamiliar and difficult for them, such as handling finances and doing home repairs (see the box "Aftercare").

The death of a spouse can also result in the loss of a primary source of one's social interactions.[3] It is important for the remaining spouse to maintain a network of family and friends for social support and interaction. This social support will be crucial in determining how well the survivor will adjust to his or her new situation. Fortunately, there are support groups for recently widowed persons. These can be found in local communities through churches or social support agencies. Support groups also exist on the Internet for those who wish to seek an online form of support.

Death of a Sibling The death of a brother or a sister can be very difficult for the surviving sibling(s). It is common for children to feel great guilt for outliving their sibling. They may wonder why the death happened to the sibling rather than them. They may start to question their own mortality and feel more vulnerable to death themselves. Survivors may feel overwhelmed with guilt and believe that they, in some strange way, caused the death. For example, the surviving child who frequently had wished "that his brother was dead" (a common sibling rivalry wish) may believe that his wish caused the car accident that killed his brother.

The manner in which parents communicate and respond to the situation can help the surviving child come to terms with the sibling death. Parents need to keep the lines of communication open, listen to the child's concerns, avoid becoming overly protective of the child, and avoid attempting to re-create in the living child certain qualities of the deceased child.[3] Children must be allowed to express their feelings. Talking with mental health experts in the field of grief and bereavement can be especially helpful to children. Individual counseling sessions and group sessions are available in most communities.

Rituals of Death

Our society has established many rituals associated with death that help the survivors accept the reality of death, ease the pain associated with the grief process, and provide a safe disposal of the body. Our rituals give us the chance to formalize our good-byes to a person and to receive emotional support and strength from family members and friends (see the box "Cultural Differences in Death Rituals"). In recent years, more of our rituals seem to be celebrating the life of the deceased. In doing this, our rituals also reaffirm the value of our own lives.

Most of our funeral rituals take place in funeral homes, churches, and cemeteries. Funeral homes (or mortuaries) are business establishments that provide a variety of services to the families and friends of the deceased. The services are carried out by funeral directors, who are licensed by the state in which they operate. Most funeral directors are responsible for preparing the bodies for viewing, filing death certificates, preparing obituary notices, establishing calling hours, assisting in the

There are cultural differences in the rituals associated with death. Day of the Dead, which originated in Mexico, is a celebration of the dead and the continuation of life, characterized by both sadness and joy. Graves may be decorated with orange marigolds, the deceased's favorite foods, sugared skulls, and figurines of skeletons.

preparation and details of the funeral, selecting a casket, transporting mourners to and from the cemetery, and counseling the family. Although licensing procedures vary from state to state, most new funeral directors must complete one year of college, one year of mortuary school, and one year of internship with a funeral home before taking a state licensing examination.

Full Funeral Services

An ethical funeral director will attempt to follow the wishes of the deceased's family and provide only the services requested by the family. Most families want traditional, **full funeral services.** Three significant components of the full funeral services are as follows.

Embalming *Embalming* is the process of using formaldehyde-based fluids to replace the blood components.

Learning from Our Diversity

Cultural Differences in Death Rituals

Death rituals vary considerably among ethnic and religious groups. Even within the broad categories of ethnic, racial, or religious distinction, differences exist in how groups of people dispose of their deceased. For example, funeral rituals may differ between Orthodox Jews and Conservative Jews. Furthermore, groups of people living in the United States may not be able to follow the traditional funeral rituals of their home countries because they lack the necessary resources and community support. However, some general cultural differences in funeral rituals can be seen in the following examples.

According to Purnell and Paulanka, funeral rituals by the Amish are carried out in the deceased person's home. The church community takes care of the arrangements for visitors, relieving the grieving family of these tasks. In some Amish communities, a wakelike "sitting up" takes place in which family members are supported by friends throughout the night. The funeral itself is simple, with burial in an unadorned wooden coffin, often made by the local Amish carpenter. Children are encouraged to see death as a transition to a better life. Although the Amish clearly feel the pain of their loss, they often may not express this grief openly.

Muslim death rituals are based on their belief that death is the result of God's will. Death is foreordained. For Muslims (and for members of many other religious groups), life in this world is seen as a preparation for eternal life. At death, the deceased's bed is turned to face the Holy City of Mecca, and verses of hope and acceptance are read from the *Qur'an*. The dead body is washed three times by a Muslim of the same sex as the deceased and then it is wrapped in white material and buried as soon as possible, usually in a brick or cement-lined grave facing Mecca. Prayers are offered for the dead at the cemetery, at the mosque, or at the home. Unless the deceased is a husband or close relative, women usually do not attend the burial. Cremation is not practiced among Muslims.

In Judaism, death is seen as part of the life cycle. Traditional Jews believe in an afterlife in which a person's soul continues to flourish. In this afterlife, people are judged by their actions in life. People who have lived righteous lives are likely to be rewarded in the next world. Judaism does not have a form of last rites; any Jew may ask for God's forgiveness.

At traditional Jewish funerals, the body is rarely embalmed, unless there are unusual circumstances causing burial to be delayed. Burial routinely takes place within a short time after death. Cosmetic restoration is used minimally, if at all. The body is wrapped in a shroud and placed in an unadorned wooden casket. Traditionally, flowers are not displayed at the funeral or at the cemetery. The funeral service is directed at honoring the deceased, while praising God and encouraging people to reaffirm their faith. Traditionally, a 7-day period of immediate mourning (*shiva*) takes place after the burial. After this period there are established mourning periods. For example, mourning for a relative typically lasts 30 days; for a parent, 1 year.

Source: LD Purnell and BJ Paulanka, *Transcultural Healthcare* (Philadelphia: F.A. Davis, 1998).

Embalming helps preserve the body and return it to a natural look. Embalming permits friends and family members to view the body without being subjected to the odors associated with tissue decomposition. Embalming is often an optional procedure, except when death results from specific communicable diseases or when body disposition (disposal) is delayed.

Calling Hours Sometimes called a *wake* or *visiting hours,* this is an established time when friends and family members can gather in a room to share their emotions and common experiences about the deceased. Generally in the same room, the body will be in a casket, with the lid open or closed. Open caskets help some people to confirm that death truly did occur. Some families prefer not to have any calling hours.

Funeral Service *Funeral services* vary according to religious preference and the emotional needs of the survivors. Although some services are held in a church, most funeral services today take place in a funeral home, where a special room might serve as a chapel. Some services are held at the graveside. Families may also choose to have a simple memorial service within a few days after the funeral. Completing the Personal Assessment at the end of this chapter will help you think about what kind of funeral arrangements, if any, you would prefer for yourself.

Memorial Service

Some families prefer to have a **memorial service** in addition to (or instead of) the full funeral services. The memorial service is usually a celebration of the life of the deceased person. This service may have elements of a religious service, with eulogies spoken by friends and relatives of the dead person. Frequently, the public is invited to attend a memorial service. A memorial service typically takes place weeks or months after a person's death, and may follow an earlier, private funeral service. Thus, the body of the deceased person is rarely present at a memorial service.

> **Key Terms**
>
> **full funeral services** All the professional services provided by funeral directors.
>
> **memorial service** A broad term for a ceremony that honors the life of a person who has died.

Table 21.2 Estimated Funeral Costs

Services	
Professional service charges	$392–$2,890
Embalming	$185–$990
Other preparations (cosmetology, hair, etc.)	$25–$500
Visitation/viewing	$50–$1,085
Hearse (local)	$65–$458
Funeral at mortuary	$75–$3,075
Memorial service	$75–$2,625
Graveside service	$50–$3,440
Direct cremation	$300–$3,000
Immediate burial	$270–$5,000
Merchandise	
Caskets	$299–$8,000
Burial vaults	$252–$17,800

Source: General Price List Survey, National Funeral Directors Association, Research and Information Department, Brookfield, Wisconsin.

Disposition of the Body

Ground Burial   We dispose of bodies in one of four ways. Ground burial is the most common method. About 70 percent of all bodies undergo ground burial. The casket is almost always placed in a metal or concrete *vault* before being buried. The vault serves to further protect the body (a need only of the survivors) and to prevent collapse of ground because of the decaying of caskets. Most cemeteries require the use of a vault. See Table 21.2 for the costs involved in this type of burial.

Entombment   A second type of disposition is *entombment*. Entombment refers to nonground burial, most often in structures called **mausoleums.** A mausoleum contains a series of shelves where caskets or urns of cremated remains can be sealed in vaultlike spaces called **niches.** Entombment also can take place in the floors, walls, or basements of buildings, especially in large, old churches. For example, the bodies of many famous British religious, cultural, and government leaders are entombed in the **crypts** of Westminster Abbey in London.

Cremation   *Cremation* is a third type of body disposition. In the United States, 30 percent of all bodies are cremated.[15] This practice is increasing. Generally, both the body and casket (or cardboard cremation box) are incinerated so that only the bone ash from the body remains. The body of an average adult produces about 5–7 pounds of bone ash. These ashes then are placed in containers called *urns,* and then buried, entombed, or scattered, if permitted by state law (see the box "State-of-the-Art and High-Tech Ways of Dealing with Death"). The itemized crematory fee ($500–$850) is much less than the fee for ground burial. Some families choose to cremate after having full funeral services.[16]

Anatomical Donation   A fourth method of body disposition is *anatomical donation*. Separate organs (such as corneal tissue, kidneys, or the heart) can be donated to a medical school, research facility, or organ donor network. Some people choose to donate their entire body to medical science. Often this is done through prior arrangements with medical schools. Bodies still require embalming. After they are studied, the remains are often cremated and returned to the family, if requested. Just as with an organ donation, those who wish to donate their bodies should discuss their wishes with family members beforehand so that their wishes can be carried out at the time of death.

Costs

The full funeral services offered by a funeral home cost upward of $4,000, with other expenses added to this price. Casket prices vary significantly, with the average cost between $1,500–$2,500. If the family chooses an especially fancy casket, then the costs could spiral up to $10,000 or more. Costs that extend beyond these expenses include (should one choose them) those shown in Table 21.2. When all the expenses associated with a typical funeral are totaled, the average cost is approximately $6,500.[17]

Regardless of the rituals you select for the handling of your body (or the body of someone in your care), you may want to make prearrangements. You can ease your survivors' burden by putting your wishes in writing. *Funeral prearrangements* relieve the survivors of many of the details that must be handled at the time of your death and can better ensure that your wishes will be carried out. You can gather much of the information for your obituary notice and your wishes for the disposition of your body. You can make prearrangements with a funeral director, family member, or attorney. Many individuals also prepay the costs of their funeral. By making arrangements before the need arises, you can improve your own peace of mind. Currently, about 30–40 percent of funerals are preplanned and prepaid. In the 1960s nearly all funerals were planned by relatives at the time of a person's death.

Personal Preparation for Death

We hope that this chapter helps you to develop a new framework about death and form your own personal perspective on death and dying. Remember that the ultimate goal of death education is a positive one—to help you best use and enjoy your life. Becoming aware of the reality of your own mortality is a step in the right direction. Reading about the process of dying, grief resolution, and the rituals surrounding death can also help you accept that someday you too will die.

You can prepare for the reality of your own death in some additional ways. Preparing a will, purchasing a

People cope with death in many individual ways. Collectively, these serve the diverse needs of society. As our society becomes more culturally diverse, funeral directors are becoming more familiar (and accommodating) with rituals used not only by dozens of Christian denominations but also with rituals for Buddhist, Hindu, and Muslim groups.

Increasingly, funeral directors indicate that there is no longer a set "conventional funeral service." Families mourn the loss of loved ones by developing their own customized funerals. For example, soft music, classical music, rap music, folk music, rock music, or ethnic music may be heard at calling hours (body visitation). Food and drinks (including alcoholic drinks) might be served during calling hours or after the service is performed. More and more families are choosing to display collages of pictures of the deceased person to allow the mourners to remember the life of the dead person.

One unconventional practice that is gaining popularity is the use of the "drive-through mortuary." Mourners can save time by driving up to a funeral home's drive-through window. Without getting out of their car, they can view the body, sign the guest register, and pay their "respects." Although viewed by many as a callous approach, this option was probably inevitable in a society that seems to value squeezing more activities into less time.

With cremation on the rise in the United States, some companies are starting to capitalize on ways to use or display the cremated remains (ashes). Some of these approaches can only be characterized as high-tech. For example, one company will rocket into space a small container of your loved one's ashes. Other companies manufacture and sell display urns for ashes. These urns can be shaped into almost anything, including a motorcycle gas tank, a fiddle, a stuffed animal, a heart, or a car. Jewelry artisans are even producing customized "cremation jewelry" that allows you to carry the ashes of the deceased in a pendant around your neck. Some of this jewelry can cost up to $10,000. Ashes can also be compressed into diamonds for jewelry or crushed into balls and placed in the ocean.

Another high-tech approach to death is the use of "electronic" memorials. These are Internet websites that people create to memorialize their deceased loved ones. They usually contain pictures of the person who died, a written life story or family history, and notes and written remembrances from relatives or friends. Some websites allow cybermourners to post condolence messages and share their grief online. "Virtual cemeteries" are websites that feature the posting of pictures and biographical information of the deceased, a chance for mourners to sign the guest book, and the option of leaving "digital flowers." Blogs, MySpace, Facebook, and instant messages are also used to post condolences and pay tribute to loved ones who have died. It is also a way for mourners to connect and gain support.

Some cemeteries even are offering high-tech choices. Special grave markers store a small video monitor that can display up to 250 pages of information about the deceased person. Thus, while standing at the grave site, a mourner can study the entire life of the person buried beneath his or her feet.

Other high-tech influences reflect the variety of ways that people cope with death. Many funeral homes now make video recordings that are sold to friends and relatives who cannot attend the funeral service. In some cases, digital cameras are used to transmit live video images of a funeral service over the Internet. As the world rapidly changes, so do the ways we handle death rituals.

Sources: L. A. DeSpelder and A. L. Strickland, *The Last Dance*, 7th ed. (New York: McGraw-Hill, 2005); New Creations Personalize Cremation, *USA Today*, October 20, 2006.

---

life insurance policy, making funeral prearrangements, preparing a living will, and considering an anatomical or organ donation are measures that help you to prepare for your death. At the appropriate time, you might also wish to talk with family and friends about your death. You may discover that an upbeat, positive discussion about death can help relieve some of your apprehensions and those of others around you.

Another suggestion to help you emotionally prepare for your death is to prepare your *obituary notice* or **eulogy.** Include all the things you would like to have said about you and your life. Now compare your obituary notice and eulogy with the current direction your life seems to be taking. Are you doing the kinds of activities for which you want to be known? If so, great! If not, perhaps you will want to consider why your current direction does not reflect how you would like to be remembered. How do you want to restructure your life to better fit your life's goals, meaning, and purpose?

Another suggestion to help make you aware of your eventual death is to write your own **epitaph,** an inscription on a grave marker or monument. Before doing this, you might want to visit a cemetery. Reading the epitaphs of others may help you develop yours.

Key Terms

mausoleum (moz oh **lee** um) An above-ground structure, which frequently resembles a small stone house, into which caskets can be placed for disposition.

niche A recessed area in a mausoleum where a casket can be placed.

crypts Burial locations generally in the walls, floors, or basements of churches.

eulogy A composition or speech that praises someone; often delivered at a funeral or memorial service.

epitaph An inscription on a grave marker or monument.

To assist you in expanding and accepting your awareness of your own mortality, consider answering the following questions: (1) If I had only one day to live, how would I spend it? (2) What one accomplishment would I like to achieve before I die? (3) After I am dead, what two or three things will people miss most about me? By answering these questions and accomplishing a few of the tasks suggested in this section, you will have a good start on accepting your own death and understanding the value of life itself.

Taking Charge of Your Health

- Start considering how you might plan for your funeral by completing the Personal Assessment at the end of this chapter.

- Consider completing a living will and designating a health care agent or proxy. Discuss your wishes with your family and friends.

- Consider completing an organ donor card, purchase life insurance, and/or prepare a will.

- If you don't already know, ask your family about their end-of-life wishes.

- Write your own eulogy, epitaph, or obituary.

- If you have experienced a loss, where would you place yourself in the psychological stages of grief? If appropriate, explore with a trusted friend, family member, spiritual leader, or counselor how you can move closer to a sense of acceptance of this loss.

SUMMARY

- Death is determined primarily by clinical and legal factors.
- Euthanasia can be performed through either direct or indirect measures.
- Currently, physician-assisted suicide is legal in only one state, Oregon.
- The most current advance health care directives are the living will and the durable power of attorney for health care.
- Denial, anger, bargaining, depression, and acceptance are the five classic psychological stages that dying people commonly experience, according to Kübler-Ross.
- When a parent dies, a child needs support and the truth, especially two crucial pieces of information: that the dead parent will never return and that the body has been buried in the ground or cremated.
- Death in our society is associated with many rituals to help survivors cope with the loss of a loved one and to ensure proper disposal of the body.
- The shortage of organ donations is the biggest problem facing people who need a transplant to save their lives.
- Hospice care is an alternative end-of-life health care option for terminally ill patients and their families.
- We dispose of bodies in four ways: ground burial, entombment, cremation, and anatomical donation.

REVIEW QUESTIONS

1. Identify and explain the clinical and legal determinants of death, and identify who establishes each of them.
2. Explain the difference between direct and indirect euthanasia.
3. What is physician-assisted suicide, and in what states is it legal?
4. How does a living will differ from a durable power of attorney as a health care document? Why are these advance health care directives becoming increasingly popular?
5. Identify and explain the five psychological stages that dying people tend to experience. Explain each stage.
6. Identify and explain the four strategies that form the basis of hospice care. What are the advantages of hospice care for the patient and the family?
7. Define the term *grief*. Identify and explain the sensations and emotions most people have when they experience grief. When does the grieving process end?
8. What purposes do the rituals of death serve? What are the significant components of the full funeral service?
9. What are the four ways in which bodies are disposed?
10. Define these terms: *mausoleum, niche, crypt, vault, urn, eulogy, obituary,* and *epitaph.*

ANSWERS TO THE "WHAT DO YOU KNOW?" QUIZ

1. False   2. False   3. True   4. True   5. True   6. True   7. False

Ordering Organs Online

Patients can wait as long as 10 years for organ transplants through the federal government's United Network for Organ Sharing (UNOS) list, and sometimes they do not receive them in time. Today there is a new way to obtain healthy body organs—online. The nonprofit website known as MatchingDonors.com is a nonprofit website that matches donors with those in need of transplants. Individuals seeking organs pay $49 weekly, or $595 for unlimited usage; potential donors use the site free of charge. While some say the originators of this site, Dr. Jeremiah Lowney and Paul Dooley, have created a great service, others argue that it has serious faults—for instance, this system is not regulated, and organs might be distributed by favoritism or fraud or to the highest bidder, and not everyone who needs a transplant has access to the Internet. However, for some people it has been a lifesaver.

Source: "Kidneys Online," *People Magazine,* March 26, 2007.

ENDNOTES

1. Leming MR, Dickinson GE. *Understanding Dying, Death and Bereavement* (5th ed.). New York: Harcourt, 2001.
2. Kastenbaum RJ. *Death, Society, and Human Experience* (6th ed.). Boston: Allyn & Bacon, 1998.
3. DeSpelder L, Strickland A. *The Last Dance: Encountering Death and Dying,* 7th ed. New York: Mc-Graw-Hill, 2005.
4. Kübler-Ross E. *On Death and Dying* (reprint ed.). Collier Books, 1997.
5. Kübler-Ross E. *To Live Until We Say Goodbye* (reprint ed.). Upper Saddle River, NJ: Prentice Hall, 1997.
6. Moody RA. *The Last Laugh: A New Philosophy of Near Death Experiences, Apparitions, and the Paranormal.* Hampton Roads, 1999.
7. Ring K. *Life at Death: A Scientific Investigation of the Near-Death Experience.* Coward, McCann and Geoghegan, 1980.
8. Bendiksen R, Fulton R (Eds). *Death and Identity* (3rd ed.). Charles Press, 1994.
9. Staudacher, C. *Beyond Grief.* Oakland, CA: New Harbinger Publications, 1987.
10. National Hospice and Palliative Care Organization. *Facts and Figures on Hospice Care in America,* 2005, www.nhpco.org, November 2006.
11. Doctor of Death to Be Paroled Soon, *The Star Press,* December 14, 2006.
12. Partnership for Caring. *Facts about Advance Directives,* www .partnershipforcaring.org, October 10, 2000.
13. Organ donors lives on the line, *St. Louis Post,* May 22, 2005.
14. United Network for Organ Sharing. *The Critical Organ Shortage,* www.unos.org, February 23, 2007.
15. New Creations Personalize Cremation, *USA Today,* October 20, 2006.
16. Bowman J (Licensed Funeral Director). Personal correspondence, November 15, 2000.
17. Plan funeral now to make sure you have the final word. *USA Today,* July 28, 2006.

Personal Assessment

Planning Your Funeral

In line with this chapter's positive theme of the value of personal death awareness, here is a funeral service assessment that we frequently give to our health classes. This inventory can help you assess your reactions and thoughts about the funeral arrangements you would prefer for yourself.

After answering each of the following questions, you might wish to discuss your responses with a friend or close relative.

1. Have you ever considered how you would like your body to be handled after your death?

    _____ Yes _____ No

2. Have you already made funeral arrangements for yourself?

    _____ Yes _____ No

3. Have you considered a specific funeral home or mortuary to handle your arrangements?

    _____ Yes _____ No

4. If you were to die today, which of the following would you prefer?

    _____ Embalming _____ Ground burial
    _____ Cremation _____ Entombment
    _____ Donation to medical science

5. If you prefer to be cremated, what do you want done with your ashes?

    _____ Buried _____ Entombed
    _____ Scattered
    _____ Other; please specify _____

6. If your funeral plans involve a casket, which of the following do you prefer?

    _____ Plywood (cloth covered)
    _____ Hardwood (oak, cherry, mahogany, maple, etc.)
    _____ Steel (sealer or nonsealer type)
    _____ Stainless steel
    _____ Copper or bronze
    _____ Other; please specify _____

7. How important is a funeral service for you?

    _____ Very important
    _____ Somewhat important
    _____ Somewhat unimportant
    _____ Very unimportant
    _____ No opinion

8. What kind of funeral service do you want for yourself?

    _____ No service at all
    _____ Visitation (calling hours) the day before the funeral service; funeral held at church or funeral home
    _____ Graveside service only (no visitation)
    _____ Memorial service (after body disposition)
    _____ Other; please specify _____

9. How many people do you want to attend your funeral service or memorial service?

    _____ I do not want a funeral or memorial service
    _____ 1–10 people
    _____ 11–25 people
    _____ 26–50 people
    _____ Over 51 people
    _____ I do not care how many people attend

10. What format would you prefer at your funeral service or memorial service? Select any of the following that you like:

	Yes	No
Religious music	_____	_____
Nonreligious music	_____	_____
Clergy present	_____	_____
Flower arrangements	_____	_____
Family member eulogy	_____	_____
Eulogy by friend(s)	_____	_____
Open casket	_____	_____
Religious format	_____	_____
Other; please specify _____		

11. Using today's prices, how much do you expect to pay for your total funeral arrangements, including cemetery expenses (if applicable)?

    _____ Less than $4,500
    _____ Between $4,501 and $6,000
    _____ Between $6,001 and $7,500
    _____ Between $7,501 and $9,000
    _____ Between $9,001 and $13,000
    _____ Above $13,000

TO CARRY THIS FURTHER . . .

Which items had you not thought about before? Were you surprised at the arrangements you selected? Will you share your responses with anyone else? If so, whom?

First Aid

Accidents are the leading cause of death for people ages 1 to 37. Injuries sustained in accidents can often be tragic. They are grim reminders of our need to learn first aid skills and to practice preventive safety habits.

First aid knowledge and skills allow you to help people who are in need of immediate emergency care. They also can help you save yourself if you should become injured. We recommend that our students enroll in American Red Cross first aid and safety courses, which are available in local communities or through colleges or universities. In this appendix, we briefly present some information about common first aid emergencies. (Please note that our information is *not* a substitute for comprehensive American Red Cross first aid instruction.)

First Aid

- Keep a list of important phone numbers near your phone (your doctor, ambulance service, hospital, poison control center, police, and fire departments).
- In case of serious injury or illness, call the appropriate emergency service immediately for help (if uncertain, call "911" or "0").

Common First Aid Emergencies

Specific Problem	What to Do
Asphyxiation Victim stops breathing and skin, lips, tongue, and fingernail beds turn bluish or gray.	Tip head back with one hand on forehead and other lifting the lower jaw near the chin. Look, listen, and feel for breathing. If the victim is not breathing, place your mouth over victim's mouth, pinch the nose, get a tight seal, and give 2 slow breaths. Do a pulse check. If no pulse is detected, CPR must be administered. (Note: some states require CPR training for those who administer CPR.) If there is a pulse but no breathing, give breaths once every 5 seconds for an adult, once every 3 seconds for a child, once every 3 seconds for infants (do not exaggerate head tilt for babies). Recheck pulse and breathing every 2 minutes.
Bleeding Victim bleeding severely can quickly go into shock and die within 1 or 2 minutes.	Use universal precautions. With the palm of your hand, apply firm, direct pressure to the wound with a clean dressing or pad. Elevate the body part if possible. Do not remove blood-soaked dressings; use additional layers, continue to apply pressure, and elevate the site.
Choking Accidental ingestion or inhalation of food or other objects causes suffocation that can quickly lead to death. There are over 3,000 deaths annually, mostly of infants, small children, and the elderly.	The procedure of giving 5 back blows followed by 5 abdominal thrusts is easy to learn; however, the correct technique must be learned from a qualified instructor. The procedure varies somewhat for infants, children, adults, pregnant women, and obese people.
Hyperventilation A situation in which a person breathes too rapidly; often the result of fear or anxiety; may cause confusion, shortness of breath, dizziness, or fainting. Intentional hyperventilation before an underwater swim is especially dangerous, since it may cause a swimmer to pass out in the water and drown.	Have the person relax and rest for a few minutes. Provide reassurance and a calming influence. Having the victim take a few breaths from a paper bag (not plastic) may be helpful. Do not permit swimmers to practice hyperventilation before attempting to swim.

Common First Aid Emergencies *continued*

Specific Problem	What to Do
Bee Stings Not especially dangerous except for people who have developed an allergic hypersensitivity to a particular venom. Those who are not hypersensitive will experience swelling, redness, and pain. Hypersensitive people may develop extreme swelling, chest constriction, breathing difficulties, hives, and shock signs.	For nonsensitive people: Scrape stinger from skin and apply cold compresses or over-the-counter topical preparation for insect bites. For sensitive people: Get professional help immediately. Scrape the stinger from skin; position the person so that the stung body part is below the level of the heart; help administer prescribed medication (if available); apply cold compresses.
Poisoning Often poisoning can be prevented with adequate safety awareness. Children are frequent victims.	Call the poison control center immediately; follow the instructions provided. Keep syrup of ipecac on hand.
Shock A life-threatening depression of circulation, respiration, and temperature control; recognizable by a victim's cool, clammy, pale skin; weak and rapid pulse; shallow breathing; weakness; nausea; or *unconsciousness*.	Keep the victim calm; loosen tight clothing. Help the victim to a comfortable, reclining position with legs elevated 8–12 inches (*if there are head, neck, back, or internal injuries, do not move the person at all;* if breathing is difficult, help the person to sit or semi-recline). Prevent loss of body heat; cover if necessary. Do not give food or fluids. Seek further emergency assistance.
Burns Burns can cause severe tissue damage and lead to serious infection and shock.	Minor burns: immerse in cold water 10–15 minutes; dry; apply antibiotic agent and loose sterile dressing; do not apply butter or grease to burns. Major burns: immerse in cold water; cover affected area with sterile or clean dressings; do not try to clean the burn area or break blisters. Seek medical attention. Chemical burns: flood the area with running water.
Broken Bones Fractures are a common result of car accidents, falls, and recreational accidents.	Do not move the victim unless absolutely necessary to prevent further injury. Immobilize the affected area. Give care for shock while waiting for further emergency assistance.

Source: American Red Cross. *First Aid: Responding to Emergencies*, 4th ed. Staywell Publishers, 2006.

Epilepsy: Recognition and First Aid

Seizure Type	What It Looks Like	Often Mistaken for	What to Do	What Not to Do
Convulsive Generalized tonic-clonic (also called grand mal)	Sudden cry, fall, rigidity, followed by muscle jerks, frothy saliva on lips, shallow breathing or temporarily suspended breathing, bluish skin, possible loss of bladder or bowel control, usually last 2–5 minutes; normal breathing then starts again; there may be some confusion and/or fatigue, followed by return to full consciousness	Heart attack Stroke Unknown but life-threatening emergency	Protect from nearby hazards Loosen ties or shirts collars Place folded jacket under head Turn on side to keep airway clear; reassure when consciousness returns Look for medical identification *after* seizure subsides or protective steps have been taken If single seizure lasted less than 5 minutes, ask if hospital evaluation wanted If multiple seizures, or if one seizure lasts longer than 5 minutes, seek medical attention	Don't put any hard implement in the mouth Don't try to hold tongue; it can't be swallowed Don't try to give liquids during or just after seizure Don't use artificial respiration unless breathing is absent after muscle jerks subside, or unless water has been inhaled Don't restrain
Nonconvulsive	This category includes many different forms of seizures, ranging from temporary unawareness (petit mal) to brief, sudden, massive muscle jerks (myoclonic seizures)	Daydreaming, acting out, clumsiness, poor coordination, intoxication, random activity, mental illness, and many others	Usually no first aid necessary other than to provide reassurance and emotional support If behavior during seizure places person in potentially hazardous situation (e.g., traffic, machinery), gently guide person away from hazard Medical evaluation is recommended	Do not shout at, restrain, or grab a person having a nonconvulsive seizure (unless danger threatens); do not expect verbal instructions to be obeyed

A

abortion Induced premature termination of a pregnancy.

absorption The passage of nutrients or alcohol through the walls of the stomach or intestinal tract into the bloodstream.

abuse Any use of a legal or illegal drug in a way that is detrimental to health or well-being.

Acceptable Macronutrient Distribution Range (AMDR) The range of intakes for energy sources associated with adequate nutrient intake and reduced risk of chronic disease.

acquired immunity (AI) A form of immunity resulting from exposure to foreign protein (most often wild, weakened, or killed pathogenic organisms).

acupuncture The insertion of fine needles into the body to alter electroenergy fields and treat disease.

acute Having a sudden onset and a prompt resolution.

acute alcohol intoxication A potentially fatal elevation of BAC, often resulting from heavy, rapid consumption of alcohol.

acute rhinitis The common cold; the sudden onset of nasal inflammation.

adaptive thermogenesis The physiological response of the body to adjust its metabolic rate to the presence of food.

addiction Compulsive, uncontrollable dependence on a substance, habit, or practice to such a degree that cessation causes severe emotional or physiological reactions.

additive effect The combined (but not exaggerated) effect produced by the concurrent use of two or more drugs.

adipose tissue Tissue made up of fibrous strands around which specialized cells designed to store liquefied fat are arranged.

aerobic energy production The body's primary means of energy production, used when the respiratory and circulatory systems can process and transport sufficient oxygen to muscle cells to convert fuel to energy.

agent The causal pathogen of a particular disease.

agoraphobia A fear of being in situations from which there is no escape or where help would be unavailable should an emergency arise; often associated with panic disorder.

air pollution Substances found in the atmosphere that can have adverse effects on human health, crop productivity, and natural communities.

air toxics A class of 188 toxic air pollutants identified by the U.S. Environmental Protection Agency as known or suspected causes of cancer or other serious health effects, such as reduced fertility, birth defects, or adverse environmental effects.

alarm stage The first stage of the stress response involving physiological, involuntary changes that are controlled by the hormonal and nervous system; the fight or flight response is activated in this stage.

alcohol abuse Patterns of alcohol use that create problems for the drinker's school and job performance, other responsibilities, and interpersonal relationships. Individuals persist in drinking even though they are having legal problems and know that their drinking is causing them problems. Also called problem drinking.

alcohol dependence Tolerance, withdrawal, and a pattern of compulsive use of alcohol. A primary, chronic disease with genetic, psychosocial, and environmental factors affecting its development. Also called *alcoholism.*

allopathy (ah **lop** ah thee) A system of medical practice in which specific remedies (often pharmaceutical agents) are used to produce effects different from those produced by a disease or injury.

alveoli (al **vee** oh lie) Thin, saclike terminal ends of the airways; the site at which gases are exchanged between the blood and the lungs.

Alzheimer's disease Adult-onset form of dementia resulting from loss of acetylcholine production within specific areas of the brain.

amenorrhea The absence of menstruation.

amino acids The building blocks of protein; manufactured by the body or obtained from dietary sources.

anabolic steroids (ann uh **bol** ick) Drugs that function like testosterone to produce increases in muscle mass, strength, endurance, and aggressiveness.

anaerobic energy production The body's alternative means of energy production, used when the available oxygen is insufficient for aerobic energy production. Anaerobic energy production is a much less efficient use of stored energy.

anal intercourse A sexual act in which the erect penis is inserted into the rectum of a partner.

androgyny (an **droj** en ee) The blending of both masculine and feminine qualities.

andropause Significant decrease in androgenic hormone production in aging men; also called male menopause.

anorexia nervosa An eating disorder in which the individual weighs less than 85 percent of the expected weight for his or her age, gender, and height, has an intense fear of gaining weight, and, in females, ceases to menstruate for at least three consecutive months. People with anorexia perceive themselves as overweight, even though they are underweight.

angina pectoris (an **jie** nuh **peck** tor is) Chest pain that results from impaired blood supply to the heart muscle.

antagonistic effect The effect produced when one drug reduces or offsets the effects of a second drug.

antibodies Chemical compounds produced by the body's immune system to destroy antigens and their toxins.

antioxidants Substances that may prevent cancer by interacting with and stabilizing unstable molecules known as free radicals.

artificially acquired immunity (AAI) A type of acquired immunity resulting from the body's response to pathogens introduced into the body through immunizations.

asbestos A class of minerals that have a fibrous crystal structure; inhalant carcinogens.

asphyxiation Death resulting from lack of oxygen to the brain.

atherosclerosis The buildup of plaque on the inner wall of arteries.

attention deficit hyperactivity disorder (ADHD) An above-normal rate of physical movement; often accompanied by an inability to concentrate on a specified task; also called *hyperactivity.*

autoimmune disorders Disorders caused by the immune system's failure to recognize the body as "self"; thus the body mounts an attack against its own cells and tissues.

axon The portion of a neuron that conducts electrical impulses to the dendrites of adjacent neurons; neurons typically have one axon.

B

ballistic stretching A "bouncing" form of stretching in which a muscle group is lengthened repetitively to produce multiple, quick, forceful stretches.

basal metabolic rate (BMR) The amount of energy, expressed in calories, that the body requires to maintain basic functions.

basic needs Deficiency needs that are viewed as essential and fundamental, including physiological safety, belonging, and love and esteem needs.

behavior therapy A behavior modification therapy based upon the learning principles of reinforcement therapy, stimulus-response, and conditioning responses to change behavior.

benign Noncancerous; localized non-malignant tumors contained within a fibrous membrane.

beta blockers Drugs that reduce the workload of the heart, which results in angina pectoris.

beta endorphins Mood-enhancing, pain-reducing, opiatelike chemicals produced within the smoker's body in response to the presence of nicotine.

bias and hate crimes Criminal acts directed at a person or group solely because of a specific characteristic, such as race, religion, ethnic background, sexual orientation, or other attribute.

bigorexia An obsession with getting bigger and more muscular, and thinking that your body is never muscular enough.

binge drinking The consumption of five or more drinks on the same occasion (or in the span of a couple of hours) on at least one day.

binge eating disorder An eating disorder formerly referred to as compulsive overeating disorder; binge eaters use food to cope in the same way that bulimics do and also feel out of control, but do not engage in compensatory purging behavior.

biological air pollutants Living organisms or substances produced by living organisms that cause disease or allergic reactions, including bacteria, molds, mildew, viruses, dust mites, plant pollen, and animal dander, urine, or feces.

biological water pollutants Disease-causing organisms that are found in water.

biopsychological model A model that addresses how biological, psychological, and social factors interact and affect psychological health.

bipolar disorder A mood disorder characterized by alternating episodes of depression and mania.

birth control All of the methods and procedures that can prevent the birth of a child.

blackout A temporary state of amnesia experienced by an alcoholic; an inability to remember events that occur during a period of alcohol use.

blastocyst Early stage of the developing life form that imbeds into the endometrial lining of the uterus.

blood alcohol concentration (BAC) The percentage of alcohol in a measured quantity of blood; BAC can be determined directly, through the analysis of a blood sample, or indirectly, through the analysis of exhaled air.

body dysmorphic disorder (BDD) A secret preoccupation with an imagined or slight flaw in one's appearance.

body image One's subjective perception of how one's body appears to oneself and others.

body mass index (BMI) A mathematical calculation based on weight and height; used to determine desirable body weight.

bolus theory A theory of nicotine addiction based on the body's response to the bolus (ball) of nicotine delivered to the brain with each inhalation of cigarette smoke.

bonding Important initial recognition established between the newborn and those adults on whom the newborn will depend.

bradycardia Slowness of the heartbeat, as evidenced by a resting pulse rate of less than 60 beats per minute.

brand name The specific patented name assigned to a drug by its manufacturer.

bulimia nervosa An eating disorder in which individuals engage in episodes of binging, consuming unusually large amounts of food and feeling out of control, and then engaging in some compensatory purging behavior to eliminate the food.

C

calcium channel blockers Drugs that reduce the workload of the heart; used in the long-term management of angina pectoris.

calendar method A form of periodic abstinence in which the variable lengths of a woman's menstrual cycle are used to calculate her fertile period.

calipers A device used to measure the thickness of a skinfold from which percentage of body fat can be calculated.

caloric balance Caloric intake and caloric expenditure are equal and body weight remains constant.

calories Units of heat (energy); specifically, 1 calorie (used here to mean *kilocalorie*) equals the heat required to raise 1 kg of water 1 degree C.

carbohydrates Chemical compounds composed of sugar units; the body's primary source of energy.

carbon monoxide A gaseous byproduct of the incomplete combustion of natural gas, kerosene, heating oil, wood, coal, gasoline, and tobacco; a compound that can "inactivate" red blood cells.

carcinogens Environmental agents, including chemical compounds within cigarette smoke, that stimulate the development of cancerous changes within cells.

cardiac arrest Immediate death resulting from a sudden change in the rhythm of the heart causing loss of heart function.

cardiac muscle Specialized muscle tissue that forms the middle (muscular) layer of the heart wall.

cardiorespiratory endurance The ability of the heart, lungs, and blood vessels to process and transport oxygen required by muscle cells so that they can contract over a period of time. Cardiorespiratory endurance is produced by exercise that requires continuous, repetitive movements.

cardiovascular Pertaining to the heart (*cardio*) and blood vessels (*vascular*).

catabolizing The metabolic process of breaking down tissue for the purpose of converting it to energy.

cell-mediated immunity Immunity provided principally by the immune system's T cells both working alone and in combination with highly specialized B cells; also called *T cell–mediated immunity*.

cellulite Tissue composed of fat cells intertwined around strands of fibrous connective tissue.

cerebrovascular occlusions Blockages to arteries supplying blood to the cerebral cortex of the brain; cause of the most common type of stroke.

cesarean delivery (si **zare** ee an) Surgical removal of a fetus through the abdominal wall.

chemical name The name used to describe the molecular structure of a drug.

chemoprevention Cancer prevention using food, dietary supplements, or medications thought to bolster the immune system or reduce the damage caused by carcinogens.

child maltreatment The act or failure to act by a parent or caregiver that results in abuse or neglect of a child or that places the child in imminent risk of serious harm.

chiropractic Manipulation of the vertebral column to relieve malalignment and cure illness.

chlamydia The most prevalent sexually transmitted disease; caused by a nongonococcal bacterium.

cholesterol A primary form of fat found in the blood; lipid material manufactured within the body, as well as derived from dietary sources.

chronic Develops slowly and persists for an extended period of time.

chronic bronchitis Persistent inflammation and infection of the smaller airways within the lungs.

chronic fatigue syndrome (CFS) An illness that causes severe exhaustion, fatigue, aches, and depression; mostly affects women in their 30s and 40s.

chronic stress A high level of physiological arousal for an extended period of time; it can also occur when an individual is not able to immediately react to a real or perceived threat.

cilia (**sill** ee uh) Small, hairlike structures that extend from cells that line the air passages.

circadian rhythms The internal, biological clock that helps coordinate physiological processes to the 24-hour light/dark cycle.

clinical depression A psychological disorder in which individuals experience a lack of motivation, decreased energy level, fatigue, social withdrawal, sleep disturbance, disturbance in appetite, diminished sex drive, feelings of worthlessness, and despair.

club drug One of a variety of psychoactive drugs typically used at raves, bars, and dance clubs.

cognitive-behavioral therapy An action-oriented form of therapy that assumes that maladaptive, or faulty, thinking patterns cause maladaptive behavior and negative emotions; treatment focuses on changing an individual's thoughts or cognitive patterns in order to change his or her behavior and emotional state.

cohabitation Sharing of a residence by two unrelated, unmarried people; living together.

coitus (**co** ih tus) Penile-vaginal intercourse.

coitus interruptus (withdrawal) (**co** ih tus in ter **rup** tus) A contraceptive practice in which the erect penis is removed from the vagina before ejaculation.

cold turkey Immediate, total discontinuation of use of a drug; associated withdrawal discomfort.

colonoscopy (co lun **os** ko py) Examination of the entire length of the colon, using a flexible fiberoptic scope to inspect the structure's inner lining.

compliance Willingness to follow the directions provided by another person.

computerized axial tomography (CT) scan An x-ray procedure designed to illustrate structures within the body that would not normally be seen through conventional x-ray procedures.

condom A latex shield designed to cover the erect penis and retain semen upon ejaculation; "rubber."

congestive heart failure Inability of the heart to pump out all the blood that returns to it; can lead to dangerous fluid accumulations in veins, lungs, and kidneys.

consumer fraud The marketing of unreliable and ineffective services, products, or information under the guise of curing disease or improving health; quackery.

contraception Any method or procedure that prevents fertilization.

contraceptive sponge A small, pillow-shaped contraceptive device that contains a spermicide; placed deep in the vagina to cover the cervical opening.

contraceptive patch Contraceptive skin patch containing estrogen and progestin; replaced each week for a three-week period.

contraceptive ring Thin, polymer contraceptive device containing estrogen and progestin; placed deep within the vagina for a three-week period.

contraindications Factors that make the use of a drug inappropriate or dangerous for a particular person.

coronary arteries Vessels that supply oxygenated blood to heart muscle tissues.

coronary artery bypass surgery A surgical procedure designed to improve blood flow to the heart by providing alternate routes for blood to take around points of blockage.

corpus luteum (kore pus **loo** tee um) The cellular remnant of the graafian follicle after the release of an ovum.

cross-tolerance Transfer of tolerance from one drug to another within the same general category.

cruciferous vegetables (crew **sif** er us) Vegetables that have flowers with four leaves in the pattern of a cross.

crypts Burial locations generally in the walls, floors, or basements of churches.

crystal methamphetamine A dangerous form of methamphetamine that quickly produces intense physical and psychological exhilaration when smoked.

cunnilingus (cun uh **ling** gus) Oral stimulation of the vulva or clitoris.

curette A metal scraping instrument that resembles a spoon, with a cup-shaped cutting surface on its end.

current use At least one drink in the past 30 days.

cyanosis Blue coloration of the lips, skin, and nail beds caused by inadequate oxygenation of the blood.

D

degenerative A slow but progressive deterioration of the body's structure or function.

dehydration Abnormal depletion of fluids from the body; severe dehydration can be fatal.

delirium tremens (DTs) Uncontrollable shaking, combined with irrational hallucinations, caused by abstinence from alcohol following habitual alcohol use.

dementia The loss of cognitive abilities, including memory and reason.

dendrite The portion of a neuron that receives electrical stimuli from adjacent neurons; neurons typically have several such branches or extensions.

dependence A physical and/or psychological need to continue using a drug.

depressants A category of drugs that sedate the user by slowing central nervous system function; they produce tolerance and strong psychological and physical addiction in users.

designated driver A person who abstains from or carefully limits alcohol consumption to be able to safely transport other people who have been drinking.

desirable weight The weight range deemed appropriate for people, taking into consideration gender, age, and frame size.

diaphragm A soft rubber cup designed to cover the cervix.

diastolic pressure (**dye** uh stol ick) The blood pressure against blood vessel walls when the heart relaxes.

Dietary Reference Intakes (DRIs) Measures that refer to three types of reference values: Estimated Average Requirement, Recommended Dietary Allowance, and Tolerable Upper Intake Level.

dilation The gradual expansion of an opening or passageway, such as the cervix.

dilation and suction curettage (D&C) (kyoo re **taage**) A surgical procedure in which the cervical canal is dilated to allow the uterine wall to be scraped; vacuum aspiration.

dilation and evacuation (D&E) Second-trimester abortion procedure that requires greater dilation, suction, and curettage than first-trimester vacuum aspiration procedures.

direct (active) euthanasia Intentionally causing death.

dissonance A feeling of uncertainty that occurs when a person believes two equally attractive but opposite ideas.

distillation The process of heating an alcohol solution and collecting its vapors into a more concentrated solution.

distress Stress that diminishes the quality of life; commonly associated with disease, illness, and maladaptation.

dose-response curve The size of a drug's effect on the body related to the amount of the drug administered.

drink 12 ounces of beer, 5 ounces of wine, or 1.5 ounces of liquor.

drug Any natural or artificial substance, other than food, that by its chemical or physical nature alters structure or function in the living organism.

durable power of attorney for health care A legal document that designates who will make health care decisions for people unable to do so.

duration The length of exercise time of each training session; for aerobic fitness, 20–60 minutes is recommended.

dynamic therapy An intensive therapy based upon the belief that effective treatment must focus on the psychological forces underlying the individual's problems.

E

ectopic pregnancy A pregnancy in which the fertilized ovum implants at a site other than the uterus, typically in the fallopian tubes.

electrical impedance A method used to measure the percentage of body fat using a harmless electrical current.

embolism A potentially fatal condition in which a circulating blood clot lodges in a smaller vessel.

embryo Developmental stage from the end of the second week after conception until the end of the eighth week.

emergency contraception Contraceptive measures used to prevent pregnancy within five days after unprotected intercourse; also called post-coital or morning after contraception.

emotional intelligence The ability to understand others and act wisely in human relations and measure how well you know your emotions, manage your emotions, motivate yourself, recognize emotions in others, and handle relationships.

empowerment The nurturing of an individual's or group's ability to be responsible for their own health and well-being.

endocrine-disrupting chemicals Substances that interact with the glands, hormones, and tissues that regulate many physiological processes in humans, including growth, development from fetus to adult, metabolism, reproduction, and development of the brain and nervous system.

enriched Foods that have been resupplied with some of the nutritional elements (B vitamins and iron) removed during processing.

enucleated egg An ovum with the nucleus removed.

environment The physical conditions (temperature, humidity, light, presence of substances) and other living organisms that exist around your body.

environmental tobacco smoke Tobacco smoke, regardless of source, that stays within a common source of air.

enzymes Organic substances that control the rate of physiological reactions but are not altered in the process.

epidemic A highly significant increase in the number of cases of an infectious illness in a given time period in a given geographical area.

epitaph An inscription on a grave marker or monument.

erection The engorgement of erectile tissue with blood; characteristic of the penis, clitoris, nipples, labia minora, and scrotum.

erotic dreams Dreams whose content elicits a sexual response.

Estimated Average Requirement (EAR) The intake value that is estimated to meet the requirement in 50 percent of an age- and gender-specific group.

eulogy A composition or speech that praises someone; often delivered at a funeral or memorial service.

eustress (**yoo** stress) Stress that enhances the quality of life.

excitement stage Initial arousal stage of the sexual response pattern.

exercise A subcategory of physical activity; it is planned, structured, repetitive, and purposive in the sense that an improvement or maintenance of physical fitness is an objective (Casperson et al., 1985).

exhaustion stage The point at which the physical and psychological resources used to deal with stress have been consumed.

exocrine glands Glands whose secretions are released through tubes or ducts, such as sweat glands.

F

false labor Conditions that resemble the start of true labor; may include irregular uterine contractions, pressure, and discomfort in the lower abdomen.

family violence The use of physical force by one family member against another, with the intent to injure or otherwise cause harm.

fat density The percentage of a food's total calories that are derived from fat; above 30 percent reflects higher fat density.

FDA Schedule 1 A list of drugs that have a high potential for abuse but have no medical use.

fecal coliform bacteria A category of bacteria that live within the intestines of warm-blooded animals; the presence of these bacteria is used as an indicator that water has been contaminated by feces.

fellatio (feh **lay** she oh) Oral stimulation of the penis.

fermentation A chemical process whereby plant products are converted into alcohol by the action of yeast cells on carbohydrate materials.

fertility The ability to reproduce.

fetal alcohol syndrome (FAS) The characteristic birth defects noted in the children of some women who consume alcohol during their pregnancies.

fetus Developmental stage from the beginning of the ninth week after conception until birth.

fiber The plant material that cannot be digested; found in cereal, fruits, and vegetables.

fight or flight response The physiological reaction to a stressor that prepares the body for confrontation or avoidance.

fistula A fissure, break, or hole in the wall of an organ.

flaccid (**fla** sid) Nonerect; the state of erectile tissue when vasocongestion is not occurring.

flexibility The ability of joints to function through an intended range of motion.

food allergy A reaction in which the immune system attacks an otherwise harmless food or ingredient; allergic reactions can range from mildly unpleasant to life-threatening.

food intolerance An adverse reaction to a specific food that does not involve the immune system; usually caused by an enzyme deficiency.

foreplay Activities, often involving touching and caressing, that prepare individuals for sexual intercourse.

formaldehyde A chemical widely used in glues, adhesives, paints, and numerous household products; also a byproduct of combustion. Readily evaporates at room temperature; a major indoor pollutant.

frequency The number of exercise sessions per week; for aerobic fitness, 3–5 days are recommended.

FSH (follicle-stimulating hormone) A gonadotrophic hormone required for initial development of ova (in the female) and sperm (in the male).

full funeral services All the professional services provided by funeral directors.

functional foods Foods capable of contributing to the improvement/prevention of specific health problems.

G

gaseous phase The portion of tobacco smoke containing carbon monoxide and many other physiologically active gaseous compounds.

gateway drug An easily obtainable legal or illegal drug that represents a user's first experience with a mind-altering drug; this drug can serve as the "gateway" to the use of other drugs.

gender The general term reflecting a biological basis of sexuality; the male gender or the female gender.

gender adoption The long process of learning the behavior that is traditional for one's gender.

gender identification The achievement of a personally satisfying interpretation of one's masculinity or femininity.

gender identity Recognition of one's gender.

gender preference Emotional and intellectual acceptance of one's own gender.

general adaptation syndrome (GAS) Sequenced physiological responses to the presence of a stressor, involving the alarm, resistance, and exhaustion stages of the stress response.

generalized anxiety disorder (GAD) An anxiety disorder that involves experiencing intense and nonspecific anxiety for at least six months, in which the intensity and frequency of worry is excessive and out of proportion to the situation.

gene replacement therapy An experimental therapy in which a healthy human gene is incorporated into a harmless virus to be delivered to cells that have an abnormal version of the gene.

generic name The common or nonproprietary name of a drug.

green space Areas of land that are dominated by domesticated or natural vegetation, including rural farmland, city lawns and parks, and nature preserves.

greenhouse gases A category of gases in the atmosphere that allow solar radiation to pass through the atmosphere to the Earth, but then trap the heat that is radiated from the Earth back toward space; greenhouse gases include water vapor, carbon dioxide, methane, nitrous oxide, and tropospheric ozone.

H

hallucinogens Psychoactive drugs capable of producing hallucinations (distortions of reality).

health One's ability to use the *intrinsic* and *extrinsic* resources related to each dimension of our holistic makeup to participate fully in the activities that contribute to growth and development, with the goal of feeling a sense of well-being as one evaluates one's progress through life.

health claims The liable statements attesting to a food's contribution to the improvement/prevention of specific health problems.

health promotion A movement in which knowledge, practices, and values are transmitted to people for use in lengthening their lives, reducing the incidence of illness, and feeling better.

herbalism An ancient form of healing in which herbal preparations are used to treat illness and disease.

high-density lipoprotein (HDL) The type of lipoprotein that transports cholesterol from the bloodstream to the liver, where it is eventually removed from the body; high levels of HDL are related to a reduction in heart disease.

high-risk health behavior A behavioral pattern, such as smoking, associated with a high risk of developing a chronic illness.

high sensitivity C-reactive protein (hsCRP) A chemical compound found in the blood that is associated with inflammation; high levels are related to increased risk of coronary heart disease.

holistic health A view of health in terms of its physical, emotional, social, intellectual, spiritual, and occupational makeup.

homeopathy (hoe mee **op** ah the) The use of minute doses of herbs, minerals, or other substances to stimulate healing.

homicide The intentional taking of one person's life by another person.

homocysteine An amino acid found in the bloodstream; high levels of homocysteine are thought to be related to an increased risk of coronary heart disease.

hormone replacement therapy (HRT) Medically administered hormones to replace hormones lost as the result of menopause; also called postmenopausal hormone therapy (PHT).

hospice care (**hos** pis) An approach to caring for terminally ill patients that maximizes the quality of life and allows death with dignity.

host negligence A legal term that reflects the failure of a host to provide reasonable care and safety for people visiting the host's residence or business.

hot flashes Temporary feelings of warmth experienced by women during and after menopause, caused by blood vessel dilation.

human cloning The replication of a human being.

human papillomavirus (HPV) Sexually transmitted viruses, some of which are capable of causing precancerous changes in the cervix; causative agent for genital warts.

humanistic therapy A treatment approach based on the belief that people, left to their own devices, will naturally grow in positive and constructive ways.

humoral immunity Immunity responsible for the production of critically important immune system elements known as *antibodies*; also called *B cell–mediated immunity.*

hydrostatic weighing Weighing the body while it is submerged in water.

hypercellular obesity A form of obesity that results from having an abnormally high number of fat cells.

hyperglycemia The condition of having an abnormally high blood glucose level.

hypertonic saline solution A salt solution with a concentration higher than that found in human fluids.

hypervitaminosis Excessive accumulation of vitamins within the body; associated with the fat-soluble vitamins.

hypoglycemia The condition of having an abnormally low blood glucose level.

hypertrophic obesity A form of obesity in which there is a normal number of fat cells, but the individual fat cells are enlarged.

hypothyroidism A condition in which the thyroid gland produces an insufficient amount of the hormone thyroxin.

hypoxia Oxygenation deprivation at the cellular level.

I

ICSH (interstitial cell stimulating hormone) A gonadotropic hormone of the male required for the production of testosterone.

identity theft A crime involving the fraudulent use of a person's name, Social Security number, credit line, or other personal, financial, or identifying information.

immune system The system of cellular chemical elements that protects the body from invading pathogens and foreign protein and abnormal cells.

indirect (passive) euthanasia Allowing people to die without the use of life-sustaining procedures.

indoor air quality Characteristics of air within homes, workplaces, and public buildings, including the presence and amount of oxygen, water vapor, and a wide range of substances that can have adverse effects on your health.

infatuation An often shallow, intense attraction to another person.

inhalants Psychoactive drugs that enter the body through inhalation.

inhibitions Inner controls that prevent a person from engaging in certain types of behavior.

insulin A hormone produced by the islet cells of the pancreas that is necessary for the normal utilization of glucose.

intensity The level of effort put into an activity; for aerobic fitness, 50–80 percent of heart rate range is recommended.

intentional injuries Injuries that are purposefully inflicted, either by the victim or by another person.

intervention An organized process that involves encouraging a chemically addicted individual to enter into drug treatment; usually coordinated by family and friends along with a mental health professional.

intimacy Any close, mutual, verbal, or nonverbal behavior within a relationship.

intimate partner violence Violence committed against a person by a current or former spouse, date, or cohabiting partner.

intoxication Dysfunctional and disruptive changes in physiological and psychological functioning, mood, and cognitive processes, resulting from the consumption of a psychoactive substance.

intrapsychic stressors Our internal worries, self-criticisms, and negative self-talk.

intrauterine device (IUD) A small, plastic, medicated or unmedicated contraceptive device that prevents pregnancy when inserted in the uterus.

in vitro Outside the living body, in an artificial environment.

ionizing radiation Electromagnetic radiation that is capable of breaking chemical bonds, such as x-rays and gamma rays.

isokinetic exercises (eye so kin **et** ick) Muscular strength training exercises in which machines are used to provide variable resistances throughout the full range of motion at a fixed speed.

isometric exercises (eye so **met** rick) Muscular strength training exercises in which the resistance is so great that the object cannot be moved.

isotonic resistance exercises Muscular strength training exercises in which traditional barbells and dumbbells are used to provide variable resistances throughout the full range of motion.

L

learned helplessness A theory of motivation explaining how individuals can learn to feel powerless, trapped, or defeated.

learned optimism An attribution style regarding permanence, pervasiveness, and personalization; how people explain both positive and negative events in their lives, accounting for success and failure.

living will A legal document that requires physicians or family members to carry out a person's wishes to die naturally, without receiving life-sustaining treatments.

low-density lipoprotein (LDL) The type of lipoprotein that transports the largest amount of cholesterol in the bloodstream; high levels of LDL are related to heart disease.

lumpectomy A surgical treatment for breast cancer in which a minimal amount of breast tissue is removed; when appropriate, this procedure is an alternative to mastectomy, in which the entire breast and underlying tissue are removed.

luteinizing hormone (LH) (**loo** ten eye zing) A gonadotropic hormone of the female required for fullest development and release of ova; ovulating hormone.

Lyme disease A bacterial infection transmitted by deer ticks.

M

magnetic resonance imaging (MRI) scan An imaging procedure that uses a powerful magnet to generate an image of body tissue.

mainstream smoke Smoke inhaled and then exhaled by a smoker.

mania An extremely excitable state characterized by excessive energy, racing thoughts, impulsive and/or reckless behavior, irritability, and being prone to distraction.

probiotics Living bacteria ("good bugs") that help prevent disease and strengthen the immune system.

problem drinking An alcohol use pattern in which a drinker's behavior creates personal difficulties or difficulties for other people.

Prochaska's Transtheoretical Model of Health Behavior Change Six predictable stages—precontemplation, contemplation, preparation, action, maintenance, and termination—people go through in establishing new habits and patterns of behavior.

procrastination A tendency to put off completing tasks until some later time, sometimes resulting in increased stress.

procreation Reproduction.

prophylactic mastectomy Surgical removal of the breasts to prevent breast cancer in women who are at high risk of developing the disease.

prophylactic oophorectomy Surgical removal of the ovaries to prevent ovarian cancer in women at high risk of developing the disease.

prostate-specific antigen (PSA) test A blood test used to identify prostate-specific antigen, an early indicator that the immune system has recognized and mounted a defense against prostate cancer.

prosthodontics A dental specialty that focuses on the construction and fitting of artificial appliances to replace missing teeth.

proteins Compounds composed of chains of amino acids; primary components of muscle and connective tissue.

proto-oncogenes (pro toe **on** co genes) Normal regulatory genes that may become oncogenes.

psychiatrist A medical doctor with specialized training in the diagnosis and treatment of psychological disorders through the use of biological and medical interventions.

psychoactive drug Any substance capable of altering one's feelings, moods, or perceptions.

psychological dependence Craving a drug for emotional reasons and to maintain a sense of well-being; also called *habituation.*

psychological health A broadly based concept pertaining to cognitive functioning in conjunction with the way people express their emotions, cope with stress, adversity,

and success, and adapt to changes in themselves and their environment.

psychologist A doctoral-level practitioner with specialized training in the diagnosis and treatment of psychological disorders through the use of psychotherapy.

psychosocial sexuality Masculine and feminine aspects of sexuality.

pulmonary emphysema An irreversible disease process in which the alveoli are destroyed.

purging Using vomiting, laxatives, diuretics, enemas, or other medications, or means such as excessive exercise or fasting to eliminate food.

Q

quack A person who earns money by purposely marketing inaccurate health information, unreliable health care, or ineffective health products.

quackery The practice of disseminating or supplying inaccurate health information, unreliable health care, or ineffective health products for the purposes of defrauding another person.

R

radon A naturally occurring radioactive gas that is emitted during the decay of uranium in soil, rock, and water.

recessive inheritance pattern The inheritance of traits whose expression requires that they be carried by both biological parents.

Recommended Dietary Allowance (RDA) The dietary intake level sufficient to meet the nutrient requirements of nearly all individuals in an age- and gender-specific group.

refractory errors Abnormal patterns of light wave transmission through the structures of the eye.

refractory phase That portion of the male's resolution stage during which sexual arousal cannot occur.

regulatory genes Genes that control cell specialization replication, DNA repair, and tumor suppression.

resistance stage The second stage of a response to a stressor, during which the body attempts to reestablish its equilibrium or internal balance.

resolution stage The fourth stage of the sexual response pattern; the return of the body to a preexcitement state.

retinal hemorrhage Uncontrolled bleeding from arteries within the eye's retina.

rheumatic heart disease Chronic damage to the heart (especially the heart valves) resulting from a streptococcal infection within the heart; a complication of rheumatic fever.

risk factor A biomedical index such as serum cholesterol level, or a behavioral pattern such as smoking, associated with a chronic illness.

S

salt sensitive The term used to describe people whose bodies overreact to the presence of sodium by retaining fluid, thus increasing blood pressure.

sarcopenia A reduction in the size of muscle fibers, related to aging.

satiety (suh **tie** uh tee) The feeling of no longer being hungry; a diminished desire to eat.

saturated fats Fats that promote cholesterol formation; they are in solid form at room temperature; primarily animal fats.

schizophrenia One of the most severe mental disorders, characterized by profound distortions in one's thought processes, emotions, perceptions, and behavior. Symptoms may include hallucinations, delusions, disorganized thinking, and/or maintaining a rigid posture and not moving for hours.

sclerotic changes (skluh **rot** ick) Thickening or hardening of tissues.

seasonal affective disorder (SAD) A form of depression that develops in relation to the changes in the seasons.

secondary prevention Measures aimed at early detection, intervention, and treatment of drug abuse before severe physical, psychological, emotional, or social consequences can occur.

secondary virginity The discontinuation of sexual intercourse after initial exploration.

self-actualization The highest level of psychological health—at which one reaches his or her highest potential and values truth, beauty, goodness, spirituality, love, humor, and ingenuity.

self-antigens The cells and tissues that stimulate the immune system's autoimmune response.

self-care movement The trend toward individuals taking increased responsibility for prevention or management of certain health conditions.

self-concept An individual's internal picture of himself or herself; the way one sees oneself.

self-esteem An individual's sense of pride, self-respect, value, and worth.

self-fulfilling prophecy The tendency to inadvertently make something more likely to happen as a result of your own expectations and attitudes.

semen A secretion containing sperm and nutrients discharged from the urethra at ejaculation.

semivegetarian diet A diet that significantly reduces but does not eliminate meat consumption and allows consumption of dairy products and eggs.

serial monogamy A pattern of dating in which a person is involved in a series of exclusive relationships, one after the other.

set point A genetically programmed range of body weight, beyond which a person finds it difficult to gain or lose additional weight.

sex chromosomes The X and Y chromosomes that determine sex; chromosomes other than the autosomes.

sex flush The reddish skin response that results from increasing sexual arousal.

sexual fantasies Fantasies with sexual themes; sexual daydreams or imaginary events.

sexually transmitted diseases (STDs) Infectious diseases that are spread primarily through intimate sexual contact.

shingles Painful fluid-filled skin erruptions along underlying sensory nerve pathways—due to reactivation of once-sequestered herpes zoster (chicken pox) viruses.

shock The profound collapse of many vital body functions; evident during acute alcohol intoxication and other serious health emergencies.

sidestream smoke The smoke that comes from the burning end of a cigarette, pipe, or cigar.

sigmoidoscopy Examination of the sigmoid colon (lowest section of the large intestine), using a short, flexible fiberoptic scope.

skinfold measurement A measurement to determine the thickness of the fat layer that lies immediately beneath the skin; used to calculate body composition.

sleep apnea A condition in which abnormalities in the structure of the airways lead to periods of greatly restricted air flow during sleep, resulting in reduced levels of blood oxygen and placing greater strain on the heart to maintain adequate tissue oxygenation.

smegma Cellular discharge that can accumulate beneath the clitoral hood or the foreskin of an uncircumcized penis.

social phobia A phobia characterized by feelings of extreme dread and embarrassment in situations in which public speaking or social interaction is involved.

social worker A professional with a master's degree in social work. Social workers provide both mental health and social services to the community and are the largest group of professionals to provide psychological services.

sodomy Generally refers to anal or oral sex; a legal term whose definition varies from state to state.

solid waste Pollutants that are in solid form, including nonhazardous household trash, industrial wastes, mining wastes, and sewage sludge from wastewater treatment plants.

solution-focused therapy A goal-oriented counseling approach that helps clients change by looking for solutions rather than dwelling on problems.

specific phobia An excessive and unreasonable fear that causes anxiety and distress and interferes with a person's functioning.

spermatogenesis (sper mat oh **jen** uh sis) The process of sperm production.

spermicides Chemicals capable of killing sperm.

spontaneous abortion Any cessation of pregnancy resulting from natural causes; also called a miscarriage.

stalking Repeated visual or physical proximity, nonconsensual communication, or threats that would cause fear in a reasonable person.

static stretching The slow lengthening of a muscle group to an extended stretch; followed by a holding of the extended position for a recommended time period.

stem cells Premature (pleurepotent) cells that have the potential to turn into any kind of body cell.

stent A device inserted inside a coronary artery during a percutaneous coronary intervention (PCI) to prevent the artery from narrowing at this site.

sterilization Generally permanent birth control techniques that surgically disrupt the normal passage of ova or sperm.

stimulants Psychoactive drugs that stimulate the function of the central nervous system.

stress The physiological and psychological state of disruption caused by the presence of an unanticipated, disruptive, or stimulating event.

stress response The physiological and psychological responses to positive or negative events that are disruptive, unexpected, or stimulating.

stressors Factors or events, real or imagined, that elicit a state of stress.

synapse (**sinn** aps) The location at which an electrical impulse from one neuron is transmitted to an adjacent neuron; also referred to as a *synaptic junction*.

synergistic effect A heightened, exaggerated effect produced by the concurrent use of two or more drugs.

synesthesia A sensation of combining of the senses, such as perceiving color by hearing or perceiving taste by touching.

systemic (sis **tem** ic) Distributed or occurring throughout the entire body system.

systolic pressure (sis **tol** ick) The blood pressure against blood vessel walls when the heart contracts.

T

tachycardia Excessively rapid heartbeat, as evidenced by a resting pulse rate of greater than 100 beats per minute.

tar A chemically rich, syrupy, blackish-brown material obtained from the particulate matter within cigarette smoke when nicotine and water are removed.

target heart rate (THR) The number of times per minute the heart must contract to produce a cardiorespiratory training effect.

teratogenic agent Any substance that is capable of causing birth defects.

terrorism Any actions intended to harm or kill civilians in order to intimidate a populace or force a government to take some action.

tertiary prevention The treatment and rehabilitation of drug-dependent people to limit physical, psychological, emotional, and social deterioration or prevent death.

test anxiety A form of performance anxiety that generates extreme feelings of distress in exam situations.

therapeutic cloning The use of certain human replication techniques to reproduce body tissues and organs.

thermic effect of food (TEF) The amount of energy our bodies require for the digestion, absorption, and transportation of food.

thorax The chest; the portion of the torso above the diaphragm and within the rib cage.

threshold dose The smallest amount of a drug to have an observable effect on the body.

titration (tie **tray** shun) The particular level of a drug within the body; adjusting the level of nicotine by adjusting the rate of smoking.

Tolerable Upper Intake Level (UL) The maximum level of daily nutrient intake that is unlikely to pose risks of adverse health effects for almost all of the individuals in the group for whom it is designed.

tolerance An acquired reaction to a drug in which the continued intake of the same dose has diminishing effects.

toxic pollutants Substances known to cause cancer or other serious health effects.

toxic shock syndrome (TSS) A potentially fatal condition caused by the proliferation of certain bacteria in the vagina whose toxins enter the general blood circulation.

trace elements Minerals whose presence in the body occurs in very small amounts; micronutrient elements.

transcervical balloon tuboplasty The use of inflatable balloon catheters to open blocked fallopian tubes; a procedure used for some women with fertility problems.

trans-fatty acid An altered form of an unsaturated fat molecule in which the hydrogen atoms on each side of the double bond(s) are on opposite sides. Also called *trans fat.*

transgendered Refers to persons whose appearance and behaviors do not conform to society's traditional gender role expectations.

transient ischemic attack (TIA) (**tran** see ent iss **key** mick) Strokelike symptoms caused by the temporary spasm of cerebral blood vessels.

transsexualism A sexual variation in which a person rejects his or her biological sexuality.

transvestism Atypical behavior in which a person derives sexual pleasure from dressing in the clothes of the opposite gender.

trimester A three-month period; human pregnancies encompass three trimesters.

tropospheric ozone Ozone is composed of three oxygen atoms that are bound into a single molecule. Tropospheric ozone refers to this substance as it occurs in the lower layer of the atmosphere, close to the ground.

tumor A mass of abnormal cells; may be cancerous (malignant) or noncancerous (benign).

type A personality A personality type that tends to be competitive, ambitious, and impatient; often associated with heart attacks and other stress-related conditions.

type B personality A personality type that tends to be more relaxed and patient.

U

underweight A condition in which the body is below the desirable weight.

unintentional injuries Injuries that have occurred without anyone's intending that harm be done.

urethra (yoo **ree** thra) The passageway through which urine leaves the urinary bladder.

V

vasectomy A surgical procedure in which the vasa deferens are cut to prevent the passage of sperm from the testicles; the most common form of male sterilization.

vegan vegetarian diet A vegetarian diet that excludes all animal products, including eggs and dairy products.

virulent (**veer** yuh lent) Capable of causing disease.

vitamins Organic compounds that facilitate the action of enzymes.

volatile organic compounds A wide variety of chemicals that contain carbon and readily evaporate into the air.

W

wellness The promotion and achievement of optimal health, including physical, emotional, social, spiritual, intellectual, and occupational well-being.

Wernicke-Korsakoff syndrome A syndrome that results from vitamin B_1 deficiency, often as the result of alcoholism. Symptoms include impaired short-term memory, psychosis, impaired coordination, and abnormal eye movements.

withdrawal illness An uncomfortable, perhaps toxic response of the body as it attempts to maintain homeostasis in the absence of a drug; also called *abstinence syndrome.*

X

xenotransplant A transplant of tissue from an animal, such as a pig, to a human recipient.

Y

Yerkes-Dodson Law A bell-shaped curve demonstrating that there is an optimal level of stress for peak performance. This law states that too little or too much stress is not helpful, while a moderate level of stress is positive and beneficial.

young adult years The segment of the life cycle from ages 18 to 24; a transitional period between adolescence and adulthood.

Z

zero-tolerance laws Laws that severely restrict the right to operate motor vehicles for underage drinkers who have been convicted of driving under the influence of alcohol or any other drug.

zygote A fertilized ovum.

Chapter 1

page 1: © Javier Pierini/Getty Images; **page 3:** © BananaStock/Jupiterimages; **page 6:** © Colin Paterson/Getty Images; **page 12:** © Jack Star/PhotoLink/Getty Images; **page 15:** © The McGraw-Hill Companies, Inc./Gary He, photographer; **page 18:** © Brand X Pictures/PunchStock

Chapter 2

page 19: © Comstock/PictureQuest; **page 34:** © Getty Images; **page 41:** © Royalty-Free/Corbis; **page 44:** © BananaStock/Jupiterimages; **page 52:** © The McGraw-Hill Companies, Inc./Gary He, photographer; **page 57:** © Comstock Images/PictureQuest

Chapter 3

page 64: © Brand X Pictures/PunchStock; **page 69:** © The McGraw-Hill Companies, Inc./Gary He, photographer; **page 74:** © The McGraw-Hill Companies, Inc./Andrew Resek, photographer; **page 86:** © Jupiterimages (left), © Royalty-Free/Corbis (right)

Chapter 4

page 98: © Ryan McVay/Getty Images; **page 103:** © The McGraw-Hill Companies, Inc./Gary He, photographer; **page 107:** Courtesy Leonard Kaminsky (all three photos); **page 111:** © The McGraw-Hill Companies, Inc./Andrew Resek, photographer; **page 116:** © The McGraw-Hill Companies, Inc./Lars A. Niki, photographer; **page 125:** Courtesy Stewart Halperin (both photos); **page 127:** Courtesy Stewart Halperin (all four photos)

Chapter 5

page 127: © Nick Rowe/Getty Images; **page 132:** © The McGraw-Hill Companies, Inc./Andrew Resek, photographer; **page 144:** © Royalty-Free/Corbis; **page 146:** © RubberBall Productions/Getty Images; **page 150:** © Mitch Hrdlicka/Getty Images; **page 161:** © The McGraw-Hill Companies, Inc./Andrew Resek, photographer

Chapter 6

page 167: © Royalty-Free/Corbis; **page 170:** © The McGraw-Hill Companies, Inc./John Flournoy, photographer; **page 174:** Courtesy Life Measurement, Inc.; **page 178:** © The McGraw-Hill Companies, Inc./Lars A. Niki, photographer; **page 183:** © The McGraw-Hill Companies, Inc./John Flournoy, photographer (left), © Royalty-Free/Corbis (right); **page 190:** © The McGraw-Hill Companies, Inc./Jill Braaten, photographer; **page 194:** © BananaStock/PunchStock

Chapter 7

page 206: © Getty Images; **page 209:** © The McGraw-Hill Companies, Inc./Gary He, photographer; **page 211:** © The McGraw-Hill Companies, Inc./Gary He, photographer (top), © Royalty-Free/Corbis (middle), © The McGraw-Hill Companies, Inc./Gary He, photographer (bottom); **page 214:** © BananaStock/PunchStock; **page 222:** U.S. Drug Enforcement Administration; **page 227:** © BananaStock/PunchStock

Chapter 8

page 235: © Dynamic Graphics/Jupiterimages; **page 237:** © Royalty-Free/Corbis; **page 240:** © The McGraw-Hill Companies, Inc./Jill Braaten, photographer; **page 246:** Courtesy Mothers Against Drunk Driving; **page 252:** © D. Falconer/PhotoLink/Getty Images

Chapter 9

page 260: © Royalty-Free/Corbis; **page 265:** © The McGraw-Hill Companies, Inc./Gary He, photographer; **page 268:** © The McGraw-Hill Companies, Inc./Christopher Kerrigan, photographer; **page 276:** Courtesy Wayne Jackson; **page 277:** © The McGraw-Hill Companies, Inc./Christopher Kerrigan, photographer; **page 278:** © Medioimages/PictureQuest; **page 279:** National Cancer Institute; **page 282:** © Royalty-Free/Corbis; **page 287:** © Stockbyte/PictureQuest

Chapter 10

page 294: © Getty Images; **page 299:** © BananaStock/PunchStock; **page 305:** © Keith Brofsky/Getty Images; **page 314:** © The McGraw-Hill Companies, Inc./Ken Karp, photographer

Chapter 11

page 319: National Cancer Institute; **page 328:** The Skin Cancer Foundation; **page 330:** © Kerry-Edwards 2004, Inc./Sharon Farmer, photographer; **page 344:** National Cancer Institute/Bill Branson, photographer

Chapter 12

page 351: © Royalty-Free/Corbis; **page 355:** © Custom Medical Stock Photo; **page 358:** © Custom Medical Stock Photo; **page 359:** © Custom Medical Stock Photo; **page 372:** © Rufus F. Folkks/Corbis

Chapter 13

page 379: © The McGraw-Hill Companies, Inc./Jill Braaten, photographer; **page 391:** © Janis Christie/PhotoDisc/Getty Images; **page 397:** Courtesy of the Centers for Disease Control and Prevention; **page 399:** © The McGraw-Hill Companies, Inc./Christopher Kerrigan, photographer; **page 401:** © The McGraw-Hill Companies, Inc./Christopher Kerrigan, photographer; **page 406:** © Phototake; **page 407:** © Custom Medical Stock Photo

Chapter 14

page 416: © The McGraw-Hill Companies, Inc./Jill Braaten, photographer; **page 420:** © Thinkstock Images/Jupiterimages (left), © Brand X Pictures/Jupiterimages (right)

Chapter 15

page 435: © Burke/Triolo Productions/Getty Images; **page 443:** © The McGraw-Hill Companies, Inc./Christopher Kerrigan, photographer; **page 444:** © Ryan McVay/Getty Images; **page 449:** © Ryan McVay/Getty Images; **page 452:** © Buccina Studios/Getty Images; **page 453:** © Thinkstock

Chapter 16

page 459: © The McGraw-Hill Companies, Inc./Kirstan Price, photographer; **page 467:** © The McGraw-Hill Companies, Inc./Kirstan Price, photographer; **page 468:** Courtesy Stewart Halperin; **page 470:** © The McGraw-Hill Companies, Inc./Kirstan Price, photographer; **page 471:** Courtesy Stewart Halperin; **page 474:** Courtesy Organon USA; **page 475:** © The McGraw-Hill Companies, Inc./Christopher Kerrigan, photographer

Chapter 17

page 482: © Trinette Reed/Brand X Pictures/Jupiterimages; **page 484:** © E. Dygas/Getty Images; **page 486:** © Science Photo Library/Photo Researchers, Inc.; **page 488:** © Science Photo Library/Photo Researchers, Inc.; **page 489:** © Brand X Pictures/